Drug Transport in Antimicrobial and Anticancer Chemotherapy

INFECTIOUS DISEASE AND THERAPY

Series Editors

Brian E. Scully, M.B., B.Ch.
Harold C. Neu, M.D.

College of Physicians & Surgeons
Columbia University
New York, New York

Additional Volumes in Production

Drug Transport in Antimicrobial and Anticancer Chemotherapy

edited by
Nafsika H. Georgopapadakou

Roche Research Center
Nutley, New Jersey

Marcel Dekker, Inc.   New York•Basel•Hong Kong

Library of Congress Cataloging-in-Publication Data

Drug transport in antimicrobial and anticancer chemotherapy / edited
    by Nafsika H. Georgopapadakou.
        p.   cm. — (Infectious disease and therapy ; 17)
    Includes bibliographical references and index.
    ISBN 0-8247-9399-4 (hardcover : alk. paper)
    1. Anti-infective agents—Physiological transport.
  2. Antineoplastic agents—Physiological transport.
  I. Georgopapadakou, Nafsika H.   II. Series.
    [DNLM: 1. Anti-Infective Agents—pharmacokinetics.   2. Biological
Transport—drug effects.   3. Antineoplastic Agents—
pharmacokinetics.   4. Drug Resistance.   W1 IN406HMN v. 17 1995 / QV
250 D795   1995]
    RM267.D78   1995
    615'.7—dc20
    DNLM/DLC
    for Library of Congress   95-12771
                                                                        CIP

The publisher offers discounts on this book when ordered in bulk quantities. For
more information, write to Special Sales/Professional Marketing at the address
below.

This book is printed on acid-free paper.

Marcel Dekker, Inc.
270 Madison Avenue, New York, New York 10016

Current printing (last digit):
10   9   8   7   6   5   4   3   2   1

PRINTED IN THE UNITED STATES OF AMERICA

To
Daniel Bennahmias
(1923–1994)
Sonderkommando,
Unique friend

Series Introduction

Marcel Dekker, Inc., has for many years specialized in the publication of high-quality monographs in tightly focused areas in a variety of medical disciplines. These have been of great value to both the practicing physician and the research scientist as sources of detailed and up-to-date information presented in an attractive format. During the last decade, there has been a veritable explosion in knowledge in the various fields related to infectious diseases and clinical microbiology. Antimicrobial resistance, antibacterial and antiviral agents, AIDS, Lyme disease, infections in immunocompromised patients, and parasitic diseases are but a few of the areas in which an enormous amount of significant work has been published. The Infectious Disease and Therapy series covers carefully chosen topics that should be of interest and value to the practicing physician, the clinical microbiologist, and the research scientist.

Brian E. Scully, M.B., B.Ch.
Harold C. Neu, M.D.

Preface

The development and use of antimicrobial agents have been key factors in the control of infectious diseases and constitute perhaps the major medical success of this century. Their use has been most effective in the control of bacterial diseases, and less so for viral, fungal, and parasitic ones. Parasitic diseases, traditionally regarded as a third-world problem, are no longer contained there because of the homogenization of the world population, as shown by the recent import of leishmaniasis by soldiers returning from the Gulf war. In the past several years the number of drug-resistant pathogens has increased, in some cases dramatically—for example, methicillin-resistant *S. aureus*, multidrug-resistant *M. tuberculosis*, and chloroquine-resistant *P. falciparum*. Resistance has been associated with altered target/pathway or drug-inactivating enzymes, with altered transport often a major contributing factor. Understanding microbial transport, its contribution to drug action and resistance, and its potential as a drug target has been the object of intensive research in both industry and academia.

Cancer chemotherapy, a development of the second half of this century, has been less successful than antimicrobial chemotherapy. Although childhood and hematological cancers generally respond well to treatment, many common solid tumors respond only partially. Resistance, intrinsic or acquired, is a major stumbling block to effective treatment. Like its microbial counterpart, mammalian cell resistance to anticancer drugs is associated with altered target/pathway or inactivating metabolic enzymes, with altered transport often a contributing factor. Understanding the role of transport in anticancer drug action and resistance and exploiting it in drug design—relatively recent developments—have spurred explosive multidisciplinary research.

There is a vast and growing literature on drug transport and its role in resistance. This book aims to provide a current, balanced, clear, and readable introduction to this complex topic for students and investigators in infectious diseases, oncology, pharmacology, and toxicology. It is organized into four sections: the first section (Chaps. 1–4) serves as an introduction and establishes the biochemical and clinical framework for a diverse audience; each of the next three sections focuses specifically on the transport of antibacterial (Chaps. 5–10), antifungal/antiparasitic (Chaps. 11–14), and anticancer (Chaps. 15–20) agents.

Chapter 1 focuses on the clinical relevance of transport in the activity of major classes of antibacterial agents. The role of transport in the clinical effectiveness of anticancer agents is the topic of Chapter 2. Chapter 3 concerns the composition and properties of cell membranes, generally protein-rich, lipid bilayers that function both as barriers and as conduits for transport. Cellular transport is a multifactorial process and may involve passage across more than one membrane in either direction (influx, efflux). Certain structural and mechanistic motifs, discussed in Chapter 4, are found in both prokaryotes and eukaryotes. Drug transport itself is an elaboration of the transport motifs involved in the uptake of nutrients (influx) and the exclusion or elimination of waste or toxic products (efflux).

The simplest case of transport involves the passage of β-lactam antibiotics through the bacterial outer membrane to their targets in the periplasmic space (Chap. 5). In combination with β-lactamases, reduced penetration is responsible for the vast majority of gram-negative resistance to β-lactams. A further level of complexity is introduced when the target is in the cytoplasm, as is the case for most other antibacterials. Thus, aminoglycoside accumulation, the topic of Chapter 6, is impeded by a combination of decreased uptake and inactivating enzymes. Both β-lactam and aminoglycoside transport are thought to involve influx exclusively, although this has recently been questioned, at least for β-lactams in *Pseudomonas*. The transport of tetracyclines (Chap. 7) and quinolones (Chap. 8) introduces still another level of complexity, drug efflux. It is significant that neither class of antibiotics undergoes enzymatic inactivation. Diminished drug transport without concomitant inactivation may contribute to the initial, low levels of resistance, a recurring theme in the role of efflux in eukaryotes.

Nowhere is the effect of the barrier function of the cell envelope on antibiotic activity as dramatic as in mycobacteria (Chap. 9), organisms that have stigmatized people throughout history with the diseases of leprosy and tuberculosis. Tuberculosis, which had been relegated to the dust bin of medical history, has recently undergone a renaissance of sorts with the advent of AIDS and, perhaps, the global south-to-north migration of people. Its resurgence in the large cities of the western world presents a social as well as a medical challenge.

Bacterial transport systems can be exploited to increase the uptake of antibacterials, as discussed in Chapter 10. Although clinical candidates have yet to emerge, significant progress has been made, and chemical leads (catechol cephalosporins, cationic peptides) are still under investigation.

Fungal infections have acquired a new urgency as their frequency and number of pathogenic species have increased. Amphotericin, a discovery of the 1950s, remains the "gold standard." In fungi, it complexes with the membrane sterols, thereby compromising membrane integrity, while in mammalian cells, it may become internalized, with serious implications for toxicity (Chap. 11). Azoles, a major class of antifungals that inhibit sterol biosynthesis, have an intracellular target, and are thus subject to transport constraints, including efflux (Chap. 12). Transport is also important in the resistance to antiparasitic agents. Both antimalarial (Chap. 13) and antileishmanial (Chap. 14) agents may be substrates for efflux systems leading to resistance.

Nucleosides are among the oldest anticancer agents, and some (cytarabine, 5-fluorouracil) still have important clinical applications. Their transport may be equilibrative or concentrative, and involves several mediated transport systems (Chap. 15). Antifolates are also widely used in cancer chemotherapy, and their carrier-mediated transport has been more thoroughly studied than any other class of anticancer drugs (reviewed in Chap. 16).

The possibility that efflux may be an important component of anticancer drug resistance was first recognized in the early 1970s, shortly after the discovery of anthracyclines, one of the most successful and enduring classes of anticancer agents. Since the realization that increased efflux may lead to simultaneous resistance to several drug classes, known as multidrug resistance (MDR), it has attracted interest both as a functional barrier (Chap. 17) and as a chemotherapeutic target (Chap. 18). Its regulation through signal transduction has added to the possibilities for intervention. However, its physiological presence in the adrenal and blood–brain barrier, with toxicity implications, and its controversial role in resistance have dampened enthusiasm for its modulation, at least in the pharmaceutical industry.

Another pump with broad substrate specificity, associated with glutathione conjugation, may be responsible for resistance to cisplatin and other nucleophilic agents (Chap. 19). Like MDR, it is a normal detoxification system, highlighting a central problem in anticancer chemotherapy: the limited selectivity of drugs for cancer cells. Yet there is hope, even on the anticancer front. Chapter 20 discusses ways of overcoming transport-associated resistance and introduces the complex subject of drug delivery through conjugates and liposomes.

The impetus for creating this book came when I changed fields from infectious diseases to cancer research and, in so doing, saw the similarities in the transport mechanisms between microbial and cancer cells. Thanks are due to Roy Cleeland, former director of the Department of Infectious Diseases at Roche, who countered my initial reluctance to proceed with this project by urging me to "go for it." I am also grateful to the contributors, who, with enthusiasm and diligence, covered complex and often rapidly evolving topics in their fields of expertise. They made this book possible and, without knowing it, helped me maintain scientific perspective in the corporate turmoil. I thank them for both. Daniel Bennahmias, a very close friend who developed leukemia and eventually succumbed to a *Pseudomonas* infection, was a source of encouragement and inspiration throughout the project. The successes and failures of his treatment provided a sobering perspective. Finally, my thanks to the staff of Marcel Dekker—Sandra Beberman, Tami Booth, Tanja Noren, and Elyce Misher—for their support and efficiency which ensured that the project was always on track.

Nafsika H. Georgopapadakou

Contents

Contributors

Francis Ali-Osman, D.Sc.   Department of Experimental Pediatrics, The University of Texas M.D. Anderson Cancer Center, Houston, Texas

Suresh V. Ambudkar, Ph.D.   Division of Nephrology, Departments of Medicine and Physiology, The Johns Hopkins University School of Medicine, Baltimore, Maryland

Adolf Bauernfeind, M.D. Department of Medical Microbiology, Max von Petenkofer Institute, University of Munich, Munich, Germany

Patrick Boiron, Ph.D.   Unité de Mycologie, Centre National de Référence des Mycoses et des Antifongiques, Institut Pasteur, Paris, France

Jacques Bolard, Ph.D., D.Sc. Laboratoire de Physique et Chimie Biomoléculaires, Université Pierre et Marie Curie, Paris, France

Patrick G. Bray, Ph.D.   Department of Pharmacology and Therapeutics, University of Liverpool, Liverpool, England

Henk J. Broxterman, Ph.D.   Department of Medical Oncology, Free University Hospital, Amsterdam, The Netherlands

Karen Bush, Ph.D. Infectious Disease Section, Lederle Laboratories, Pearl River, New York

Carol E. Cass, Ph.D. Department of Biochemistry, University of Alberta, Edmonton, Alberta, Canada

Dennis Chapman, Ph.D., D.Sc., F.R.S. Department of Protein and Molecular Biology, Royal Free Hospital School of Medicine, University of London, London, England

Ian Chopra, Ph.D., D.Sc. Microbiology Research, SmithKline Beecham Pharmaceuticals, Brockham Park, Surrey, England

Saibal Dey, Ph.D. Department of Biochemistry, Wayne State University School of Medicine, Detroit, Michigan

Nafsika H. Georgopapadakou, Ph.D. Department of Oncology, Roche Research Center, Nutley, New Jersey

Michael M. Gottesman, M.D. Laboratory of Cell Biology, National Cancer Institute, National Institutes of Health, Bethesda, Maryland

Katherine Grondin Service d'Infectiologie, Centre Hospitalier de l'Université Laval, Laval, Quebec, Canada

Annas Haimeur Service d'Infectiologie, Centre Hospitalier de l'Université Laval, Laval, Quebec, Canada

Robert E. W. Hancock, Ph.D. Department of Microbiology and Immunology, University of British Columbia, Vancouver, British Columbia, Canada

Toshihisa Ishikawa, Ph.D. Department of Experimental Pediatrics, The University of Texas M.D. Anderson Cancer Center, Houston, Texas

Gerrit Jansen, Ph.D. Department of Medical Oncology, Free University Hospital, Amsterdam, The Netherlands

Jan Lankelma, Ph.D. Department of Medical Oncology, Free University Hospital, Amsterdam, The Netherlands

Eric Leblanc Service d'Infectiologie, Centre Hospitalier de l'Université Laval, Laval, Quebec, Canada

Danielle Légaré Service d'Infectiologie, Centre Hospitalier de l'Université Laval, Laval, Quebec, Canada

Sabine C. Linn, Ph.D. Department of Medical Oncology, Free University Hospital, Amsterdam, The Netherlands

Larry H. Matherly, Ph.D. Developmental Therapeutics Program, Michigan Cancer Foundation, Detroit, Michigan

Michael H. Miller, M.D. Division of Infectious Diseases, Department of Medicine, Albany Medical College, Albany, New York

Mikihiko Naito, Ph.D. Institute of Molecular and Cellular Biosciences, The University of Tokyo, Tokyo, Japan

Marc Ouellette, Ph.D. Service d'Infectiologie, Centre Hospitalier de l'Université Laval, Laval, Quebec, Canada

Barbara Papadopoulou, Ph.D. Service d'Infectiologie, Centre Hospitalier de l'Université Laval, Laval, Quebec, Canada

Ira Pastan, M.D. Laboratory of Molecular Biology, National Cancer Institute, National Institutes of Health, Bethesda, Maryland

Graeme Y. Ritchie, Ph.D. Department of Pharmacology and Therapeutics, University of Liverpool, Liverpool, England

Barry P. Rosen, Ph.D. Department of Biochemistry, Wayne State University School of Medicine, Detroit, Michigan

Gaétan Roy Service d'Infectiologie, Centre Hospitalier de l'Université Laval, Laval, Quebec, Canada

Alain R. Thierry, Ph.D. Laboratory of Tumor Cell Biology, National Cancer Institute, National Institutes of Health, Bethesda, Maryland

Joaquim Trias, Ph.D. Department de Microbiologia i Parasitologia Sanitàries, Facultat de Farmacia, Universitat de Barcelona, Barcelona, Spain

Takashi Tsuruo, Ph.D.   Institute of Molecular and Cellular Biosciences, University of Tokyo, Tokyo, Japan

Aline Vertut-Doï, Ph.D.   Laboratoire de Physique et Chimie Biomoléculaires, Université Pierre et Marie Curie, Paris, France

Stephen Andrew Ward, Ph.D.   Department of Pharmacology and Therapeutics, University of Liverpool, Liverpool, England

Drug Transport in Antimicrobial and Anticancer Chemotherapy

1

Clinical Significance of Antibacterial Transport

Adolf Bauernfeind
*Max von Pettenkofer Institute, University of Munich,
Munich, Germany*

Nafsika H. Georgopapadakou
Roche Research Center, Nutley, New Jersey

I. INTRODUCTION

Antibacterial chemotherapy began with the introduction of sulfonamides in the 1930s. It progressed rapidly with the development of penicillin and streptomycin in the 1940s; chloramphenicol, tetracycline, and vancomycin in the 1950s; erythromycin, the antistaphylococcal penicillins, and broad-spectrum cephalosporins in the 1960s; gentamicin, clindamycin, trimethoprim, sulfamethoxazole, and second-generation cephalosporins in the 1970s; quinolones, third-generation cephalosporins, and other β-lactams (carbapenems, monobactams, and β-lactamase inhibitors) in the 1980s. Although it is too early to take inventory and assess the antibacterial drug discoveries of the 1990s, they will most likely include novel β-lactams active against methicillin-resistant staphylococci (MRS) (see Chap. 5), quinolones (see Chap. 8), tetracyclines (glycylcyclines) (see Chap. 6), macrolides, and other protein synthesis inhibitors.

Bacterial resistance to antibiotics, relentlessly Darwinian, has shadowed the introduction of every class of new agent. For example, β-lactamase-mediated resistance was recognized as early as 1944, and by 1947, most staphylococci were resistant to penicillin. Similarly, early resistance to macrolides and chloramphenicol severely limited their use. In the real world, as in the laboratory, resistance has simply emerged in response to antibiotic pressure (1–3). Obvious underlying factors are the very large numbers of bacteria involved, their genetic versatility, and their short doubling time. Resistance continues to be a major concern in the treatment of infectious diseases affecting both patients (increased morbidity and mortality, more toxic drugs) and society (reduced antibiotic options, more expensive drugs) (4,5). As a result, there is renewed interest in multiresistant, "problem pathogens" [vancomycin-resistant enterococci (VRE); MRS, mycobacteria] in terms of hitting the new target [penicillin-binding protein (PBP) 2a of MRS], identifying new targets (VRE), or gaining access to the targets (mycobacteria). This brings up the two central issues in antibacterial chemotherapy in the 1990s: the (re)emergence of bacterial pathogens and the emergence of bacterial resistance.

Resistance mechanisms include preventing an antibiotic from reaching its target through (1) altered transport or (2) enzymatic inactivation; (3) altering the target so that it is no longer sensitive to the antibiotic; (4) overproducing or altogether bypassing the target (Table 1). There are several excellent reviews on bacterial resistance (4–7). This chapter will focus on transport-associated resistance to five major antibiotic classes: β-lactams, aminoglycosides, tetracyclines, quinolones, and macrolides.

The clinical impact of a mechanism of resistance to antibiotics is mainly determined by its relevance to the treatment of infections. From this point of view, the incidence of a resistance mechanism among major pathogens is of particular interest. Knowledge about the distribution of a resistance mechanism depends on the availability of data necessary for its identification. Inhibition zones (disk-diffusion assay) or minimum inhibitory concentrations (MICs; serial dilution assay) of therapeutically relevant antibiotics are collected routinely in laboratories of clinical bacteriology (8). The zone diameters or MICs that are obtained are then translated into "susceptible," "intermediate," or "resistant" categories by referring to standardized values for the particular antibiotic: a species is considered susceptible if 90% or more of the strains tested are sensitive to the drug.

The resistance phenotype allows one to assess the underlying mechanism of resistance of specific pathogens (9). However, this is mainly applicable for enzyme-mediated resistance mechanisms. For example, it may reveal PBP-mediated resistance in *Staphylococcus* spp., *Streptococcus pneumoniae*, *Haemophilus influenzae*, *Neisseria* spp., or β-lactamase-mediated resistance in *Staphylococcus* spp. and other bacteria. The approach is less reliable for the detection of resistance mechanisms related to reduced intracellular concentrations of antibiotics, which may be caused by reduced permeability or by an active efflux mechanism.

The identification of transport-associated resistance is not possible by data from routine antibiotic susceptibility testing, but instead, relies on

Table 1 Mechanisms of Resistance to Major Antibiotic Classes

General mechanism Antibiotic class	Specific mechanism
1. Enzymatic inactivation/modification	
β-Lactams	β-lactamase (chromosomal or plasmid-mediated)
Aminoglycosides	N-Acetyltransferase, O-adenylyltransferase, O-phosphotransferase
Macrolides	Esterase, phosphorylase, 2′-glycosylase
Chloramphenicol	O-Acetyltransferase
2. Decreased binding to target/additional target	
β-Lactams	Novel, altered PBP
Aminoglycosides	Protein S12
Tetracyclines	Ribosomal protection
Macrolides	rRNA methylation
Quinolones	Altered DNA gyrase
Glycopeptides	Altered peptidoglycan precursor
Rifampicin	Altered RNA polymerase
3. Decreased intracellular accumulation	
a. Decreased uptake	
β-Lactams	Altered porins
Aminoglycosides	Altered active transport
b. Increased efflux	
Tetracyclines	
Quinolones	
Macrolides	
4. Overproduced/bypassed target	
Glycopeptides	Ligase with altered specificity
Sulfonamides	Resistant dihydropteroate synthetase (plasmid-mediated)
Trimethoprim	Resistant dihydrofolate reductase (plasmid-mediated)

specific studies. A further complication arises from the observation that more than one mechanism of resistance may be operating simultaneously in a single pathogen. These mechanisms may interact with each other; for example, resistance owing to reduced permeability may be enhanced by an enzymatic mechanism (10,11). Thus, the relevance of a resistance mechanism to the overall resistance depends on the incidence of other mechanisms that may also be present. It is often difficult to dissect antimicrobial resistance into components, or to assess precisely the contribution of a transport mechanism to overall resistance.

II. β-LACTAMS AND AMINOGLYCOSIDES: IMPAIRED INFLUX AND ASSOCIATED RESISTANCE

A. β-Lactams

For the past 50 years β-lactams have been the most widely used group of antibiotics (see Chap. 5). Their common structural feature, the β-lactam ring, is the biologically active moiety, its reactivity and selectivity toward the target cell wall-synthesizing enzymes being influenced by substituents or fused rings (12). β-Lactams are characterized by high bactericidal activity, clinical efficacy, versatile spectrum (antistaphylococcal penicillins, gram-negative monobactams, broad-spectrum imipenem) and administration (oral, parenteral), good tolerance, and safety.

Resistance to β-lactams in clinical isolates results preponderantly from their inactivation by β-lactamases, bacterial enzymes that hydrolyze the β-lactam ring (Table 2). In gram-negative bacteria, β-lactamases are plasmid-mediated and constitutive or chromosomal and inducible (to different extent by different β-lactams), and strategically positioned in the periplasm. In conjunction with the outer membrane, they effectively decrease the concentration of active β-lactam available to bind to the target penicillin-binding proteins (PBPs) on the cytoplasmic membrane. In gram-positive bacteria, β-lactamases are plasmid-mediated and inducible, are produced in large amounts, and are released extracellularly. The diffuse capsular material and the lattice peptidoglycan layers of gram-positive bacteria allow the nonspecific passage of large molecules, such as lysozyme (M_r 14.4 kDa) and do not constitute a barrier to antibiotic entry (13). β-Lactam antibiotics thus have free access to their targets at the cytoplasmic membrane, and their activity against gram-positive bacteria is determined solely by their binding to essential PBPs (staphylococci, enterococci, *S. pneumoniae*) and stability to β-lactamases.

Accordingly, the role of permeation in resistance of human pathogens to β-lactams is limited mainly to gram-negative organisms (14,15). They are surrounded by an outer membrane that is rather impermeable to small hydrophilic molecules such as β-lactams, except for nonspecific transmembrane channels formed by porins (see Chap. 5). These channels (OmpF and OmpC in *Escherichia coli*) exclude molecules above a certain size (800 Da in *E. coli*) and preferentially allow the passage of hydrophilic molecules like the majority of β-lactams (sieving effect). Resistance to β-

Table 2 Major Therapeutic Indications for β-Lactams and Bacterial Resistance

Organism	Infection/disease	Penam	Cephem	Penem[b]	Comb[c]
			Resistance[a]		
Enterobacteriaceae					
E. coli	UTI, gallbladder	+ +	±	±	±
K. pneumoniae	Nosocomial pneumonia	+ + +	+	±	±
P. mirabilis	Diarrhea, sepsis	+	±	±	±
E. cloacae		+ + +	+ + +	±	+ + +
Pseudomonas					
P. aeruginosa	UTI, cystic fibrosis, nosocomial pneumonia	+ +	+ +	+	+ +
Haemophilus					
H. influenzae	RTI, meningitis	+ +	±	±	±
Neisseriaceae					
N. gonorrhoeae	Gonorrhea	+ +	±	±	±
M. catarrhalis	Bronchitis	+ + +	±	±	±
Staphylococci					
S. aureus MS	Skin infections, sepsis	+ + +	+	±	±
S. aureus MR		+ + +	+ + +	+ + +	+ + +
Streptococci					
S. pneumoniae	RTI (upper and lower)	+	+	±	±
S. pyogenes	Angina, tonsilitis	±	±	±	±
Enterococci					
E. faecalis	Endocarditis, UTI	+	+ + +	±	±
E. faecium		+	+ + +	±	±
Bacteroides					
B. fragilis	Abdominal infections	+ + +	+ + +	±	+
Clostridium					
C. difficile	Antibiotic-associated colitis	±	+ +	±	±

[a] ±, ≤5%; +, ≤15%; + +, ≤30%; + + +, >30% of clinical isolates.
[b] Includes carbapenems.
[c] β-Lactam–β-lactamase inhibitor combination.
Abbreviations: RTI, respiratory tract infections; UTI, urinary tract infections; MS, methicillin-sensitive; MR, methicillin-resistant.

lactams is associated with reduced permeation, usually in combination with enzymatic hydrolysis of the antibiotic. With a single, notable exception (16), there are no reports on active efflux mechanisms being involved in resistance to β-lactams.

The diffusion of β-lactams follows Fick's first law of diffusion: the rate of diffusion is proportional to the concentration gradient across the outer membrane, the total area of channels in the outer membrane, and the physicochemical nature of the β-lactam and channel properties (17). Briefly, hydrophobic β-lactams penetrate more slowly than hydrophilic ones. Dianionic β-lactams penetrate more slowly than monoanionic compounds, which penetrate more slowly than zwitterionic compounds. Imipenem is the most rapidly permeating zwitterionic β-lactam. Compounds with bulky side chains (piperacillin, cefoperazone) penetrate slower than expected from their hydrophobicity. The substituted oxime side chain on the α-carbon of the substituent group at position 7 of the cephem nucleus (cefuroxime, ceftizoxime, cefotaxime) decreases the permeation rate. Further reduction of permeability of β-lactams impairs their activity, particularly if their intrinsic rate of permeation is low. Thus, laboratory mutants of *E. coli* were resistant only to compounds with high hydrophobicity or with two negative charges (18).

The in vivo role for porins in the uptake of β-lactam antibiotics across the outer membrane of enteric bacteria is suggested by reports on reduced β-lactam susceptibility of porin-deficient mutants, in comparison with their isogenic wild-type strains (19). Higher MICs for mutants were observed mainly for cefoxitin, cefazolin, and ampicillin and, to a lesser extent, for all other β-lactams, except imipenem.

In *Enterobacter cloacae*, alterations in outer-membrane porins were associated with a moderate level of resistance to only those β-lactam compounds that were unaffected by derepression of β-lactamases (20). It was concluded that alterations in both outer membrane proteins and β-lactamase can affect susceptibility of *E. cloacae* to β-lactams. The interplay between the two resistance mechanisms was examined by Marchou et al. (21). They demonstrated that resistance of *E. cloacae* to ceftriaxone and other β-lactams is associated, at least in some strains, with an altered OmpF-like porin (37–38 kDa). Most of the mutant R1 and R2 clones showed lower amounts of 37- to 38-kDa membrane proteins, often concomitantly with higher amounts of 42-kDa protein. Incorporation of the radiolabeled β-lactam Sch 34343 proceeded slower in the R2 clone than in R1, and intact cells of mutant R2 hydrolyzed ceftriaxone more slowly than R1 clones. However, alterations in β-lactamase alone (derepression of β-lactamase production) were sufficient to produce multiple β-lactam resistance in *E. cloacae*.

Pseudomonas aeruginosa, a major pathogen in immunocompromised patients, lacks the permeability pores of enteric bacteria, such as the OmpF channel. The rates of diffusion of β-lactam antibiotics through its outer membrane are about 100–500 times lower than for *E. coli* (22). This has been attributed to the smaller size of its diffusion pores (proteins C and E), except for protein F, which, however, seems to be mostly in a closed state (22). Outer membrane permeability plays a major role in the resistance of *P. aeruginosa*. Thus, *P. aeruginosa* wild-type strains are resistant to most β-lactams, except ceftazidime, cefoperazone, piperacillin, aztreonam, and imipenem. Resistance to imipenem, so far rare in *Enterobacteriaceae* (e.g., *Klebsiella pneumoniae*, *E. cloacae*), is rather frequent in clinical isolates of *P. aeruginosa*. Such mutants lack the outer membrane protein D2 (OprD2), which transports basic amino acids, but not protein C, which allows diffusion of anionic antipseudomonal β-lactams, or protein E (22).

B. Aminoglycosides

The aminoglycosides are among the older antibacterials: streptomycin and neomycin were discovered in the 1940s, kanamycin in the 1950s, and gentamicin and tobramycin in the 1960s. They are broad-spectrum, bactericidal agents and, in spite of their toxicity (nephrotoxicity, ototoxicity), are still used in the treatment of life-threatening gram-negative infections, often in combination with other agents (β-lactams, quinolones; Table 3). Currently, clinically important aminoglycosides are gentamicin, tobramycin, kanamycin, amikacin, isepamicin, sisomicin, and its *N*-ethyl derivative, netilmicin (see Chap. 6).

Aminoglycosides diffuse through the porin channels very efficiently, as rapidly as hexoses and disaccharides. The susceptibility of *E. coli* mutants that produce 3–4% of the porins was not significantly different from that of strains producing wild-type levels of porins (23). Therefore, the diffusion of aminoglycosides through the outer membrane is not a rate-limiting step for aminoglycoside influx or action (23). Diffusion through the plasma membrane, on the other hand, is energy-dependent and far more complex (see Chap. 6).

Clinically, the most significant mechanism of aminoglycoside resistance is enzymatic modification. The modifying enzymes, named according to the reaction they catalyze (*N*-acetyltransferases, *O*-phosphoryltransferases, and *O*-adenyltransferases), have broad-substrate specificity and can catalyze more than one reaction (24). Impaired uptake may contribute to resistance (25).

Table 3 Major Therapeutic Indications for Aminoglycosides and Bacterial Resistance

Organism	Infection/disease	Resistance[a]
Enterobacteriaceae		
E. coli	UTI, gallbladder	±
K. pneumoniae	Nosocomial pneumonia	±
P. mirabilis	Diarrhea, sepsis	±
E. cloacae		±
Pseudomonas		
P. aeruginosa	UTI, cystic fibrosis, nosocomial pneumonia	+ +
Haemophilus		
H. influenzae	RTI, meningitis	±
Neisseriaceae		
N. gonor-	Gonorrhea	+ +
rhoeae	Bronchitis	±
M. catarrhalis		
Staphylococci		
S. aureus MS	Skin infections, sepsis	±
S. aureus MR		+ + +
Streptococci		
S. pyogenes	Angina, tonsilitis	+ + +
S. pneumoniae		+ + +
Enterococci		
E. faecalis	Endocarditis, UTI	+ + +
E. faecium		+ + +
Bacteroides		
B. fragilis	Abdominal infections	+ + +

[a] ±, ≤5%; +, ≤15%; + +, ≤30%; + + +, >30% of clinical isolates.

Abbreviations: RTI, respiratory tract infections; UTI, urinary tract infections; MS, methicillin-sensitive; MR, methicillin-resistant.

III. TETRACYCLINES, MACROLIDES, QUINOLONES: EFFLUX-ASSOCIATED RESISTANCE

Active efflux mechanisms contributing to antimicrobial resistance have so far been described mainly for tetracyclines, macrolides, and quinolones (26).

A. Tetracyclines

Tetracyclines have been widely used as antibacterials since the discovery of chlortetracycline in 1948. Their application has not been limited to human infections, but has extended to bacterial infections in animals. Tetracycline use (primarily, doxycycline and minocycline) still persists, although there are alternative drugs for the therapy of infections treatable by tetracyclines. Major reasons for their continued use are (1) the broad-spectrum, oral activity of tetracyclines, which covers both gram-positive and gram-negative, aerobic and anaerobic bacteria, including intracellular pathogens; (2) the extensive clinical experience in their use, including side effects; and (3) their low cost. Currently, there are only a few first-line indications for tetracyclines, mainly infections caused by intracellular pathogens (Table 4).

Some bacteria, such as *Proteus* spp., *Providencia* spp., *Serratia* spp., and *P. aeruginosa*, are intrinsically resistant to tetracyclines. Among the susceptible species, a variable percentage of clinical isolates have MICs above the concentration achievable at the site of infection and, therefore, are classified as resistant to tetracyclines. Resistance against established tetracyclines is found in a broad range of human and animal pathogens, both gram-positive and gram-negative, including mycoplasmas. The incidence of tetracycline resistance among clinical isolates varies regionally and with time, depending on the selective pressure exerted by the amount

Table 4 Major Therapeutic Indications for Tetracyclines and Bacterial Resistance

Organism	Infection/disease	Resistance[a]
Chlamydia	Pneumonia, trachoma, ornithosis	±
Mycoplasma	Pneumonia, pyelonephritis, pelvic inflammatory disease	+
Ureaplasma urealyticum	Bartholinitis, prostatitis	±
Rickettsia	Q-fever, typhoid fever	±
Coxiella burnetii	Pneumonia	±
Francisella tularensis	Tularemia	±
Borrelia	Lyme disease, relapsing fever	±
Brucella	Brucellosis	+
Pseudomonas		
P. mallei	Glanders	±
P. pseudomallei	Melioidosis	±

[a] ±, ≤5%; +, ≤15%; + +, ≤30%; + + +, >30% of clinical isolates.

of tetracyclines used in human and veterinary medicine. Resistance to tetracycline implies resistance to all compounds with the tetracycline structure in a therapeutic sense (parallel resistance). This means that although a tetracycline, such as minocycline, may be slightly superior to another (doxycycline) in its in vitro activity against staphylococci or *Acinetobacter* spp., it does not represent an alternative for infections caused by tetracycline-resistant strains.

A major mechanism of tetracycline resistance was first thought to be reduced permeation through the cell envelope, in particular the cytoplasmic membrane, as indicated by a reduced concentration of tetracycline in resistant cells compared with susceptible organisms. However, as reviewed in Chapter 7, the major mechanism for tetracycline resistance involves an inducible active efflux system. Several genes encoding for components of this system, located mostly on plasmids, have been identified. In addition, there is resistance associated with a protein protecting the ribosomes (e.g., in mycoplasmas) (27). Although reduced tetracycline accumulation through active efflux is not high enough to account for all tetracycline resistance in bacteria, it appears to be the major contributing factor and is of clinical concern.

The use of the established tetracyclines is limited mainly by the incidence of resistant strains (e.g., in *Enterobacteriaceae* and gram-positive cocci). Is there a prospect to reduce the effect of tetracycline efflux as a mechanism of resistance? A comparison of tetracyclines of different structures indicates that they are not equally recognized by tetracycline-transport proteins; for example, TetA(K) does not recognize the structure of minocycline and doxycycline. Recently, a more promising prospect for overcoming efflux-associated tetracycline resistance has emerged: novel tetracycline derivatives, the glycylcyclines [*N*,*N*-dimethylglycylamino-derivatives of minocycline (CL 329,998) and 6-dimethyl-6-deoxytetracycline (CL 331,002); (28)], which are not recognized by the tetracycline-transporters TetA, TetB, TetC, TetD, and TetK (29,30). Most tetracycline-resistant strains appear to transport tetracyclines by these proteins, as their MICs are much lower for the glycylcyclines relative to tetracycline or minocycline; these compounds remain active against tetracycline-resistant strains (see Chap. 7).

Prerequisites for tetracycline efflux are recognition of the compound by the transporter protein(s), an exportable tetracycline, and a functional transporter protein. Two possibilities to circumvent tetracycline resistance are being explored; namely, changing tetracycline structures so that they are no longer exportable, and screening for inhibitors of the tetracycline transport proteins. The second approach, inhibiting the function of the efflux pump by tetracycline analogues, is in an early stage. Tetracycline derivatives that inhibit the TetA(B) efflux pump have been identified, and further screening for active compounds is in progress (31).

Such developments may, in the future, reduce the results of active efflux on tetracycline resistance and remove a major limitation in the clinical use of tetracyclines. Recently, new structural modifications of tetracycline and minocycline seem to overcome the so far obligatory parallel resistance, since the bacterial ribosome appears not to be the primary target for their mechanism of action (32,33; see Chap. 7). However, these compounds have increased host toxicity.

B. Quinolones

Quinolones have potent, broad-spectrum bactericidal activity (including intracellular pathogens), good pharmacokinetic properties, few side effects, and oral activity. They are highly effective in many common outpatient infections and have been widely used in the past 10 years (Table 5). This has led to resistance development, particularly in staphylococci and pseudomonas (34). Resistance is exclusively chromosomal, spreading along with the resistant organism (clonal spread).

At this time, the effect of active efflux on quinolone resistance appears to be minor in comparison with *gyrA* mutations and reduced permeability. Active efflux, however, may act in concert with reduced outer membrane permeability in gram-negative bacteria to facilitate the emergence of fluoroquinolone-resistant strains.

A carrier-mediated active efflux for norfloxacin was detected in everted inner membrane vesicles of wild-type *E. coli* strains (35). Nevertheless, these strains were susceptible to norfloxacin. The efficiency of the efflux may, however, be increased; for example, by increasing gene dosage or phenotypic expression of the carrier protein, or by higher affinity of the transporter for the fluoroquinolones.

Reduced accumulation of quinolones has been observed in resistant mutants of other gram-negative rods [e.g., *P. aeruginosa* (36) and *Proteus vulgaris* (37)]. It was reversible by the energy inhibitor carbonylcyanide-*m*-chlorophenylhydrazone (CCCP), indicating an energy-dependent efflux mechanism as well.

In *Staphylococcus aureus* the *norA* gene encodes for a hydrophobic protein that contains 12 membrane-spanning domains (38,39). This gene confers fluoroquinolone resistance to both *S. aureus* and *E. coli* (40). Accumulation of enoxacin and norfloxacin is reduced and can be abolished by CCCP (41). Therefore, the *norA* gene most likely encodes for a quinolone efflux transporter, driven by the proton gradient across the cell membrane. Its amino acid sequence is similar to a group of a transporter pro-

Table 5 Major Therapeutic Indications for Quinolones and Bacterial Resistance

Organism	Infection/disease	Resistance[a]
Enterobacteriaceae		
E. coli	UTI, gallbladder	±
K. pneumoniae	Nosocomial pneumonia	±
P. mirabilis	Diarrhea, sepsis	±
E. cloacae		±
Haemophilus		
H. influenzae	RTI, meningitis	±
Neisseriaceae		
N. gonorrhoeae	Gonorrhea	±
M. catarrhalis	Bronchitis	±
Pseudomonas		
P. aeruginosa	UTI, cystic fibrosis, nosocomial pneumonia	+ +
Staphylococci		
S. aureus MS	Skin infections, sepsis	±
S. aureus MR		+ + +
Streptococci		
S. pyogenes	Angina, tonsilitis	±
S. pneumoniae	RTI (upper and lower)	±
Enterococci		
E. faecalis	Endocarditis, UTI	±
E. faecium		±
Bacteroides		
B. fragilis	Abdominal infections	±

[a] ±, ≤5%; +, ≤15%; + +, ≤30%; + + +, >30% of clinical isolates.
Abbreviations: RTI, respiratory tract infections; UTI, urinary tract infections; MS, methicillin-sensitive; MR, methicillin-resistant.

teins related to the plasmid-encoded proteins that mediate active efflux of tetracyclines (42).

C. Macrolides

Macrolide antibiotics, such as erythromycin, have been important oral drugs for over 40 years. Among the safest of antimicrobial agents, they have been traditionally used to treat upper respiratory infections caused by gram-positive cocci, particularly in children (Table 6). They are primarily bacteriostatic; they inhibit protein synthesis by binding to the 50S ribosomal subunit and preventing the formation of new peptide chains.

Table 6 Major Therapeutic Indications for Macrolides and Bacterial Resistance

Organism	Infection/disease	Resistance[a]
Staphylococci		
S. aureus MS	Skin infections, sepsis	±
S. aureus MR		+ + +
Streptococci		
S. pneumoniae	RTI (upper and lower)	±
S. pyogenes	Angina, tonsillitis	±
Enterococci		
E. faecalis	Endocarditis, UTI	+ +
E. faecium		+ + +
Haemophilus		
H. influenzae	RTI, meningitis	±
Neisseriaceae		
N. gonorrhoeae	Gonorrhea	±
M. catarrhalis	Bronchitis	±

[a] ±, ≤5%; +, ≤15%; + +, ≤30%; + + +, >30% of clinical isolates.
Abbreviations: RTI, respiratory tract infections; UTI, urinary tract infections; MS, methicillin-sensitive; MR, methicillin-resistant.

Within the last 15 years, macrolides have undergone a renaissance (43). This is due to the increasing incidence of some childhood infections (otitis media, respiratory infections) and the growing importance of certain intracellular pathogens (*Chlamydia*, *Legionella*, and *Mycoplasma* spp.). Numerous new compounds have been synthesized and found their way into therapy (Fig. 1). Recent entries include azithromycin (CP 62,993, XZ-450), clarithromycin (A-56268, TE-031), roxithromycin (RU 28965, RU-965), and dirithromycin (AS-E 136).

Macrolides are lipophilic molecules, with a 12- to 16-membered lactone ring, without nitrogen, except for azithromycin. The newer macrolides are superior to erythromycin in their pharmacokinetics (e.g., roxithromycin has a half-life of 12 h, azithromycin 4 days, and can be thus administered less frequently), and in the reduction of gastrointestinal side effects owing to their stability in the low pH of the stomach. Their antibacterial activity and spectrum are qualitatively similar to the older compounds; they are active against most gram-positive and gram-negative cocci, but inactive against gram-negative rods. There is also complete cross-resistance between old macrolides and the new compounds.

Resistance to macrolides is due to several mechanisms: altered target, antibiotic inactivation, and decreased accumulation (44). Clinically, the

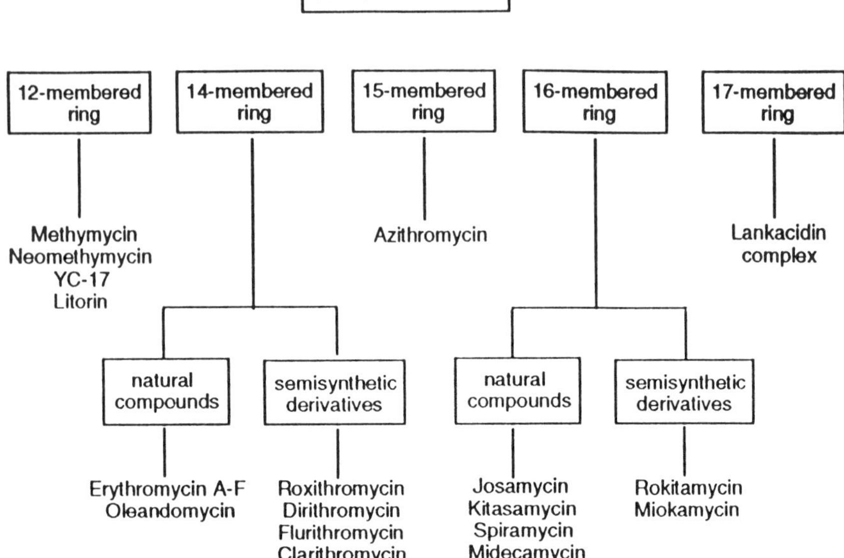

Figure 1   Classification of macrolides. (Adapted from Ref. 53.)

most common form of macrolide resistance includes resistance to the functionally similar, but structurally different, lincosamides and streptogramins (MLS-resistance). The MLS-resistant strains produce a methylase that dimethylates adenine 2058 in the 28S RNA (45). Consequently, MLS antibiotics can no longer bind to the ribosomes, and protein synthesis proceeds unhindered. In addition, sole resistance to macrolides can result from hydrolysis of the macrolide ring by esterases (46), phosphorylation (47,48), or glycosylation at the 2'-position (49).

Reduced antibiotic entry into the cell has been recently described as a possible mechanism of resistance to macrolides (50). It was found in *Staphylococcus epidermidis* and in producers of macrolides (*Streptomyces fradiae*). A strain of *S. epidermidis* resistant to erythromycin (MIC 25 µg/ml) was able to maintain an intracellular macrolide concentration below the level necessary for binding to ribosomes and inhibiting protein synthesis. This strain became susceptible to erythromycin (MIC 0.04 µg/ml) after exposure to CCCP, which is known to dissipate the membrane proton motive force (pmf). In parallel, the intracellular erythromycin concentration increased to a level indistinguishable from that in an erythromycin-susceptible strain (Fig. 2). The energy-dependent efflux pump was linked to a plasmid, pNE24, present only in the resistant strain. This novel mechanism of macrolide resistance appears to recognize specific structures, since it is confined to 14-membered macrolides and azithromycin only.

The impact of this mechanism on the resistance to macrolides at present and in future development is difficult to assess. So far, an energy-dependent efflux pump was identified only in four *S. epidermidis* strains: one by Lampson in the United States in 1986 (51) and three in Japan in 1970 (30). This may indicate no or slow spread, although the genes for the

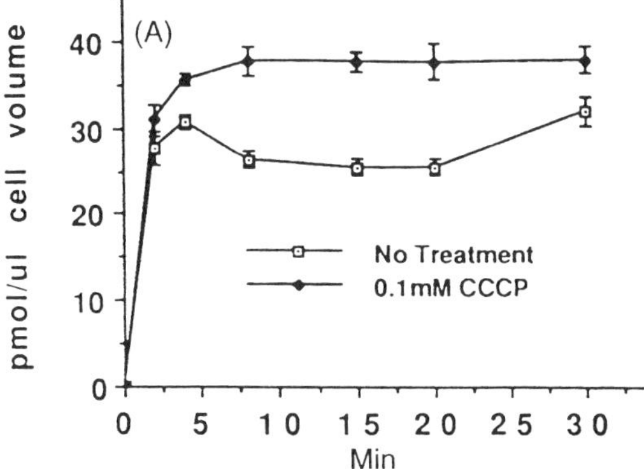

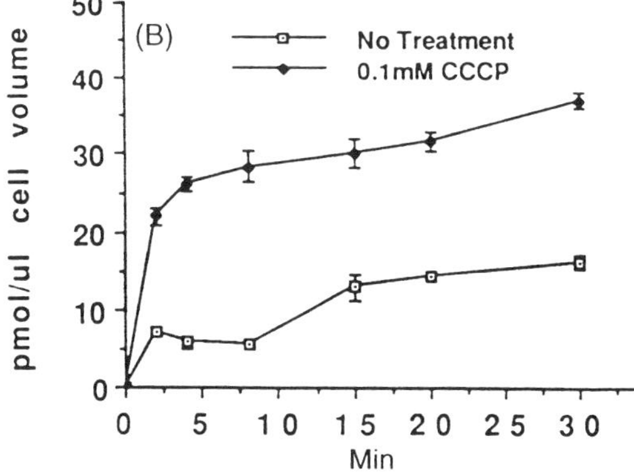

Figure 2 Intracellular erythromycin concentration after pretreatment with CCCP in *Staphylococcus epidermidis*. (A) Erythromycin-susceptible; (B) Erythromycin-resistant strain. (Adapted from Ref. 50.)

efflux pump are located on a plasmid. However, macrolide resistance mechanisms other than MLS-resistance are not easily recognized, and reduced permeability may be confused in a significant number of strains with energy-dependent efflux. Further spread of the latter to 14- and 15-membered macrolides may thus proceed unrecognized.

IV. CONCLUSIONS AND FUTURE DIRECTIONS

Although several classes of antibacterial agents currently exist, all are vulnerable to resistance in some bacteria. Even though most resistant pathogens (staphylococci, enterococci, or pseudomonas) are hospital-based, some (*S. pneumoniae* and *M. tuberculosis*) are, alarmingly, community acquired. β-Lactam antibiotics, the centerpiece of antibacterial chemotherapy for the past 50 years, have encountered perhaps the greatest diversity of resistance mechanisms: enzymatic inactivation; altered, new, or overproduced targets; and altered transport. Other antibiotics, the quinolones, macrolides, tetracyclines, and aminoglycosides, have faced less diverse, although equally effective, resistance mechanisms. Altered transport has played a primary role in the resistance to tetracyclines (active efflux) and β-lactams (impaired transport through the outer membrane, combined with β-lactamase), and a secondary role in the resistance to quinolones, macrolides, and aminoglycosides. Transport, by its very nature, has potential for cross-resistance between unrelated antibiotics: quinolones and tetracyclines, or quinolones and β-lactams (imipenem). Yet, its challenge also presents opportunities: to specifically block antibiotic efflux, or to increase uptake through the outer membrane and, thereby, enhance the activity of several antibiotics (see Chap. 10). Other possibilities include exploiting additional transport pathways through the outer membrane (a feat serendipitously achieved with catechol cephalosporins, although none has yet become a drug), or bypassing the efflux pump altogether, possibly by increasing hydrophobicity.

Clearly, our understanding of transport-associated resistance mechanisms has progressed to a point where they can be approached rationally as chemotherapeutic targets. The recently reported mechanism-based screens for detecting inhibitors of tetracycline efflux pumps (52) and structure–activity relations of inhibitors of the tetracycline efflux pump (31) are steps in that direction.

REFERENCES

1. Parry MF. Epidemiology and mechanisms of antimicrobial resistance. Am J Infect Control 1989; 17:286–294.

2. Levy SB. Confronting multidrug resistance: a role for each of us. JAMA 1993; 269:1840–1842.
3. Kunin CM. Resistance to antimicrobial drugs—a worldwide calamity. Ann Intern Med 1993; 118:557–561.
4. Neu HC. The crisis in antibiotic resistance. Science 1992; 257:1064–1073.
5. Jacoby GA, Archer GL. New mechanisms of bacterial resistance to antimicrobial agents. N Engl J Med 1991; 324:601–612.
6. Amyes SGB, Gemmell CG. Antibiotic resistance in bacteria. J Med Microbiol 1992; 36:4–29.
7. Bryan LE. General mechanisms of resistance to antibiotics. J Antimicrob Chemother 1988; 22 (suppl A):1–15.
8. Schmidt LH. The MIC_{50}/MIC_{90} assessments of in vitro activities of antimicrobial agents that facilitate comparative agent–agent and agent–species susceptibility comparisons. Antimicrob Newslett 1987; 4:1–8.
9. Courvalin P. Interpretive reading of antimicrobial susceptibility tests. ASM News 1992; 58:368–375.
10. Hiraoka M, Okamoto R, Inoue M, Mitsuhashi S. Effects of β-lactamases and *omp* mutation on susceptibility to β-lactam antibiotics in *Escherichia coli*. Antimicrob Agents Chemother 1989; 33:382–386.
11. Jarlier V, Gutmann L, Nikaido H. Interplay of cell wall barrier and β-lactamase activity determines high resistance to β-lactam antibiotics in *Mycobacterium chelonae*. Antimicrob Agents Chemother 1991; 35:1937–1939.
12. Neuhaus FC, Georgopapadakou NH. Strategies in β-lactam design. In: Sutcliffe JA, Georgopapadakou NH, eds. Emerging Targets in Antibacterial and Antifungal Chemotherapy. New York: Chapman & Hall, 1992:205–273.
13. Livermore DM. Antibiotic uptake and transport by bacteria. Scand J Infect Dis [Suppl] 1991; 74:15–22.
14. Nikaido H, Vaara M. Molecular basis of outer membrane permeability. Microbiol Rev 1985; 49:1–32.
15. Georgopapadakou NH. Antibiotic permeation through the bacterial outer membrane. J Chemother 1990; 2:275–279.
16. Li X-Z, Ma D, Livermore DM, Nikaido H. Role of efflux pump(s) in intrinsic resistance of *Pseudomonas aeruginosa*: active efflux as a contributing factor to β-lactam resistance. Antimicrob Agents Chemother 1994; 38:1742–1752.
17. Yoshimura F, Nikaido H. Diffusion of β-lactam antibiotics through the porin channels of *Escherichia coli* K-12. Antimicrob Agents Chemother 1985; 27:84–92.
18. Harder KJ, Nikaido H, Matsuhashi M. Mutants of *Escherichia coli* that are resistant to certain β-lactam compounds lack the *ompF* porin. Antimicrob Agents Chemother 1981; 20:549–552.
19. Hancock REW, Bell A. Antibiotic uptake into gram-negative bacteria. Eur J Clin Microbiol Infect Dis 1988; 7:713–720.
20. Werner V, Sanders CC, Sanders E Jr, Goering RV. Role of β-lactamases and outer membrane proteins in multiple β-lactam resistance of *Enterobacter cloacae*. Antimicrob Agents Chemother 1985; 27:455–459.
21. Marchou B, Bellido F, Charnas R, Lucain C, Pechère J-C. Contribution of β-lactamase hydrolysis and outer membrane permeability to ceftriaxone

resistance in *Enterobacter cloacae*. Antimicrob Agents Chemother 1987; 31:1589–1595.

22. Satake S, Yoshihara E, Nakae T. Diffusion of β-lactam antibiotics through liposome membranes reconstituted from purified porins of the outer membrane of *Pseudomonas aeruginosa*. Antimicrob Agents Chemother 1990; 34:685–690.

23. Nakae R, Nakae T. Diffusion of aminoglycoside antibiotics across the outer membrane of *Escherichia coli*. Antimicrob Agents Chemother 1982; 22:554–559.

24. Shaw KJ, Rather PM, Hare RS, Miller GH. Molecular genetics of aminoglycoside resistance genes and familial relationships of the aminoglycoside-modifying enzymes. Microbiol Rev 1993; 57:138–163.

25. Perlin MH, Lerner SA. High-level amikacin resistance in *E. coli* due to phosphorylation and impaired aminoglycoside uptake. Antimicrob Agents Chemother 1986; 29:216–224.

26. Levy SB. Active efflux mechanisms for antimicrobial resistance. Antimicrob Agents Chemother 1992; 36:695–703.

27. Burdett V. Purification and characterization of Tet(M), a protein that renders ribosomes resistant to tetracycline. J Biol Chem 1991; 266:995–1004.

28. Testa RT, Petersen PJ, Jacobus NV, Sum P-E, Lee VJ, Tally FP. In vitro and in vivo antibacterial activities of the glycylglycines, a new class of semisynthetic tetracyclines. Antimicrob Agents Chemother 1993; 37:2270–2277.

29. Eliopoulos GM, Wennerstein CB, Cole G, Moellering RC. In vitro activities of two glycylcyclines against gram-positive bacteria. Antimicrob Agents Chemother 1994; 38:534–541.

30. Omura S, Namiki S, Shibata M, Mura T, Sawada J. Studies on the antibiotics from *Streptomyces spinichromogenes* var. *kujimyceticus*. V. Some antimicrobial characteristics of kujimycin A and kujimycin B against macrolide resistant staphylococci. J Antibiot 1970; 9:448–460.

31. Nelson ML, Park BH, Levy SB. Molecular requirements for the inhibition of the tetracycline antiport protein and the effect of potent inhibitors on the growth of tetracycline-resistant bacteria. J Med Chem 1994; 37:1355–1361.

32. Rasmussen BA, Noller HF, Daubresse G, Oliva B, Misulovin Z, Rothstein DM, Ellestad GA, Gluzman Y, Tally FP, Chopra I. Molecular basis of tetracycline action: identification of analogs whose primary target is not the bacterial ribosome. Antimicrob Agents Chemother 1991; 35:2306–2311.

33. Chopra I. Tetracycline analogs whose primary target is not the bacterial ribosome. Antimicrob Agents Chemother 1994; 38:637–640.

34. Wolfson JS, Hooper DC. Bacterial resistance to quinolones: mechanisms and clinical importance. Rev Infect Dis 1989; 11(suppl 5):S960–S968.

35. Cohen SP, Hooper DC, Wolfson JS, Souza KS, McMurry LM, Levy SB. An endogenous active efflux of norfloxacin in *Escherichia coli*. Antimicrob Agents Chemother 1988; 32:1187–1191.

36. Chamberland S, Bayer AS, Schollaardt T, Wong SA, Bryan LE. Characterization of mechanisms of quinolone resistance in *Pseudomonas aeruginosa*

strains in vitro and in vivo during experimental endocarditis. Antimicrob Agents Chemother 1989; 33:624–634.

37. Ishii H, Sato K, Hoshino K, Sato M, Yamaguchi A, Sawai T, Osada Y. Active efflux of ofloxacin by a highly quinolone-resistant strain of *Proteus vulgaris*. J Antimicrob Chemother 1991; 28:827–836.

38. Yoshida H, Bogaki M, Nakamura S, Ubukata K, Konno M. Nucleotide sequence and characterization of the *Staphylococcus aureus norA* gene, which confers resistance to quinolones. J Bacteriol 1990; 172:6942–6949.

39. Neyfakh AA, Bidnenko VE, Chen LB. Fluoroquinolone resistance protein NorA of *Staphylococcus aureus* is a multidrug efflux transporter. Antimicrob Agents Chemother 1993; 37:128–129.

40. Kaatz GW, Seo SM, Ruble CA. Efflux-mediated fluoroquinolone resistance in *Staphylococcus aureus*. Antimicrob Agents Chemother 1993; 37:1086–1094.

41. Kaatz GW, Seo SM, Ruble CA. Mechanisms of fluoroquinolone resistance in *Staphylococcus aureus*. J Infect Dis 1991; 163:1080–1086.

42. Nikaido H, Saier MH Jr. Transport proteins in bacteria: common themes in their design. Science 1992; 258:936–942.

43. Fernandes P. The macrolide revival: thirty-five years after erythromycin. Antimicrob Newslett 1987; 4:25–34.

44. Eady EA, Ross JI, Cove JH. Multiple mechanisms of erythromycin resistance. J Antimicrob Chemother 1990; 26:461–465.

45. Skinner R, Cundliffe E, Schmidt FJ. Site of action of a ribosomal RNA methylase responsible for resistance to erythromycin and other antibiotics. J Biol Chem 1983; 258:12702–12706.

46. Arthur M, Brisson-Noel A, Courvalin P. Origin and evolution of genes specifying resistance to macrolide, lincosamide and streptogramin antibiotics: data and hypotheses. J Antimicrob Chemother 1987; 20:783–802.

47. Wiley PF, Baczynskyj L, Dolak LA, Cialdella JI, Marshall VP. Enzymatic phosphorylation of macrolide antibiotics. J Antibiot 1987; 40:195–201.

48. Leclerq R, Courvalin P. Intrinsic and unusual resistance to macrolide, lincosamide, and streptogramin antibiotics in bacteria. Antimicrob Agents Chemother 1991; 35:1273–1276.

49. Duval J. Evolution and epidemiology of MLS resistance. J Antimicrob Chemother 1985; 16(suppl A):137–149.

50. Goldman RC, Capobianco JO. Role of an energy-dependent efflux pump in plasmid pNE24-mediated resistance to 14- and 15-membered macrolides in *Staphylococcus epidermidis*. Antimicrob Agents Chemother 1990; 34:1973–1980.

51. Lampson BC, von David W, Parisi JT. Novel mechanism for plasmid-mediated erythromycin resistance by pNE24 from *Staphylococcus epidermidis*. Antimicrob Agents Chemother 1986; 30:653–658.

52. Rothstein DM, McGlynn M, Bernan V, et al. Detection of tetracyclines and efflux pump inhibitors. Antimicrob Agents Chemother 1993; 37:1624–1629.

53. Bryskier A, Agouridas C, Chantot J-F. Relation structure activity of 14- and 15-membered macrolides. Chemotherapie 1993; 2(suppl 2):2–11.

2

The Impact of Transport-Associated Resistance in Anticancer Chemotherapy

Henk J. Broxterman, Gerrit Jansen, Sabine C. Linn, and Jan Lankelma
Free University Hospital, Amsterdam, The Netherlands

I. INTRODUCTION

A. Cancer Incidence and Response to Chemotherapy

1. Cancer Chemotherapy Resistance Associated with Age and Site

Cancer treatment consists of three modalities: surgery, radiotherapy, and systemic therapy. Systemic therapy includes treatment with cytotoxic agents, hormones, and, in experimental settings, immunomodulators, monoclonal antibodies, or genes. Although surgery, sometimes combined with radiotherapy, is still the mainstay of cancer treatment, the application of chemotherapy has a definite influence on overall cancer survival statistics and has become the curative treatment of choice for some malignancies. In general, the most chemosensitive tumors are those characterized by rapid growth rates, which are rapidly lethal in the absence of effective systemic treatment (1). The treatment of childhood cancer by chemotherapy has had the largest effect on patient survival rates, with a 5-year survival increase from 28% in 1960 to 67% in 1985 (2). However, the most common forms of cancer in adults, mainly cancers of epithelial origin, are rarely curable by chemotherapy. These cancers, for the most part, comprise lung, gastrointestinal (colorectal), breast, and prostate cancer, which are responsible for 50–60% of all cancer deaths (2). This less responsive group of tumors, with generally low growth rates that result in long clinical doubling times relative to childhood cancer, shows a sharp rise in incidence between 25 and 50 years of age. The poor response of these tumors to chemotherapy is now generally thought to reflect the duration of exposure to environmental carcinogenic factors. These considerations point to relationships between age, tumor growth, and drug resistance (1).

2. Cancer Chemotherapy Resistance: Concepts

The concept of resistance is as old as cytotoxic chemotherapy itself (3). As with antimicrobial chemotherapy, failure of cancer chemotherapy may be due to overgrowth of resistant cells. Therefore, doses of antitumor drugs needed to kill those cells are then intolerable to the host. This points to an essential, clinical observation that, whereas cancers become chemoresistant, the toxicity to normal cells or tissues remains.

The study of clinical drug resistance in cancer patients is still in the early days, with key mechanisms just now beginning to be discovered. The ideas on the mechanisms (and their development) responsible for resistance have changed over the years. Originally, the major postulated resistance mechanism was kinetic: the most resistant tumor cells were considered to be nonproliferating (G_0 phase) (3), and new drugs able to kill those quiescent cells were sought.

The second major mechanism of resistance is based on pharmacological and pharmacokinetic considerations: a drug would not kill cancer cells unless it reached the tumor at adequate concentrations for an appropriate time period (3). This postulated resistance mechanism includes all aspects of drug distribution, excretion, poor perfusion of drug into the tumor, blood–brain barrier, metabolism, or other, and provoked extensive pharmacokinetic studies. A major obstacle to improving cancer therapy following this line is that tumor tissue concentrations of drugs are usually difficult to assess.

Later, the concept of biochemical resistance developed, building on the postulated biochemical mechanisms of action of antitumor agents such as methotrexate and fluorouracil. It allowed testable hypotheses for cellular resistance, based on biochemical alterations in the cells. It is this third mechanism that is currently the subject of intense experimentation. The start for such studies was the work of Goldie and Coldman in 1979 (4), who developed mathematical models that related curability to the probability of occurrence of singly or doubly resistant cell clones. Their work was analogous to the observations of Luria and Delbruck in 1943, which indicated that bacteria have an inherent ability to mutate toward resistance to agents they have never encountered. Thus, the Goldie–Coldman model emphasized genetic mechanisms of drug resistance and assumed spontaneous mutation rates toward resistance, similar to natural mutation frequencies, in the order of 10^{-6}.

More recently, tumor development is thought to be a multistep process, requiring several mutations to occur for a cell to become a tumor ("stem") cell. Moreover, for most tumors, it is thought that a high genetic instability exists during the long growth period before they become clinically manifest and detectable by their size and before metastasizing. Thus, tumor cell populations develop that are highly heterogeneous genetically and biologically (5). At the time of diagnosis, most cancers, especially in older persons, consist of subpopulations of cells differing in such basic features as growth rates or hormone production. In addition, the possibility of mutations affecting susceptibility to cytotoxic drugs is great. Such concepts, although not excluding all other factors, such as low tumor cell growth fraction, may partly explain why larger tumor masses (having undergone more doubling times and mutations) are generally less curable.

In terms of the genetics involved in tumor drug resistance, the selection of preexisting subpopulations with resistance to drugs ("intrinsic resistance"), or mutations occurring in the presence of drug ("acquired resistance"), are not basically different. The latter, however, is more easily studied in cell culture, by increasing drug concentrations stepwise to select highly resistant cell lines suitable for biochemical analysis (5). Since, in principle, mutations are irreversible, the resistance is retained if the cells are grown without drug. In fact, this type of approach has led to the identification of several biochemical resistance mechanisms responsible for in vitro resistance (e.g., to methotrexate and anthracyclines).

A genetic basis for cancer drug resistance was established by Biedler and Spengler (6) and Schimke and collegues (7), who found that amplified DNA in cell lines resistant to methotrexate contained extra copies of the gene coding for the target enzyme dihydrofolate reductase. The ability to clone and sequence genes has led to the identification of other such genetic changes underlying several forms of drug resistance. In particular, the cloning of the drug transporter protein, P-glycoprotein (Pgp), discussed in Chapters 17 and 18 of this volume, has generated much research.

3. Cancer Chemotherapy Resistance and Tumor Classes

Cancers in the elderly are generally less responsive to chemotherapy than are juvenile cancers. Part of this difference could be related to the generally low growth fraction of these cancers, making them less susceptible to cytostatic drugs, or to the long growth period during which "resistance mutations" could have activated drug resistance mechanisms.

Childhood tumors generally well responsive to chemotherapy are mainly hematological; in childhood leukemias and lymphomas chemotherapy is capable of cures. Another sensitive tumor is childhood nephroblastoma, an embryonal tumor of the kidney; adult renal cell carcinoma, however, is one of the most chemoresistant tumors (8).

Some tumor types show moderate to high response rates to chemotherapy. In this category belong frequently occurring tumor types, such as breast, ovarian, and small-cell lung cancer (SCLC), as well as acute myeloid leukemia. Almost invariably, however, tumors regrow, and these recurring tumors do not respond to chemotherapy. Typically, ovarian cancer is now treated with cisplatin-based combination chemotherapy, leading to an improvement in long-term survival of patients with advanced-stage ovarian cancer. Nevertheless, most patients relapse and die of their chemotherapy-refractory disease (9). An even more dramatic example is SCLC, which has a very high initial clinical complete response rate of 90% to combination chemotherapy, including doxorubicin and etoposide. However, despite this high sensitivity, patients with SCLC relapse, and subsequent resistance to all chemotherapeutic agents develops in most patients. This type of cancer resistance may be called acquired resistance, although it is not known whether, in fact, selection of preexisting subclones or mutation during chemotherapy has occurred. The most unfortunate characteristic of this resistance, however, is that it extends to all standard agents available and, thus, is termed multidrug resistance.

A third group of tumors are already largely resistant to chemotherapy at diagnosis. Although some of these tumors initially do respond to chemotherapy, the 5-year survival has not improved. Therefore, no standard chemotherapy is available for this group of patients. These cancers include renal cell cancer, carcinomas of the gastrointestinal tract and lung, non–small-cell lung cancer, pancreatic cancer, and malignant melanoma. Nevertheless, even in this group, an individual patient may occasionally show complete tumor remission (10). The causes for such rapid or complete clinical drug resistance, such as in non–small-cell lung cancer, malignant melanoma, or renal cell cancer, are still largely unknown. It is interesting, though, that many such cancers arise from epithelial tissues, in contact with the environment, that have lifelong exposure to carcinogenic chemicals or radiation. Such tissues have "normal" defense mechanisms against cytotoxic insults, which may still be expressed in the malignant cells arising from them. An interesting hypothesis, put forward by Harris (11), is that the primary resistant state of tumor cells may be the normal state, reflecting the resistance of most normal, nondividing tissues to chemotherapy, requiring mutations to become sensitive. Experimental evidence to support this hypothesis is largely lacking.

B. Antitumor Drug Classes, Structures, and Targets

Approximately 65 chemicals are now approved products for treatment of cancer in the United States. We will briefly discuss the major classes of antitumor agents that are currently in clinical use. Resistance to all these classes of agents is common in clinical practice and, in fact, is the cause of failing therapy for many disseminated forms of cancer. For more complete information and entries to specific literature we refer to the volume by DeVita et al. (12).

1.　Alkylating Agents

The alkylating agents were the first useful drugs in cancer chemotherapy and still remain important as single agents, or in combination therapy. Although a structurally heterogeneous group of compounds, alkylating agents have in common that they produce a positively charged electrophilic (alkyl) group that attacks biological molecules. Their antitumor action is thought to result from their ability to form DNA adducts that interfere with DNA function. Two such conventional alkylators are melphalan and cyclophosphamide (Fig. 1). Melphalan is used in the treatment of multiple myeloma and some solid tumors, and cyclophosphamide is used in breast cancer and other tumors.

2.　Platinum Complexes

Platinum complexes, mainly cisplatin (see Fig. 1) and carboplatin, are curative in combination therapies for testicular cancer and play an important role in the treatment of lung, bladder, and head and neck cancer. Although not an "alkylator," cisplatin can bind covalently to all DNA bases, and also to RNA, and less to proteins. The formation of platinum–DNA adducts changes the DNA conformation and is thought to be primarily responsible for the cytotoxic action.

3.　Antimetabolites

The most important antimetabolites in cancer treatment are methotrexate, fluorouracil, and cytarabine (cytosine arabinoside; AraC; see Fig. 1). The basis for the mechanism of action of these compounds is that they are structural analogues of molecules essential for DNA or RNA synthesis. Methotrexate inhibits de novo purine synthesis by blocking the enzyme dihydrofolate reductase, which ultimately results in blockade of DNA synthesis.

4.　Vinca Alkaloids and Taxol

Many anticancer agents are natural products derived from plants or slightly modified derivatives thereof. The vinca alkaloids, vincristine and

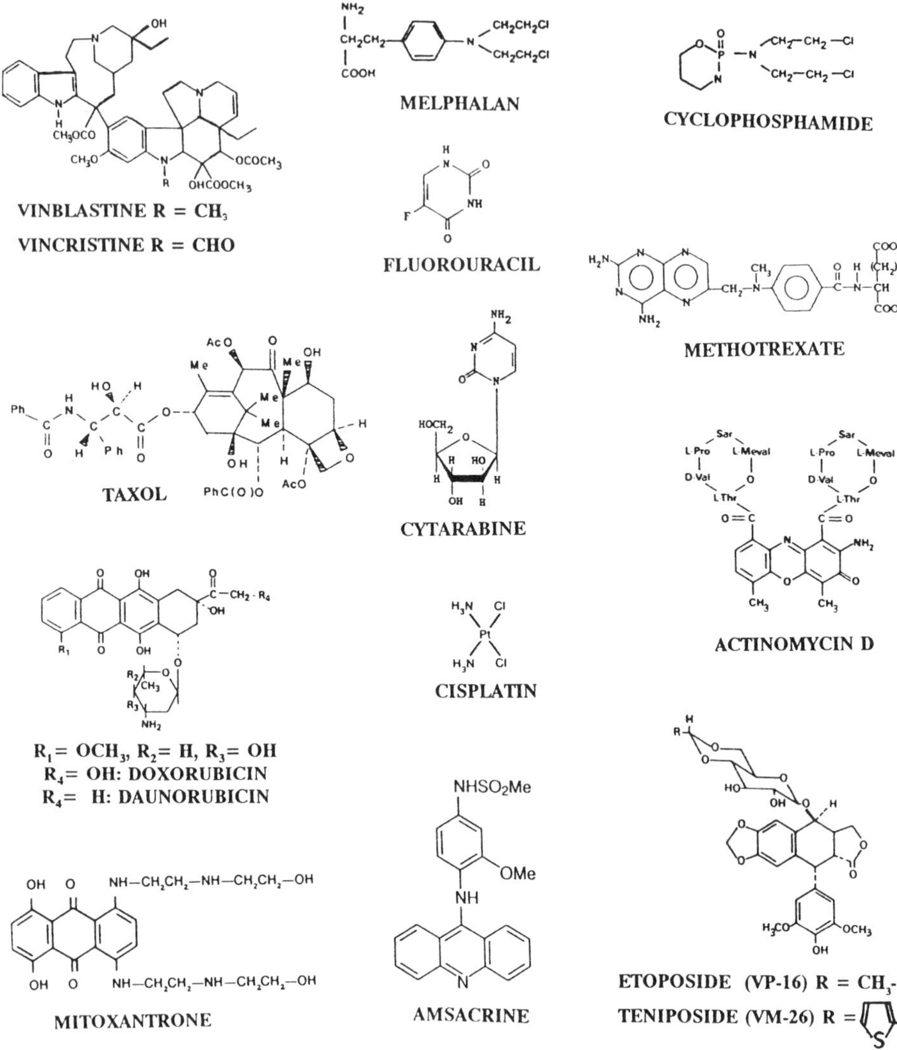

Figure 1   Major classes of antitumor agents.

vinblastine, as well as the investigational agent taxol (see Fig. 1) are such plant-derived alkaloids. Taxol is a very complex molecule with 11 optically active sites and a side chain at C-13 essential for antitumor activity. The vinca alkaloids have broad-spectrum antitumor activity in childhood as well as adult cancers. The development of taxol as a clinically useful agent has been hampered for about 20 years, since its first isolation in 1971, by a lack of clearly superior activity relative to other drugs, low water solubility, and a shortage in the supply of the drug. In recent years, however, taxol has been shown to have definite activity against ovarian cancer. The cytotoxic action of vinca alkaloids is due to inhibition of microtubule assembly, whereas that of taxol is due to inhibition of microtubule disassembly. In either event, the dynamic instability of microtubules is perturbed, which is critical in essential cellular functions, such as intracellular transport, motility, and mitosis. Both vinca alkaloids and taxol inhibit mitosis in eukaryotic cells.

5. *Dactinomycin and Anthracyclines*

Dactinomycin (actinomycin D) is a natural product isolated from *Streptomyces* spp. and is the only member of its class used clinically in the treatment of relatively rare cancers, such as nephroblastoma (Wilms' tumor) and Ewing's sarcoma. It is composed of a phenoxazone ring system to which are attached two cyclic peptide moieties (see Fig. 1). The drug acts by intercalating in a specific manner in the DNA double-helix, thereby inhibiting synthesis of RNA and DNA. The anthracyclines are one of the most widely used classes of antitumor agents. Daunorubicin is most effective in the treatment of leukemias, whereas doxorubicin is used mainly in solid tumors, such as breast and lung cancer. The anthracyclines (see Fig. 1) are produced by *Streptomyces* and have a planar anthraquinone nucleus, with an amino sugar attached to it. Daunorubicin and doxorubicin intercalate between DNA base pairs and trap topoisomerase II in a cleavable complex with DNA. The cleavable complex is eventually transformed into a permanent DNA break that is lethal to the cell.

6. *Epipodophyllotoxins and Amsacrine*

The epipodophyllotoxins etoposide (VP-16) and teniposide (VM-26) (see Fig. 1) are glycosidic derivatives of podophyllotoxin from the mandrake plant (*Podophyllum peltatum*). They have highly significant clinical activity against many cancer types, such as non-Hodgkin's lymphomas, leukemias, and SCLC. Similar to anthracyclines, their mechanism of action involves interference with the DNA cleavage–resealing reaction of topoisomerase II. Unlike anthracyclines, neither compound intercalates in DNA.

Amsacrine (*m*-AMSA) (see Fig. 1) is an acridine dye that intercalates between both DNA strands and produces single- and double-stranded breaks, a process involving topoisomerase II. It is also cytotoxic. Amsacrine is used in combination with cytarabine (Ara-C) in the treatment of acute myeloid leukemia refractory to anthracyclines. Resistance to all topoisomerase II-interactive drugs, such as mitoxantrone, anthracyclines, and especially, VP-16 and m-AMSA, generally involves alterations in topoisomerase II expression or activity (13).

II. CLINICAL MULTIDRUG RESISTANCE (MDR)

A. Definition of MDR

1. Criteria for MDR

The basis for what we presently call multidrug resistance of tumor cells was provided by the work of Biedler and of Ling and colleagues, who selected Chinese hamster cells for resistance to the cytotoxic agents dactinomycin (14,15) and colchicine (16), respectively. Both groups obtained cells that were cross-resistant to a broad group of drugs and found that overexpression of a 170-kDa plasma membrane protein to be associated with the resistant phenotype. This protein is now known as P-glycoprotein (Pgp) (17).

In the present overview, we confine ourselves to the type of MDR defined as cross-resistance to several structurally and mechanistically unrelated antitumor agents, typically the anthracyclines and taxol (see Sec. I.B), which have different targets. Therefore, cross-resistance to such a wide variety of agents is most likely caused by a decrease in drug concentration at the intracellular target sites. The decrease in activity may be due to a decrease in active drug uptake, enhanced drug efflux, or altered metabolism, resulting in increased detoxification of the drug in the cell.

If cells are exposed to a drug for a relatively short period, before steady state is reached, increased rapid drug trapping in (exocytotic) vesicles could, theoretically, also contribute to resistance (18).

Significant progress has been made in understanding MDR, with the cloning of the human *MDR1* gene, and the identification of its protein product Pgp as a drug-transporter molecule, causing drug transport out of cells (17).

The pharmacological criteria for identifying the MDR phenotype, established in cultured tumor cell lines, are as follows:

1. Decreased steady-state accumulation of several unrelated drugs
2. Energy-dependent drug accumulation
3. Reduced drug influx or increased drug efflux
4. Altered intracellular distribution of anthracyclines (decreased drug concentration at nuclear target sites)
5. Transport of drug out of the cell against a concentration gradient
6. Transport is saturable after increasing drug concentration
7. Reversal of the phenotype by inhibitors of the drug transporter

2. Genes and Proteins Involved in MDR

The identification of a transporter molecule causing drug transport has been established by transfection experiments for *MDR1*/Pgp (19). The Pgp has been identified as a member of the ATP-binding cassette (ABC) superfamily and has been shown to render cells resistant to a large number of mostly lipophilic drugs by effluxing these drugs in an ATP-dependent process (17,19). Vulnerable drugs include clinically important agents, such as the anthracyclines, doxorubicin and daunorubicin, the vinca alkaloids, vincristine and vinblastine, taxol, mitoxantrone, and etoposide. Not affected are alkylating agents, the antimetabolites, and cisplatin. Furthermore, the resistance to many MDR drugs in cell lines, as well in the clinic, is probably multifactorial, involving in addition target-associated mechanisms, such as topoisomerase II-mediated resistance for doxorubicin or etoposide (see following) (20).

A second ABC transporter postulated to be involved in MDR has been cloned recently by Cole and colleagues (21). The gene was designated as multidrug resistance-associated protein (*MRP*) and encodes a 190-kDa protein. Transfection experiments have shown that *MRP* is able to confer MDR to a sensitive cell line (22). It is not yet clear by which mechanism and to which drugs *MRP* causes resistance, but such drugs include at least doxorubicin, daunorubicin, etoposide, and vincristine. Also, *MRP* expression can be up-regulated after selection with low doses of doxorubicin (23).

A few other proteins have been found to be overexpressed in MDR cell lines that do not express *MDR1*/Pgp (p110, p95; 24,25), but their structures or functions are unknown. Other proteins potentially involved in clinical MDR must be mentioned here for completeness, although they will not be further discussed, since they do not involve active drug transport.

A frequent mechanism of resistance to topoisomerase II-targeted drugs (anthracyclines, etoposide, *m*-AMSA, mitoxantrone), at least in cell lines, is the occurrence of altered topoisomerase II or decreased topoisomerase II expression. This target-related form of resistance probably contributes to resistance to doxorubicin at early selection steps, with possibly clinically relevant concentrations. For a recent review on drug resistance associated with altered DNA topoisomerase II we refer to Beck et al. (26).

Another form of MDR not associated with drug transport may be blockade of the pathway leading to cell death downstream from the primary interaction with the target. This process of active cell death, called *apoptosis*, is suggested to be triggered by various stimuli, including cytotoxic drugs, such as topoisomerase II inhibitors or alkylating agents, and it is now rapidly unraveled in molecular terms. At least two genes have been identified to be involved in apoptosis: *bcl-2* and *p53*. As a protooncogene involved in a chromosomal translocation frequently found in human malignant lymphomas, *bcl-2* inhibits apoptosis by an unknown mechanism (27). Thus, overexpression of *bcl-2* would make tumor cells resistant to chemotherapy by inhibiting apoptotic cell death (28).

In contrast, the *p53* tumor suppressor gene product seems to be required for efficient execution of the apoptotic cell death program, induced by, for example, fluorouracil, etoposide, and doxorubicin (29). Since oncogene expression can stabilize p53 protein and, thereby, lower the threshold for apoptosis, this would give an explanation for the rather high vulnerability of tumor cells to anticancer agents (29). The prevalence of *p53* mutations in several tumor types that are inherently chemoresistant (malignant melanoma, and colon, bladder, or prostate cancer) would be consistent with this hypothesis (30,31).

3.   *Diagnostics of MDR*

The diagnostics of MDR in human cancers rely mainly on the detection of Pgp or *MDR1* (over)expression. In human tumor samples, *MDR1* mRNA expression has been initially analyzed by Northern blots and is heterogeneous among tumor samples, without evidence for gene amplification. Later, the more sensitive polymerase chain reaction has been used to quantify *MDR1* mRNA. With this method, *MDR1* expression was detectable in many, but not all, human normal tissues and tumors (32). Earlier immunohistochemical analyses with monoclonal antibodies had already established that many normal human epithelial cells lining the gastrointestinal tract and in kidney tubules, in endothelial cells in blood vessels (brain) and in the adrenal cortex had a particularly high Pgp expression, suggesting a role for Pgp in protection of tissues against environmental toxins (8,33,34). Expression of Pgp in tumors was highest in those tumors originating from the colon or kidney, but was very low in lung cancer. Thus, although some of the most chemoresistant tumor types have a relatively high Pgp expression, a correlation between prognosis of patient groups and Pgp expression has been established clearly in only a very few tumor types, particularly childhood sarcomas and neuroblastomas (35). Correlation between prognosis of treatment and *MDR1*/Pgp expression in acute myeloid leukemias has been suggested by several studies, but its causal relation has never been proved (36).

Interpretation of the many studies published on *MDR1*/Pgp expression in human tumors is complicated by the variety in techniques, probes, and antibodies used, which have led to a sometimes confusing picture. Many of these studies do not allow definite conclusions on the significance of Pgp expression for the resistance phenotype of the tumors.

Critical technical factors include the following:

1. When bulk RNA or protein techniques (Northern or Western blot-

ting) are used, it must be remembered that these may not be sensitive enough and that many normal stromal or blood components are likely to contribute to the signal.

2. In situ techniques, such as immunocytochemical and in situ hybridization, have, until now, been largely inconclusive because of lack of sensitivity, cross-reactions of antibodies, or technical problems.
3. Flow cytometric detection of Pgp is sensitive and, in principle, feasible for hematological malignancies, but has not yet been developed for solid tumors.
4. Interlaboratory standardization studies are still in an early phase.

Furthermore, when applying RNA or protein measurements to predict an "MDR index" or response of a patient's tumor to chemotherapy, several other factors must be taken into account. These are posttranslational modification of Pgp (mainly phosphorylation), heterogeneity of expression, relative contribution of Pgp-mediated transport to total (passive plus active) drug transport, as well as the presence of other resistance mechanisms (other transporters or detoxification).

For the determination of drug transporters, the development of functional assays may partly circumvent these problems. The fact that drugs, such as the anthracyclines, as well as other highly fluorescent molecules, such as the rhodamines (37–39), are transported by Pgp offers unique possibilities to combine functional assays with Pgp (or other transporter) detection by using flow cytometry or laser scan microscopy (40). An example of the potential of such methodology is given in Figure 2. It shows a model experiment, in which three cell populations are mixed: a sensitive tumor cell line (KB3-1), a Pgp-expressing cell line (KB8-5), and a Pgp-negative, MRP-overexpressing cell line (GLC$_4$/ADR). After loading the cells with daunorubicin and staining with the Pgp-specific monoclonal antibody MRK-16, the intracellular daunorubicin fluorescence and Pgp expression in the plasma membrane is visualized and can be quantified by two-parameter flow cytometric analysis. The effects of two different modulators, one inhibiting Pgp-mediated daunorubicin transport in KB8-5 cells (PSC833), and another inhibiting the pump, probably the MRP-protein, in the GLC$_4$/ADR cells (genistein; 41) are compared. It can be seen that PSC833 increases only the mean cellular daunorubicin uptake (y-axis is daunorubicin fluorescence) in the Pgp-expressing KB8-5 cells (shift to the right on the x-axis is MRK16). Genistein increases drug uptake in the GLC$_4$/ADR cells, but decreases it in the KB8-5 cells, possibly owing to stimulation of Pgp action (41). Similar experiments to determine the MDR phenotype of tumor cells can be done by fluorescence quantification of intranuclear anthracycline with laser scan microscopy (42), which has been applicable in acute myeloid leukemia (43).

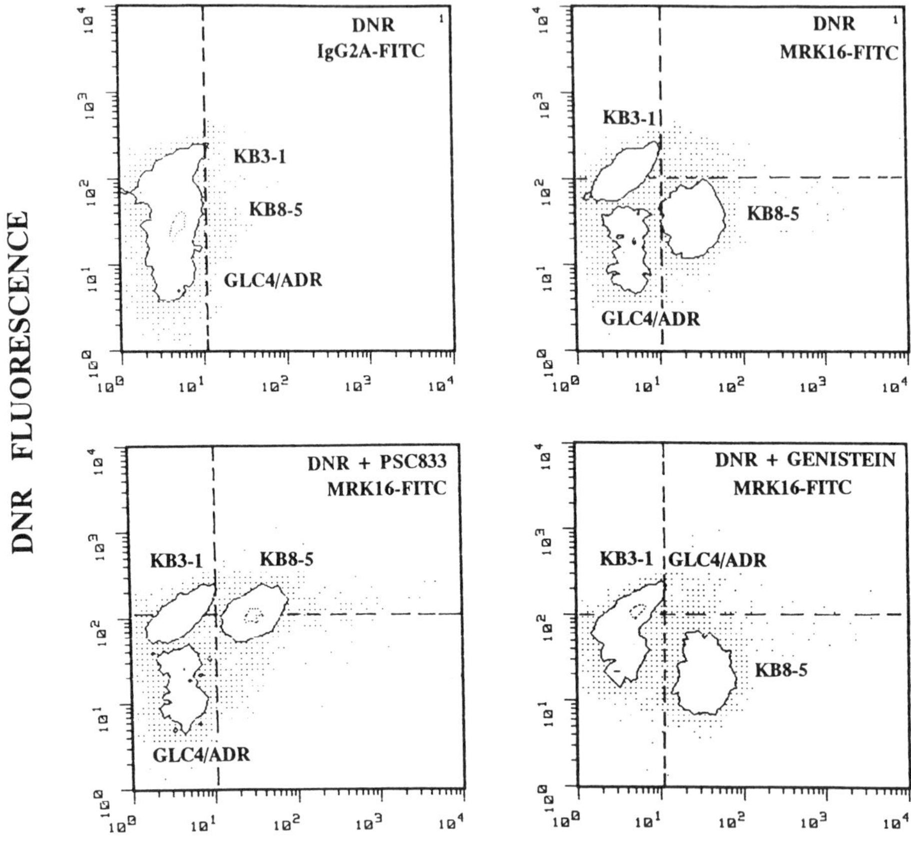

Figure 2 Detection of *MDR1* and *MRP* overexpressing tumor cells by flow cytometry. (Experiment and artwork by Karin Kuiper.)

Apart from the presence of an MDR drug pump, the transport of a drug to the target in a tumor cell in a patient can be affected by other factors, such as blood flow rate, extra- and intracellular pH, and passive membrane leakage (see also next section). It will be difficult to dissect the role of Pgp in vivo from other processes when whole-tumor concentrations of cytostatics are measured, and even that is usually not possible in clinical practice. Ideally, the cytosolic free-drug concentration (or a direct derivative thereof) in a patient's tumor cells in vivo should be measured with a noninvasive method, before and after administration of a Pgp modulatory agent. The application of an organotechnetium complex, already in use for cardiac imaging, represents a potential approach for the functional imaging of Pgp (44). Whatever method is used to estimate the effect of an MDR drug pump in vivo, it should be remembered that, for the therapeutic result, it is necessary that the drug reaches the site where it should do its work. To assess this, doxorubicin would, again, be a good candidate (e.g., with needle aspirates of tumor tissue after doxorubicin administration). However, data representative of the whole tumor must be obtained.

B. Cellular Pharmacokinetics of MDR Drugs

1. Drug Target Concentration

The presence of an MDR pump in the plasma membrane will lower the intracellular concentration of those antitumor drugs that are substrates for that particular pump. For vincristine and doxorubicin, the target is likely to be intracellular, although doxorubicin has been suggested to act additionally at the level of the plasma membrane, as it is still cytotoxic when coupled to agarose beads (45). That MDR cells with a pump for doxorubicin became resistant to the same extent as the nuclear drug concentration was decreased (46,47) argues in favor of the nucleus being the main target at cytotoxic doxorubicin concentrations. When the change in cellular drug accumulation is not in accordance with the measured change in growth mean inhibitory concentration (IC_{50}), the conclusion "drug resistance is multifactorial" is often stated, without considering cellular drug distribution (42,48,49). However, if the drug is present in cellular compartments having no relation with its cytotoxicity, the change of the drug concentration *at target* may change much more than is reflected in the total cellular drug content. Especially for low levels of MDR (comparable with clinically induced resistance, see Ref. 5), the mechanism may be less multifactorial than is sometimes suggested. When the decrease in drug concentration at a target site is known, the increase in drug plasma concentration required to overcome this MDR effect can be calculated. For the relatively widely used drugs, doxorubicin and daunorubicin, studies on concentration at target are facilitated by their intense natural fluorescence and high cellular drug accumulation. Recent developments in sensitive (confocal) laser microscopy technology are helpful in here. Another advantage in estimating the relevance of MDR for these drugs is the extensive literature available on several aspects of the pharmacology of doxorubicin and daunorubicin, such as the physicochemical properties (aggregate formation, free radical formation, interaction with membranes, DNA, and so forth). For other MDR drugs, such as vincristine or taxol, cellular pharmacokinetic studies with intact cells are more difficult to perform; the lack of intense fluorescence necessitates indirect measurements.

2. *Free Cytosolic Drug Concentration*

For doxorubicin and daunorubicin, the free cytosolic drug concentration is in equilibrium with the nuclear-bound drug. For daunorubicin, the effect of Pgp on the free cytosolic drug concentration was measured by Spoelstra et al. (50). By rapidly inhibiting the Pgp-mediated daunorubicin pumping after steady state had been reached, a net drug influx could be measured, driven by a concentration gradient. Since the permeability coefficient for passive leak across the plasma membrane was also known, the free cytosolic drug concentration could be calculated from this influx (50). This concentration is supposed to be critical for determining drug concentrations in other cellular compartments (17). The plasma membrane, however, may form a special compartment from which the drug might be pumped directly ("vacuum cleaner" model, see next section).

On increasing the free cytosolic daunorubicin concentration, saturation of Pgp-mediated transport was found (50). When the substrate concentration rises above the K_m of the drug pump, the passive leak would become more important, compared with the active pumping rate, whereas the latter approaches its V_{max}. Thus, the role of this resistance mechanism in the clinic could be potentially affected by adjusting the peak drug concentration. However, the extracellular concentration range at which daunorubicin reached saturation is mostly above plasma concentrations obtained after bolus injections in patients (51). For vinblastine, Horio et al. (52) reported a K_m for drug pumping of about 1 μM, which is higher than the drug plasma concentrations found in patients (53,54). In another study, using membrane vesicles, two K_m values of 0.14 and 24.8 μM were reported for vincristine (55), whereas published plasma concentrations in patients were largely lower than these values (54,56,57). Therefore, it is reasonable to suggest that Pgp pump capacity for daunorubicin, vincristine, and vinblastine is not overcome by passive drug efflux in clinical situations. However, for other drugs or metabolites with low K_m values for efflux, this consideration may be important. In Figure 3 the effect of different K_m values is illustrated using a model simulation of the free cytosolic drug concentration along the lines presented in the foregoing for daunorubicin and moderately resistant, Pgp-expressing cells (50).

Another point for consideration is the choice of MDR-reversing agents in the clinic. We found that daunorubicin pumping by Pgp in intact cells is inhibited by verapamil in a noncompetitive way (58). In contrast, in another study that used membrane vesicles, competitive inhibition of Pgp was reported (59). In the case of a competitive inhibitor (increases in K_m

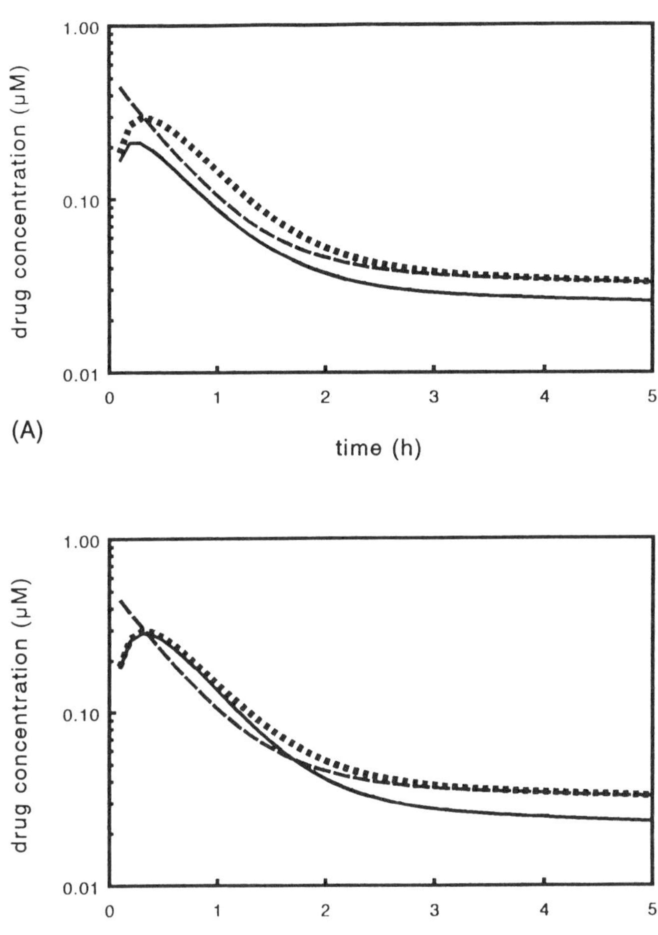

Figure 3 Computer simulation of intracellular free-drug concentration in moderately multidrug-resistant cells without (solid line) or with (dotted line) an inhibitor completely blocking drug pumping when the K_m of the drug efflux pump is (A) above or (B) below the extracellular free-drug concentration (dashed line). The extracellular concentration was taken to equal the plasma concentration. The K_m was (A) 1 μM and (B) 0.01 μM, respectively. At a K_m of 0.01 μM (B) the V_{max} was adapted to obtain a similar drug-pumping rate at the lowest drug concentrations compared with the simulation at a K_m of 1 μM (A). Calculations were based on kinetics and parameter values descriptive of P-glycoprotein-mediated daunorubicin pumping (50).

of drug), its inhibitory effect may be overcome by the rising (competing) free cytosolic drug concentration that results from inhibition of the Pgp-pumping rate of the latter. Then a noncompetitive inhibitor would be preferable (no rise of K_m, only lowering of V_{max}). However, below the K_m, the inhibitory effect of a modulator becomes independent of the substrate concentration, for competitive as well as noncompetitive inhibition. As already pointed out for vincristine, vinblastine, and daunorubicin, saturation of Pgp in patient's tumor cells is expected to be minimal. However, for other drugs or metabolites for which saturation is indicated, rational decisions could be made in favor of a noncompetitive inhibitor. In the near future, kinetic data for Pgp-mediated drug transport of more drugs and metabolites are likely to become available. This will be of help in understanding the link between plasma concentrations and drug concentrations present at their intracellular targets.

3. Vacuum Cleaner Model for P-Glycoprotein

It has been suggested that an MDR drug pump, such as Pgp, can pump hydrophobic drugs directly from a plasma membrane compartment, acting as a vacuum cleaner (60). The presence of a vacuum cleaner would cause a larger decrease in initial drug uptake than would be calculated from measured half-life times of cellular drug disappearance by a drug efflux pump (61). In a kinetic analysis, a "membrane compartment" from which the drug is removed has to be introduced. We obtained evidence for the existence of such a separate compartment in a non-Pgp MDR cell line, SW1573/2R120, by showing decreased daunorubicin plasma membrane concentration in these cells, when compared with the drug-sensitive parental cell line (62). Whether the pump acts as a vacuum cleaner or as a cytosolic drug pump will affect the shape of the free cytosolic drug concentration versus time curve. Theoretically, the effect on this curve will be most pronounced if a drug has a shorter half-life extracellularly relative to intracellularly.

4. The Effect of MDR Drug Pumps In Vivo

Reports on the effect of an MDR drug pump on cytostatic drug concentration in tumor cells in situ in cancer patients are not yet available. In mice, transplanted MDR tumor cells have caused drug resistance, which could be decreased with an MDR modifier (63–65). Also in mice, Houghton et al. found a correlation between response and retention of vincristine in rhabdomyosarcoma xenografts (66). However, they also found a correlation of drug sensitivity with intracellular-binding affinity, which could point to a pharmacokinetically higher distribution volume, rather than to reduced active drug efflux. Doxorubicin concentrations in tumors grown in nude mice from MDR cells lines, were lower when compared with tumors grown from wild-type cells (65; H. J. Broxterman and J. Lankelma, unpublished data). These results underscore the importance of the plasma membrane as a barrier for drugs in vivo and that, in principle, Pgp could have substantial influence on intracellular drug concentrations in vivo. Since, in animal experiments, a steep dose–response curve was measured (see Ref. 12 Chap. 16; 67) a twofold change of the intracellular concentration may have a dramatic effect on therapeutic response.

C. Clinical Modulation of MDR

1. Selection of Cancer Types for MDR Modulation in the Clinic

A major reason for chemotherapeutic failure is thought to be the occurrence of drug resistance. Although laboratory studies, extensively reviewed in this book, have focused on cellular drug resistance, other factors may make a tumor appear resistant in the clinical setting. These factors include resistance caused by poor drug absorption, unfavorable tumor pH, or poor vascularization or localization (blood–brain barrier). Such factors might be circumvented in certain patients by changing the route of administration or drug dose, or by changing to another drug (68). However, many human tumors are resistant to all available chemotherapeutic agents.

The purpose of clinical trials to overcome MDR is to test ways to diminish the potential negative effect of drug transporters on therapy outcome. Such trials have been stimulated to a great extent by the identification of the *MDR1*/Pgp gene as a drug transporter and the in vitro identification of many modulators of the Pgp drug pump activity (see Chap. 18). The first resistance-modifying agent (RMA) to be identified was verapamil, a calcium channel blocker and well-known antiarrhythmic agent (69). Verapamil blocks the Pgp-mediated efflux of several anticancer drugs from tumor cells (69). Numerous compounds have been subsequently identified with MDR-reversing potential (70). These include calcium channel blockers, steroids and hormonal analogues, calmodulin inhibitors, and cyclosporine and derivatives. Only few of these compounds have reached the clinic as experimental drugs for MDR modulation (71).

A key question is whether Pgp expression is contributing to MDR in the clinical setting. Numerous studies have examined Pgp expression in several cancer types, comparing untreated patients with chemotherapy-treated patients (72,73). The results suggest that Pgp expression increases in most tumor types in relapse after chemotherapy. This is not true, however, in those cancers derived from Pgp-expressing normal human tissues (72,73). Although this is suggestive that Pgp plays a role in the development of clinical MDR, another possibility might be that Pgp is a marker of a more aggressive tumor phenotype (74). The analysis of repeated tumor biopsies from the same patient, matching the emergence of Pgp expression with lack of response, may clarify the clinical relevance of Pgp.

Probably the best candidates for a trial of MDR modulation are tumors with acquired MDR. Most of these tumors are Pgp-negative at diagnosis, whereas at relapse, Pgp expression is found more often and is frequently associated with chemoresistance. Examples are acute lymphoid leukemia (73,75), multiple myeloma (76), lymphoma (77,78), neuroblastoma (35), sarcoma (79), and breast cancer (80,81). Acute myeloid leukemia (AML) may also be a good candidate for MDR modulation (82), although recent reports suggest that other resistance mechanisms (e.g., non-Pgp MDR) might be equally important in AML (83,84). Further studies are needed to establish whether non-Pgp MDR plays a role in clinical chemoresistance. Research for modulators of non-Pgp MDR is still limited to the laboratory (41).

2. MDR Modulation in Hematological Malignancies and Solid Tumors

Since the first MDR modulation studies in 1985 (85,86), numerous phase I or II, pilot, and pharmacokinetic studies have been carried out with several different RMAs. Tables 1 and 2 summarize the results of most of these studies. Generally, promising results have been reported for hematological malignancies, in contrast to solid tumors (see Table 2), although most of these studies are difficult to interpret. For example, some studies have included patients who had not been proved refractory to MDR drugs (90,91,94,95). Theoretically, these patients may have responded to MDR drugs alone, and treatment outcome might thus erroneously be attributed to the addition of an RMA. Furthermore, in only one (118) of these studies were the pharmacokinetics examined, to exclude a possible interaction between RMA and anticancer drug(s), leading to a higher area under the plasma concentration versus time curve (AUC) of the anticancer drug. Lum et al. (123) found that the AUC of etoposide increased 1.5–2 times after addition of cyclosporine to the regimen, by measuring etoposide pharmacokinetics before and after addition of the RMA in the same patient. Similar increases in AUC have been reported for verapamil with doxorubicin and D-verapamil with epidoxorubicin (124). It has been reported that a higher dose of the anticancer agent may overcome temporary resistance to it, especially in hematological malignancies (125). Thus, the pharmacological interaction between cytotoxic agent and RMA, leading to dose intensification rather than to an MDR modulation, may explain improved treatment outcome. Another drawback of most studies is the lack of information on *MDR1*/Pgp expression in tumors selected for MDR

Table 1 Clinical MDR Modulation in Hematological Malignancies

RMA and cancer type	Anticancer drug(s)	Administration route[a]	RMA median plasma level[b]	Dose-limiting toxicity	Response			Ref.
					CR	PR	NR	
Diltiazem								
ALL (childhood)	Vincristine	p.o.	Not reported	Cardiac arrhythmia, renal failure	0	4	2	85
Verapamil								
Miscellaneous[c] (childhood)	Vinblastine and VP-16	IV	1,954 (at 15 min) 468.1 (at 24 h) 422.8 (at 120 h)	Hematological, cardiac arrhythmia, hypotension	0	6[d]	1	87
Multiple myeloma, Non-Hodgkin's lymphoma	VAD[e]	IV	257	Cardiac arrhythmia, hypotension	1	2	5	88
Multiple myeloma	VAD	IV	Not reported	Hypotension, nausea, angina pectoris	0	1	9	89
Malignant lymphoma	CVAD[f]	IV	1,022 (2.5 μM)	Congestive heart failure, cardiac arrhythmia, hypotension	5	8	5	90
Quinine								
Acute leukemia	Mitoxantrone and Ara-C	IV	11,700 (peak) 8,500 (median lowest level during infusion)	Hematological, nausea/vomiting, cardiac arrhythmia, tinnitus, vertigo, mild hearing loss, hyperbilirubinemia	8	2	4	91
Cyclosporine								
AML[g]	Daunorubicin	IV	3.2–0.5 μM (peak and trough level)	Hematological, no toxicity attributable to RMA	1	0	0	92
Multiple myeloma	VAD	IV	(steady state) 706 (5 mg/kg/d) 971 (7.5 mg/kg/d) 1,010 (10 mg/kg/d)	Musculoskeletal pain, peripheral neuropathy, hypertension, hyperbilirubinemia	1	9	10	93
CML (blast phase) AML	Daunorubicin and Ara-C	IV	≥1,500 (16–20 mg/kg/d)	Nausea/vomiting, hypomagnesemia, burning dysesthesias, hyperbilirubinemia, prolonged myelosuppression	26	3	13	94
Acute leukemia	Mitoxantrone and VP-16	IV	2,775 (15 mg/kg/d)	Hyperbilirubinemia, prolonged myelosuppression, stomatitis, somnolence	2	4	8	95

RMA, resistance-modifying agent; CR, complete remission; PR, partial response; NR, no response; ALL, acute lymphoid leukemia; AML, acute myeloid leukemia.
[a] Route of administration of RMA: IV, intravenously; p.o., per os.
[b] In nanograms per milliliter, unless stated otherwise.
[c] Including solid tumors.
[d] PR defined as ≥25% reduction of tumor diameters in solid tumors, or complete disappearance of peripheral blasts in leukemia.
[e] VAD, vincristine, doxorubicin, dexamethasone.
[f] CVAD, cyclophosphamide, vincristine, doxorubicin, dexamethasone.
[g] Case report.

Table 2 Clinical MDR Modulation in Solid Tumors

RMA[a] and cancer type	Anticancer drug(s)	Administration route	Median plasma level[b]	Dose-limiting toxicity	Response CR	PR	NR	Ref.
Verapamil								
Miscellaneous	Vinblastine	IV	290	Cardiac arrhythmia	Not reported			86
Miscellaneous	Doxorubicin	p.o.	455 (1 μM)[c]	Cardiac arrhythmia, hypotension	0	1	9	96
Miscellaneous[f]	Epidoxorubicin	p.o.	301[c]	Hypotension	0	3	10	97
Ovarian	Doxorubicin	IV	1,273	Congestive heart failure, cardiac arrhythmia	0	0	8	98
Ovarian	Mitoxantrone	p.o.	455[c]	Cardiac arrhythmia, hypotension	0	0	14	99
Colorectal	Doxorubicin	p.o.	656 (1.44 μM)	Cardiac arrhythmia, hypotension, dizziness	0	2	19	100
NSCLC[d]	Vindesine/ ifosfamide	p.o.	455 (1μM)	Peripheral neuropathy, constipation, cardiac arrhythmia	2	11	19	101
SCLC[d]	Cyclophosphamide/ doxorubicin/ vincristine/ etoposide	p.o.	387 (0.85 μM)	Hematological	37	43	9	102
Hepatocellular Carcinoma	Doxorubicin	p.o.	Not reported	Not reported	1[e]	4	16	103
Verapamil (Vp) + tamoxifen (Txn)								
SCLC	Doxorubicin/ vincristine/ etoposide	p.o. (both RMA)	Vp: 100–500[c] Txn: 400[c]	Hematological	14	20	24	104
D-Verapamil								
Miscellaneous	Doxorubicin	p.o.	861 (1.89 μM)	Cardiac arrhythmia/Hypotension	0	1	9	105
Bepridil								
Miscellaneous	(Epi)doxorubicin	IV	1943	Hematological, congestive heart failure	0	0	14	106
Colorectal	Vinblastine	IV	1320	Cardiac arrhythmia, constipation	1	0	14	10
Quinidine								
Breast cancer	Epidoxorubicin	p.o.	5.6 μM	Cinchonism (visual disturbance, ringing in the ears, dizziness), lethargy	0	1	17	107
Quinine								
Miscellaneous[f]	Doxorubicin	IV and p.o.	4,400–10,100	Not reported	Not reported			108
Nifedipine								
Miscellaneous	Etoposide	p.o.	0.45–0.66 μM	Hematological	0	0	15	109
Dipyridamole								
Gynecological	Etoposide	IP	0.4 μM 69.0 μM (i.p.) 15.4 μM (nonprotein-bound i.p.)	Hematological	1	0	15	110

					CR	PR	NR	
Amiodarone								
Miscellaneous	Doxorubicin	p.o. and IV	10 μM	Hematological, cardiac arrhythmia	0	1	13	111
Hepato-carcinoma	Doxorubicin	IV and p.o.	Not reported	Hematological	0	0	15	112
Trifluoperazine								
Miscellaneous[f]	Doxorubicin	p.o.	84.65	Extrapyramidal side effects	1	6	29	113
Breast cancer	Doxorubicin	p.o.	Not reported	Extrapyramidal side effects	0	9	11	114
Prochlorperazine								
Miscellaneous	Doxorubicin	IV	1,151	Hypotension, muscle spasms, chills, sedation	0	1	10	115
Cyclosporine								
Colorectal	Epidoxorubicin	IV	6,248 (peak) 1,012 (at 18 h)	Flushing,[g] hematological	0	1	23	116
Renal cell cancer	Vinblastine	IV	5,668 (peak) 753 (at 18 h)	Flushing,[g] nausea/vomiting	0	0	15	117
Miscellaneous	Etoposide	IV	2,860–3,512[h]	Hematological, nausea/vomiting, headache, hyperbilirubinemia, hypertension, hypomagnesemia, stomatitis, diarrhea, nephrotoxicity, tumor pain, anaphylactoid reactions[g]	0	2	23 (in patients with RMA levels $\geq$ 2000 ng/ml & bilirubin $\geq$ 1.5 mg/100 ml)	118
Miscellaneous	Doxorubicin	IV	2,210	Hematological, nausea/vomiting, hyperbilirubinemia, fluid retention, nephrotoxicity	0	0	23	119
Miscellaneous[f]	Vinblastine	IV	0.97 μM	Hematological, nausea/vomiting, hyperbilirubinemia, constipation, muscle cramps, hypertension, nephrotoxicity, hyponatremia, hypomagnesemia, azotemia, anaphylactoid reactions[g]	0	0	60	120
Tamoxifen								
Miscellaneous	Etoposide	p.o.	984 (2.65 μM)	Hematological, vomiting, thromboembolic events	2	4	52	121
Miscellaneous	Vinblastine	p.o.	4.0 μM	Neurotoxicity, grand mal seizure, unsteady gait, "wooziness," cardiac arrhythmia	0	3	44	122

RMA, resistance-modifying agent; CR, complete remission; PR, partial response; NR, no response.

[a] Route of administration of RMA: IV intravenously; p.o., per os; IP, intraperitoneal.

[b] In nanograms per milliliter, unless stated otherwise.

[c] Derived from other studies.

[d] Randomized trial: verapamil versus no verapamil.

[e] CR defined as complete disappearance of palpable liver.

[f] Including hematological malignancies.

[g] Probably related to the vehicle of cyclosporine.

[h] At recommended dose level for phase II.

modulation. In addition, the use of different *MDR1*/Pgp assays by different investigators makes data comparison difficult (see Sec. II.A.3). Nevertheless, responses of a refractory, Pgp-negative tumor on an MDR drug–RMA regimen are rare (88,91,93). Another often raised issue is the question of whether the RMA concentration *at the site of the cancer cells* is high enough to block Pgp-mediated drug efflux. Determinations of RMA plasma levels are more or less sufficient to answer this question for hematological malignancies and to give an indication for solid tumors. The RMA plasma concentrations reached in the patient are compared with those needed in vitro to reverse MDR. It would be more elegant if one could demonstrate RMA-mediated increased drug uptake in Pgp-expressing cancer cells directly in the patient by a noninvasive-imaging technique. Such techniques are currently being developed (44). As long as these techniques are not clinically available, other indicators of adequate modifier activity are being sought. P-glycoprotein is also expressed in several normal human tissues, and impairment of Pgp activity in tumor cells may go along with impairment of normal physiological function of Pgp. Some studies, in which adequate RMA plasma levels have been reached in patients to reverse MDR in vitro, suggest that hyperbilirubinemia might be an in vivo marker for sufficient Pgp functional impairment (95,118,120). However, it is not yet clear that hyperbilirubinemia is caused by inhibition of bilirubin excretion through impairment of Pgp function (94,119). It has been proposed that inhibition of Pgp in normal human tissues might lead to unacceptable toxicities when anticancer drugs are combined with MDR modulators (71,122). Indeed, several side effects have been related to possible interference with normal Pgp function, such as nephrotoxicity (kidney proximal tubules; 122), nausea–vomiting and somnolence (blood–brain barrier; 91,94,95,118,121,122), and increased myelosuppression (CD34$^+$ hematopoietic stem cells; 91,94,95,118,119,120; see Tables 1 and 2). Future MDR modulation trials will have to address the question of whether the use of systemic RMAs with MDR drugs can selectively eradicate tumor cells. The relative protection of Pgp-expressing normal tissues could, for instance, be due to a lower growth rate, or to the presence of additional resistance mechanisms to the cytotoxic agent (71).

For most RMAs, it is virtually impossible to reach adequate plasma levels owing to prohibitive toxicity, such as congestive heart failure with verapamil (98). Currently, several phase I/II trials are studying new RMAs with a much higher MDR-reversing potential in vitro and a more favorable toxicity profile, such as the cyclosporine analogue PSC 833 (64), which lacks immunosuppressive and nephrotoxic side effects.

Several other mechanisms have been recently associated with the MDR phenotype in vitro (see Sec. II.A.2). The clinical significance of these mechanisms is as yet largely unknown. Theoretically, these mechanisms might play a role in failures of clinical MDR modulation in Pgp-positive tumors.

In conclusion, carefully designed studies are needed to clarify whether Pgp is contributing to MDR and whether adequate reversal can be obtained by the addition of a modifying agent to therapy. First, we should prove that patients are refractory to MDR drugs. Then, we should determine if Pgp is expressed in their tumor. A treatment combining MDR drugs with a modifier should be administered, while monitoring the pharmacokinetics of both MDR drugs and modifier. Pharmacokinetics of MDR drugs given in combination with an RMA should be comparable with those of MDR drugs given alone, and RMA plasma levels should be at least equal to those needed in vitro to reverse MDR. Treatment outcome will decide if MDR modulation regimens are feasible. Finally, randomized phase III trials will provide insight into the possible benefit of MDR modulation. A hematological malignancy, such as multiple myeloma, may be most suitable for this type of study, since Pgp expression in multiple myeloma is associated with acquired resistance, and myeloma is often treated with MDR drugs only (vincristine, doxorubicin, dexamethasone). Moreover, tumor cells are readily obtainable for determining Pgp expression, and no problems are expected with tumor accessibility to cytotoxic agents and RMA owing to poor tumor vascularization.

3. Future Candidates for Clinical Testing of MDR Modulation

Two alternative approaches for circumventing Pgp-mediated MDR are still under preclinical investigation, but may soon enter phase I clinical trials. One of these is the addition of liposomes to doxorubicin (126) to enhance cytotoxic activity in MDR tumor cells (see Chap. 20). Liposomes may potentiate cytotoxicity three- to ninefold in MDR cell lines (depending on the cell line studied), whereas cytotoxicity in parental cell lines is unaltered (126). The lack of in vivo toxicity of liposomes (127) makes them interesting MDR-reversing agents for clinical testing, competing favorably with the RMAs currently in clinical trials. Another approach is the use of *MDR1*-specific anti–Pgp-directed monoclonal antibodies in combination with MDR drugs. This approach appeared feasible for the MRK16 monoclonal antibody in transgenic mice, the bone marrow cells of which express the human *MDR1* gene at a level approximately equal to that found in many human cancers (128). An increased bone marrow toxicity was observed after addition of the monoclonal antibody to MDR drugs (128). Results of future clinical trials exploring these modalities are eagerly awaited.

III. OTHER ANTICANCER DRUG TRANSPORT-ASSOCIATED RESISTANCE

Although the experimental literature on MDR transport has been overwhelming during recent years after the cloning of the *MDR1*/Pgp gene, other drug transport systems possibly relevant to cancer treatment still await discovery. Two systems on which a considerable amount of data have already been accumulated are the antifolate transport, responsible for antifolate (methotrexate) uptake into cells (see Chap. 16), and the glutathione–conjugate export pump (see Chap. 19).

A. Antifolate Transport

1. Introduction

The essential role of reduced folate cofactors as one-carbon donors in various biosynthetic processes (e.g., amino acid, purine, and thymidylate synthesis for DNA) has been exploited in the development of folate antagonistic drugs with antiproliferative potential. One of the best known folate antagonists is methotrexate (MTX), which has had an accepted role in cancer chemotherapy for over 30 years, both as a single agent and in combination regimens. Methotrexate is included in the treatment modalities of (childhood) leukemia, head and neck cancer, breast cancer, choriocarcinoma, colon cancer, and gastric cancer (129). At least three critical factors determine the clinical effectiveness of folate-based chemotherapy: (1) transport across the plasma membrane (to be discussed in more detail hereafter); (2) level of the intracellular target enzyme, dihydrofolate reductase (DHFR) (129); and (3) polyglutamylation of MTX, a process catalyzed by the enzyme folylpolyglutamate synthetase (FPGS) and involving the addition of multiple glutamate residues (up to seven to the γ-carboxyl group of MTX (130). Polyglutamylation of MTX has two effects: it prolongs the intracellular retention of MTX by preventing efflux, and polyglutamates of MTX are also potent inhibitors of key enzymes in folate metabolism other than DHFR; namely, thymidylate synthase (TS) and glycinamide ribonucleotide formyltransferase (GARTFase) (131,132).

Two pathways are considered to be of importance in the internalization of naturally occurring folates and folate antagonists. One membrane transport route is by an active *carrier*-mediated process (133) (designated hereafter as reduced folate carrier; RFC). Another route is by a *receptor*-mediated process, involving a membrane receptor with a high affinity for folic acid and reduced folates (134; designated hereafter as membrane folate receptor; MFR).

2. Reduced Folate Carrier

The transport kinetic properties of RFC have been documented in a variety of tumor cells of different origin (133,135). The physiological substrate for RFC is the serum folate 5-methyltetrahydrofolate (5-CH$_3$THF) which is internalized with a relatively high affinity (K_m = 1–5 μM). Although the rate of transport (V_{max}) of 5-CH$_3$THF by RFC (1–12 pmol min^{-1} mg^{-1} protein) is several orders of magnitude lower than for other nutrient transport systems (e.g., amino acids or nucleosides), the capacity is more than sufficient to meet the cellular folate requirements for optimal cell growth (133). Folate antagonists, such as MTX, can be transported by RFC with almost the same efficiency as 5-CH$_3$THF. Affinity-labeling techniques have demonstrated that the RFC in murine leukemia cells is a 46- to 48-kDa glycoprotein (136). In human leukemia cells, a higher relative molecular mass (M$_r$ of 80–100 kDa) has been observed for the carrier protein as a result of more extensive glycosylation (137,138). It is unclear how transport activity by RFC is regulated, although there is some preliminary evidence that the intracellular levels of reduced folate cofactors and purine metabolites play a role in this process (135,138).

3. Membrane Folate Receptor

The membrane folate receptors (MFRs) are characterized by a high-binding affinity for natural folates, such as folic acid or 5-CH$_3$THF (K_d = 1–3 nM), but a low affinity for folate-based inhibitors of DHFR such as MTX (K_d = 50–100 nM) (134). The glycosylated receptor protein has an M$_r$ of 40–50 kDa and is linked to the membrane by a glycosylphosphatidylinositol anchor (139). The mechanism of folate and antifolate uptake by MFRs is not clearly established. In some tissues, MFR-mediated uptake proceeds by the classic receptor-mediated endocytosis pathway (140), involving clustering of receptors in clathrin-coated pits, internalization of the coated vesicles, and fusion of vesicles to form endosomes. After entry into an acidic endosome, the ligand is dissociated from the receptor, which then recycles to the cell surface. Recently, another mechanism, termed potocytosis (141), has been postulated for folate transport by MFR. Potocytosis involves clustering of MFRs in specialized membrane invaginations, termed caveolae (142), that have cavaeolin as coat protein, instead of clathrin. The caveolae remain associated with the plasma membrane, but can temporarily close from the extracellular space. Following this process, the lumen of the caveolae is acidified, and the ligand is dissociated from the receptor. The ligand is then translocated across the membrane by a specific carrier protein, after which caveolae open for a new cycle of uptake.

4. *Cellular Expression of MFR/RFC*

The purification of the MFR protein and the cloning of its gene (143,144) has allowed the use of immunological and molecular techniques to examine MFR expression in normal and malignant cells and tissues (145). Substantial amounts of receptor have been observed in the choroid plexus, lung, thyroid, and kidney. Among neoplastic tissues, high MFR expression has been demonstrated in ovarian carcinoma (146), along with variable expression (10–50% of cases) in lung, kidney, brain, breast, and colorectal carcinomas (147).

Unlike MFR, the tissue distribution of RFC is relatively unexplored, mainly because of the lack of immunological or molecular probes. However, transport kinetic data obtained from neoplastic cells maintained in vitro suggest that RFC is expressed in the majority of tumor cells (133). Moreover, RFC can also be coexpressed in MFR-expressing cells (148).

5. *Transport-Related Drug Resistance*

Largely, on the basis of in vitro model systems, it has been established that quantitative (decreased amounts) or qualitative (increased K_m or decreased V_{max}) defects of RFC and MFR are associated with intrinsic or acquired tumor cell resistance to MTX and cross-resistance to other antifolates (133,149–151). Cases of clinical resistance to MTX resulting from a membrane transport defect by RFC have been documented, although the number of patients in these studies was small. Nevertheless, within a group of patients with acute lymphocytic leukemia, defective transport of MTX appeared to be quite common (up to 50% of cases) (152). A basal level of functional RFC is required so that the uptake of folates for cell growth is not compromised. On the other hand, expression of MFRs may provide a molecular basis for the uptake of reduced folate cofactors for cell growth and for resistance to MTX. Given the high affinity of MFR for 5-CH$_3$THF and the low affinity for MTX, a relatively high molar ratio of MTX will be required to compete with 5-CH$_3$THF for the receptor (153).

Current research is focused on obtaining immunological (154) and molecular probes for RFC. Along with the probes available for MFR, a more systematic analysis with a larger number of patients may delineate the tissue distribution of RFC and MFR and the levels of expression in normal and neoplastic cells. The importance of this type of studies for folate-based chemotherapeutics is evident: it may have predictive value in identifying potential sites of drug toxicity to normal cells and potential drug sensitivity–resistance profiles of neoplastic cells. The early recognition of intrinsic drug resistance, or the onset of acquired drug resistance before or during treatment, will provide an opportunity for alternative treatment regimens.

6.　*Circumvention of Transport-Associated Drug Resistance*

The development of new antifolate drugs that may be more effective than MTX, or may circumvent resistance to MTX, is an area of intensive research. New folate-based inhibitors have been discovered not only of DHFR, but also of other key enzymes in folate metabolism such as TS, GARTFase, and FPGS. The chemical structures of three novel antifolates which have promising activity in phase I/II clinical trials are shown in Figure 4. They are 10-ethyl-10-deaza-aminopterin (10-EdAM), a DHFR inhibitor (133,155); ICI-D1694 (a TS inhibitor) (156); and 5,10-dideazatetrahydrofolate (DDATHF), a GARTFase inhibitor (157). The chemical

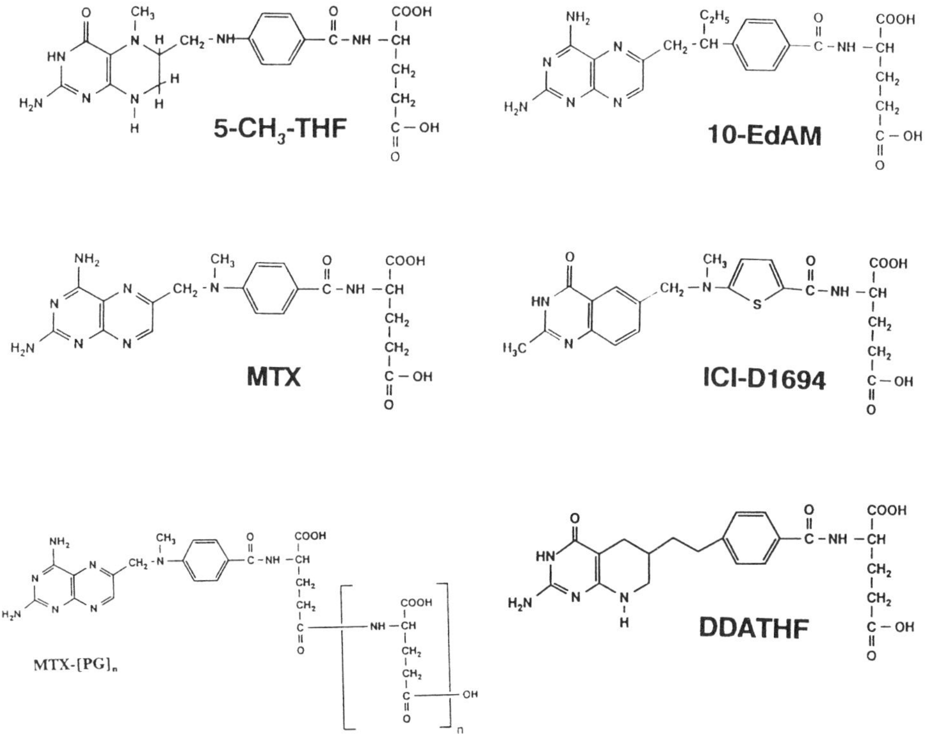

Figure 4　Chemical structures of the natural reduced folate 5-CH$_3$THF, MTX (polyglutamates), and some novel folate antagonists.

structures of 5-CH$_3$THF and MTX are also given for comparison. An important aspect of these novel antifolates is that they are more efficiently transported by RFC, and are better substrates for FPGS than MTX. Moreover, in contrast with folate-based DHFR inhibitors, MFR may be a potential route of internalization of ICI-D1694 and DDATHF, since the affinity of MFR for these drugs is almost as high as for folic acid. It cannot yet be predicted whether one of these novel antifolates will be superior to MTX in chemotherapeutic regimens of leukemia or solid tumors, or effective against MTX-resistant cells.

B. Transport of Platinum-Based Cytotoxics and of Melphalan

A drug not affected by the MDR drug transporter Pgp is cisplatin. Nevertheless, clinical reistance to platinum-based compounds is a frequent event, with intrinsic resistance (non–small-cell lung and colon cancer) and acquired resistance (testicular and ovarian cancer) probably playing some role. Resistance to cisplatin appears to be multifactorial in cell lines with acquired resistance, involving reduced drug accumulation, increased detoxification, and increased repair of Pt–DNA adducts (158).

Studies of cellular cisplatin transport have provided some evidence for small decreases of cisplatin accumulation in resistant cancer cells. However, because of methodological problems, the mechanism, clinical significance, or even relevance in cell lines remains unclear. Typically, most cisplatin-selected, resistant cell lines exhibit a 50% decrease in drug accumulation. Cisplatin is thought to enter cells passively, since uptake is not saturable nor inhibited by analogues. Furthermore, drug concentration is a rate-limiting factor for cisplatin uptake. Evidence for protein-mediated cisplatin transport is scarce. A monoclonal antibody has been developed against an overexpressed plasma membrane protein (159), but its significance is still unclear. Circumvention of reduced cisplatin accumulation by a more lipophilic platinum compound, JM244, has been shown in a cisplatin-uptake mutant from an ovarian cancer cell line (160).

A putative mechanism for cisplatin export from cells is conjugation with glutathione and transport by the glutathione-S–conjugate export pump (161; see also Chap. 19). A recent interesting study reports the selection with cisplatin of a human ovarian cancer cell line, cross-resistant to melphalan, but also to doxorubicin, mitoxantrone, and taxol. The MDR phenotype of this cell line was not a result of *MDR1*/Pgp or *MRP* overexpression, but was correlated with increased intracellular glutathione levels, leading the authors to suggest that an ATP-dependent glutathione-

S–conjugate export pump might be partly responsible for the resistance (162).

Resistance to the alkylating drug melphalan has been frequently associated with glutathione metabolism, especially increased levels of glutathione (163). However, conflicting results have been reported on the putative involvement of the glutathione-S–conjugate pump in melphalan export. Alternative models implicate a decreased capacity of melphalan uptake by the L-amino acid transporter system (164).

IV. CONCLUSIONS AND FUTURE DIRECTIONS

From molecular biology studies and studies of the cellular pharmacology of cytotoxic drugs, it has been established during the past decade that transport systems mediating the uptake and efflux of cytostatic drugs are present in the plasma membrane of mammalian cancer cells. In in vitro cell systems, these transporters may contribute significantly to the overall uptake of many antitumor agents and to the concentration at their target sites.

An important, largely unexplored, feature of anticancer drug transport is that it may be influenced by signal transduction pathways. In vitro Pgp activity is altered by its phosphorylation state by protein kinase C inhibition or activation. This may suggest that in vivo Pgp is regulated in a dynamic way by protein kinase C, opening the possibility that certain combination of modulators might be more effective in achieving blockade of anticancer drug efflux (165). Also, certain protein tyrosine kinase inhibitors may affect drug transporters in a complex, sometimes opposite way, such as has been discussed in this chapter for the action of (iso)flavonoids on daunorubicin transport in MRP and Pgp overexpressing cells, respectively. Since many anticancer agents have membrane-related activity, possible interactions with signal transduction pathways, involving systems such as drug transporter activity, topoisomerase II activity, and the apoptotic pathway, are conceivable (166). Moreover, it has recently become clear that, following selection with certain drugs at low, clinically relevant concentrations, drug transport defects can be induced in lung cancer cells in vitro (23). It can now be investigated whether sudden up-regulation of drug transporter activities by exposure to cytotoxic drugs can also occur (167).

This work has already stimulated clinical trials designed to circumvent Pgp-mediated drug resistance. Newer antifolates are being tested in the clinic that are more efficiently transported into the cell. The complexity of such trials is just beginning to appear, and any conclusion concerning the effect that any individual drug transporter will have on cancer chemotherapy may be premature. However, optimism is based on the increasing knowledge we have on the basal defense mechanisms against harmful chemicals, such as anticancer agents, that play a role in human physiology and pathology. The development of more specific modulators, monoclonal antibody-based technology, or non–cross-resistant drugs may be expected to impinge on some clinical situations in the future.

ACKNOWLEDGMENT

Dr. H. V. Westerhoff is gratefully acknowledged for performing computer simulations of intracellular drug concentrations.

REFERENCES

1. Goldie JH, Coldman AJ. The genetic origin of drug resistance in neoplasms: implications for systemic therapy. Cancer Res 1984; 44:3643–3653.
2. Fraumeni JF Jr, Devesa SS, Hoover RN, Kinlen LJ. Epidemiology of cancer. In: DeVita VT Jr, Hellman S, Rosenberg SA, eds. Cancer. Principles and Practice of Oncology. Vol 1. 4th ed. Philadelphia: Lippincott, 1993:150–181.
3. Carter SK. Some thoughts on resistance to cancer chemotherapy. Cancer Treat Rev 1984; 11(S):3–7.
4. Goldie JH, Coldman AJ. A mathematical model for relating the drug sensitivity of tumors to their spontaneous mutation rate. Cancer Treat Rep 1979; 63:1727–1733.
5. Borst P. Genetic mechanisms of drug resistance. Rev Oncol 1991; 4:87–105 (in Acta Oncol Vol. 30 No. 1).
6. Biedler JL, Spengler BA. Metaphase chromosome anomaly association with drug resistance and specific cell products. Science 1976; 191:185–187.
7. Alt FW, Kellems RE, Bertino JR, Schimke RT. Selective multiplication of dihydrofolate reductase genes in methotrexate-resistant variants of cultured murine cells. J Biol Chem 1978; 253:1357–1370.
8. van Kalken CK, van der Valk P, Hadisaputro MMN, Pieters R, Broxterman HJ, Kuiper CM, Scheffer GL, Veerman AJP, Meyer CJLM, Scheper RJ, Pinedo HM. Differentiation dependent expression of P-glycoprotein in the normal and neoplastic human kidney. 1991; Ann Oncol 2:55–62.
9. Ozols RF, Young RC. Chemotherapy of ovarian cancer. Semin Oncol 1984; 11:251–263.
10. Linn SC, van Kalken CK, van Tellingen O, van der Valk P, van Groeningen CJ, Kuiper CM, Pinedo HM, Giaccone G. A clinical and pharmacological study of multidrug resistance reversal with vinblastine and bepridil. 1994; J Clin Oncol 12:812–819.

11. Harris AL. DNA repair and resistance to chemotherapy. Cancer Surv 1985; 4:601–624.
12. DeVita VT Jr, Hellman S, Rosenberg SA, eds. Cancer. Principles and practice of oncology. Vol. 1. 4th ed. Philadelphia: Lippincott, 1993.
13. Gudkov AV, Zelnick CR, Kazarov AR, Thimmapaya R, Parker Suttle D, Beck WT, Roninson IB. Isolation of genetic suppressor elements, inducing resistance to topoisomerase II-interactive cytotoxic drugs, from human topoisomerase II cDNA. Proc Natl Acad Sci USA 1993; 90:3231–3235.
14. Peterson RHF, Biedler JL. Plasma membrane proteins and glycoproteins from Chinese hamster cells sensitive and resistant to actinomycin D. J Supramol Struct 1978; 9:289–298.
15. Bosmann HB. Mechanism of cellular drug resistance. Nature 1971; 233:566–569.
16. Juliano RL, Ling V. A surface glycoprotein modulating drug permeability in Chinese hamster ovary cell mutants. Biochim Biophys Acta 1976; 455:152–162.
17. Juranka PF, Zastawny RL, Ling V. P-glycoprotein: multidrug-resistance and a superfamily of membrane-associated transport proteins. FASEB J 1989; 3:2583–2592.
18. Demant EJF, Sehested M, Jensen PB. A model for computer simulation of P-glycoprotein and transmembrane ΔpH-mediated anthracycline transport in multidrug-resistant tumor cells. Biochim Biophys Acta 1990; 1055:117–125.
19. Chen C, Chin JE, Ueda K, Clark DP, Pastan I, Gottesman MM, Roninson IB. Internal duplication and homology with bacterial transport proteins in the *MDR1* (P-glycoprotein) gene from multidrug-resistant human cells. Cell 1986; 47:381–389.
20. Zijlstra JG, De Vries EGE, Mulder NH. Multifactorial drug resistance in an Adriamycin-resistant human small cell lung carcinoma cell line. Cancer Res 1987; 47:1780–1784.
21. Cole SPC, Bhardwaj G, Gerlach JH, Mackie JE, Grant CE, Almquist KC, Stewart AJ, Kurz EU, Duncan AMV, Deeley RG. Overexpression of a transporter gene in a multidrug-resistant human lung cancer cell line. Science 1992; 258:1650–1654.
22. Grant CE, Valdimarsson G, Hipfner DR, Almquist KC, Cole SPC, Deeley RG. Overexpression of multidrug resistance-associated protein (MRP) increases resistance to natural product drugs. Cancer Res 1994; 54:357–361.
23. Versantvoort CHM, Withoff S, Broxterman HJ, Mulder NH, Kuiper CM, Center MS, de Vries EGE. Resistance associated factors in human small cell lung carcinoma cell line GLC$_4$ sublines with increasing Adriamycin resistance. Int J Cancer (in press).
24. Scheper RJ, Broxterman HJ, Scheffer GL, Kaaijk P, Dalton WS, van Heijningen THM, van Kalken CK, Slovak ML, de Vries EGE, van der Valk P, Meijer CJLM, Pinedo HM. Overexpression of a M_r 110,000 vesicular protein in non–P-glycoprotein mediated multidrug resistance. Cancer Res 1993; 53:1475–1479.

25. Chen Y-N, Mickley LA, Schwartz AM, Acton EM, Hwang J, Fojo AT. Characterization of Adriamycin-resistant human breast cancer cells which display overexpression of a novel resistance-related membrane protein. J Biol Chem 1990; 265:10073–10080.

26. Beck WT, Danks MK, Wolverton JS, Kim R, Chen M. Drug resistance associated with altered DNA topoisomerase II. Adv Enzyme Regul 1993; 33:113–127.

27. Kamesaki S, Kamesaki H, Jorgensen TJ, Tanizawa A, Pommier Y, Cossman J. Bcl-2 protein inhibits etoposide-induced apoptosis through its effects on events subsequent to topoisomerase II-induced DNA strand breaks and their repair. Cancer Res 1993; 53:4251–4256.

28. Korsmeyer SJ. *bcl-2* initiates a new category of oncogenes: regulators of cell death. Blood 1992; 80:879–886.

29. Lowe SW, Ruley HE, Jacks T, Housman DE. *p53* Dependent apoptosis modulates the cytotoxicity of anticancer agents. Cell 1993; 74:957–967.

30. Stretch JR, Gatter KC, Ralfkiaer E, Lane DP, Harris AL. Expression of mutant *p53* in melanoma. Cancer Res 1991; 51:5976–5979.

31. Fearon ER, Vogelstein B. A genetic model for colorectal tumorigenesis. Cell 1990; 61:759–767.

32. Noonan KE, Beck C, Holzmayer TA, Chin JE, Wunder JS, Andrulis IL, Gazdar AF, Willman CL, Griffith B, von Hoff DD, Roninson IB. Quantitative analysis of *MDR1* (multidrug resistance) gene expression in human tumors by polymerase chain reaction. Proc Natl Acad Sci USA 1990; 87:7160–7164.

33. Cordon-Cardo C, O'Brien JP, Casals D, Rittman-Grauer L, Biedler JL, Melamed MR, Bertino JR. Multidrug-resistance (P-glycoprotein) is expressed by endothelial cells at blood–brain barrier sites. Proc Natl Acad Sci USA 1989; 86:695–698.

34. van der Valk P, van Kalken CK, Ketelaars H, Broxterman HJ, Scheffer GL, Kuiper CM, Tsuruo T, Lankelma J, Meijer CLJM, Pinedo HM, Scheper RJ. Distribution of multidrug resistance-associated P-glycoprotein in normal and neoplastic human tissues. Ann Oncol 1990; 1:56–64.

35. Chan HSL, Haddad G, Thorner PS, De Boer G, Lin YP, Ondrusek N, Yeger H, Ling V. P-glycoprotein expression as a predictor of the outcome of therapy for neuroblastoma. N Engl J Med 1991; 325:1608–1614.

36. Pirker R, Wallner J, Geissler K, Linkesch W, Haas OA, Bettelheim P, Hopfner M, Scherrer R, Valent P, Havelec L, Ludwig H, Lechner K. *MDR1* gene expression and treatment outcome in acute myeloid leukemia. JNCI 1991; 83:708–712.

37. Lampidis TJ, Castello C, Del Giglio A, Pressman BC, Viallet P, Trevorrow KW, Valet GK, Tapiero H, Savaraj N. Relevance of the chemical charge of rhodamine dyes to multiple drug resistance. Biochem Pharmacol 1989; 38:4267–4271.

38. Neyfakh AA. Use of fluorescent dyes as molecular probes for the study of multidrug resistance. Exp Cell Res 1988; 174:168–176.

39. Homolya L, Hollo Z, Germann UA, Pastan I, Gottesman MM, Sarkadi B.

Fluorescent cellular indicators are extruded by the multidrug resistance protein. J Biol Chem 1993; 268:21493–21496.

40. Broxterman HJ, Schuurhuis GJ, Lankelma J, Baak JPA, Pinedo HM. Towards functional screening for multidrug resistant cells in human malignancies. In: Mihich E, ed. Pezcoller Found Symposium. Vol. 1. Drug Resistance: Mechanisms and Reversal. Roma: John Libbey CIC, 1990:309–319.

41. Versantvoort CHM, Schuurhuis GJ, Pinedo HM, Eekman CA, Kuiper CM, Lankelma J, Broxterman HJ. Genistein modulates the decreased drug accumulation in non–P-glycoprotein mediated multidrug resistant tumour cells. Br J Cancer 1993; 68:939–946.

42. Schuurhuis GJ, Broxterman HJ, Cervantes A, van Heijningen THM, de Lange JHM, Baak JPA, Pinedo HM, Lankelma J. Quantitative determination of factors contributing to doxorubicin resistance in multidrug-resistant cells. JNCI 1989; 81:1887–1892.

43. Schuurhuis GJ, Broxterman HJ, Ossenkoppele GJ, Baak JPA, Lankelma J, Eekman JK, Pinedo HM. Functional detection of MDR phenotype in acute myeloid leukemia. Correlation with clinical response. Exp Hematol 1993; 21:1079.

44. Piwnica-Worms D, Chiu ML, Kronauge JF, Kramer RA, Croop JM. Functional imaging of multidrug-resistant P-glycoprotein with an organotechnetium complex. Cancer Res 1993; 53:977–984.

45. Tritton TR, Yee G. The anticancer agent Adriamycin is actively cytotoxic without entering the cells. Science 1982; 217:248–250.

46. Gigli M, Rasoanaivo TWD, Millot J-M, Jeannesson P, Rizzo V, Jardillier J-C, Arcamone F, Manfait M. Correlation between growth inhibition and intranuclear doxorubicin and 4′-deoxy-4′-iododoxorubicin quantitated in living K562 cells by microspectrofluorometry. Cancer Res 1989; 49:560–564.

47. Schuurhuis GJ, Van Heijningen THM, Cervantes A, Pinedo HM, de Lange JHM, Keizer HG, Broxterman HJ, Baak JPA, Lankelma J. Changes in intracellular doxorubicin distribution and accumulation can largely account for doxorubicin resistance in SW-1573 lung cancer and MCF-7 breast cancer multidrug resistant tumor cells. Br J Cancer 1993; 68:898–908.

48. Hindenburg AA, Gervasoni JE Jr, Krishna S, Stewart VJ, Rosado M, Lutzky J, Bhanna K, Baker MA, Taub RN. Intracellular distribution and pharmacokinetics of daunorubicin in anthracycline-sensitive and -resistant HL-60 cells. Cancer Res 1989; 49:4607–4614.

49. Lankelma J, Mülder HS, van Mourik F, Wong Fong Sang HW, Kraayenhof R, van Grondelle R. Cellular daunomycin fluorescence in multidrug resistant 2780[AD] cells and its relation to cellular drug localisation. Biochim Biophys Acta 1991; 1093:147–152.

50. Spoelstra EC, Westerhoff HV, Dekker H, Lankelma J. Kinetics of daunorubicin transport by P-glycoprotein of intact cancer cells. Eur J Biochem 1992; 207:567–579.

51. Speth PAJ, Linssen PCM, Boezeman JBM, Wessels HMC, Haanen C. Leu-

kemic cell and plasma daunomycin concentrations after bolus injection and 72 h infusion. Cancer Chemother Pharmacol 1987; 20:311–315.

52. Horio M, Pastan I, Gottesman MM, Handler JS. Transepithelial transport of vinblastine by kidney-derived cell lines. Application of new kinetic model to estimate in situ K_m of the pump. Biochim Biophys Acta 1990; 1027:116–122.

53. Owellen RJ, Hartke CA, Hains FO. Pharmacokinetics and metabolism of vinblastine in humans. Cancer Res 1977; 37:2597–2602.

54. Nelson RL, Dyke RW, Root MA. Comparative pharmacokinetics of vindesine, vincristine and vinblastine in patients with cancer. Cancer Treat Rev 1980; 7:17–24.

55. Tamai I, Safa AR. Competitive interaction of cyclosporins with the vinca alkaloid-binding site of P-glycoprotein in multidrug-resistant cells. J Biol Chem 1990; 265:16509–16513.

56. Owellen RJ, Root MA, Hains FO. Pharmacokinetis of vindesine and vincristine in humans. Cancer Res 1977; 37:2603–2607.

57. Jackson DV, Sethi VS, Spurr CL, White DR, Richards FR, Stuart JJ, Muss HB, Cooper MR, Castle MC. Pharmacokinetics of vincristine infusion. Cancer Treat Rep 1981; 65:1043–1048.

58. Spoelstra EC, Westerhoff HV, Pinedo HM, Dekker H, Lankelma J. The multidrug resistance reverser verapamil interferes with cellular P-glycoprotein-mediated pumping of daunorubicin as a non-competing substrate. Eur J Biochem 1994; 221:363–373.

59. Sinicrope FA, Dudeja PK, Bissonnette BM, Safa AR, Brasitus TA. Modulation of P-glycoprotein-mediated drug transport by alterations in lipid fluidity of rat liver canalicular membrane vesicles. J Biol Chem 1992; 267:24995–25002.

60. Gottesman MM. How cancer cells evade chemotherapy: sixteenth Richard and Hinda Rosenthal Foundation award lecture. Cancer Res 1993; 53:747–754.

61. Versantvoort CHM, Broxterman HJ, Pinedo HM, de Vries EGE, Feller N, Kuiper CM, Lankelma J. Energy-dependent processes involved in reduced drug accumulation in multidrug-resistant human lung cancer cell lines without P-glycoprotein expression. Cancer Res 1992; 52:17–23.

62. Mülder HS, van Grondelle R, Westerhoff HV, Lankelma J. A plasma membrane "vacuum cleaner" for daunorubicin in non–P-glycoprotein multidrug-resistant SW-1573 human non-small cell lung carcinoma cells. A study using fluorescence resonance energy transfer. Eur J Biochem 1993; 218:871–882.

63. Shinoda H, Inaba M, Tsuruo T. In vivo circumvention of vincristine resistance in mice with P388 leukemia using a novel compound, AHC-52. Cancer Res 1989; 49:1722–1726.

64. Boesch D, Gaveriaux C, Jachez B, Pourtier-Manzanedo A, Bollinger P, Loor F. In vivo circumvention of P-glycoprotein-mediated multidrug resistance of tumor cells with SDZ PSC 833. Cancer Res 1991; 51:4226–4233.

65. Niwa K, Yamada K, Furukawa T, Shudo N, Seto K, Matsumoto T, Takao S, Akiyama S-I, Shimazu H. Effect of a dihydropyridine analogue, 2-[Benzyl(phenyl)amino]ethyl 1,4-dihydro-2,6-dimethyl-5-(5,5-dimethyl-2-oxo-1,3,2-dioxaphosphorinan-2-yl)-1-(2-morpholino-ethyl)-4-(3-nitrophenyl)-3-pyridinecarboxylate on reversing in vivo resistance of tumor cells to Adriamycin. Cancer Res 1992; 52:3655–3660.

66. Houghton JA, Williams LG, Dodge RK, George SL, Hazelton BJ, Houghton PJ. Relationship between binding affinity, retention and sensitivity of human rhabdomyosarcoma xenografts to vinca alkaloids. Biochem Pharmacol 1987; 36:81–88.

67. Houghton JA, Williams LG, Torrance PM, Houghton PJ. Determinants of intrinsic sensitivity to vinca alkaloids in xenografts of pediatric rhabdomyosarcomas. Cancer Res 1984; 44:582–590.

68. McVie JG. Drug disposition and pharmacology. In: Fox BW, Fox M, eds. Antitumor Drug Resistance. Berlin: Springer-Verlag, 1984:39–66.

69. Tsuruo T, Iida H, Tsukagoshi S, et al. Overcoming of vincristine resistance in P388 leukemia in vivo and in vitro through enhanced cytotoxicity of vincristine and vinblastine by verapamil. Cancer Res 1981; 41:1967–1972.

70. Ford JM, Hait WN. Pharmacology of drugs that alter multidrug resistance in cancer. Pharmacol Rev 1990; 42:155–199.

71. Sikic BI. Modulation of multidrug resistance: at the threshold. J Clin Oncol 1993; 11:1629–1635.

72. Goldstein LJ, Galski H, Fojo A, et al. Expression of a multidrug resistance gene in human cancers. JNCI 1989; 81:116–124.

73. Linn SC, Giaccone G, van Kalken CK, Pinedo HM. P-glycoprotein mediated multidrug resistance and its clinical relevance in cancer treatment. Forum 1992; 2:642–657.

74. Twentyman PR. *MDR1* (P-glycoprotein) gene expression—implications for resistance modifier trials. JNCI 1992; 84:1458–1460.

75. Goasguen JE, Dossot J-M, Fardel O, Le Mee F, Le Gall E, Leblay R, LePrise PY, Chaperon J, Fauchet R. Expression of the multidrug resistance-associated P-glycoprotein (P-170) in 59 cases of de novo acute lymphoblastic leukemia: prognostic implications. Blood 1993; 81:2394–2398.

76. Grogan TM, Spier CM, Salmon SE, Matzner M, Rybski J, Weinstein RS, Scheper RJ, Dalton WS. P-glycoprotein expression in human plasma cell myeloma: correlation with prior chemotherapy. Blood 1993; 81:490–495.

77. Moscow JA, et al. Expression of anionic glutathione-*S*-transferase and P-glycoprotein genes in human tissues and tumors. Cancer Res 1989; 49:1422–1428.

78. Pileri SA, et al. Immunohistochemical detection of the multidrug transport protein P170 in human normal tissues and malignant lymphomas. Histopathology 1991; 19:131–140.

79. Chan HSL, Thorner PS, Haddad G, Ling V. Immunohistochemical detection of P-glycoprotein: prognostic correlation in soft tissue sarcoma of childhood. J Clin Oncol 1990; 8:689–704.

80. Sanfilippo O, Ronchi E, de Marco C, et al. Expression of P-glycoprotein

in breast cancer tissue and in vitro resistance to doxorubicin and vincristine. Eur J Cancer 1991; 27:155–158.

81. Verelle P, Meissonnier F, Fonck Y, et al. Clinical relevance of immunohistochemical detection of multidrug resistance of P-glycoprotein in breast carcinoma. JNCI 1991; 83:111–116.

82. Marie J-P, Zittoun R, Sikic BI. Multidrug resistance (*MDR1*) gene expression in adult acute leukemias: correlations with treatment outcome and in vitro drug sensitivity. Blood 1991; 78:586–592.

83. Marie J-P, Faussat-Suberville A-M, Zhou D, Zittoun R. Daunorubicin uptake by leukemic cells: correlations with treatment outcome and *MDR1* expression. Leukemia 1993; 7:825–831.

84. Ross DD, Wooten PJ, Sridhara R, Ordóñez JV, Lee EJ, Schiffer CA. Enhancement of daunorubicin accumulation, retention and cytotoxicity by verapamil or cyclosporin A in blast cells from patients with previously untreated acute myeloid leukemia. Blood 1993; 82:1288–1299.

85. Bessho F, Kinumaki H, Kobayashi M, Habu H, Nakamura K, Yokota S, Tsuruo T, Kobayashi N. Treatment of children with refractory acute lymphocytic leukemia with vincristine and diltiazem. Med Pediatr Oncol 1985; 13:199–202.

86. Benson AB III, Trump DL, Koeller JM, Egorin MI, Olman EA, Witte RS, Davis TE, Tormey DC. Phase I study of vinblastine and verapamil given by concurrent iv infusion. Cancer Treat Rep 1985; 69:795–799.

87. Cairo MS, Siegel S, Anas N, Sender L. Clinical trial of continuous infusion verapamil, bolus vinblastine, and continuous infusion VP-16 in drug resistant pediatric tumors. Cancer Res 1989; 49:1063–1066.

88. Dalton WS, Grogan TM, Meltzer PS, et al. Drug-resistance in multiple myeloma and non-Hodgkin's lymphoma: detection of P-glycoprotein and potential circumvention by the addition of verapamil to chemotherapy. J Clin Oncol 1989; 7:415–424.

89. Trümper LH, Ho AD, Wulf G, Hunstein W. Addition of verapamil to overcome drug resistance in multiple myeloma: preliminary clinical observations in 10 patients [letter]. J Clin Oncol 1989; 7:1578.

90. Miller TP, Grogan TM, Dalton WS, et al. P-glycoprotein expression in malignant lymphoma and reversal of clinical drug resistance with chemotherapy plus high dose verapamil. J Clin Oncol 1991; 9:17–24.

91. Solary E, Caillot D, Chauffert B, Casasnovas R-O, Dumas M, Maynadie M, Guy H. Feasibility of using quinine, a potential multidrug resistance-reversing agent, in combination with mitoxantrone and cytarabine for the treatment of acute leukemia. J Clin Oncol 1992; 10:1730–1736.

92. Sonneveld P, Nooter K. Reversal of drug-resistance by cyclosporin-A in a patient with acute myelocytic leukaemia. Br J Haematol 1990; 75:208–211.

93. Sonneveld P, Durie BGM, Lokhorst HM, et al. Modulation of multidrug-resistant multiple myeloma by cyclosporin. Lancet 1992; 340:255–259.

94. List AF, Spier C, Greer J, Wolff S, Hutter J, Dorr R, Salmon S, Futscher B, Baier M, Dalton W. Phase I/II trial of cyclosporine as chemotherapy-resistance modifier in acute leukemia. J Clin Oncol 1993; 11:1652–1660.

95. Marie J-P, Bastie J-N, Coloma F, Faussat Suberville A-M, Delmer A, Rio B, Delmas-Marsalet B, Leroux G, Casassus P, Baumelou E, Catalin J, Zittoun R. Cyclosporin A as a modifier agent in the salvage treatment of acute leukemia. Leukemia 1993; 7:821–824.

96. Presant CA, Kennedy PS, Wiseman C, Gala K, Bouzaglou A, Wyres M, Naessig V. Verapamil reversal of clinical doxorubicin resistance in human cancer. Am J Clin Oncol 1986; 9:355–357.

97. Demicheli R, Jirillo A, Bonciarelli G, Lonardi F, Balli M, Bandello A. 4′-Epidoxorubicin plus verapamil in anthracycline-refractory cancer patients. Tumori 1989; 75:245–247.

98. Ozols RF, Cunnion RE, Klecker RW, Hamilton TC, Ostchega Y, Parrillo JE, Young RC. Verapamil and Adriamycin in the treatment of drug-resistant ovarian cancer patients. J Clin Oncol 1987; 5:641–647.

99. Hendrick AM, Harris AL, Cantwell BMJ. Verapamil with mitoxantrone for advanced ovarian cancer: a negative phase II trial. Ann Oncol 1991; 2:71–72.

100. Dalmark M, Pals H, Johnsen AH. Doxorubicin in combination with verapamil in advanced colorectal cancer. Acta Oncol 1991; 30:23–26.

101. Millward MJ, Cantwell BMJ, Munro NC, Robinson A, Corris PA, Harris AL. Oral verapamil with chemotherapy for advanced non-small cell lung cancer: a randomised study. Br J Cancer 1993; 67:1031–1035.

102. Milroy R, on behalf of the West of Scotland Lung Cancer Research Group, and the Aberdeen Oncology Group. A randomised clinical study of verapamil in addition to combination chemotherapy in small cell lung cancer. Br J Cancer 1993; 68:813–818.

103. Lai ECS, Choi TK, Cheng CH, Mok FPT, Fan ST, Tan ESY, Wong J. Doxorubicin for unresectable hepatocellular carcinoma. Cancer 1990; 66:1685–1687.

104. Figueredo A, Arnold A, Goodyear M, Findlay B, Neville A, Normandeau R, Jones A. Addition of verapamil and tamoxifen to the initial chemotherapy of small cell lung cancer. A phase I/II study. Cancer 1990; 65:1895–1902.

105. Bissett D, Kerr DJ, Cassidy J, Meredith P, Traugott U, Kaye SB. Phase I and pharmacokinetic study of D-verapamil and doxorubicin. Br J Cancer 1991; 64:1168–1171.

106. van Kalken CK, van der Hoeven JJM, de Jong J, Giaccone G, Schuurhuis GJ, Maessen PA, Blokhuis WMD, van der Vijgh WJF, Pinedo HM. Bepridil in combination with anthracyclines to reverse anthracycline resistance in cancer patients. Eur J Cancer 1991; 27:739–744.

107. Jones RD, Kerr DJ, Harnett AN, Rankin EM, Ray S, Kaye SB. A pilot study of quinidine and epirubicin in the treatment of advanced breast cancer. Br J Cancer 1990; 62:133–135.

108. Chauffert B, Pelletier H, Corda C, Solary E, Bedenne L, Caillot D, Martin F. Potential usefulness of quinine to circumvent the anthracycline resistance in clinical practice. Br J Cancer 1990; 62:395–397.

109. Philip PA, Joel S, Monkman SC, Dolega-Ossowski, Tonkin K, Carmichael J, Idle JR, Harris AL. A phase I study on the reversal of multidrug resistance

(MDR) in vivo: nifedipine plus etoposide. Br J Cancer 1992; 65:267–270.
110. Isonishi S, Kirmani S, Kim S, Plaxe SC, Braly PS, McClay EF, Howell SB. Phase I and pharmacokinetic trial of intraperitoneal etoposide in combination with the multidrug-resistance-modulating agent dipyridamole. JNCI 1991; 83:621–626.
111. van der Graaf WTA, de Vries EGE, Uges DRA, Nanninga AG, Meijer C, Vellenga E, Mulder POM, Mulder NH. In vitro and in vivo modulation of multidrug resistance with amiodarone. Int J Cancer 1991; 48:616–622.
112. Chauffert B, Seitz J-F, Bedenne L, Renard P, Conroy T, Rougier P. Phase II evaluation of doxorubicin plus amiodarone in advanced hepatocarcinoma. Gastroenterol Clin Biol 1991; 15:774–775.
113. Miller RL, Bukowski RM, Budd GT, Purvis J, Weick JK, Shepard K, Midha KK, Ganapathi R. Clinical modulation of doxorubicin resistance by the calmodulin-inhibitor, trifluoperazine: a phase I/II trial. J Clin Oncol 1988; 6:880–888.
114. Budd GT, Bukowski RM, Lichtin A, Bauer L, van Kirk P, Ganapathi R. Phase II trial of doxorubicin and trifluoperazine in metastatic breast cancer. Invest New Drugs 1993; 11:75–79.
115. Sridhar KS, Krishan A, Samy TSA, Sauerteig A, Wellham LL, McPhee G, Duncan RC, Anac SY, Ardalan B, Benedetto PW. Prochlorperazine as doxorubicin-efflux blocker: phase I clinical and pharmacokinetics studies. Cancer Chemother Pharmacol 1993; 31:423–430.
116. Verweij J, Herweijer H, Oosterom R, van der Burg MEL, Planting AST, Seynaeve C, Stoter G, Nooter K. A phase II study of epidoxorubicin in colorectal cancer and the use of cyclosporin-A in an attempt to reverse multidrug resistance. Br J Cancer 1991; 64:361–364.
117. Rodenburg CJ, Nooter K, Herweijer H, Seynaeve C, Oosterom R, Stoter G, Verweij J. Phase II study of combining vinblastine and cyclosporin-A to circumvent multidrug resistance in renal cell cancer. Ann Oncol 1991; 2:305–306.
118. Yahanda AM, Adler KM, Fisher GA, et al. Phase I trial of etoposide with cyclosporine as a modulator of multidrug resistance. J Clin Oncol 1992; 10:1624–1634.
119. Erlichman C, Moore M, Thiessen JJ, Kerr IG, Walker S, Goodman P, Bjarnason G, DeAngelis C, Bunting P. Phase I pharmacokinetic study of cyclosporin A combined with doxorubicin. Cancer Res 1993; 53:4837–4842.
120. Samuels BL, Mick R, Vogelzang NJ, Williams SF, Schilsky RL, Safa AR, O'Brien SM, Ratain MJ. Modulation of vinblastine resistance with cyclosporine: a phase I study. Clin Pharmacol Ther 1993; 54:421–429.
121. Millward MJ, Cantwell BMJ, Lien EA, Carmichael J, Harris AL. Intermittent high-dose tamoxifen as a potential modifier of multidrug resistance. Eur J Cancer 1992; 28A:805–810.
122. Trump DL, Smith DC, Ellis PG, Rogers MP, Schold SC, Winer EP, Panella TJ, Jordan VC, Fine RL. High-dose oral tamoxifen, a potential multidrug-resistance-reversal agent: phase I trial in combination with vinblastine. JNCI 1992; 84:1811–1816.

123. Lum BL, Kaubisch S, Yahanda AM, et al. Alteration of etoposide pharmacokinetics and pharmacodynamics by cyclosporine in a phase I trial to modulate multidrug resistance. J Clin Oncol 1992; 10:1635–1642.

124. Scheithauer W, Schenk T, Czejka M. Pharmacokinetic interaction between epirubicin and the multidrug resistance reverting agent D-verapamil. Br J Cancer 1993; 68:8–9.

125. Henderson IC, Hayes DF, Gelman R. Dose-response in the treatment of breast cancer: a critical review. J Clin Oncol 1988; 6:1501–1515.

126. Thierry AR, Vigé D, Coughlin SS, Belli JA, Drithschilo A, Rahman A. Modulation of doxorubicin resistance in multidrug-resistant cells by liposomes. FASEB J 1993; 7:572–579.

127. Treat J, Greenspan A, Forst D, Sanchez AJ, Ferrans VJ, Potkul LA, Woolley PV, Rahman A. Anti-tumor activity of liposome-encapsulated doxorubicin in advanced breast cancer: phase II study. JNCI 1990; 82:1706–1710.

128. Mickisch GH, Pai LH, Gottesman MM, Pastan I. Monoclonal antibody MRK16 reverses the multidrug resistance of multidrug-resistant transgenic mice. Cancer Res 1992; 52:4427–4432.

129. Bertino JR. Ode to methotrexate. J Clin Oncol 1993; 11:5–14.

130. Barredo J, Moran RG. Determinants of antifolate cytotoxicity: folylpolyglutamate synthetase activity during cell proliferation and development. Mol Pharmacol 1992; 42:687–694.

131. Allegra CJ, Chabner BA, Drake JC, Lutz R, Rodbard D, Jolivet J. Enhanced inhibition of thymidylate synthase by methotrexate polyglutamates. J Biol Chem 1985; 260:9720–9726.

132. Allegra CJ, Drake JC, Jolivet J, Chabner BA. Inhibition of phosphoribosylaminoimidazolecarboxamide transformylase by methotrexate and dihydrofolic acid polyglutamates. Proc Natl Acad Sci USA 1985; 82:4881–4885.

133. Sirotnak FM. Obligate genetic expression in tumor cells of a fetal membrane property mediating "folate" transport: biological significance and implications for improved therapy of human cancer. Cancer Res 1985; 45:3992–4000.

134. Antony AC. The biological chemistry of folate receptors. Blood 1992; 79:2807–2820.

135. Jansen G, Westerhof GR, Jarmuszewski MJA, Kathmann I, Rijksen G, Schornagel JH. Methotrexate transport in variant human CCRF-CEM leukemia cells with elevated levels of the reduced folate carrier. J Biol Chem 1990; 265:18272–18277.

136. Price EM, Ratnam M, Rodeman K, Freisheim JH. Characterization of the methotrexate transport pathway in murine L1210 leukemia cells: involvement of a membrane receptor and a cytosolic protein. Biochemistry 1988; 27:7853–7858.

137. Matherly LH, Czajkowski CA, Angeles SM. Identification of a highly glycosylated methotrexate membrane carrier in K562 human erythroleukemia cells up-regulated for tetrahydrofolate cofactor and methotrexate transport. Cancer Res 1991; 51:3420–3426.

138. Freisheim JH, Ratnam M, McAlinden TP, Prasad KMR, Williams FE,

Westerhof GR, Schornagel JH, Jansen G. Molecular events in the membrane transport of methotrexate in human CCRF-CEM leukemia cell lines. Adv Enzyme Regul 1992; 32:17–31.

139. Lacey SW, Sanders JM, Rothberg K, Anderson RGW, Kamen BA. Complementary DNA for the folate binding protein correctly predicts anchoring to the membrane by glycosyl-phosphatidylinositol. J Clin Invest 1989; 84:715–720.

140. Hjelle JT, Christensen EI, Carone FA, Selhub J. Cell fractionation and electron microscope studies of kidney folate binding protein. Am J Physiol 1991; 260:C338–C346.

141. Anderson RGW, Kamen BA, Rothberg, KG, Lacey SW. Potocytosis: sequestration and transport of small molecules by caveolae. Science 1992; 255:410–411.

142. Anderson RGW. Caveolae: where incoming and outcoming messengers meet. Proc Natl Acad Sci USA 1993; 90:10909–10913.

143. Ratnam M, Marquardt H, Duhring JL, Freisheim JH. Homologous membrane folate binding proteins in human placenta: cloning and sequence of a cDNA. Biochemistry 1989; 28:8249–8254.

144. Elwood PC. Molecular cloning and characterization of the human folate binding protein cDNA from placenta and malignant tissue culture (KB) cells. J Biol Chem 1989; 28:14893–14901.

145. Weitman SD, Lark RH, Coney LR, Fort DW, Frasca V, Zurawski VA Jr, Kamen BA. Distribution of the folate receptor GP38 in normal and malignant cell lines and tissues. Cancer Res 1992; 52:3396–3401.

146. Campbell IG, Jones T, Trowsdale J. High-affinity folate binding protein is a marker for ovarian cancer. Cancer Res 1991; 51:5329–5338.

147. Garin-Chesa P, Campbell I, Saigo PE, Lewis JL, Old LJ, Rettig WJ. Trophoblast and ovarian cancer antigen LK26. Sensitivity and specificity in immunopathology and molecular identification as a folate-binding protein. Am J Pathol 1993; 142:557–567.

148. Westerhof GR, Jansen G, van Emmerik N, Kathmann I, Rijksen G, Jackman AL, Schornagel JH. Membrane transport of antifolate compounds in L1210 cells: the role of carrier- and receptor-mediated transport systems. Cancer Res 1991; 51:5507–5513.

149. Saikawa Y, Knight CB, Saikawa T, Page ST, Chabner BA, Elwood PC. Decreased expression of the human folate receptor mediates transport defective methotrexate resistance in KB cells. J Biol Chem 1993; 268:5293–5301.

150. Trippett T, Schlemmer S, Elisseyeff Y, Goker E, Wachter M, Steinherz P, Tan C, Berman E, Wright JE, Rosowsky A, Schweitzer B, Bertino JR. Defective transport as a mechanism of acquired resistance to methotrexate in patients with acute lymphocytic leukemia. Blood 1992; 80:1158–1162.

151. Jansen G, Westerhof GR, Kathmann I, Rademaker BC, Rijksen G, Schornagel JH. Identification of a membrane-associated folate-binding protein in human leukemic CCRF-CEM cells with transport related methotrexate resistance. Cancer Res 1989; 49:2455–2459.

152. Assaraf YG, Schimke RT. Identification of methotrexate transport deficiency in mammalian cells using fluoresceinated methotrexate and flow cytometry. Proc Natl Acad Sci USA 1987; 84:7154–7158.

153. Schuetz JD, Matherly LH, Westin EH, Goldman ID. Evidence for a functional defect in the translocation of the methotrexate transport carrier in a methotrexate-resistant L1210 leukemia cell line. J Biol Chem 1988; 263:9840–9847.

154. Matherly LH, Angeles SM, Czajkowski CA. Characterization of transport-mediated methotrexate resistance in human tumor cells with antibodies to the membrane carrier for methotrexate and tetrahydrofolate cofactors. J Biol Chem 1992; 267:23253–23260.

155. Schornagel JH, Verweij J, de Mulder PHM, Cognetti F, Vermorken JB, Cappelaere P, Armand JP, Wildiers J, Clavel M, Kirkpatrick A, Lefebvre JL. A phase II trial of 10-ethyl-10-deaza-aminopterin, a novel antifolate, in patients with advanced and/or recurrent squamous cell carcinoma of the head and neck. Ann Oncol 1992; 3:223–226.

156. Jackman AL, Taylor GA, Gibson W, Kimbell R, Brown M, Calvert AH, Judson IR, Hughes LR. ICI-D1694, a quinazoline antifolate thymidylate synthase inhibitor that is a potent inhibitor of L1210 tumor cell growth in vitro and in vivo: a new agent for clinical studies. Cancer Res 1991; 51:5579–5586.

157. Beardsley GP, Moroson BA, Taylor EC, Moran RG. A new folate antimetabolite, 5,10-dideaza-5,6,7,8-tetrahydrofolate is a potent inhibitor of de novo purine synthesis. J Biol Chem 1989; 264:328–333.

158. Scanlon KJ, Kashani-Sabet T, Tone T, Funato T. Cisplatin resistance in human cancers. Pharmacol Ther 1991; 52:385–406.

159. Kawai K, Kamatani N, Georges E, Ling V. Identification of a membrane glycoprotein overexpressed in murine lymphoma sublines resistant to *cis*-dichloroplatinum(II). J Biol Chem 1990; 265:13137–13142.

160. Kelland LR, Mistry P, Abel G, Loh SY, O'Neill CF, Murrer BA, Harrap KR. Mechanism-related circumvention of acquired *cis*-diamminedichloroplatinum(II) resistance using two pairs of human ovarian carcinoma cell lines by ammine/amine platinum(IV) dicarboxylates. Cancer Res 1992; 52:3857–3864.

161. Ishikawa T, Ali-Osman F. Glutathione-associated *cis*-diamminedichloroplatinum(II) metabolism and ATP-dependent efflux from leukemia cells. J Biol Chem 1993; 268:20116–20125.

162. Hamaguchi K, Godwin AK, Yakushiji M, O'Dwyer PJ, Ozols RF, Hamilton TC. Cross-resistance to diverse drugs is associated with primary cisplatin resistance in ovarian cancer cell lines. Cancer Res 1993; 53:5225–5232.

163. Ahmad S, Okine L, Wood R, Aljian J, Vistica DT. gamma-Glutamyl transpeptidase and maintenance of thiol pools in tumor cells resistant to alkylating agents. J Cell Physiol 1987; 131:240–246.

164. Moscow JA, Swanson CA, Cowan KH. Decreased melphalan accumulation in a human breast cancer cell line selected for resistance to melphalan. Br J Cancer 1993; 68:732–737.

165. Bates SE, Lee JS, Dickstein B, Spolyar M, Fojo AT. Differential modulation of P-glycoprotein transport by protein kinase inhibition. Biochemistry 1993; 32:9156–9164.
166. Tritton TR, Hickman JA. How to kill cancer cells: membranes and cell signalling as targets in cancer chemotherapy. Cancer Cells 1990; 2:95–105.
167. Chaudhary PM, Roninson IB. Induction of multidrug resistance in human cells by transient exposure to different chemotherapeutic drugs. JNCI 1993; 85:632–639.

3

Composition and Properties of Cellular Membranes

Dennis Chapman
Royal Free Hospital School of Medicine,
University of London, London, England

I. INTRODUCTION

A. General Overview

All cells possess biomembranes composed of lipids and proteins. Electron microscopy was particularly valuable in showing the extensive biomembrane systems that occur in various cells. In gram-positive bacteria, only a single plasma membrane is present. The membrane acts as a barrier for the passage of inorganic ions and hydrophilic molecules. Gram-negative bacteria, however, have a second outer membrane (discussed in Chap. 5). In eukaryotic cells, additional membranes envelop the organelles inside the cell, such as the nucleus, the endoplasmic reticulum, and mitochondria.

During the 1960s, there was much debate concerning the structure of biomembranes. The various arguments emphasized the preponderance of the protein or the lipid components until, finally, a concensus view was reached; namely, all biomembranes are built on a lipid matrix (with few exceptions, a bimolecular sheet) into which the membrane proteins are either embedded (integral proteins) or associated with the membrane surface, usually by electrostatic interactions with the lipid polar head groups (peripheral proteins). For awhile there was a lull in research activity in biomembranes and their dynamic character, but that has changed in recent years. The renewed interest is related to the technological advances made in determining the detailed structure of the membrane proteins and the use of molecular biology techniques for cloning and protein manipulation. There is also renewed interest in the extrinsic proteins, the receptor proteins, and the processes of protein translocation. Furthermore, signaling through the membrane by transmembrane receptor proteins and lipids, such as phosphatidylinositol, is now an area of intense research activity.

In this chapter we review some of the basic characteristics of biomembranes as well as the techniques commonly used for their study.

B. Membrane Components

1. Lipids

Lipids are key structural components of membranes, and they often function as essential messengers that trigger important physiological processes. Typically, biomembranes contain over 100 different lipid species (1). These are often based on glycerol (phosphoglycerides) or sphingosine (sphingolipids). The structures of some of the common phospholipids are shown in Table 1 (for a review, see Ref. 2). The lipids found in biological membranes are almost invariably amphiphilic, possessing a hydrophilic polar head-group and a hydrophobic hydrocarbon region. It is the amphiphilic character of the lipids that leads them to assume the basic bilayer organization, which provides a permeability barrier between the exterior and interior compartments.

Variations in the hydrophilic and hydrophobic regions give rise to the structural diversity found in membrane lipids. The most abundant lipids are the phospholipids, phosphatidylcholine (PC) being preponderant in animal membranes, phosphatidylethanolamine (PE) in bacterial membranes, and glycolipids in plant membranes. Glycosphingolipids and gangliosides differ from sphingomyelin in having a short carbohydrate chain in place of the PC head group. Gangliosides act as receptors for some hormones and toxins on the cell surface. Sterols are found exclusively in eukaryotic cells. Cholesterol is the major sterol of mammalian plasma membranes, lysosomal membranes, and Golgi membranes; ergosterol is preponderant in fungal membranes, whereas sitosterol and stigmasterol are preponderant in plant plasma membranes.

The fluidity of biomembranes depends largely on the nature of the acyl chains of membrane lipids (see Sec. IV.A.2). The acyl chains of natural membrane lipids are mostly even-numbered, with the proportion of odd-numbered fatty acyl chain substituents usually below 2 mol%. The C_{16}, C_{18}, and C_{20} substituents constitute 80% of the acyl chains. Unsaturated

Table 1 Some Typical Lipids of Cellular Membranes

Neutral lipids	Glycolipids	Phospholipids			
Sterols		Sphingomyelins	Phosphatidyl-		
			choline	ethanolamine	serine
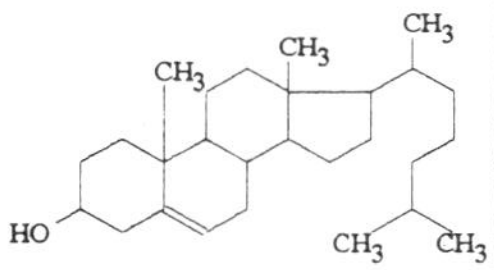 cholesterol 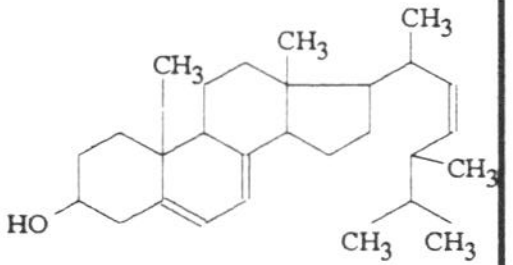 ergosterol	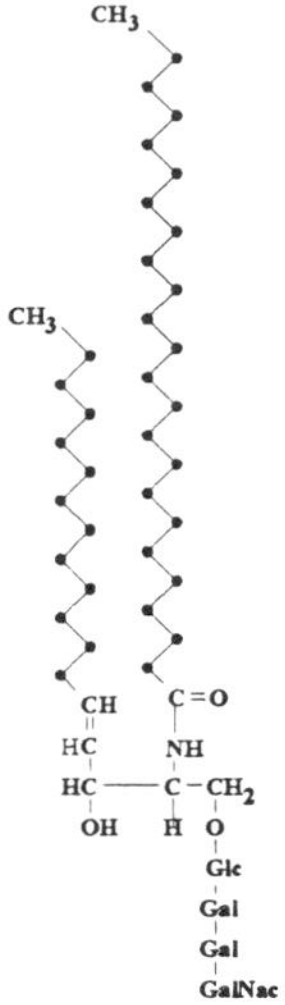 Glc Gal Gal GalNac	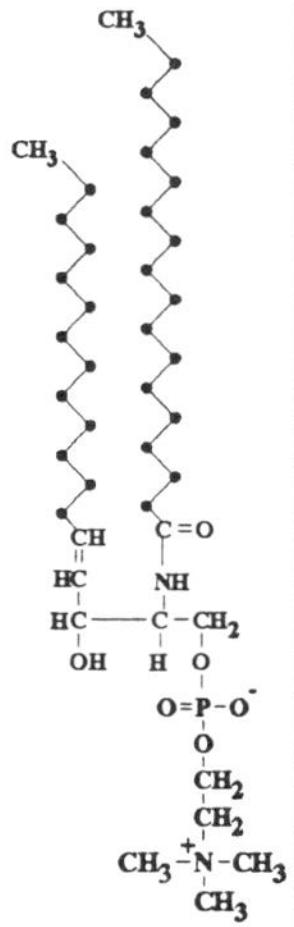	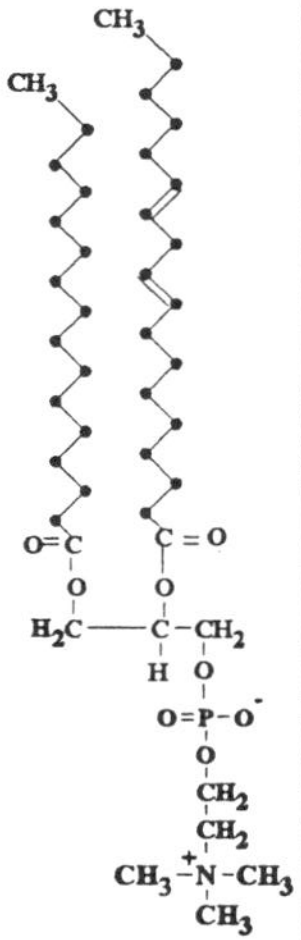	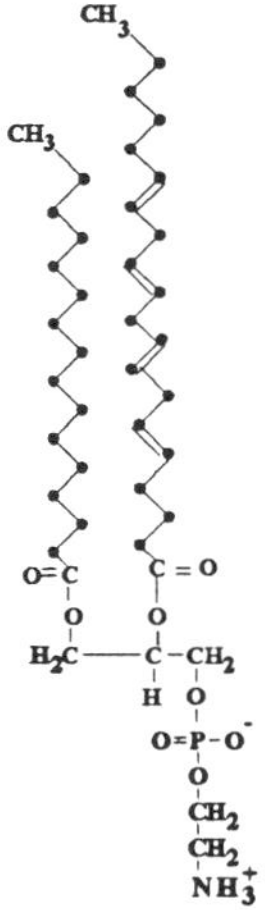	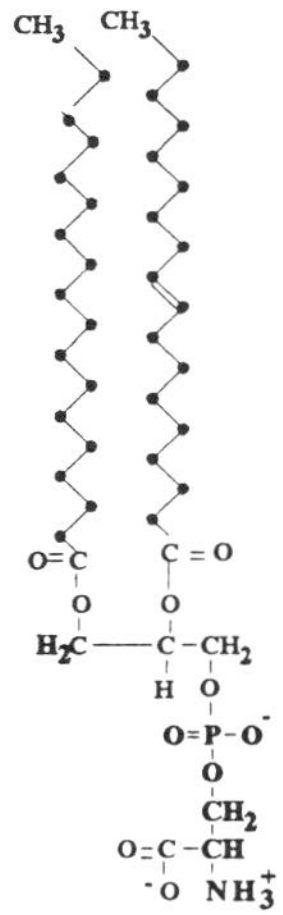

chains are present in many membranes; the $C_{18:1}$, $C_{18:2}$, and $C_{20:4}$ lipids are the major unsaturated species.

Unusual lipid molecules occur in thermophilic prokaryotic organisms, which may be either *Eubacteria* or *Archaeobacteria*. The distinction between *Eubacteria* and *Archaeobacteria* is based on phylogenetic criteria—sequence of ribosomal RNAs, subunit composition of RNA polymerase, size and shape of ribosomes—or on the chemical composition of the lipids. Thermophilic *Eubacteria* belong to different genera that comprise a wide variety of microorganisms—aerobic, anaerobic, spore-forming, gram-positive, gram-negative—capable of growing over a wide pH range (2.0–9.0).

Archaeobacteria constitute a novel family of prokaryotic microorganisms, recently identified as the third kingdom of life. They are found in exceptional ecological niches and are classified according to their habitat into halophiles, thermophiles, and methanogens. The lipids extracted from *Archaeobacteria* are characterized by remarkable structural features. First, these lipids are based exclusively on *ether* linkages; second, the molecules are formed by condensation of glycerol, or of more complex polyols, with isoprenoid alcohols containing 20, 25, or 40 carbon atoms; third, the glycerol ethers (3) contain a 2,3-di-*O*-*sn*-glycerol.

2. *Proteins*

The ratio of protein to lipid present in a biomembrane ranges considerably from one cell system to another. It is high in the bacterial purple membrane, with bacteriorhodopsin as the major protein, and lower in the myelin membranes (Table 2). Investigations into membrane proteins led to a broad division of these molecules into two classes: integral (intrinsic) and peripheral (extrinsic) membrane proteins. The latter are easily dissociated from the membrane, often with little or no effect on either the structure or function of the protein. Thus, they behave much like cytoplasmic proteins. Integral membrane proteins are intimately associated with the hydrophobic interior of the lipid bilayer; their dissociation from membranes requires complete physical disruption of the membrane. The integral proteins contain large hydrophobic regions, whereas the extrinsic proteins resemble soluble enzymes. The integral proteins are synthesized somewhat differently, with signal or localization sequences determining their final location. The integral proteins are concerned with transmembrane functions, such as membrane transport and transmembrane signaling.

3. *Glycoproteins*

In addition to proteins and lipids, cells contain sugar residues on their surface. These have an important role in cell recognition processes, anti-

Table 2 Composition of Various Membranes Expressed as
Their Protein/Lipid Weight Ratio (P/L)

Membrane	P/L
Bovine myelin	0.28
Human erythrocyte	1.11
Outer mitochondrial membrane	1.22
Retinal rod outer segment	1.44
Hepatocyte plasma membrane	1.50
Micrococcus lysodeikticus	1.91
Saccharomyces cerevisiae plasma membrane	1.98
Chloroplast lamella	2.22
Acholeplasma laidlawii	2.33
Halophilic bacteria	3.14

genic properties, and hormone reception. Some of the sugar residues are
attached to lipids, mainly sphingolipids. Many are covalently linked to
proteins. In some animal cells, this is the major part of the so-called glyco-
calyx.

The sugars are either O-linked or N-linked to proteins. The first type
bind by serine or threonine (and, rarely, hydroxylysine); the second type
do so by asparagine. The O-linked glycoproteins obligatorily contain N-
acetyl-D-galactosamine (GaINAc) as the first and often the second sugar;
the N-linked ones always bind to N-acetyl-D-glycosamine (GlcNAc) and
always contain the sequence:

$$\overset{1,4}{\text{Man}} \rightarrow \overset{1,4}{\text{GlcNAc}} \rightarrow \text{GlcNAc} \rightarrow \text{Asn}$$

(where Man is D-mannose)

A typical glycoprotein is glycophorin A of erythrocytes, with 131-amino
acid residues, plus a full 60% of total weight in sugar residues, 15 of the
oligosaccharide chains O-linked, one N-linked.

II. ORGANIZATION OF LIPID COMPONENTS INTO BIOMEMBRANES

The first suggestion that a lipid bilayer was the core of a biological membrane was proposed in 1925 by Gorter and Grendel (4). These workers
extracted the lipid from erythrocyte membranes, compressed it at an
air–water interface, and showed that it occupied a surface area equal to
twice the external area of the cells. (Later workers showed that there
were compensating errors in these deductions; 5.) Danielli and Davson

further developed this model in 1935 to include proteins, but suggested that the lipid polar groups were coated with layers of protein, to account for the low membrane tension (6). The development of the electron microscope appeared to support this concept, giving rise to the "unit membrane" hypothesis. At this time, electron microscopic studies required fixing cells, often with osmium tetroxide, dehydration, and embedding; a particular difficulty was to be sure of the location of the osmium material. Work on myelin, using X-ray defraction methods, also appeared to fit the unit membrane structure. Other workers argued against this model emphasizing the high amount of protein present in certain membrane systems.

A. Lipid Matrix

The current consensus is that the phospholipids in biomembranes are organized in a bilayer structure. The *Archaeobacteria*, which have only a single lipid spanning the lipid matrix, are an exception to this rule. Perhaps the best proof of the existence of a lipid bilayer structure is based on freeze-fracture electron microscopy. The fracture takes place along the center of the bilayer (i.e., the fracture plane) and particles can be seen representing the embedded integral proteins. There have been many suggestions and attempts to demonstrate nonlamellar structures as permanent structures in biomembranes, but this is not yet proven. Lipids extracted from biomembranes often form hexagonal or cubic phases at physiological temperatures, but this does not mean that these are present in natural membranes when protein is present.

The fluid–mosaic model proposed in 1972 by Singer and Nicholson (7) was based on the work of several scientists. The model emphasized the concept of a fluid lipid sheet of varying composition and fluidity. The concept of lipid membrane fluidity had been proposed in 1966 by Chapman and co-workers (8). Embedded in the sheet are the integral proteins, which are able to undergo lateral and rotational diffusion. The integral proteins were suggested to have α-helical structures.

This model is a useful summary of the scientific studies of many workers in the biomembrane field. There are exceptions to the model; for example, the bacteriorhodopsin protein is fixed in position within the lipid sheet and does not undergo rotational or lateral diffusion. The lipids are also particularly rigid and immobile. Some biomembranes contain regions of crystalline lipid and fluid lipid (e.g., *Acholeplasma laidlawii* membranes). Some membrane proteins, notably the porins (see Chap. 5), have a β-barrel structure (see Sec. III.B).

B. Static and Dynamic Lipid Asymmetry
in Cell Membranes

The asymmetrical distribution of lipid classes was first observed in human erythrocyte membranes by Bretscher (9). Most biological membranes appear to have a different phospholipid composition in their inner and outer leaflets. In erythrocytes, phosphatidylserine (PS), phosphatidylethanolamine (PE), and probably, phosphatidylinositol (PI), are located mainly in the inner layer, whereas phosphatidylcholine (PC) and sphingomyelin (SM) are essentially in the outer layer.

Various techniques have been used to determine lipid asymmetry in biomembranes. These techniques include chemical labeling with nonpenetrating agents [e.g., with trinitrobenzenesulfonic acid (TNBS) or fluorescamine], immunological methods, phospholipase digestion of membrane phospholipids, use of phospholipid-exchange proteins, and physicochemical methods such as x-ray diffraction and nuclear magnetic resonance (NMR).

Lipid asymmetry was thought to be the consequence of asymmetrical membrane biogenesis and asymmetrical lipid turnover by endogenous phospholipases and reacylases, together with the asymmetrical insertion of lipid constituents. The differences in potential or pH between the two surfaces could also explain the stability of the asymmetrical distribution (negatively charged phospholipids on the cytosolic half of the lipid bilayer). However, in 1984, the existence of an ATP-requiring mechanism responsible for the specific translocation of aminophospholipids (PS and PE) was demonstrated in human red cells and, later, in other plasma membranes (see review, Ref. 10).

C. Protein and Glycoprotein Arrangements

The proteins associated with biomembranes can be arranged in different ways relative to the lipid bilayer matrix. Some of these arrangements are shown in Figure 1.

1. Integral Proteins

Occasionally, the protein is fully submerged in the lipid matrix (e.g., in myelin), whereas integral membrane proteins that span the lipid matrix are abundant, particularly those associated with transport and energy transduction. Sometimes the membrane-spanning helical polypeptide arrangements have been directly demonstrated by using electron diffraction techniques, as with bacteriorhodopsin. In other instances, hydropathy

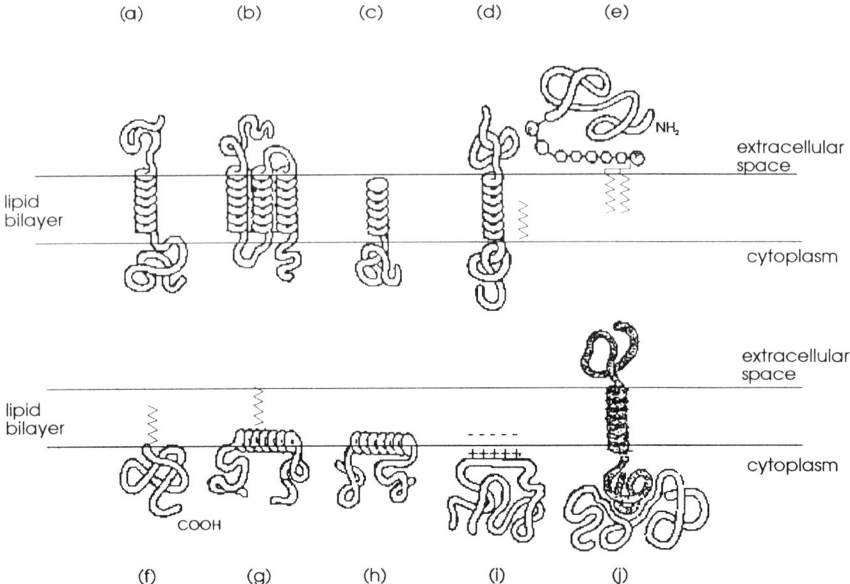

Figure 1 Different ways in which membrane proteins can be associated with membranes. Transmembrane proteins extend across the bilayer as single α-helices, (a) and (b). Other membrane proteins are attached to the bilayer by a hydrophobic polypeptide anchor (c), or solely by a covalently linked lipid such as a glycophospholipid (e) or a fatty acid (f). In some cases, a combination of both hydrophobic segments of the polypeptide and covalently attached lipids are responsible for membrane attachment of the protein (d,g). Still other proteins contain hydrophobic domains on their surface that favor a direct protein–membrane association (h,g). Finally, many proteins are attached to the membrane only by noncovalent interactions with the polar head groups of the membrane lipids (i) or with other membrane proteins (j).

plots have been used to create models that give rise to various spanning segments.

2. Extrinsic Proteins

The extrinsic proteins can be removed from the biomembrane structure by manipulating the ionic strength; for instance, with the erythrocyte membrane, exposure to a low salt concentration and a chelating agent removes an extrinsic protein, spectrin. Other extrinsic proteins include those located on the outer surface of plasma membranes and anchored to the surface by a phospholipase-sensitive lipid component. These anchor-type proteins are discussed in the following.

A large number of proteins have been discovered that are anchored to plasma membranes by a glycosylphosphatidylinositol (GPI) grouping. This appears to be an alternative-anchoring mechanism for those proteins that have a single-pass, hydrophobic transmembrane domain (11). It appears to be the preponderant form of anchoring cell surface proteins in protozoa. The lipid portions vary depending on their source.

There now are also several examples of covalent attachment of fatty acids to proteins; for example, the amino-terminus of the outer-membrane lipoprotein in gram-negative bacteria is modified mainly by palmitic acid. Those proteins that utilize fatty acid moieties appear to use them primarily as a localization mechanism.

III. METHODS FOR STUDYING MEMBRANE COMPONENTS

A. Lipids

A range of physical techniques have been used to study the lipids of biomembranes. These include calorimetry, nuclear magnetic resonance (NMR) and electron spin resonance (ESR) spectroscopy, infrared (IR) spectroscopy, as well as several techniques involving fluorescent probes.

1. Calorimetry

From calorimetric studies, Chapman and co-workers showed that the phospholipids of biomembranes can undergo an endothermic phase transition (12). They also suggested that the fluid character of the bilayer matrix of biomembranes is different from that of a simple paraffinic melt. This contrasted with the view, based on x-ray diffraction studies, that the interior chains were in a random chaotic state. The ΔH values associated with the gel to liquid-crystal transition are lower, in fact, than the ΔH values from melting of pure hydrocarbons. The same holds true for the entropy change in the process. The incremental ΔS per CH_2 group is only about 1 entropy unit (e.u.) for the gel to liquid-crystal transition of bilayers, but is almost twice as large for the melting of simple paraffins. These thermodynamic results show that the hydrocarbon chains in the bilayer core are not as disordered as they are in a pure liquid hydrocarbon.

The introduction of double bonds into the lipid hydrocarbon chain decreases the melting point, the enthalpy, and the entropy of the main chain transition (i.e., hexagonally packed chains to liquidlike chains). For example, the introduction of a single double bond at the 9–10 position of octadecanoic acid decreases the chain melting point by 39°C for a single-chain substitution (e.g., distearoyl lecithin, 54°C; stearoyl-oleoyl lecithin, 15°C), and substitutions in both chains lower it even farther (dioleoyl lecithin,

$-20°C$); *trans* double bonds have less of an effect. The addition of a single, double bond in one of the fatty acids lowers the melting temperature, and the addition of two double bonds in a single chain decreases the chain melting point by about the same (70°C) extent as does the addition of a single, double bond in both chains. The addition of a third or fourth double bond has little or no further effect (13). The position of the double bond also appears to be a critical factor in determining the transition temperature and enthalpy of the lipid main endothermic phase transition.

2. *Nuclear Magnetic Resonance*

Although the early studies with proton NMR were valuable in establishing the mobility of the lipid molecules, another useful innovation was the introduction of nonperturbing deuterium probes for deuterium magnetic resonance studies, by Oldfield et al. (14). This has been particularly valuable for studying the details of lipid dynamics within model and natural biomembranes. Deuterium probes have been particularly exploited by Seelig and co-workers (15) to examine the order parameter. They found that *gauche* conformations can occur only in complementary pairs, leaving the hydrocarbon chains essentially parallel to each other. The deuterium probe results differ from those obtained using spin-labeled molecules; for example, the spin labels detect a continuous decrease of the order parameter, whereas the deuterium probe shows that the order parameter remains approximately constant for the first nine segments.

The deuterium magnetic resonance technique has also been applied to the study of lipid dynamics of natural biomembranes. This was first carried out by Stockton et al. (16) with *A. laidlawii* cells. Similar studies have also been performed with *Escherichia coli* membranes. The characteristic order parameter signature of model membranes is carried over into biological membranes. The agreement between the order profile of *A. laidlawii* and those of the pure phospholipid membranes is striking.

3. *Infrared Spectroscopy*

Infrared spectroscopic studies of the main endothermic phase transition of the phospholipid–water systems results in an abrupt change in the band parameters of both methylene bands (17,18). The frequency of the band maximum has been used to monitor changes in the lipid conformation. As has been observed by the use of other different physical techniques, such as calorimetry, slight impurities in the samples make the main transition less sharp. Studies of the symmetrical stretching vibrations at about 2850 cm^{-1} give practically the same results. The minor overall change of the band maximum frequencies for the symmetrical vibration (only 3–4 cm^{-1}) during the lipid chain melting transition make it less suitable for these types of studies because of the greater relative influence of the experimental error in the band position ($\sim$0.5 cm^{-1}).

The results obtained with the pure lipid–water systems are in accord with those of various workers, using a variety of physical techniques, including calorimetry and NMR spectroscopy. The way in which the abrupt endothermic lipid-phase transition is indicated by the shift of the asymmetrical methylene band at the appropriate T_c temperature (the main endothermic lipid phase transition temperature) is reassuring for the application of this technique.

Cameron et al. (18) have also used infrared spectroscopy to study the pretransition observed in calorimetric studies of saturated lecithins. They used Fourier transform infrared (FTIR) spectroscopy to study the infrared-active acyl chain vibrational modes of fully hydrated multibilayers of 1,2-dipalmitoyl-*sn*-glycero-3-phosphocholine (L-DPPC) over the temperature range 0–55°C. Frequencies, bandwidths, and other spectral parameters were measured as a function of temperature for the methylene-scissoring, -rocking, and -wagging modes, as well as for the C–H-stretching modes, and were used to monitor the packing of the acyl chains. Particular emphasis was placed on determining the nature of the pretransition event. They showed that between 36° and 38°C the spectral changes are indicative of a phase change in the acyl chain packing from an orthorhombic to a hexagonal subcell. It was concluded that, in the gel phase, at all temperatures below the main transition, the acyl chains are preponderantly in an all-*trans* conformation and that the temperature-dependent variations of spectral parameters result from changes in interchain interactions.

B. Membrane Protein Structures

Crystallographic techniques that reveal the greatest structural detail for soluble proteins are now being applied to studies of membrane protein structure. A major problem in the application of these techniques to membranes is that integral proteins are in contact with both polar and nonpolar environments. This bipolar environment must be reproduced in the crystal to maintain conformation and, thereby, complicates crystallization (see Ref. 19 for a discussion of crystallization of membrane proteins). As yet, only matrix porin (20) and photosynthetic reaction centers from a purple bacterium have been crystallized in forms suitable for high-resolution analyses.

Matrix porin, a major component of the outer membrane of *E. coli*, in which ordered, two-dimensional arrays are formed, was crystallized from detergent solutions (21). Large quantities of detergent remained associated with the crystalline protein; however, the structural resolution was to within 0.29 nm and reproduced the hexagonal arrangement found for the protein in phospholipid bilayers. Much more complex crystals were obtained for the reaction centers of *Rhodopseudomonas viridis* (22). The isolated and crystallized complexes contain four different protein subunits. The complexity of this reaction center, two copies of which are present in each asymmetrical unit of the tetragonal unit cell, posed a formidable crystallographic challenge. Three-dimensional crystals of bacteriorhodopsin have also been obtained (23,24), although their small size and the presence of structural defects preclude high-resolution x-ray crystallographic studies. The results of crystallographic attempts suggest that only those proteins that are known to form two-dimensional crystal-like arrays within membranes have a sufficient propensity toward self-ordering to form three-dimensional crystals.

For those proteins that do not form ordered arrays, x-ray diffraction has been used to obtain a profile of electron density in the direction perpendicular to the membrane plane. Such profiles are generally prepared from wet pellets. In the absence of three-dimensional crystals, a great deal of effort has been focused on the study of preformed two-dimensional arrays of membrane proteins. Some of these arrays occur naturally in differentiated membrane regions (e.g., bacteriorhodopsin in purple membrane), whereas others have been induced in model systems [e.g., vesicles isolated from sarcoplasmic reticulum (25) and an acetylcholine receptor (26)]. The diffraction of x rays, which are scattered by electrons, is not possible with such a thin crystal. Under these circumstances, diffraction patterns are best obtained from neutrons and electrons, for which the scattering centers are the atomic nuclei. The three-dimensional image reconstruction of the purple membrane, obtained by Fourier analysis of electron micrographs prepared from unstained samples, has contributed greatly to our knowledge of the static structure of a membrane protein (27,28).

The amount of structural detail revealed by this method is dependent on structural preservation of the sample while in the electron beam. The use of electron-opaque stains must be avoided to access the nonsurface structure of the protein. Extremely low electron doses limit the damage induced by the electron beam. The damage associated with dehydration of membranes in vacuo is prevented by immersion of the sample in a glucose solution before dehydration. This is essential, as x-ray diffraction patterns showed that drying causes shrinking as well as disordering of the purple membrane lattice (29).

The electron-density contour maps for bacteriorhodopsin show seven rods of density 3.5–4.0 nm long (i.e., sufficient to extend completely through the membrane), which may be recognized as the α-helical segments identified by x-ray diffraction (30). Three of the rods are perpendicular to the plane of the lipid bilayer, whereas the other four are tilted slightly. Their relative tilts are consistent with a structural stabilization by helix–helix interactions: this notion finds support in the capacity to regenerate the native structure from proteolytic fragments of bacteriorhodopsin (31). Attempts have been made to fit the amino acid sequence (32,33) to the three-dimensional structure, and a better-resolved projection map has been obtained. Despite these advances, the available data do not permit an unequivocal description of the structure of this protein, or of its mechanism of proton translocation.

The necessity of a well-ordered, two-dimensional lattice has limited the number of structures studied by these techniques. Three-dimensional reconstructions have also been prepared for negatively stained gap junctions (34), crystalline lattices of cytochrome oxidase (35), the acetylcholine receptor (36), and reconstituted vesicles of matrix porin (37). Micrographs of negatively stained specimens yield information about the stain-excluding portions of the structures. Crystallographic analyses of protein structures reflect static structures; positional assignments of individual amino acid side chains must await improvements in the isolation of three-dimensional crystals. When interpreted in the light of crystallographic results, dynamic spectroscopic studies may soon provide detailed views of the structural fluctuations that are associated with the function of membrane proteins.

A recent structural model for the Ca^{2+}-ATPase of sarcoplasmic reticulum, prepared from the amino acid sequence determined from a DNA clone (38,39), is considered to contain transmembrane α-helices, together with domains of parallel and antiparallel β-sheet on the outside of the membrane. According to a proposed structure of the Ca^{2+}-ATPase (Fig. 2), there are ten helical segments embedded in the lipid matrix. There is also a considerable portion of the protein outside the lipid and connected by a polypeptide stalk. Nucleotide phosphorylation and transactivation domains are also indicated.

Recent studies of the acetylcholine receptor have modified the model of its structure, particularly the membrane-spanning region. Previously, each subunit was considered to consist of a bundle of four transmembrane helices. Now, it is believed that only one transmembrane helix per subunit is present. The central pore is still lined by five helices, but these are surrounded by a continuous rim of density, presumed to consist of a β-barrel structure. A model showing a section through the nicotinic acetylcholine receptor channel is shown in Figure 3 (40; see also review, Ref. 41). Sansom comments on the uncritical use of hydropathy plots for generating models of transmembrane topology (41). The folding diversity of

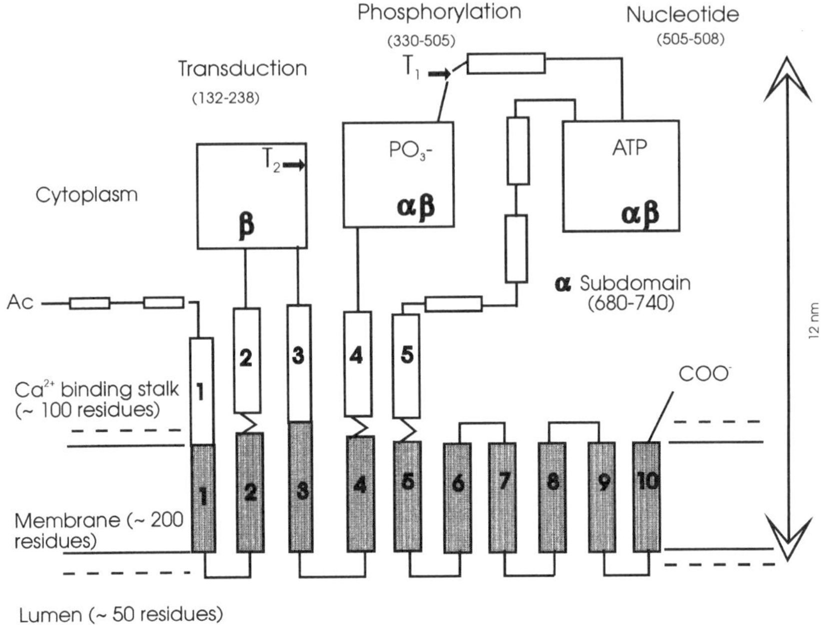

Figure 2 Assembly of Ca^{2+}-ATPase domains. The predicted arrays are laid out in a planar diagram. (From Ref. 38.)

integral membrane proteins has also been recently discussed (42), and the need to be cautious in the use of hydropathy plots for predicting membrane protein structure was again pointed out (42).

1. NMR and IR Spectroscopy

The application of NMR spectroscopy for the study of membrane proteins has met several technical difficulties. The protein is an anisotropic environment within the lipid bilayer and often has a high relative molecular mass. Some of these difficulties can be overcome by a combination of methods. Thus, high-resolution NMR techniques can be applied to the membrane proteins in solution in micelles, and solid-state NMR spectroscopy applied to the proteins in lipid bilayers. An example of this is recent studies of the membrane-bound bacteriophage Pf1 coat protein. In this example, extensive use was made of isotopically labeled proteins (43). The secondary structure of the protein was deduced from distance measurements in the micelles, and the arrangement of these secondary struc-

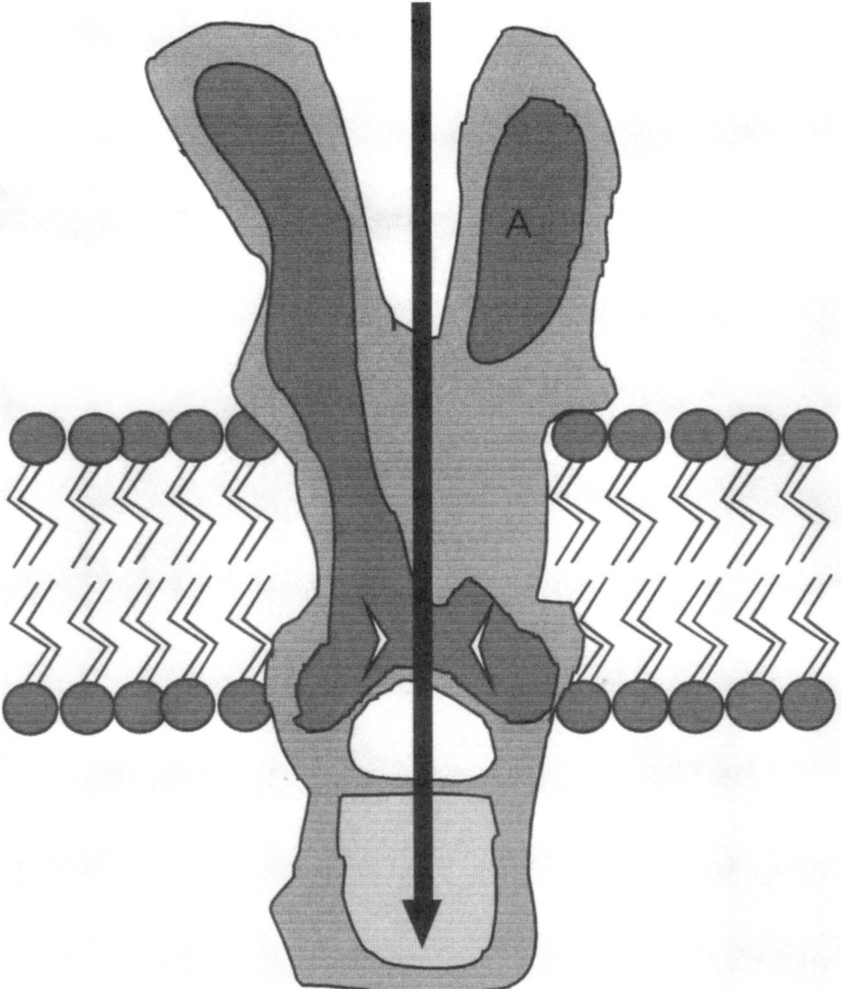

Figure 3   Section through the nAChR showing the receptor channel, the 43-kDa protein, and the lipid bilayer. The dark and light colors represent density contours. The two shapes represent the positions of the M_2 helices. A indicates the acetylcholine-binding cavity. The arrow shows the path taken by permeant cations. (From Ref. 41.)

tures was deduced from angular measurements with oriented layers. The dynamics of the protein was determined from motional narrowing of line shapes in solid-state experiments.

The distance information on proteins in solution was obtained from ^{1}H–^{1}H homonuclear nuclear Overhauser effect (NOE) measurements and used to determine secondary and tertiary structure. With the bacteriophage protein, labeling took place with ^{2}H (80%) on all carbon sites, ^{15}N (98%) on all nitrogen sites, and ^{2}H (50%) on all exchangeable sites; ^{1}H–^{15}N heteronuclear correlation was then combined with ^{1}H–^{1}H NOE spectroscopy.

Another spectroscopic technique that has been applied to the study of biomembrane systems is FTIR. This technique has become quite popular, since technical developments have made it possible to obtain good infrared spectra of biomolecules in H_2O. Previously, the strong absorption of water had made it difficult to obtain information about the protein structure owing to overlap of the water absorption with that of the protein. Experiments have been carried out with both model membranes consisting of lipid–water systems, and reconstituted systems containing polypeptides or proteins, as well as with natural biomembranes. The phase transition of the lipid–water systems are readily studied using this technique, and the effects of cholesterol or polypeptides on the phase transition have been examined (18). The results are in agreement with those obtained with techniques such as calorimetry or NMR spectroscopy. Studies of the secondary structure of various proteins have also been reported (44).

The major band in the FTIR spectra of proteins is the amide I band. This absorption arises preponderantly from the C=O stretch of the peptide bonds and, as such, is sensitive to the hydrogen-bonding state of the protein. The different secondary structures present in a protein are each associated with a characteristic hydrogen-bonding pattern; thus, each is associated with a characteristic amide I frequency. The presence of a range of secondary structures in membrane proteins results in the production of multiple amide absorptions. The half-width of each absorption is such that they cannot be resolved instrumentally, and a composite band results. Recently developed mathematical resolution enhancement techniques, such as second-derivative and deconvolution analysis, have been used to detect the presence of individual components beneath the broad amide I contour of several proteins. These enhancement techniques, coupled with hydrogen–deuterium exchange studies, have been used to detect small changes in protein structure (45,46).

The FTIR spectra of a large number of membrane proteins obtained in both H_2O and ^2H_2O reveal that the proteins are preponderantly α-helical in structure. Furthermore, the amide I maxima for the α-helical structure in membrane protein spectra differ from the corresponding maxima in the spectra of soluble proteins (44).

Bacteriorhodopsin and rhodopsin are two light-transducing transmembrane proteins. Bacteriorhodopsin is found in the purple membrane of *Halobacterium halobium*. The protein contains a chromophore, all-*trans*-retinal, which isomerizes to 13-*cis*-retinal after absorption of a photon. The pioneering work of Henderson and Unwin, using electron diffraction and electron microscopy (27), has contributed greatly to our knowledge of the structure of bacteriorhodopsin. It has been suggested that rhodopsin, the primary intrinsic protein of vertebrate photoreceptor disk membranes, has a structure in the membrane similar to that shown for bacteriorhodopsin. The supposed structural similarities are striking. For example, the two proteins occupy roughly the same cross-sectional area in the membrane, and the retinal attachment lysine is located in approximately the same vertical position on the COOH-terminal transmembrane helix. The FTIR spectroscopic studies reveal differences in the amide I maxima of these two proteins. The high-frequency (1662 cm^{-1}) amide I band of bacteriorhodopsin is unusual. Some workers suggest that it is due to the presence of α_{II}-helices. On the other hand, the band maximum for rhodopsin is observed at 1657 cm^{-1}, at a frequency similar to the ATPases (Na$^+$/K$^+$, H$^+$/K$^+$, Ca^{2+}), glucose transporter, cytochrome c oxidase, bacterial and higher plant reaction centers (47).

The comparison between the infrared spectra of porin and bacteriorhodopsin in H$_2$O (Fig. 4) reveals marked differences, corresponding to the different folding of these membrane proteins. Porin has a β-barrel structure, whereas bacteriorhodopsin is preponderantly α-helical.

2. *Site-Directed Antibodies*

Another method used to provide information on the topology of membrane proteins is based on site-directed antibodies. This method arises from the fact that antibodies raised against short, synthetic peptides frequently recognize the same sequence in native proteins. Thus, antibodies can be produced against proteins of known sequence, even when they have not been isolated. These site-directed antibodies are commonly raised in the form of polyclonal sera. In proteins of known three-dimensional structure, the best sequences to give useful antibodies (i.e., which bind to the native proteins) appear to be those with the segmental mobility. Typically, peptides 15–20 residues in length are chosen for the production of site-directed antibodies. It is usually necessary to couple the peptide to a carrier protein, such as keyhole limpet hemocyanin, to obtain a good immune response (e.g., with rabbits).

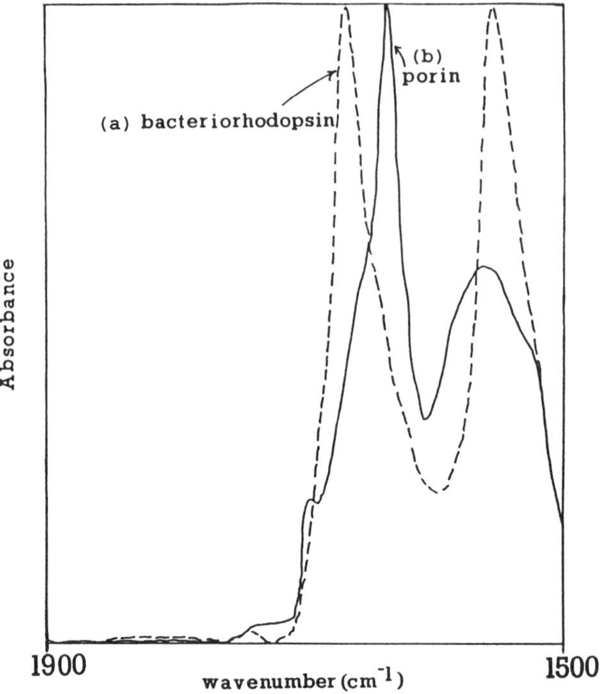

Figure 4   An FTIR spectra showing the amide I region of two membrane proteins: (a) bacteriorhodopsin and (b) porin. (From Ref. 45.)

This technique has been applied by Davies et al. for probing the topology of the human erythrocyte glucose transport protein (48). Antibodies raised against peptides from a large central extramembranous loop recognize the native protein. By examining the ability of antibodies to bind the right-side-out and inside-out membrane vesicles, these workers were able to show which sequence is located on the cytoplasmic side of the membrane. Recent studies using antibodies have suggested that facilitative glucose transporters may fold as β-barrel structures, rather than the previously suggested 12-helix model (49).

Chemical cross-linking processes have also been useful for studying the associations between subunits of oligomeric membrane proteins and cytoskeletal proteins (see Ref. 50).

3. *Molecular Biology Techniques*

There is considerable interest in the structure of voltage-gated ion channels (51). These ion channels are the plasma proteins responsible for the

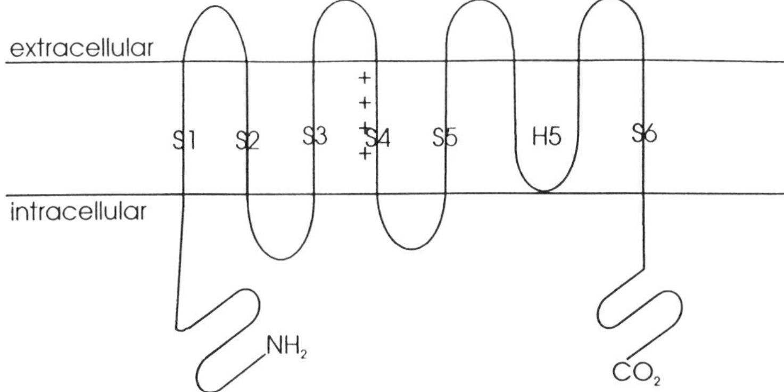

Figure 5 Transmembrane-folding model for a voltage-activated K^+ channel subunit. Hydropathy profiles show six hydrophobic stretches (S1 through S6). H5 reaches across the membrane and lines the ion conduction pore. The plus symbols in S4 indicate the presence of basic residues at every third position in an otherwise hydrophobic region (51).

propagation of electrical signals in excitable cells, such as nerve and muscle. There are three types of voltage-gated channels: namely, K^+, Na^+, and Ca^{2+}. A typical K^+ channel is considered to be built as a tetramer of a 600-residue subunit. The Na^+ and Ca^{2+} channels are formed from a single polypeptide of about 2000 residues, containing four homologous domains.

The use of molecular biology techniques, including site-directed mutagenesis and probe molecules that bind specifically to the proteins of K^+ channels, has led to a model shown in Figure 5. Three types of ligand were known to interact specifically with the pore of K^+ channels: scorpion venom peptides, tetraethylammonium (TEA), and the ions themselves. A localized region linking the fifth and sixth membrane-spanning helical stretches of amino acids (S_5 and S_6) is thought to form the K^+-channel pore (51).

IV. MODELS FOR CELLULAR MEMBRANES

A. Membrane Models

A variety of model systems have been used to study cellular membrane properties. These include monolayer systems, lamellar systems, as well as black lipid film techniques. Here we briefly discuss some of these model systems.

1. Monolayer Systems

The use of monolayer systems as models for biomembranes is based on the idea that the monolayer is half of a lipid bilayer, the bilayer being the basic lipid matrix for biomembrane structures. The area per molecule can be defined, the pressure area curves can be obtained, and expanded and condensed films can also be obtained. Phillips and Chapman pointed out that a correlation exists between the lipid monolayer properties at the air–water interface of lipids and the properties of the lipid bilayers in aqueous dispersions (52). The "condensed monolayer" corresponds to the "fluid" or melted state that occurs above the lipid transition temperature. Thermotropic phase changes occur with the monolayers similar to those that occur with lipid bilayers (53).

All monolayer states are possible with the saturated lecithin and PE homologues. It is apparent that, if the hydrocarbon chains are sufficiently long, condensed monolayers are formed, whereas with shorter chains, liquid-expanded films occur. These two limiting states are sufficiently well defined such that at any particular temperature only one of the homologues studied exhibits the transition state. The data indicated that variations in hydrocarbon chain length that do not give rise to change in monolayer state do not have a significant effect on the pressure–area (Π-A) curves. Temperature changes can also give rise to the condensed state, whereas at higher temperatures it is fully expanded. Monolayers in the two limiting states are more or less invariant with temperature, and it is the sensitivity of the phase transition to temperature that leads to the variety of isotherms. The molecules in a completely condensed PE monolayer are much more closely packed than are those in the equivalent lecithin monolayer.

2. Lamellar Systems

Biomembrane structures are built on a lipid bilayer matrix into which the proteins are inserted. The properties of the lamellar phase of the lipid–water systems, therefore, are of direct relevance (Fig. 6). These include movement of the lipids within the fluid bilayer and the possibility of triggering phase changes by temperature or dehydration during which the lipid chains may crystallize or, in some cases, cause the production of hexagonal or cubic phases. Biological membranes pose additional complexities; they contain complex mixtures of lipids and, in addition, the lipid composition is normally asymmetrical across the bilayer structure.

From an examination of the various lipid–water phase diagrams, the degree of biomembrane fluidity is a direct reflection of the transition temperature of the lipids; that is, the fluidity is greatest when highly unsaturated lipids are present and less when more-saturated lipids are present. Occasionally, the transition temperature of the lipids will be below or at

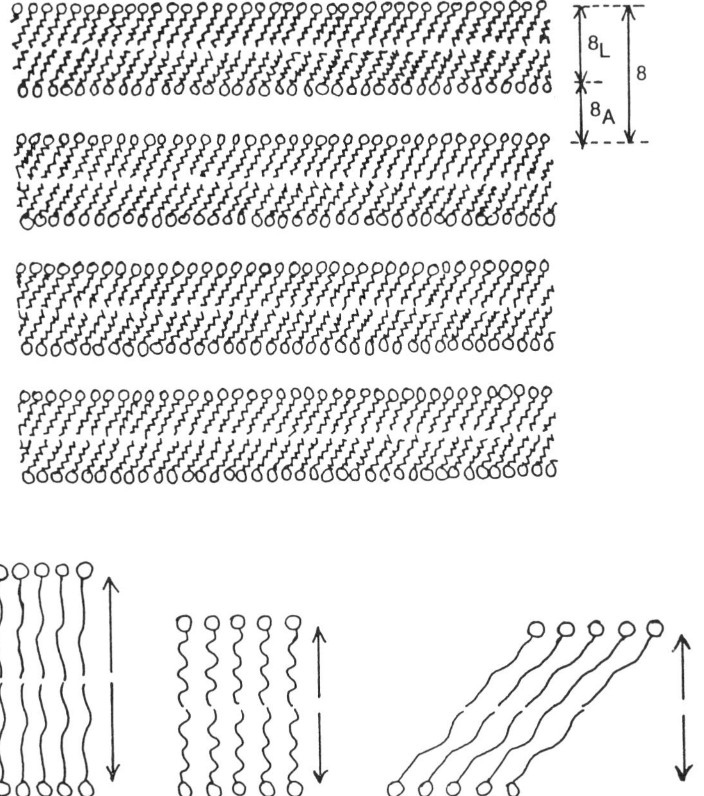

Figure 6 Lipid bilayers that can spontaneously form in water with lecithin molecules. The chain organizations showing tilted, vertical, and "melted" arrangements are indicated.

growth temperature, whereas on other occasions, it may be above it. The appropriate phase transition characteristic of the lipids present, therefore, determines the appropriate fluidity of the particular cell membrane and also the correct lipid-phase separation characteristic. These in turn can affect membrane elasticity; the insertion, aggregation, and diffusional movements of the protein and the lipid components; as well as the permeability characteristics.

In certain practical situations, it is important to freeze cells and tissues, as in the various requirements in the field of cryobiology, so that major changes of temperatures are involved. When cells or membranes are frozen to very low temperatures, lipid-phase characteristics and phase separation need to be considered. Whether the lipid crystallizes before the ice melting point, or at a lower temperature, could be important in determining freeze damage. The various phenomena of lipid-phase separation and protein aggregation are relevant to this situation (54).

Studies have been made of permeability characteristics for water and various other molecules above and below the lipid-phase transition temperature; for example, the kinetics of water permeability through lipid systems have been studied and related to lipid fluidity. Thus, there is a marked increase in water permeability as the lipid chains become more unsaturated. This is also true with nonelectrolytes such as glycerol and erythritol. The self-diffusion rate of $^{22}Na^+$ through lecithin bilayers also shows a marked increase when the lipid is in the fluid state; the effect of cholesterol is to decrease water permeability. Black lipid membranes also show the same effect. These results are consistent with a reduction in the fluidity characteristics of the lipid. On the other hand, the presence of cholesterol is to enhance the rate of water permeability of liposomes derived from saturated liposomes.

Triggering mechanisms may occur as a result of interactions with the biomembrane by metal ions, proteins, or drugs, so that local changes of fluidity, phase separation and, hence, changes of permeability characteristics, can take place.

The first studies on phase separation of lipid–water systems were discussed by Ladbrooke and Chapman, who reported studies of binary mixtures of lecithins using calorimetry (55). These authors examined mixtures of distearoyl lecithin and dipalmitoyl lecithin (DSL–DPL) and also distearoyl lecithin and dimyristoyl lecithin (DSL–DML).

Some of these membrane model systems, such as those formed by lipids in a closed lamellar phase, have useful properties in the form of lipid capsules called liposomes (see next section). These have been used to study osmotic properties, effects of anesthetics, and are used as drug-delivery vehicles (see Chap. 20).

3. *Liposomes*

The term *liposome* is used to describe vesicles in which there is an aqueous volume enclosed by one more concentric phospholipid bilayers. Liposomes form spontaneously when certain lipids (e.g., lecithins) are heated above a critical temperature in aqueous media; the vesicles can range in size from tens of nanometers to tens of microns in diameter. They can be made of natural constituents; the liposome membrane forms a bilayer structure that is similar to the lipid portion of a natural cell membrane. The introduction of charged lipids such as stearylamine or phosphatidic acid into the liposomes increases their stability and inhibits aggregation.

Liposomes can be formed by a variety of methods used to control the size and also the number of "membranes" or bilayers associated with the vesicles (56). Liposomes of different sizes often require different methods of preparation and are classified for practical convenience according to their size (57). Small unilamellar vesicles [<400 A (40 nm) in diameter] are prone to fusion, particularly at the lipid-phase transition temperature. The permeability of a liposomal membrane depends very much on the lipid composition, and also on the solute that is entrapped. Liposomes have been shown to be permeable to water, ions, and nonelectrolytes, although the permeability depends on the chemical composition of the liposome (56). Positively charged liposomes (e.g., lecithin plus a positively charged lipid such as stearylamine) are impermeable to cations, whereas negatively charged liposomes (e.g., containing phosphatidic acid) are permeable to cations. The permeability of liposomes to protons is low. Anions diffuse rapidly through negatively and positively charged lipid membranes. Increasing the saturation or length of the phospholipid fatty acyl chains causes a decrease in the permeability of the liposomes to all solutes. This is a reflection of the transition temperature (T_c) of the lipids. General anesthetics, such as ether and chloroform, cause an increase in cation permeability, but no increase in glucose permeability.

Liposomes have been prepared with archaeobacterial lipids. Freeze-fracture studies show that the liposomes fracture crosswise, rather than through the midplane of the lipid bilayer, consistent with the formation of single lipid membranes, rather than of the normal bilayer type.

Various methods have been employed to increase the stability of liposomes: (1) by introducing large amounts of cholesterol (molar/molar) into the liposomes; (2) by covalently cross-linking membrane components; (3) by using methods, such as glutaraldehyde fixation; (4) osmification or polymerization of alkyne-containing phospholipids (e.g., using diacetylene lipids followed by irradiation with UV light or γ-irradiation). One method that does not restrict the relative mobility of adjacent phospholipids is to incorporate long aliphatic branched-chain polymers, such as polyvinyl alcohols esterified with palmitic or stearic acid. These compounds, when incorporated up to about 10% by weight into phosphatidylcholine membranes, can be substitutes for cholesterol in reducing the leakage of medium-sized solutes. The incorporation of sphingomyelin into the liposomes can also increase their stability.

The stability of liposomes and, hence, their ability to retain entrapped solvents, may also be affected by freezing and by drying. When liposomes undergo dehydration, they often crack and release their entrapped solutes. Various added materials have been used to overcome this problem. The materials are similar to those used in the cryoprotection of cells (e.g., pyrrolidone and various sugar molecules). One example of the latter is trehalose. This can produce a free-flowing, dry liposomal powder that retains the solute molecules, and the liposome can next be reconstituted by adding water to the dry powder.

4. Proteosomes

Various methods have now been developed, usually using detergent dialysis, to reconstitute membrane proteins into lipid vesicles, referred to sometimes as proteosomes. Some of the earliest studies were made by Racker, with cytochrome oxidase (58), but many other membrane proteins have been reconstituted, such as the Ca^{2+}-ATPase of the sarcoplasmic reticulum, bacteriorhodopsin, and the glucose transporter. The experiments with cytochrome oxidase were used to demonstrate respiratory control and to provide support for the Mitchell chemiosmotic hypothesis.

These reconstitution processes have been useful for the study of membrane protein transport processes (see, e.g., Chap. 5). There are a variety of methods for accomplishing this, including detergent and sonication techniques (59). Reconstituted systems are ideal for investigating the effects of bilayer fluidity and lipid composition on membrane proteins, in that the lipid environment can be controlled and the system can be investigated through the lipid chain-melting temperature (T_c). In the transport proteins, the glucose and anion transporters of the human erythrocyte membrane are two of the most extensively studied passive transport systems (i.e., transport occurs down a concentration gradient by facilitated diffusion and requires no metabolic energy). The structures of these transporters have been actively studied; both are single chains, with the glucose transporter $(M_r = 55,000)$, believed to have 12 α-helical membrane-spanning domains, and the anion transporter $(M_r = 90,000)$, 14 α-helical membrane-spanning domains.

The effects of lipid environment on the glucose transporter have been studied in some detail (60,61), reconstituted in large unilamellar vesicles prepared by reverse-phase evaporation from a range of different phospholipids. The activation energies for passive sugar transport into vesicles of phospholipids that have the same acyl chains, but different head groups, differ depending on the head group.

Maneri and Low (62) investigated the anion transporter, reconstituted in a range of phospholipid vesicles, by differential-scanning calorimetry. The experiments gave information on the structural stability of the integral domain of the transporter in terms of the temperature of maximum heat capacity (i.e., the denaturation temperature, T_d) and the enthalpy of denaturation. To focus attention on the 55-kDa membrane-spanning domain of the transporter, the 43-kDa cytoplasmic domain was removed by proteolysis. For a given phospholipid head group, the value of T_d increases markedly with acyl chain length for monosaturated symmetrical phosphotidylcholines. The change in T_d from the protein reconstituted in dimyristoleylphosphatidylcholine vesicles ($C_{14:1}$) to the dinervonylphosphatidylcholine vesicles ($C_{24:1}$) is substantial (47°–66°C), demonstrating that the stability of the transmembrane domain of the transporter is dependent on the nature of the surrounding lipid.

5. *Other Lipid Phases*

Unsaturated fatty acids are known to be fusogenic agents, and so it was of great interest when it was found that their incorporation in phospholipid bilayers, or in natural (erythrocyte) membranes, tends to induce the formation of a hexagonal (H_{II}) phase formation (Fig. 7).

Many natural membranes are rich in lipids that have strong tendencies to form H_{II} phases, and considerable effort has been spent on trying to detect such structures in biological systems. Mitochondrial inner membranes are particularly rich in cardiolipin, which forms the H_{II} phase in the presence of low levels of divalent ions.

A particular example of the relevance of these mesomorphic phases is shown by studies of *A. laidlawii*. This is a simple, cell wall-less prokaryotic microorganism that possesses several features that make it an attractive system for studying the roles of lipids in biological membrane systems. One such feature is the ability to dramatically alter its membrane lipid fatty

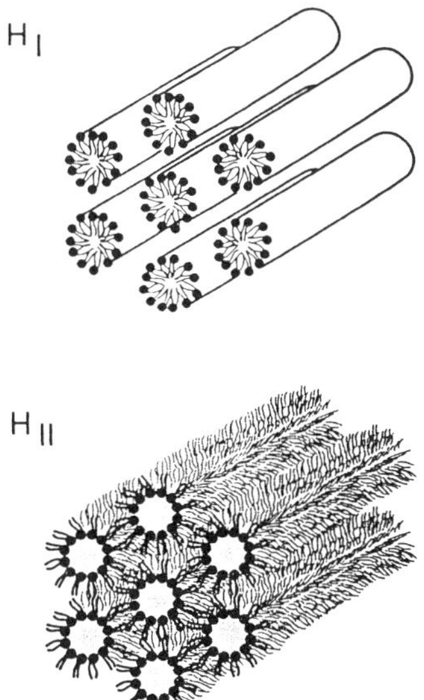

Figure 7   Hexagonal arrangements that form in water with some lipid molecules.

acid composition and cholesterol content by appropriate manipulation of the lipid composition of the growth medium. By exploiting this ability, Wieslander et al. (63) have shown that alterations in membrane lipid fatty acid composition and cholesterol content, as well as in growth temperature, induces marked changes in the quantative distribution of the major polar lipids on the limiting membranes of *A. laidlawii* strain A. These workers have postulated that, in all biological membranes, a certain balance of bilayer-preferring lipids must be maintained to ensure an optimal degree of lipid stability and functionality. For *A. laidlawii*, this requires maintaining an optimal balance between the amount of monoglycosyldiacylglycerol (MGDG) and the other membrane lipids present, in the face of alterations in growth temperature, or in the fatty acid composition or cholesterol content of the growth medium.

There are numerous reports on model systems of membrane lipids that exhibit periodic structures with electron microscopic textures, such as the cubic phases (e.g., "intramembrane particles" or "lipidic particles"). Extensive studies have shown that the lipid systems reported to give lipidic particles also form cubic phases.

Luzzati et al. have reported most interesting phase properties of lipids from the thermoresistant organism *Sulfolobus solfataricus*. These ether lipids form cubic phases under physiological conditions, and a membrane model with protein "plugs" has been proposed (3).

6. Black Lipid Films

The very useful black lipid film model system was developed by Muller and Rudin (64), to understand the electrical properties of the lipid bilayer and for the early studies of molecules such as valinomycin, gramicidin, and alamethicin. These were used to study ion transport, such as carrier and channel mechanisms, and ion discrimination between sodium and potassium ions (see, e.g., Chap. 4). The technique consists of painting a mixture of phospholipids and hydrocarbon across a small hole in a plastic sheet. The film thins down to form a single lipid bilayer, analogous to a soap film. Electrodes can be placed on each side of the film to measure resistance, capacitance, and such.

V. MEMBRANE DYNAMICS

A. Lipids

1. Lateral Diffusion

The present view of biomembrane structure is a dynamic one, in which the lipid components and protein components of many membranes are able to undergo considerable molecular motion. This includes the wagging and twisting of the CH_2 groups of the melted lipid chains above the T_c transition temperature, and also, the lateral and rotational diffusion of the lipids and the proteins within the plane of the lipid matrix.

Various measurements have been made of lipid diffusion coefficients with spin-labeled analogues within phospholipid bilayers. Träuble and Sackmann incorporated a spin-labeled steroid into dipalmitoylphosphatidylcholine–water systems and obtained a diffusion coefficient of 1×10^{-8} cm^2/s for $T > T_c$ (65). The diffusion coefficient of a spin-labeled phospholipid analogue in a sonicated egg lecithin–water system was measured and gave a value of $15 (\pm 2) \times 10^{-8}$ cm^2/s at 40°C. Devaux and McConnell (66) determined a lateral diffusion coefficient of $1.8(\pm 0.6) \times 10^{-8}$ $cm^2/$s. Other techniques have also been used, including NMR methods. Measurements of proton NMR spin-lattice relaxation times made possible the direct determination of phospholipid lateral diffusion coefficients. A diffusion coefficient of 3.8×10^{-9} cm^2/s was determined with a dipalmitoyl lecithin aqueous system, whereas studies based on ^{31}P spectral line widths gave values of 1.8×10^{-8} cm^2/s at 30°C.

Cholesterol diffusion has been measured by using a fluorescent cholesterol derivative in a dimyristoyl lecithin liposome (67). This gave diffusion coefficients, at 26°C, in the range 10^{-8} cm^2/s for this cholesterol compound—a small reduction in diffusion occurs as the molar ratio of cholesterol in the liposome is increased.

Other workers have used lipid probes and a fluorescent photobleaching technique for determining diffusion coefficients in lipid bilayer systems, whereas other workers have used triplet probes. Below the T_c temperature, when the lipid is in the gel phase, a marked reduction in lipid lateral diffusion occurs.

2. *Lipid Flip-Flop*

Yet another motion has been proposed; that lipid molecules can move from one side of the lipid bilayer to the other. This is sometimes termed flip-flop. Here, the polar moiety is considered to pass through the hydrophobic region of the bilayer. This process, in which the lipid on one side of the lipid bilayer flips to the other side, involves the polar group of the lipid moving through the hydrophobic region and, therefore, is expected to be relatively slow.

The first measurements of flip-flop were made in 1972 by Kornberg and McConnell, with a spin-labeled lecithin (68). The half-time of the process was 6.5 h at 30°C. Other experiments indicate that this lipid interchange occurs at a much slower rate; for example, some workers used a specific exchange protein that binds phosphatidylcholine and catalyzes the rapid exchange between the bound lipid and phosphatidylcholine in lipid bilayer membranes. With this approach, about two-thirds of the lipid in the phosphatidylcholine vesicles was accessible for immediate exchange. The appearance of additional exchangeable lipid (from the inside half of the bilayer), however, was not observed to take place at a measurable rate. This led to the conclusion that the half-time for lipid exchange must be greater than 11 days at 37°C. Other workers suggest that the half-life time at 23°C for exchange is as long as 16–69 days.

B. Membrane Proteins

Membrane proteins contain portions that occur in the lipid matrix, and other portions that appear in the aqueous environment. This means that a range of motions are possible. These include lateral diffusion, rotational diffusion, and also segmental motions of the amino acid groups.

1. *Lateral Diffusion*

Lateral diffusion of membrane proteins has been studied using fluorescence photobleaching. With this technique, it is necessary to be able to bleach a chromophore irreversibly with an intense light pulse. Measurements are made with a single cell, using a microscope; the chromophore is usually fluorescein or rhodamine.

In this type of measurement, a small spot some (μm^2) on a single cell is irradiated by an intense laser pulse, and the chromophores present in the spot are irreversibly bleached. The redistribution of the unbleached chromophores is then followed with the same laser beam, attenuated some 10^4-fold. Depending on how the chromophores are characterized, the experimental procedure is called fluorescence or absorption microphotolysis. These are sometimes referred to as fluorescence recovery (or redistribution) after photobleaching (FRAP) and fluorescence photobleaching recovery (FPR). A variation on the method allows bleaching and redistribution to occur simultaneously. A small area of a cell under a microscope is irradiated, this time continuously, with an intermediate intensity. The time course of the fluorescence signal originating from the irradiated area from its surroundings depends on the rate at which chromophores are decomposed and unbleached chromophores enter the irradiated area. This procedure is sometimes called continuous fluorescence (or absorption) microphotolysis.

Rhodopsin was the first system for which quantitative lateral diffusion measurements were reported (Table 3). This is because rhodopsin contains a suitable bleachable intrinsic chromophore. With an absorption microphotolysis method Poo and Cone (69) measured the lateral diffusion coefficient for rhodopsin within the frog and mudpuppy retina at 20°C and

Table 3 Lateral Diffusion Coefficient of Membrane Protein

Protein	Cell type	D_L $(m^2\ s^{-1})$
Rhodopsin	Frog retinal rod outer segment	3.5×10^{-13}
Acetylcholine receptor	Rat myotubules	10^{-16}
Epidermal growth factor receptor	Fibroblast	3×10^{-14}
Coat protein (in liposomes)	M-13 virus	7×10^{-13}
Concanavalin A receptor	Rat myotubules	3×10^{-15}
Agglutinin receptor	Wheat germ	$4\text{-}8 \times 10^{-15}$
Immunoglobulin E	Various cells	$2\text{-}7 \times 10^{-14}$
Band 3 protein	Erythrocyte	4×10^{-15}
Bacteriorhodopsin (in liposomes)		10^{-12}
Bacteriorhodopsin (in purple membranes)		10^{-14}
ADP/ATP carrier	Mitochondria	2×10^{-13}
Cytochrome c	Mitochondria	10^{-12}

found it to be $3.5(\pm 1.5) \times 10^{-9}\ cm^2\ s^{-1}$ and $3.9(\pm 1.2) \times 10^{-9}\ cm^2\ s^{-1}$, respectively.

The first lateral diffusion measurement with proteins that lack an intrinsic chromophore was performed with the human erythrocyte membrane (70). After labeling the hemoglobin-free erythrocyte ghosts with fluorescein isothiocyanate, the protein lateral diffusion was studied by the fluorescence microphotolysis method. In contrast with the rhodopsin system, the lateral diffusion of integral proteins in these ghost erythrocyte membranes at 20°C was severely restricted ($D_I^L = < 3 \times 10^{-12}\ cm^2\ s^{-1}$). The spectrin skeleton appears to restrict the lateral movement of the integral proteins by direct linkage or by trapping of proteins within the skeleton network.

Biological membranes appear to be microheterogeneous structures. A great deal of data has been collected about transmembrane and lateral nonhomogeneity of protein and lipid distribution in both eukaryotic and prokaryotic membranes. This peculiarity of membrane organization has important functional consequences.

One of the issues is how to reconcile rapid lateral diffusion of proteins in membranes, deduced from the experiments with eukaryotic cells, with the presence in the same membrane of areas differing in protein composition (especially in prokaryotic cytoplasmic membranes with relatively small total surface areas). This problem was recently debated by Kell (71) who discussed some possible reasons for hindered lateral protein mobility. It has been suggested that rapid lateral protein diffusion can coexist with the segregation of the same proteins to defined localities in the membrane.

2. Rotational Diffusion

The first measurement of the rotational diffusion of a membrane protein was carried out with rhodopsin, using the internal retinal chromophore and the technique of laser flash photolysis (72). It gave a value for the rotational correlation time of 20 μs for rhodopsin and was followed by studies on bacteriorhodopsin using the retinal internal membrane chromophore (73). The technique used a polarized pulse of light, and the decay of the induced dichroisim was determined. By contrast with rhodopsin, bacteriorhodopsin is relatively immobile within the lipid matrix.

Following these studies, the extension of measurements to other membrane proteins was made possible by the introduction of triplet probes, using molecules such as eosin (Table 4). A triplet state is necessary because of the relatively slow rotational motion of the proteins within the lipid matrix (74).

Although the rotational diffusion of macromolecules in aqueous solution has been studied by fluorescence depolarization methods, with diffusion times in the nanosecond time scale, the viscous environment of the

Table 4 Correlation Times of Rotational Diffusion of Membrane Proteins

Protein	Source	T_c (μs)
Rhodopsin	Retinal rod outer segment	20
Cytochrome a_3	Mitochondrial inner membrane	500
Cytochrome b_5	Microsomal membrane	0.4
Band 3 protein	Erythrocyte	4000
Ca^{2+}-ATPase	Sarcoplasmic reticulum	70, 130, 200
Acetylcholine receptor	*Torpedo* electroplax	0.7
Glycophorin	Erythrocyte	1–2 (monomer) 10–20 (dimer)
Epidermal growth factor receptor	Human epidermoid carcinoma cell	350
Bacteriorhodopsin	*Halobacterium* purple membrane	20,000

lipid matrix causes membrane protein rotational correlation times to be in the microsecond time scale.

3. Flippase Proteins

P-glycoproteins pump drugs out of cells by an ATP-dependent process, thereby reducing their toxicity (see Chap. 17). Recently, it has been suggested that the unusual properties of P-glycoprotein can be explained by a "flippase" model. The idea is that a drug molecule, rather than interacting with the transporter directly from the aqueous phase, interacts instead with the lipid bilayer. The protein is then envisaged to flip the drug from the inner leaflet to the outer layer (74).

The P-glycoprotein substrates are primarily cationic, lipid-soluble, planar molecules that can intercalate among the phospholipid molecules. Other flippase proteins are thought to be involved in translocating specific lipids from one leaflet of a lipid bilayer to the other to maintain lipid asymmetry within the biomembrane. The proteins responsible for flippase activity have not as yet been fully characterized, but appear to require ATP hydrolysis (75).

4. Transmembrane Signaling

In recent years, considerable progress has been made in understanding how cells, particularly eukaryotic cells, sense and respond to external stimuli (i.e., how the signals are generated and transduced across the cell membrane). A fundamental principle of transmembrane signaling is that the stimulation tends to be highly specific, even though there is a diversity of signals. Receptors for hormones, drugs, growth factors, light, and smell all have been characterized. Many transmembrane-signaling systems consist of three membrane-bound protein components: (a) a cell surface receptor; (b) an effector, such as an ion channel or the enzyme adenylate cyclase; and (c) a guanine nucleotide-binding regulatory protein or G-protein, coupled to both. Receptors mediate the action of light, peptide hormones, and neurotransmitters. Nearly all G protein-coupled receptors have sequence similarity. Given this sequence similarity, it is thought that they have a similar topological motif; that is, they consist of seven hydrophobic (possible α-helical segments) that span the lipid bilayer. This seven-helix motif is based on the analogy with the structure of bacteriorhodopsin and the presence of seven hydrophobic sequences. Currently, great activity is also centered on the role of the phosphatidylinositol lipids when they operate as second-messenger systems. The inositol group is cleaved by a phospholipase C action. This group then releases calcium from calcium storage vesicles, and the remaining diglyceride acts on protein kinase C.

5. *Protein Translocation Across Membranes*

The cell synthesizes approximately 10^3–10^4 polypeptides. Some proteins are inserted into a membrane, whereas others need to pass through one or more membranes to reach their final destination. Therefore, an important question is, what are the signals that indicate to which position in the cell these proteins should go? Certain membranes can translocate different proteins. These are termed translocation-competent membranes. Examples are the endoplasmic reticulum (ER), the peroxisomal membrane, the bacterial plasma membrane, the inner membrane of mitochondria, and the inner and thylakoid membranes of chloroplasts. The mitochondrial membrane can transport proteins in both directions, whereas the other membranes can transport in only one direction. Membranes derived from the endoplasmic reticulum, such as the Golgi complex, secretory vesicles, endosomes, lysosomes, and the smooth ER membranes, are thought to be translocation-competent.

The way in which proteins are directed to a target membrane is usually by means of a short stretch of amino acids at or near the NH_2-terminus of the protein, with the exception of many peroxisomal-targeting signals that are at the COOH-terminus. Most of these NH_2-terminal targeting signals, called leader or signal sequences, are proteolytically removed by a signal peptidase on the *trans* side of the membrane. Apparently, if the removal of the targeting side is blocked, translocation can still take place. Some translocated proteins carry targeting signals that are not proteolytically removed under normal conditions. Hydrophobic signals are used by proteins to cross the ER and bacterial membrane. These have a relatively hydrophobic NH_2-terminus, with one or two basic residues, an apolar hydrophobic core of seven or eight residues, and a relatively hydrophilic COOH-terminus, ending with an amino acid, carrying a small side chain. The hydrophobic signals are cleaved by proteases that are integral proteins (76,77).

For targeting proteins into mitochondria and chloroplasts, hydrophilic sequences occur. These are rich in basic and hydroxylated residues and contain few if any acidic residues. They are reported to have no extended polar regions. The hydrophilic signals are removed by soluble proteases that require a metal (Zn^{2+}, Mn^{2+}, or Co^{2+}) as cofactor.

6. *Signal Peptides*

For the export of a protein, whether from yeast, higher eukaryotes, or bacteria, a general requirement is a signal sequence. Part of the recognition information in a nascent chain is in a contiguous sequence for export from the cell, or a mitochondrial presequence for import into the mitochondria.

These sequences can even be transplanted from one protein to another and still retain the same localization information (78).

These targeting sequences lack primary homology, but have several properties in common. They possess

1. An NH_2-terminal region, with a net positive charge.
2. A hydrophobic core of about ten residues.
3. Six to eight residues preceding the cleavage site, which often include proline or amino acids that favor turns.
4. A cleavage site, immediately following the AXA (where X is any amino acid) motif in prokaryotes. In eukaryotes an amino acid with a small side chain replaces alanine in this motif.

A schematic diagram of a typical signal sequence (78) is shown in Figure 8.

The strong tendency for signal peptides to interact favorably with membranes, which argues for a direct membrane interaction in vivo, arises from the positive charge adjacent to a hydrophobic segment. These properties favor insertion into the endoplasmic reticulum or cytoplasmic membrane, subsequent to release of the nascent chain from the signal-recognition particle (SRP) or SecA. This insertion would facilitate subsequent interactions with membrane proteins by restricting the nascent chain to two-dimensional diffusion, and by presenting the hydrophobic portion of the signal sequence to binding sites on integral membrane proteins.

von Heine (79) has recently reviewed the secretory mechanism and how signal peptides may work, as well as the targeting peptides of mitochondria and chloroplasts. The SRP has been identified as a component involved in protein targeting to, and translocation across, the endoplasmic reticulum (ER) membrane. It is a ribonucleoprotein composed of six distinct polypeptides and an RNA molecule of 300 nucleotides (80).

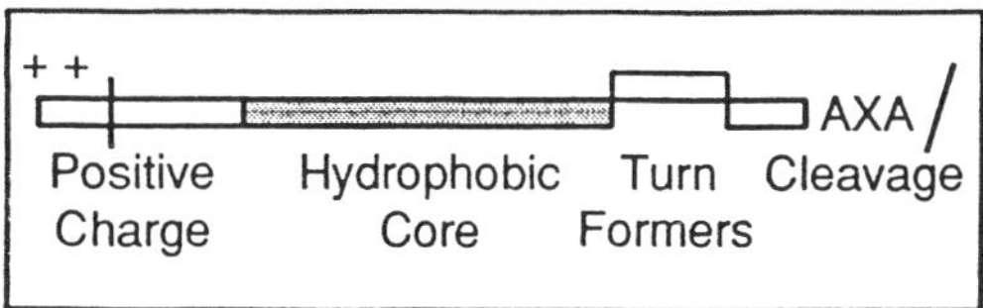

Figure 8 Suggested arrangements of charges and hydrophobic residues of signal (leader) peptide sequences. (From Ref. 78.)

7. *Chaperones*

Chaperones are a recently elucidated class of proteins that can interact with a wide array of polypeptides from the time of synthesis to the final folded state (81). They had been previously studied and are known as heat-shock proteins (Hsps), synthesized by cells in response to stress, such as an increase in temperature.

The Hsp 70 and Hsp 60 families are linked to protein folding in cells. Most members of these families are present in cells under normal non-stressful conditions. The Hsp 70 family is so named because the first member was a 70-kDa protein. The Hsp 60 proteins are organized as large assemblies arranged in two rings, each composed of seven 60-kDa subunits. This link between the Hsps and normal protein synthesis has been demonstrated in studies of the interaction of cytoplasmic Hsp 70s with the nascent polypeptide chain while it is still on the ribosome. Studies with mitochondria have shown that the proteins directed to the endoplasmic reticulum or mitochondria are bound to Hsp 70 in the cytosol. Studies of an in vitro system, consisting of *E. coli* and Hsp 70, Hsp 60 including additional Hsps, GrpE, DnaJ, and GroEs, have shown that the interaction of Hsps mimics the pathway for the interaction of Hsps in the import and folding of mitochondrial proteins. The Hsp 70 class of chaperones bind to unfolded and partially folded states of a variety of proteins, but shows little interaction with *mature* folded proteins. The release of bound protein is affected by an endogenous ATPase. In stressed cells, a plausible role for the Hsps induced by stress is to rescue unfolded or aggregated polypeptides back to an active conformation and the proteolysis of some denatured proteins.

VI. CONCLUSIONS AND FUTURE DIRECTIONS

Much attention is once again being directed at understanding the dynamics of biomembrane systems. Some of this interest is associated with the signaling mechanisms related to the phosphatidylinositol second-messenger systems and the potential for modulating these signal systems. There is also increasing attention placed on the receptors of cell membranes, including the adhesion-type molecules such as the laminins, as well as the role of the carbohydrates of the glycolipids and glycoproteins.

The methods by which proteins can translocate the biomembranes are also of increasing attention, including the structures of the signal peptides. The role of molecular biology techniques for determining both nucleotide sequence and amino acid sequences is also increasing. The ability to produce mutations in protein structures is also assisting determinations of structure, as can be seen in the recent studies of potassium ion channel proteins.

The biggest problem that remains is the present difficulty of being able to crystallize membrane proteins so that their detailed structure can be determined by x-ray diffraction methods. The use of hydropathy plots, although suggestive, can at times be confusing and completely incorrect. There is still much uncertainty in our knowledge of how ions, such as Na^+ or K^+, or molecules, such as glucose, enter or leave the cell. It may well be that a combination of (molecular) biological, biochemical, *and* biophysical methods (e.g., x-ray diffraction studies and spectroscopic techniques) will be required to obtain an understanding of the dynamics of these membrane transport processes.

REFERENCES

1. de Kruiff B. Polymorphic regulation of membrane lipid composition. Nature 1987; 329:587–588.
2. Pascher I, Lundmark M, Nyholm PG, Sundell S. Crystal structures of membrane lipids. Biochim Biophys Acta 1992; 1113:339–373.
3. Luzzati V, Gulik A, Gulik-Krzywicki T, Tardieu A. In: Lipids and Membranes Past, Present and Future. Op den Kamp JAF, Roelofsen B, Wirtz KW, eds. Elsevier, Amsterdam, 1986:137.
4. Gorter E, Grendel F. Biomolecular layers of lipids on chromatocytes of blood. J Exp Med 1925; 41:439–443.
5. Bar RS, Deamer DW, Cornwell DG. Surface area of human erythrocyte lipids: reinvestigation of experiments with plasma membrane. Science 1966; 153:1010–1012.
6. Danielli JF, Davson H. A contribution to the theory of permeability of thin films. J Cell Comp Physiol 1935; 5:483–494.
7. Singer SJ, Nicholson GL. The fluid mosaic model of the structure of cell membranes. Science 1972; 175:720–731.
8. Chapman D, Byrne P, Shipley GG. The physical properties of phospholipids. I. Solid state and mesomorphic properties of some 2,3-diacyl-DL-phosphatidyl-ethanolamines. Proc R Soc Ser A 1966; 290:115–142.
9. Bretcher MS. Phosphatidylethanolamine: differential labelling in intact cells and cell ghosts of human erythrocytes by a membrane-impermeable reagent. J Mol Biol 1972; 71:523–528.
10. Deveaux PF. Static and dynamic lipid asymmetry in cell membranes. Biochemistry 1991; 30:1163–1173.
11. Ferguson MAJ, Williams A. Cell surface anchoring of proteins via glycosyl-phosphatidylinositol structures. Annu Rev Biochem 1988; 57:258–320.
12. Phillips MC, Williams RM, Chapman D. On the nature of hydrocarbon chain motions in lipid liquid crystals. Chem Phys Lipids 1969; 3:234–244.

13. Barton PG, Gunstone FD. Hydrocarbon chain backing and molecular motion in phospholipid bilayers formed from unsaturated lecithins. Synthesis and properties of sixteen positional isomers of 1,2 dioctadecenoyl-*sn*-glycero-3-phosphocholine. J Biol Chem 1975; 250:4470–4476.

14. Oldfield E, Chapman D, Derbyshire W. Deuteron resonance. A novel approach to the study of hydrocarbon chain mobility in membrane systems. FEBS Lett 1971; 10:102–104.

15. Seelig A, Seelig J. The dynamic structure of fatty acyl chains in a phospholipid bilayer measured by deuterium magnetic resonance. Biochemistry 1974; 13:4839–4845.

16. Stockton GW, Polnaszek CF, Tulloch AP, Hasan F, Smith ICP. Molecular motion and order in single-bilayer vesicles and multilamellar dispersions of egg lecithin and lecithin-cholesterol mixtures. A deuterium magnetic resonance study of specifically labelled lipids. Biochemistry 1976; 15:954–966.

17. Asher IM, Levin IW. Effects of temperature and molecular interactions on the vibrational infrared spectra of phospholipid vesicles. Biochim Biophys Acta 1977; 468:63–73.

18. Cameron DG. Casal HL, Mantsch HH. Characterisation of the pretransition in 1,2-dipalmitoyl-*sn*-glycero-3-phosphocholine by Fourier transform infrared spectroscopy. Biochemistry 1980; 19:3665–3672.

19. Michel H. Crystallization of membrane proteins. Trends Biochem Sci 1983; 8:56–59.

20. Garavito RM, Rosenbusch JP. Three-dimensional crystals of an integral membrane protein: an initial X-ray analysis. J Cell Biol 1980; 86:327–329.

21. Garavito RM, Jenkins J, Jansonius JN, Karlsson R, Rosenbusch JP. X-ray diffraction analysis of matrix porin, an integral membrane protein from *Escherichia coli* outer membranes. J Mol Biol 1983; 164:313–327.

22. Michel H. Three-dimensional crystals of a membrane protein complex. The photosynthetic reaction centre from *Rhodopseudomonas viridis*. J Mol Biol 1982; 158:567–572.

23. Henderson R, Shotton D. Crystallization of purple membrane in three dimensions. J Mol Biol 1980; 139:99–109.

24. Michel H, Oesterhelt D. Three-dimensional crystals of membrane proteins: bacteriorhodopsin. Proc Natl Acad Sci USA 1980; 77:1283–1285.

25. Dux L, Martonosi A. Ca^{2+}-ATPase membrane crystals in sarcoplasmic reticulum. The effect of trypsin digestion. J Biol Chem 1983; 258:10111–10115.

26. Klymkowsky MW, Stroud R. Immunospecific identification and three-dimensional structure of a membrane-bound acetylcholine receptor from *Torpedo californica*. J Mol Biol 1979; 128:319–334.

27. Henderson R, Unwin P. Three-dimensional model of purple membrane obtained by electron microscopy. Nature 1975; 257:28–32.

28. Unwin P, Henderson R. Molecular structure determination by electron microscopy of unstained crystalline specimens. J Mol Biol 1975; 84:425–440.

29. Blaurock A. Bacteriorhodopsin: a transmembrane pump containing α-helix. J Mol Biol 1975; 93:139–157.

30. Henderson R. The structure of the purple membrane from *Halobacterium*

halobium: analysis of the X-ray diffraction pattern. J Mol Biol 1975; 93:123–128.

31. Liao MJ, London E, Khorana HG. Regeneration of the native bacteriorhodopsin structure from two chromotryptic fragments. J Biol Chem 1983; 258:9949–9955.

32. Ovchinnikov Y, Abdulaev N, Feigira M, Kieselev A, Labanov N. The structural basis of the functioning of bacteriorhodopsin: overview. FEBS Lett 1979; 100:219–224.

33. Khorana HG, Gerber GE, Herlihy WC, Gray CP, Andregg RJ, Bienmann K, Nihei K. Amino acid sequence of bacteriorhodopsin. Proc Natl Acad Sci USA 1979; 76:5046–5050.

34. Unwin PNT, Zampighi G. Structure of the junction between communicating cells. Nature 1982; 283:545–549.

35. Deatherage JF, Henderson R, Capaldi RA. Three-dimensional structures of cytochrome C oxidase vesicle crystals in negative stain. J Mol Biol 1982; 158:487–499.

36. Kistler J, Stroud R, Klymkowsky M, Lalancette R, Fairclough R. Structure and function of an acetylcholine receptor. Proc Natl Acad Sci USA 1981; 78:3678–3682.

37. Dorset DL, Engel A, Massalski A, Rosenbusch JP. Three-dimensional structure of a membrane pore. Electron microscopical analysis of *Escherichia coli* outer membrane matrix porin. Biophys J 1984; 45:128–129.

38. MacLennan DH, Brandl CJ, Korczak B, Green NM. Amino acid sequence of a Ca^{2+} + Mg^{2+}-dependent ATPase from rabbit muscle sarcoplasmic reticulum, deduced from its complementary DNA sequence. Nature 1985; 316:696–700.

39. Brandl CJ, Green NM, Korczak B, MacLennan DM. Two Ca^{2+}-ATPase genes: homologies and mechanistic implications of deduced amino acid sequences. Cell 1986; 44:597–607.

40. Unwin N. Nicotinic acetylcholine receptor at 9 Å resolution. J Mol Biol 1993; 230:1101–1124.

41. Sansom MSP. Peering down a pore. Curr Biol 1993; 3:239–241.

42. Cowan SW, Rosenbusch JP. Folding pattern diversity of integral membrane proteins. Science 1994; 264:914–916.

43. Shon KJ, Kimy Y, Colnago LM, Opella SJ. NMR studies of the structure and dynamics of membrane-bound bacteriophage. Science 1991; 252:1303–1305.

44. Surewicz WK, Mantsch HH, Chapman D. Determination of protein secondary structure by Fourier transform infrared spectroscopy. A critical assessment. Biochemistry 1993; 32:389–394.

45. Haris PI, Chapman D. Does Fourier transform infrared spectroscopy provide useful information on protein structures? Trends Biochem Sci 1992; 17:161–162.

46. Haris PI, Chapman D. Membrane protein conformation as determined by Fourier transform infrared spectroscopy. Biochem Soc Trans 1988; 17:328–333.

47. Haris PI, Coke M, Chapman D. Fourier transform infrared spectroscopic

investigation of rhodopsin structure and its comparison with bacteriorhodopsin. Biochim Biophys Acta 1989; 995:160–167.

48. Davies A, Ciardelli TL, Lienhard E, Boyle JM, Whetton AD, Baldwin SA. Site-specific antibodies as probes of the topology and function of the human erythrocyte glucose transporter. Biochem J 1990; 266:799–808.

49. Fischburg J, Cheung M, Czegledy F, Li J, Iserovich P, Kwang K, Hubbard J, Garner M, Rosen OM, Golde DW, Vera JC. Evidence that facilitative glucose transporters may fold as B-barrels. Proc Natl Acad Sci USA 1993; 90:11658–11662.

50. Staros JV, Anjaneyulu PS. Membrane impermeant cross-linking reagents. Methods Enzymol 1989; 172:609–628.

51. Mackinnon R, Miller C. Mutant potassium channels with altered binding of charybdotoxin, a pore-blocking peptide inhibitor. Science 1989; 245:1382–1385.

52. Phillips MC, Chapman D. Monolayer characteristics of saturated 1,2-diacylphosphatidylcholine (lecithins) and phosphatidylethanolamine at the air–water interface. Biochim Biophys Acta 1968; 163:301–313.

53. Chapman D, Williams RM, Ladbrooke BD. Physical studies of phospholipids. VI. Thermotropic and lysotropic mesomorphism of some 1,2-diacylphosphatidylcholines (lecithins). Chem Phys Lipids 1967; 1:445–475.

54. Chapman D, Benga G. Biomembrane fluidity—studies of model and natural biomembranes. In: Chapman D, ed. Biological Membranes. Vol V. London: Academic Press, 1994:1–56.

55. Ladbrooke BD, Chapman D. Thermal analysis of lipids, proteins and biological membranes. Chem Phys Lipids 1969; 3:304–367.

56. Bangham AD, Standish MM, Watkins JC. Diffusion of univalent ions across the lamellae of swollen phospholipids. J Mol Biol 1965; 13:238–252.

57. Gregoriadis G, ed. Liposomes as Drug Carriers: Recent Trends and Progress. Chichester: Wiley, 1988.

58. Kagawa Y, Racker E. Partial resolution of enzymes catalyzing oxidative phosphorylation. XXV. Reconstitution of vesicles catalysing $^{32}P_i$–adenosine triphosphate exchange. J Biol Chem 1971; 248:5841.

59. Helenius A, Sarvas M, Simons K. Asymmetric and symmetric membrane reconstitution by detergent elimination. Studies with Semliki-Forest-virus spike glycoprotein and penicillinase from the membrane of *Bacillus licheniformus*. Eur J Biochem 1981; 116:27–35.

60. Tefft RE, Carruthers A, Melchior DL. Reconstituted human sugar transporter activity is determined by bilayer lipid head groups. Biochemistry 1986; 25:3709–3718.

61. Carruthers A, Melchior DL. How bilayer lipids affect membrane protein activity. Trends Biochem Soc 1986; 11:331–335.

62. Maneri LR, Low PS. Structural stability of the erythrocyte anion transporter, band 3, in different lipid environments. J Biol Chem 1988; 263:16170–16178.

63. Wieslander A, Christiansson A, Rilfors L, Lindblom G. Lipid bilayer stability in membranes. Regulation of lipid composition in *Acholeplasma laidlawii* as governed by molecular shape. Biochemistry 1980; 17:3650–3655.

64. Muller P, Rudin DO, Tien HT, Westcott WC. Reconstitution of excitable cell membrane structure in vitro. Circulation 1962; 26:1167–1171.

65. Trauble H, Sackmann E. Studies of the crystalline–liquid phase transition of lipid model membranes. III. Structures of a steroid–lecithin system below and above the lipid phase transition. J Am Chem Soc 1972; 94:4499–4510.

66. Devaux PF, McConnell HM. Lateral diffusion in spin-labelled phosphotidyl-choline multilayers. J Am Chem Soc 1972; 94:4475–4481.

67. Veatch WR, Rando RR, Alecio MR, Colan DE. Use of a fluorescent CHOL derivative to measure lateral mobility of cholesterol. Proc Natl Acad Sci USA 1982; 79:5171–5174.

68. Kornberg RD, McConnell HM. Lateral diffusion of phospholipids in a vesicle membrane. Proc Natl Acad Sci USA 1971; 94:4475–4481.

69. Poo M, Cone RA. Lateral diffusion of rhodopsin in the photoreceptor membrane. Nature 1974; 247:438–441.

70. Peters P, Peters J, Tews KH, Bohr W. A microfluorometric study of translational diffusion in erythrocyte membranes. Biochim Biophys Acta 1974; 367:282–294.

71. Kell DB. Diffusion of protein complexes in prokaryotic membranes: fast, free, random or directed? Trends Biochem Sci 1984; 9:86–88.

72. Cone RA. Rotational diffusional of rhodopsin in the visual receptor membrane. Nature 1972; 236:39–43.

73. Razi-Naqvi J, Gonzalez-Rodriguez J, Cherry R, Chapman D. Spectroscopic technique for studying protein rotation in membranes. Nature 1973; 245:249–251.

74. Higgins CF, Gottesman MM. Is the multidrug transporter a flippase? Trends Biochem Sci 1992; 17:18–21.

75. Deveaux P. Phospholipid flippase. FEBS Lett 1988; 234:8–12.

76. Verner K, Shatz G. Protein translocations across membranes. Science 1988; 241:1307–1313.

77. Wickner W, Lodish H. Multiple mechanisms of protein insertion into and across membranes. Science 1985; 230:400–407.

78. Gierasch LM. Signal sequences. Biochemistry 1989; 28:923–930.

79. von Heine G. Transcending the impenetrable: how proteins come to terms with membranes. Biochim Biophys Acta 1988; 947:307–333.

80. Siegel V, Walter P. Functional dissection of the signal recognition particle. Trends Biochem Sci 1988; 13:314–316.

81. Graig EA. Chaperones: helpers along the pathways to protein folding. Science 1993; 260:1902–1903.

4

Mechanisms of Drug Transport in Prokaryotes and Eukaryotes

Saibal Dey and Barry P. Rosen
Wayne State University School of Medicine,
Detroit, Michigan

I. INTRODUCTION

A. Perspectives and Definitions

One of the most frequently employed strategies for drug resistance by both prokaryotes and eukaryotes is the transport of the toxic compound out of the cell, reducing the intracellular concentration to subtoxic levels (1,2; see Chaps. 1 and 2). An understanding of the molecular details of these transport systems is thus essential to the rational design of drugs for treating drug-resistant cells and microorganisms.

Operationally, transport can be divided into different classes of thermodynamic machines. This does not necessarily imply similarity in their biochemical mechanisms. At the most fundamental level, transport systems differ in their mode of coupling to biological energy. The theory behind the energetics of transport was laid down in the 1960s by Peter Mitchell (3), and the thermodynamic arguments can be found in several reviews (4,5). Primary active transport systems are engines that utilize primarily chemical or electromagnetic energy to establish chemical solute gradients or electrochemical ion gradients. Secondary active transport systems are transformers that convert the electrochemical gradients established by primary systems to gradients of other solutes. Not all transport is linked to a source of energy; facilitated or carrier-mediated transport can occur down a solute gradient, without energy. The drugs themselves can serve as transporters. Antibiotics, such as the gramicidins and amphotericin B, form membrane pores that allow solutes to pass through, and other antibiotics, such as valinomycin and nigericin, serve as mobile carriers for ions.

B. Types of Transport Systems

The major types of transport systems are as follows (Fig. 1):

1. Primary Active Transport

The sources of energy for primary transport systems vary, as do their biochemical mechanisms. Light-driven pumps were probably the first to evolve. These have photoreceptors that absorb photons, using electromagnetic energy to form ion gradients. The chlorophyll molecule is one such photoreceptor, and the photosynthetic apparatus of bacteria and chloroplasts is a primitive mechanism for channeling the light energy into formation of electrochemical gradients of protons. An equally old family of proteins, and one that couples light more directly to the formation of

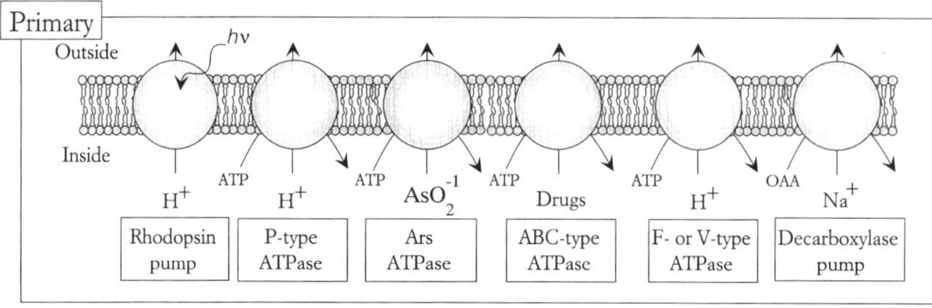

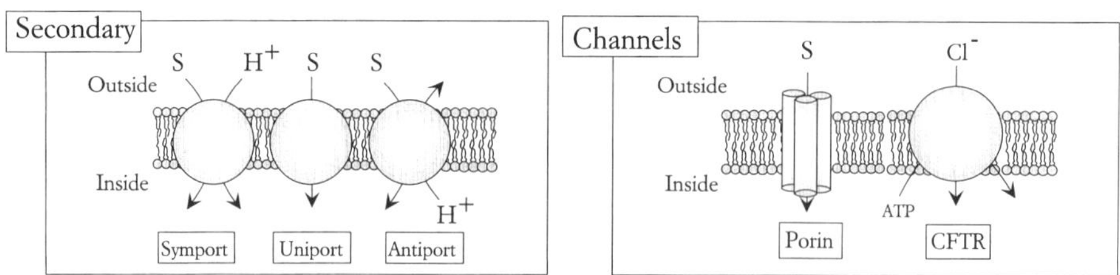

Figure 1 Schematic illustration of the types of transport systems: Shown are primary pumps, secondary porters, or channels through which solutes permeate membranes.

ion gradients, is the archaeobacterial rhodopsin-containing protein family. Bacteriorhodopsin and halorhodopsin are photonic pumps that consist of seven membrane-spanning α-helices with covalently bound rhodopsin (6). During the bacteriorhodopsin photocycle, a proton is electrogenically extruded from cells of *Halobacterium halobium*. Halorhodopsin is a homologous protein that catalyzes electrogenic chloride uptake in the halobacteria (7). The similarities and differences between these two proteins bring out an important point: the direction of substrate transport is not a basic feature built into transport proteins. Very similar proteins can function either as uptake or efflux pumps, a property that will be discussed in more detail later.

Other primary pumps use chemical energy to produce ion or solute gradients. There are several different families of such pumps, each the product of separate evolution. Decarboxylase pumps channel the energy of the decarboxylation into the formation of electrochemical sodium gradients (8). These are all biotin-dependent decarboxylase enzymes and are involved in bacterial fermentation of organic acids; none are resistance pumps.

The best-known pumps are those that couple energy from the hydrolysis of ATP into solute gradient formation. Even within this group there are at least four evolutionarily derived families. Two of the four transport only cations. The family of cation-translocating ATPases of the $E_1 E_2$ or P-type ATPase is widespread, with many members and many types of cationic substrates (9). Some are uptake systems for cations, such as the bacterial Mg^{2+} (10) and K^+ (11) transport systems. Others are exchangers or extrusion systems, for example, the sodium pump, that exchanges intracellular Na^+ for extracellular K^+ (9), or the calcium extrusion pumps of plasma membrane and sarcoplasmic reticulum (12). Some are resistance determinants, such as the plasmid- and chromosomally encoded cadmium resistance pumps of gram-positive bacteria (13). Others, such as the Na^+, K^+-ATPase, are the targets of drugs, such as ouabain, a cardiac glycoside (9). Mutations in other members can result in drug resistance. For example, hygromycin resistance was used to select mutants in the H^+-translocating ATPase of fungi (14). The rationale was that the lowered transmembrane electrochemical proton gradient would be insufficient for concentrating the drug to lethal levels.

A second family, termed the F-type ATPase, includes the $F_0 F_1$ complexes, and the H^+-translocating ATPases that are found in bacterial, mitochondrial, and chloroplast membranes, and form a family with the related V-type vacuolar pumps (9). These are mostly proton pumps, but some transport Na^+ (15). The primary functions of proteins in this family are the establishment of electrochemical proton gradients for coupling to secondary transporters or, when working in the opposite direction, for the synthesis of ATP. Thus, the electrochemical proton gradient is in equilibrium with the ATP pool. However, mutations in the genes for this enzyme can lead to drug resistance. Some of the original mutants in the *Escherichia coli unc* operon were selected for resistance to aminoglycoside antibiotics (16). Again, resistance ensued from the inability to concentrate the drug.

A third family of ATP-driven pumps is represented by a single member, the arsenical-translocating ATPase encoded by the *ars* operon of the *E. coli* plasmid R773 (17). This complex is unrelated to any of the other families. The *ars* operon was found on a clinically isolated plasmid and is responsible for resistance to a variety of chemically unrelated oxyanions, including arsenite, antimonite, arsenate, and tellurite. Although not currently in clinical use, the arsenical salvarsan, designed by Paul Ehrlich, was the first clinically valuable antimicrobial agent, and antimonials and arsenicals are still the treatment of choice for a number of tropical parasites (18; see Chap. 14). Thus, it is not surprising to find hospital-derived bacterial arsenical resistance determinants.

The fourth family, and the most relevant to antimicrobial and anticancer chemotherapy, is the ABC superfamily of transport ATPases (19,20). *ABC* stands for *ATP-b*inding *c*assette, which refers to the consensus nucleotide-binding fold (21) found in at least one subunit of each member of this family. This is somewhat of a misnomer, since the Ars ATPase and F-type and V-type ATPases all contain the same consensus nucleotide-binding sequence, but are otherwise unrelated. This illustrates an important aspect of the evolution of pumps: horizontal transfer of DNA results in similar domains that are located in otherwise unrelated proteins. Thus, three families of transport ATPases probably catalyze the hydrolysis of ATP by similar mechanisms; differences among the families will be more apparent in the mechanism of solute translocation across the membrane. This will be discussed in more detail later. The structure and function of the ABC transporters is considered in detail in Chapter 17.

2. *Secondary Active Transport*

Properly speaking, secondary systems are not active at all, since the uphill transport of one solute is always at the expense of a gradient of another, with a net decrease in the sum of the two gradients. Again, an operational definition of secondary porters includes three basic types: uniporters, symporters, and antiporters. As the names imply, these are carriers for single solutes, two or more solutes in the same direction, or multiple solutes in opposite directions, respectively. Proteins in the same families can catalyze transport in any of the three different modes: for example, the erythrocyte glucose porter is a uniporter, the tetracycline resistance protein is an antiporter or exchanger, and the bacterial arabinose and xylose permeases are H^+-linked symporters; yet all are members of the same family (22).

Most solute-uptake systems are secondary porters. Although the natural substrates of those transport systems are most likely not drugs, most drugs enter cells as analogues of natural substrates. For example, uptake of antifolates, such as methotrexate, can occur by secondary transport systems (23). Other secondary transport systems are the targets of drugs, for example, inhibition of Na^+–H^+ antiporters by amiloride.

3. *Pores and Channels*

In addition to pumps and carriers, which can catalyze concentrative transport, pores and channels allow movement of ions and solutes, usually with high specificity, down a concentration gradient. Once the pore or channel is open, it allows large numbers of molecules to pass through. In contrast, primary and secondary transporters move only one or several molecules per catalytic cycle. In the outer membrane of gram-negative bacteria there are a variety of pores formed by proteins termed porins. This topic has been recently reviewed (24; see Chap. 5) and will not be considered in detail. Porin channels allow passage of hydrophilic molecules with varying degrees of specificity. They are water filled and thus facilitate the transport of small molecules from the medium to the inner membrane, or vice versa, by simple diffusion. The diameter of the pores varies with the particular outer membrane protein, so that the mass of molecules that can permeate differ from one organism to another. In *E. coli*, monosaccharides permeate rapidly, whereas disaccharides permeate more slowly, with larger compounds, such as verbascose (828 Da), nearly completely excluded (24). However, other organisms such as *Pseudomonas aeruginosa* have different outer membrane porin channels, large enough for polysaccharides of several thousand daltons in mass. These pores are responsible for the permeation of hydrophilic drugs to their site of action or to the inner membrane. The major porins of *E. coli*, OmpF and OmpC, are rather nonspecific cation channels, but there are porins more specific for anions (PhoE) and maltose (LamB). Antibiotics, such as imipenem, require porins to enter the periplasm, and mutants of *P. aeruginosa* lacking the D2 protein become resistant to imipenem (25).

Eukaryotic cells have many more channels than bacterial cells, and their functions are quite varied (26). Depending on their structural similarity, these ion channels can be classified into several superfamilies. The voltage-gated superfamily includes K^+ channel, Na^+ channel, and Ca^{2+} channel, all of them having four homologous functional domains of six transmembrane segments. The fourth transmembrane segment functions as a voltage sensor, and the hydrophilic loop connecting the fifth and the sixth segments forms the ion-conducting pathway. A second superfamily of ligand-operated receptor channels is represented by nicotinic acetylcholine, γ-aminobutyric acid (GABA), and glutamate receptors. Members of this family are composed of five homologous subunits, each subunit with a large hydrophilic amino-terminal domain that binds ligands, followed by four transmembrane segments. Besides these two broad superfamilies there are other smaller families of ion channels. The highly homologous ryanodine receptor and the inositol-1,4,5,-triphosphate receptor can be classified as a family that catalyzes Ca^{2+} mobilization from intracellular Ca^{2+} pools. The cGMP-dependent cation channel of the vertebrate rod photoreceptor and the cAMP-operated cation channel of olfactory neuron are almost identical with each other in their polypeptide composition, and both include the remnant of the voltage sensor segment. One channel of considerable interest is the cystic fibrosis transmembrane regulator (CFTR), not because it is a drug target, but because it a close homologue of the P-glycoprotein (27). Although both proteins have sequences that suggest two nucleotide-binding sites and two groups of six membrane-spanning α-helices (2), CFTR apparently is only a chloride channel (28) and not a pump (29). On the other hand, the P-glycoprotein has chloride channel activity (30). Perhaps the common ancestor was a channel; alternatively, perhaps channel activity is a later adaptation. The latter seems reasonable, since no other ABC transporter has been shown to have channel activity.

II. ASSAY METHODS FOR DRUG TRANSPORT

Drug transport in whole cells and membrane vesicles can be efficiently measured using radiolabeled drugs or their fluorescent analogues. Identification and initial studies of a transport system can be done by monitoring accumulation of drug in whole cells, whereas biochemical characterization requires studies in isolated membrane vesicles and purification and reconstitution into proteoliposomes.

A. Intact Cells

Drugs enter cells either by passive diffusion (hydrophobic drugs) or through carrier-mediated uptake systems. Active efflux systems may extrude the drugs out of the cell faster than the entry rate, resulting in a low steady state of accumulation and, hence, resistance. Resistance associated with decreased drug accumulation may also be due to decreased drug entry, as in melarsoprol resistance in *Trypanosoma brucei* (31), or arsenate in *E. coli* (32). The differences between decreased uptake and increased efflux can be differentiated experimentally by preloading cells depleted of endogenous energy reserves with drug (Fig. 2A). The deenergized cells take up drug passively. On addition of an energy source, cells with an efflux system will extrude the preloaded drug. In contrast, cells lacking a drug-uptake system will show no effect of reenergization.

Prokaryotes such as *E. coli* can be depleted of endogenous energy reserves, such as glycogen, by treatment with the reversible inhibitor 2,4-dinitrophenol (DNP). 2,4-Dinitrophenol is a protonophoric uncoupler that dissipates the proton gradient across the inner membrane of the cell. Cells rapidly use their energy reserves to fuel a futile cycle of respiratory-driven proton extrusion and DNP-mediated proton influx (33,34). The two principal forms of cellular energy in most bacteria are chemical energy, mainly as ATP, and electrochemical energy in the form of a proton motive force (pmf). In normal cells, ATP and pmf are in equilibrium with each other through the activity of the F_0F_1 ATP synthetase. In a strain with a mutation in one of the *unc* genes encoding the F_0F_1, this equilibrium is disrupted, and differentiation between ATP- and pmf-coupled systems is possible by using combinations of energy sources and metabolic inhibitors. In these cells, glucose generates both ATP glycolytically and pmf through respiration. Formation of the proton motive force is prevented with inhibitors of the electron transport chain, such as cyanide, so that glucose metabolism in the presence of cyanide establishes intracellular conditions during which only chemical energy is available for transport. With succinate oxidation, these cells generate only a pmf. Thus, it is possible to distinguish between coupling of either of the two forms of energy (33). A similar starvation procedure can be used to deplete eukaryotic cells of endogenous energy reserves (35), although no equivalent of *unc* mutants exist to allow differentiation between chemical and electrochemical sources of coupling energy.

B. Membrane Vesicles and Reconstituted Systems

Inside-out (everted) membrane vesicles are a useful model for studying drug transport in vitro. Free from any cytoplasmic constituents, their metabolic activities are restricted to those provided by the enzymes of the membrane itself. Transport activity does not occur in everted membrane vesicles in the absence of an exogenous source of energy (see Fig. 2B). The energetics of an active efflux system can be determined by adding specific energy sources and measuring intravesicular drug accumulation.

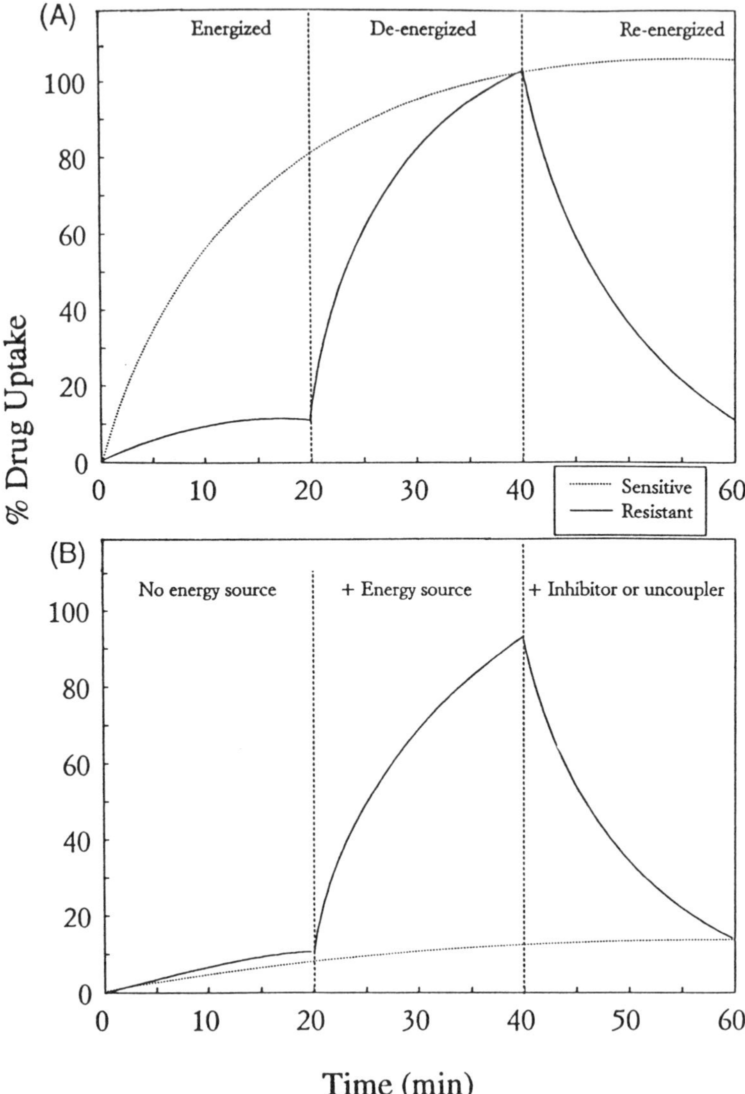

Figure 2 Determination of the mode of energy coupling of transport systems assays in whole cells and everted membrane vesicles: (A) Transport assays in resistant (——) and sensitive (····) cells. (Left panel) Drug uptake in energized cells. In the presence of an active efflux system drug accumulation in resistant cells is low compared with that of sensitive cells. (Middle panel) De-energization leads to lack of efflux activity, reflected by the same level of accumulation of drug in both resistant and sensitive cells. (Right panel) Addition of an exogenous

Everted membrane vesicles were first used for studying active Ca^{2+} extrusion in *E. coli* cells (36). Everted membrane vesicles were prepared by lysing cells under high pressure in a French pressure cell. Inside-out vesicles from eukaryotic cells competent for transport experiments can also be made by homogenization (37) or by nitrogen cavitation (38). Energy-dependent uptake of drugs into these vesicles reflects active extrusion in intact cells. By using a variety of energy sources and inhibitors, the energy requirement for transport can be determined.

In bacteria, transport systems directly coupled to the electrochemical proton gradient can be driven by addition of respiratory substrates, such as NADH or lactate, that generate a proton motive force and can be inhibited by electron transport chain inhibitors, such as cyanide, or by agents that depolarize the energized membrane, such as DNP or carbonylcyanide-*m*-chlorophenylhydrazone (CCCP). In everted membrane vesicles, ATP can generate a pmf catalyzed by the F_0F_1 ATPase. Therefore, in the presence of ATP, transport can be driven directly by ATP hydrolysis, or can be coupled secondarily to the ATP-dependent establishment of a pmf. The use of a specific F_0F_1 inhibitor, such as N,N'-dicyclohexyl-carbodiimide (DCCD), or an *unc* mutant strain, can allow discrimination between chemical and electrochemical energy. Similar problems can occur with plasma membrane vesicles of eukaryotic cells. These membranes contain the Na^+, K^+-ATPase, which generates a electrochemical sodium gradient through ATP hydrolysis. No deletion mutants in the gene for the sodium pump are available in eukaryotes, so specific inhibitors of these ATPases are required to distinguish between primary and secondary transport systems. For example, the Na^+, K^+-ATPase can be inhibited by ouabain.

Enzymes are best characterized in a homogeneous solution of purified protein. Transport proteins are the vectorial equivalent of enzymes. To preserve function, an integral membrane protein must be solubilized from the membrane with mild nonionic detergents, such as octylglucoside or dodecylmaltoside. Detergent-solubilized transport proteins do not show

---

source of energy results in rapid extrusion of the drug from resistant cells, whereas little or no efflux is observed from sensitive cells. (B) Drug uptake assay in everted membrane vesicles prepared from resistant (——) and sensitive (····) cells. (Left panel) In the absence of an energy source everted membrane vesicles exhibit no drug uptake. (Middle panel) Addition of an energy source results in accumulation of drug in everted vesicles prepared from resistant cells, but not in vesicles prepared from sensitive cells. (Right panel) Addition of inhibitors or uncouplers (in transport system coupled to electrochemical gradients) results in a decreased steady-state level of intravesicular accumulation.

activity until reconstituted into phospholipid vesicles. Osmolytes, such as glycerol, sucrose, trehalose, or glycine, added during solubilization, stabilize the conformation of the protein and prevent loss of function during the extraction step (39).

III. FAMILIES OF DRUG RESISTANCE SYSTEMS

Transport-mediated drug resistance can occur in two ways. First, mutation of a normal solute-uptake system can produce drug resistance if the drug is an alternative substrate of the uptake system. For example, fosfomycin is transported by the α-glycerolphosphate transport system encoded by the *glpT* gene in *E. coli*, and mutation in the *glpT* gene produces fosphomycin resistance (40). However, more important clinically is the emergence of new transport systems for drug extrusion. This can occur through acquisition of foreign genes, in particular plasmid-mediated drug resistance. However, expression of chromosomal genes can also be responsible for resistance. For example, resistance to daunorubicin (41) and tylosin (42) in *Streptomyces* results from the action of drug efflux systems of the ABC superfamily. *Streptomyces*, a major producer of antibiotics, requires systems to export the drug and for protection against its own poisons. It would be reasonable to consider *Streptomyces* as both the source of drugs and the source of drug resistances. However, most bacteria appear to have endogenous drug resistance efflux systems that are not normally expressed; for example, the *mar* (*m*ultiple *a*ntibiotic *r*esistance; 43) and *emr* (*E. coli m*ultidrug *r*esistance; 44) loci in *E. coli*, the *bmr* (*Bacillus m*ultidrug *r*esistance; 45) and the *norA* (46) loci in *S. aureus* and the *smr* (*Staphylococcus m*ultidrug *r*esistance; 47) locus in *S. aureus*. The normal function of any of these systems is unclear. It is possible that each has a metabolic intermediate or product as substrate, and the drug is a substrate analogue. Drug resistance would result from an increase in transport activity, usually through an increase in transcription. Alternatively, the drugs could be the real substrates of stress–response systems present in all cells. Eukaryotes have similar defenses; for example, the products of the *mdr* (*m*ultidrug *r*esistance) gene family protect cells from drugs (2). Again, the normal functions of these systems are unclear. Overexpression of *mdr* genes can occur through gene amplification or through increased transcription of an unamplified gene. Drug transporters can be primary pumps, such as the multiple drug resistance pump of mammalian cells (2), or secondary transporters, such as the multiple drug transporters of bacterial cells (48).

A. Secondary Carriers

Most bacterial drug transporters are coupled to the proton motive force. The largest family includes the tetracycline resistance determinant of gram-negative bacteria, the fluoroquinolone transporter of *S. aureus*, the multidrug resistance protein (Bmr) of *Bacillus subtilis*, and various sugar transport proteins (48,22).

1. Tetracycline Resistance

Resistance to tetracycline in gram-negative bacteria is due to active extrusion of the antibiotic (49,50), resulting in decreased intracellular accumulation (51; see Chap. 7). Five highly homologous tetracycline-resistant determinants have been identified (52). In *E. coli*, transport of tetracycline is mediated by a 43-kDa inner membrane protein, the Tet protein (53). Topological analysis of the protein suggest 12 membrane-spanning α-helices, with a large central cytoplasmic loop, dividing the protein into two complementary halves, α (NH_2-terminal) and β (COOH-terminal) (54,55). Among the homologues, the sequence of the central hydrophilic loop region is less conserved than the α- and the β-regions. Mutations in either half of the protein have been isolated. Complementation occurs between mutants in the two halves, restoring partial resistance (56,57). These results suggest that the Tet protein functions as a multimer (58,59). The α- and β-domains existing in two different polypeptides can interact in vivo to form a functional transporter (60). Rubin et al. (55) suggested that the Tet protein evolved through a gene duplication event that later evolved to develop different functions for the two domains. Everted membrane vesicles, prepared from resistant cells, exhibited energy-dependent uptake of tetracycline. Tetracycline is transported by the Tet protein as a complex with a divalent cation, such as Mg^{2+}, Co^{2+}, or Ca^{2+} (61). The tetracycline–cation complex is transported in exchange for a proton (62). The Tet protein, encoded by transposon *Tn10*, has a K_m for tetracycline of 10 μM. (63). Similar extrachromosomally encoded tetracycline-resistant determinants have also been detected in *Bacillus* spp. (64,65).

In *E. coli*, a chromosomally encoded tetracycline resistance determinant has been reported. It has a higher affinity for minocycline, the lipophilic analogue of tetracycline (66). Unlike the plasmid-encoded system, it is stimulated more by calcium than by magnesium ions (66). Tetracycline resistance can also arise from a mutation in an unrelated chromosomal gene, *marA* (43). Expression of the mutant *marA* gene resulted in active extrusion of tetracycline (67); insertional inactivation of the *marA* gene by transposon *Tn5* resulted in reversal of resistance (68).

2. *The* norA *Gene*

Fluoroquinolones are broad-spectrum antimicrobial agents effective against both gram-negative and gram-positive bacteria (see Chap. 8). Resistance to fluoroquinolones in *S. aureus* is mediated by the chromosomally encoded *norA* gene (46). The *norA* gene confers resistance to hydrophilic quinolones, such as norfloxacin, enoxacin, ofloxacin, and ciprofloxacin, in both *S. aureus* and *E. coli*, but not against hydrophobic quinolones, such as nalidixic acid, oxolinic acid, and sparfloxacin (69). The *norA* gene encodes a 388-residue hydrophobic protein, with a relative molecular mass (M_r) of about 49 kDa (70). The *norA*-mediated resistance is due to energy-dependent extrusion of quinolones (69–71). The *norA* gene from a resistant cell has a single amino acid change (72); however, it is unclear how this single amino acid difference could be responsible for the resistance phenotype. The most likely explanation is that a second mutation in the promoter sequence results in elevated expression of the *norA* gene, increasing the levels of the efflux system for quinolones.

3. *The* bmr *Gene*

In *B. subtilis* a chromosomal gene termed *bmr* confers resistance to structurally unrelated drugs such as rhodamine 6G, ethidium bromide, chloramphenicol, and puromycin (45). The phenotype is due to amplification of the *bmr* gene, with resistance resulting from active efflux of the drugs from the cell. Transport was sensitive to CCCP and to inhibitors of the mammalian multidrug resistance pump, such as verapamil and reserpine. The predicted amino acid sequence of the Bmr protein exhibits 44% identity with the *norA* gene product and is less closely related to the Tet protein (73). That it also confers resistance to quinolones suggests that the Bmr and NorA proteins belong to the Tet family of pmf-coupled efflux systems (74).

4. *The* smr *Gene*

A family of small integral membrane proteins in *S. aureus*, *E. coli*, *Ps. aeruginosa*, *Agrobacterium tumefaciens*, and *Proteus vulgaris* has been described recently (47). The *smr* gene (also known as the *qacC* gene), is a member of this family that confers resistance by pmf-coupled extrusion of lipophilic cations, such as tetraphenylphosphonium (47,75,76). The smallest transport protein thus far recognized, the *smr* gene product encodes a 107-residue, 12-kDa membrane protein, with four predicted transmembrane α-helices (47). A glutamate residue located in the first transmembrane region (E13 in Smr) is conserved in all members of the family and has been proposed to be involved in coupling exchange of lipophilic cations for protons (47).

5. *The emr Gene*

A chromosomally encoded determinant from *E. coli*, cloned into a multicopy plasmid, conferred resistance to CCCP, nalidixic acid, and several toxic hydrophobic compounds. Resistance resulted from expression of two genes: *emrA* and *emrB*. The *emrB* gene encodes a 56.2-kDa hydrophobic protein, predicted to have 14 membrane-spanning α-helices and is homologous to the QacA protein, a multidrug resistance pump of *S. aureus* (44). The product of the *emrA* gene is a 42.7-kDa membrane protein, with a single hydrophobic domain and a large periplasmic domain. The EmrA protein is homologous with the cyclosin efflux protein of *Bordetella pertussis*, the CyaD protein (44), and, to some extent, to the HlyD component of the *E. coli* hemolysin extrusion system (77). The EmrB protein has been suggested to be an inner-membrane drug transporter, and the EmrA protein an outer-membrane drug channel (44). The EmrA–EmrB system confers resistance to structurally unrelated uncouplers, such as CCCP and tetrachlorosalicylanilide, but not to more hydrophilic ones, such as pentachlorophenol or dinitrophenol, and to nalidixic acid, but not to its more hydrophilic analogues. It also mediates resistance to thiolactomycin, an inhibitor of fatty acid biosynthesis (78).

B. Primary Transporters

1. *Arsenical Pump*

Plasmid-mediated resistance to heavy metals is widespread in both gram-positive and gram-negative bacteria (1). The system encoded by plasmid R773 in *E. coli* is known to confer resistance against oxyanions of arsenic (arsenite and arsenate) and antimony (antimonite) (79). Resistance is conferred by an oxyanion-induced operon, the *ars* operon (80). The operon codes for two regulatory (ArsR and ArsD) and three structural (ArsA, ArsB, and ArsC) proteins (80–83). Resistance correlates with active extrusion of arsenite from the cell by a primary pump (84,85). The *arsA* and *arsB* gene products form a membrane-bound anion pump that confers resistance to arsenite and antimonite, whereas arsenate resistance requires expression of a third structural gene for the ArsC protein (86). The ArsC protein of both gram-positive and gram-negative bacteria reduces arsenate to arsenite, which is then extruded by the Ars pump (87,88).

The ArsA protein is a 63-kDa peripheral membrane protein that exhibits anion-stimulated hydrolysis of ATP (89,90). It has two nucleotide-binding consensus sequences, one in each homologous half of the protein (80). Both nucleotide-binding sites are required for catalytic activity (91,92). The maximal rate of antimonite-stimulated ATP hydrolysis is approximately 1 μmol mg^{-1} mm^{-1}, with a K_m for ATP of 0.1 mM. The concentrations of antimonite and arsenite that produce half-maximal ATPase activity are 10 μM and 0.1 mM, respectively (90). The active form of ArsA protein is a dimer, with dimerization favored by binding of one of the anionic substrates (93,94). The results of studies with fluorescence probes indicate conformational changes induced by binding of arsenite or antimonite (95). The sequences for the two homologous halves of the protein were subcloned, and the two halves of the ArsA protein were purified and reconstituted into an active anion-stimulated ATPase (96).

The ArsB protein is a 45-kDa integral membrane protein (97) that spans the inner membrane 12 times (98). It is the membrane anchor for the ArsA protein (99,100) and probably forms the anion-conducting pathway. The ArsB protein has been produced in large amounts as a chimeric protein, with a portion of the ArsA protein fused at the NH_2-terminus of the chimera (101). The chimeric protein retained the ability to bind the ArsA protein and to provide resistance to arsenite and antimonite. Recently, a system has been developed for the uptake of of $^{73}AsO_2^-$ into everted membrane vesicles prepared from cells that produce both the chimeric ArsB protein and a wild-type ArsA protein (101a). Transport was ATP-dependent and could not be driven by other nucleoside triphosphates, including the nonhydrolyzable ATP analogue ATPγS. In vesicles prepared from an *unc* strain, neither lactate nor NADH oxidation supported transport of $^{73}AsO_2^-$, and transport coupled to ATP was insensitive to CCCP. These results indicate that an electrochemical proton gradient is neither necessary nor sufficient for arsenite transport by the ArsA–ArsB enzyme complex. Transport had an absolute requirement for Mg^{2+} or Mn^{2+}. Uptake of $^{73}AsO_2^-$ was insensitive to NaN_3 and vanadate, inhibitors of F-type and P-type ATPases, respectively (9), but was sensitive to the sulfhydryl reagent *N*-ethylmaleimide. Antimonite, the preferred substrate of the pump, inhibited accumulation of $^{73}AsO_2^-$ with an apparent K_i tenfold less than the K_m for arsenite. No other oxyanion examined had a significant effect on $^{73}AsO_2^-$ transport.

Resistance to arsenate requires expression of the ArsC protein. The ArsC protein encoded by plasmid R773 reduces arsenate to arsenite with glutaredoxin as the direct source of reducing equivalents (101b). In contrast, thioredoxin is the reductant for the staphylococcal plasmid pI258 ArsC protein (87). The ArsC protein has been proposed to channel its product into the active site of the ArsA–ArsB complex, preventing the release of arsenate, which is more toxic than arsenate, into the cytosol (102). However, no association between the ArsC protein and the membrane-bound ArsA–ArsB complex has yet been detected.

Interestingly, the arsenical resistance operon encoded by plasmid pI258 from *S. aureus* and plasmid pSX267 from *S. xylosus*, respectively (103,104), do not have an *arsA* gene coding for the catalytic subunit of the pump. The R773 ArsB protein has recently been shown to confer an intermediate level of resistance to arsenite and antimonite in the absence of expression of the *arsA* gene (104a). Resistance was still due to active arsenite extrusion, as reflected by low intracellular accumulation of ^{73}As O_2^-. Preliminary studies on energetics of the ArsB protein-mediated arsenite extrusion indicate obligatory coupling to the electrochemical proton gradient, as opposed to the obligatory ATP coupling of the ArsA–ArsB complex.

2. *Multidrug Resistance*

Emergence of multidrug resistance (MDR) in cancer cells is one of the major causes of the failure of chemotherapy (see Chap. 2). This broad-spectrum resistance to chemotherapeutic agents is due to increased efflux, mediated by the *MDR1* gene, which encodes the P-glycoprotein (2,105). High levels of the P-glycoprotein have been found in cells of most mammals following selection for drug resistance (106). Most mammals have more than one *MDR* gene; in humans, two *MDR* genes have been identified, only one of which is related to the multidrug-resistant phenotype (107,108). The *MDR1* gene encodes a polypeptide of 1280 amino acids (106) predicted to have 10 or 12 membrane-spanning regions (109,110) in two homologous halves. Each half has a large cytoplasmic region, containing an ATP-binding site. Homology among different *MDR* genes is highest at the ATP-binding region (2). The *MDR1* gene product is a member of the ABC family (19). This family includes bacterial proteins that transport nutrients, polysaccharides, peptides, and drugs (111). It also includes eukaryotic proteins, such as the chloroquine extrusion pump of *Plasmodium falciparum* (*pfmdr*) (112,113), the transporter for the α-peptide mating factor of yeast *STE6* (114,115), and the CFTR protein, the product of cystic fibrosis transmembrane regulator gene (116). The properties of the members of this family are reviewed in Chapters 14 and 17 and will not be considered further.

C. Other Systems

1. *Oxyanion Resistance in* Leishmania

Drug resistance in parasitic protozoa has become an increasing threat to antimicrobial chemotherapy. Pentostam (sodium stibogluconate), a pentavalent antimonial compound, is the drug of choice in treating all forms of leishmaniasis. Treatment failure often results from emergence of Pentostam-resistant *Leishmania* spp. Clinically isolated Pentostam-resistant cell lines are often cross-resistant to trivalent antimony and arsenic (117). Croft et al. (118) proposed that pentavalent antimony derivatives are metabolized in vivo into trivalent antimonial compounds that may be the active form of the drug; therefore, resistance to trivalent antimonials in vitro may reflect resistance to pentavalent antimonials in vivo during drug therapy (119). Pentostam-resistant clones of *Leishmania* exhibited a fivefold lower intracellular accumulation of [^{125}Sb]Pentostam and specific binding of Pentostam to a protein similar in mass to the P-glycoprotein (120). In *L. tarentolae* and *L. major* resistance to arsenite correlated with amplification of the genes *ltpgpA* and *lmpgpA*, respectively, that encode P-glycoprotein homologues (119). Recently, in *L. tarantolae*, four different types of arsenite-resistant mutants were isolated (121). All four classes showed resistance to high concentrations of arsenite and low intracellular accumulation of ^{73}AsO$_2^-$, but only two of them had detectable amplification of the *ltpgpA* gene (121). Partial revertants of mutants that initially showed *ltpgpA* gene amplification, but lost the amplicons during growth in absence of selective pressure, retained arsenite resistance and accumulated 100-fold less ^{73}AsO$_2^-$ compared with the wild-type. Reduced accumulation of arsenite in resistant mutants could be reversed to wild-type levels by treatment with the uncoupler DNP. The reduced accumulation was due to rapid efflux of the oxyanion from resistant cells, rather than a defect in uptake, as in melarsoprol-resistant African trypanosomes (31). This indicates the presence of an arsenite efflux system in *Leishmania* independent of *pgp*-like gene amplification. The relation between amplification of the *pgp*-like genes and Pentostam resistance remains unclear. Transfection of wild-type cells with *ltpgpA* or *lmpgpA* conferred only a low level (two to fourfold) of resistance to arsenite and, at least in *L. tarantolae*, showed no alteration in the level of ^{73}AsO$_2^-$ accumulation in the cell. However, mutation in the putative nucleotide-binding fold of the *ltpgpA* gene resulted in loss of resistance in the transfectants (122). One possible explanation is that the P-glycoprotein homologue sequesters toxic anions in intracellular compartments instead of extrusion from the cell.

2. Arsenite Resistance in Chinese Hamster Cells

A stable and inducible resistance to arsenite and antimonite has been reported in Chinese hamster cell lines (123). Resistant cell lines exhibited reduced intracellular accumulation of ^{73}AsO$_2^-$ compared with that of the wild type (Z. Wang, S. Dey, B. P. Rosen, and T. G. Rossman, unpublished data). This could be the result of increased activity of an uptake system, or decreased activity of an endogenous extrusion system. A hypersensitive mutant accumulated higher levels of $^{73}AsO_2^-$. These results suggest that resistance is transport related, either through decreased uptake, or through increased efflux (123). A similar resistance to arsenite exists Chinese hamster ovary cell lines (124). Resistance was due to increased efflux of the arsenic, leading to low intracellular accumulation (125). An elevated level of the π-isozyme of glutathione S-transferase (GST-π) in the cell also correlated with resistance and active extrusion (125). Inhibitors of GST, such as Cibacron Blue or ethacrynic acid, decreased resistance to arsenite. Reelevation of GST activity by treatment with sodium arsenite, cadmium acetate, or zinc sulfate resulted in recovery of arsenite resistance (124). It has been suggested that GST-π facilitates extrusion of arsenite in a conjugated form with glutathione (125). Gyurasics et al. (126) reported that biliary excretion of arsenic is dependent on hepatobiliary transport of glutathione and suggested transport of arsenic as a glutathione conjugate. Consistent with this hypothesis, an ATP:Mg^{2+}-dependent efflux pump for glutathione S–conjugate has been characterized in vesicles from rat liver and heart cells (127; see Chap. 19). The pump is an orthovanadate-sensitive membrane ATPase that extrudes xenobiotics, such as aflatoxin B_1, and biologically active conjugated trienes, such as leukotrienes (127). However, no evidence in favor of arsenite detoxification by this system has been reported.

IV. EVOLUTION OF TRANSPORT ATPase

Of the four major families of transport ATPases discussed in Section I.B.1, three have the same type of nucleotide-binding site. The consensus sequence identified by Walker et al. (21) is found in the Ars ATPase, the F-type ATPases, and the ABC ATPases. Only the P-type ATPases have a different sequence. Again, the horizontal transfer of sequences for domains between genes allows evolution of function, independently of the overall vertical evolution of a specific gene.

The Ars system, which is normally an obligatory ATP-coupled pump, has recently been shown to function as a secondary porter in the absence of the catalytic ArsA subunit (104a). From a topological analysis of the ArsB protein, the protein has the same overall structure of two groups of six membrane-spanning α-helices, with a central cytoplasmic loop, characteristic of many secondary carriers (22,98). On the other hand, homologues of the ArsA ATPase are all soluble ATPases, with intracellular, but not transport, functions (102). For example, the *nifH* gene product is the dinitrogen reductase of the nitrogenase complex (128) and the MinD protein is an inhibitor of septum placement during *E. coli* cell division

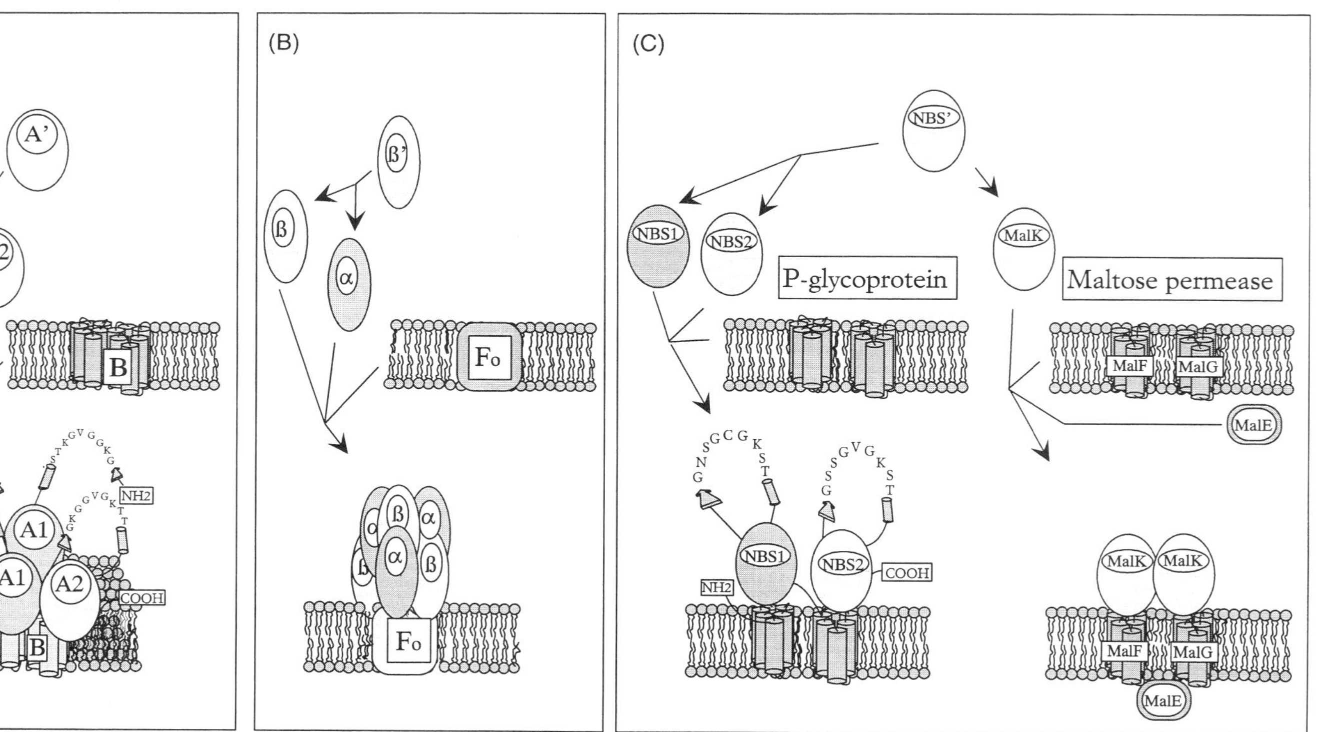

(A)
A'
A1
A2
B
A2
A1
A1
A2
NH2
COOH
COOH
NH2
(B)
β'
β
α
Fo
α
β
β
α
Fo
(C)
NBS'
NBS1
NBS2
P-glycoprotein
MalK
Maltose permease
MalF
MalG
MalE
NBS1
NBS2
NH2
COOH
MalK
MalK
MalF
MalG
MalE

(129). We have proposed a model in which the catalytic and translocation domains of primary pumps are the result of parallel evolution of genes for soluble ATPases and membrane carriers (102). The primordial soluble ATPases had nontransport functions, whereas the membrane components may have evolved as secondary carriers or channels (Fig. 3). The model implies that multicomponent, ion-translocating ATPases could not have emerged de novo, but must have evolved in discrete stages. The ancestors of the catalytic ATP-binding proteins and the membrane components may have been quite different from their present transport function. Thus, the difference between pumps and carriers is strictly operational, and homologous proteins may be have different modes of energy coupling.

Consider the way in which this hypothesis would apply to two of the other families, the F-type ATPases and the ABC proteins. The F-type H^+ transport systems can be either primary or secondary, depending on the subunit composition. The complete F_0F_1 is an obligatory ATP-coupled (or ATP synthetic) pump (130). However, in the absence of the F_1, the F_0 sector of the H^+-ATPase catalyzes $\Delta\psi$-driven H^+ movement. An ancient function of the ancestor of the F_0 may have arisen as a metabolic adaptation to allow free movement of protons in or out of the cell. The α- and

---

Figure 3 Evolution of primary pumps: The model proposes that primary pumps evolved from the separate evolution of the genes for membrane proteins and soluble ATPases. Membrane proteins, such as the ArsB protein, the F_0, or the ancestor of the membrane components of the P-glycoprotein or maltose permease, may have evolved as secondary carriers for protons, ions, or organic solutes, or as channels. Soluble proteins with ATPase activity evolved for functions involved in intracellular functions. Through duplication, the genes for the smaller nucleotide-binding proteins ancestral to the NH_2- and COOH-terminal halves of the ArsA protein or the P-glycoprotein, or to the α- and β-subunits of the F_1, would have duplicated (note, however, that some extant pumps simply use multiple copies of the same gene product; for example, the MalK protein). The duplicated genes would then evolve separate functions, sometimes fused to produce larger proteins with multiple nucleotide-binding sites (e.g., the *arsA* gene), or other times remaining separate within a single operon (e.g., the genes for the α- and β-subunits of F_1). In stages, this association would become functional, resulting in the development of (A) ion-translocating ATPases, such as the oxyanion pump, and (B) the H^+-translocating F_0F_1. In members of the ABC superfamily, gene fusions created single genes for large multifunctional proteins in eukaryotes, such as (C) the P-glycoprotein, or remained as a multisubunit complex of separate proteins, such as the maltose permease. If the genes for the membrane components of the ABC superfamily arose separately, they could have had different original functions; for example, secondary sugar transport for the MalF–G complex, or chloride channel activity for the P-glycoprotein.

β-subunits of the F_1 are related to each other and to soluble proteins with known nontransport functions (131,132). The separate, but parallel, evolution of the two components of the H^+ pump seems probable.

The members of the ABC family of transport ATPases are related only through the catalytic portions (133). The membrane components fall into several separate and unrelated families (134). For example, the *Streptomyces peucetius* daunorubicin exporter has a gene for a soluble ATPase, *drrA*, and through its sequence, the pump is classed as a member of the ABC superfamily (41). Yet the presumed membrane component, the *drrB* gene product, is unrelated to any of the membrane components of the ABC family, except for a small number of very closely related proteins (133). The membrane components of the maltose permease, the MalF and MalG proteins, are unrelated in sequence to the membrane sectors of the P-glycoprotein. The MalF protein has a quite different membrane topology from other members of the family, with eight membrane-spanning α-helices arranged in two regions of three and five helices (135), although it is similar to that of other more closely related bacterial homologues, such as the histidine permease (136). The sequence and presumed membrane topology of the membrane components of the hemolysin exporter is again quite different from either the maltose permease proteins or the P-glycoprotein (134). Thus, although the mechanism of ATP hydrolysis and energy coupling may be the same in all members of the ABC superfamily through common evolution, the mechanisms of solute translocation in the various members may differ from each other as much as any unrelated transport proteins. On the other hand, it is reasonable to consider that proteins that have homologous ATP-binding sites would bind ATP in similar ways; furthermore, the mechanism of hydrolysis and energy coupling might be similar. The differences between families (and even between members of the same superfamily) would be found in the mechanism of solute translocation through the membrane, with the translocation properties of the proteins dictated by the membrane domains. Thus, the Ars ATPase and F-type ATPases are all ABC proteins in the strictest sense. As extrusion systems, these may be good models for the function of other extrusion systems, such as the P-glycoprotein.

V. CONCLUSIONS AND FUTURE DIRECTIONS

Transport systems fall into many classes, with diverse biochemical mechanisms. Systems that have functional similarities may be evolutionarily unrelated, and related systems may transport solutes in different directions or even have different modes of energy coupling (137). Does this extreme diversity mean that no general conclusions can be drawn from the study of individual systems? On the contrary, there are many similarities in design, with common features, such as nucleotide-binding sites, found in members of evolutionarily distinct families. What is learned of mechanisms in one transport system may bear on mechanisms of others.

Future studies will likely focus on mechanistic details, broadening understanding of the fundamental aspects of membrane transport and, eventually, leading to the design of more effective drugs for the management of resistance. One pertinent question is the way in which members of a single family can have more than one mode of energy coupling; for example, the ATP-coupled pump activity of the P-glycoprotein compared with the anion channel activity of the CFTR protein.

Another enigma is the nature of the substrate site(s) of multidrug transporters. It appears that multidrug resistance proteins have evolved multiple times in various forms; the *mdr*, *mar*, *bmr*, *emr*, and *smr* gene products, all are unrelated multidrug exporters. Some are secondary porters, others are pumps; yet they recognize many of the same substrates. Transport proteins are vectorial enzymes: instead of catalyzing scalar reactions, they catalyze the movement of substrate from one compartment to another. Yet the high specificity found in enzymes is apparently absent in multidrug transporters. It is possible that primordial binding sites were less able to distinguish among molecules. Gradual evolution of binding sites with restricted substrate recognition could have led to transport proteins with narrower ranges of substrates.

Structural information is required to ascertain the details of mechanism. This is in the future for most transport proteins. Although crystallization of membrane proteins is an active field of investigation, it is still more art than science. In the near future, molecular genetics will be an informative method for identifying specific aminoacyl residues required for function. Simultaneous biochemical identification, purification, and characterization of the transport proteins will be required to relate the results of mutant studies with the function of aminoacyl residues.

ACKNOWLEDGMENTS

We thank Dr. A. Linet for suggestions and Drs. Kim Lewis and Milton Saier for discussion and preprints. This work was supported by United States Public Health Service Grants CA54141 and AI19793.

REFERENCES

1. Tisa LS, Rosen BP. Plasmid-encoded transport mechanisms. J Bioenerg Biomemb 1990; 22:493–507.
2. Gottesman MM, Pastan I. Biochemistry of multidrug resistance mediated by the multidrug transporter. Annu Rev Biochem 1993; 62:385–427.

3. Mitchell P. Coupling of phosphorylation to electron and hydrogen transfer by a chemiosmotic type of mechanism. Nature 1961; 191:141–148.

4. Rosen BP, Kashket ER. Energetics of active transport. In: Rosen BP, ed. Bacterial Transport. New York: Marcel Dekker, 1978:559–620.

5. Mitchell P. Keilin's respiratory chain concept and its chemiosmotic consequences. Science. 1979; 206:1148–1158.

6. Henderson R, Unwin PNT. Three-dimensional model of purple membrane obtained by electron microscopy. Nature 1975; 257:28–32.

7. Schobert B, Lanyi JK. Halorhodopsin is a light driven chloride pump. J Biol Chem 1982; 257:10306–10313.

8. Dimroth P. The generation of an electrochemical gradient of sodium ions upon decarboxylation of oxaloacetate by the membrane-bound and Na^+-activated oxaloacetate decarboxylase from *Klebsiella aerogenes*. Eur J Biochem 1982; 121:443–449.

9. Pedersen PL, Carafoli E. Ion motive ATPases. I. Ubiquity, properties, and significance to cell function. Trends Biochem Sci 1987; 12:146–150.

10. Maguire ME, Snavely MD, Leizman JB, Gura S, Bagga D, Tao T, Smith DL. Mg^{2+} translocating P-type ATPases of *Salmonella typhimurium*. Wrong way, wrong place enzymes. Ann NY Acad Sci 1992; 671:244–255.

11. Epstein W, Laimins L. Potassium transport in *Escherichia coli*: diverse systems with common control by osmotic forces. Trends Biochem Sci 1980; 5:21–23.

12. Carafoli E, Inesi G, Rosen BP. Calcium transport across biological membranes. In: Sigel H, ed. Metal Ions in Biological Systems. New York: Marcel Dekker, 1984:129–185.

13. Silver S, Walderhaug M. Gene regulation of plasmid- and chromosome-determined inorganic ion transport in bacteria. Microbiol Rev 1992; 56:195–228.

14. Perlin D, Brown C, Haber JE. Mutants in plasma membrane ATPase of *Saccharomyces cerevisiae* that alter membrane potential. J Biol Chem 1988; 263:18118–18122.

15. Dimroth P, Laubinger W, Kluge C, Kaim G, Ludwig W, Schleifer KH. Sodium-translocating adenosine triphosphatase of *Propionigenium modestum*. Ann NY Acad Sci 1992; 671:310–321.

16. Rosen BP. Restoration of active transport in a Mg^{2+}-adenosine triphosphatase deficient mutant of *Escherichia coli*. J Bacteriol 1973; 116:1124–1129.

17. Kaur P, Rosen BP. Plasmid-encoded resistance to arsenic and antimony. Plasmid 1992; 27:29–40.

18. Ouellette M, Borst P. Drug resistance and P-glycoprotein gene amplification in protozoan parasite *Leishmania*. Res Microbiol 1991; 142:737–746.

19. Higgins CF, Hiles ID, Salmond GP, Gill DR, Downie JA, Evans IJ, Holland IB, Gray L, Buckel SD, Bell AW, Hermodson MA. A family of related ATP-binding subunits coupled to distinct biological processes in bacteria. Nature 1986; 323:448–450.

20. Ames GFL. Bacterial periplasmic permeases as model for multidrug resistance (MDR) and the cystic fibrosis transmembrane conductance regulator (CFTR). Soc Gen Physiol Ser 1993; 48:77–94.

21. Walker JE, Saraste M, Runswick MJ, Gay NJ. Distantly related sequences in the α- and β-subunits of the ATP synthase, myosin kinases and other ATP-requiring enzymes and a common nucleotide binding fold. EMBO J 1982; 1:945–951.

22. Henderson PJ, Baldwin SA, Cairns MT, et al. Sugar–cation symport systems in bacteria. Int Rev Cytol 1992; 137:149–208.

23. Horne DW, Holloway RS, Said HM. Uptake of 5-formyltetrahydrofolate in isolated rat liver mitochondria is carrier-mediated. J Nutr 1992; 122:2204–2209.

24. Nikaido H. Transport across the bacterial outer membrane. J Bioenerget Biomembr 1993; 25:581–589.

25. Trias J, Nikaido H. Protein D2 channel of the *Pseudomonas aeruginosa* outer membrane has a binding site for basic amino acids and peptides. J Biol Chem 1992; 265:15680–15684.

26. Hirata H. Review of molecular structure and function of ion channels. Jpn J Clin Med 1993; 51:1065–1082.

27. Riordan JR, Rommens JM, Kerem BS, Alon N, Rozmahel R, Grzelczak Z, Zielenski J, Lok S, Plavsic N, Chou JL, Drumm ML, Iannuzzi MC, Collins FS, Tsui LC. Identification of the cystic fibrosis gene: cloning and characterization of complementary DNA. Science 1989; 245:1066–1073.

28. Arispe N, Rojas E, Hartman J, Sorscher EJ, Pollard HB. Intrinsic anion channel activity of the recombinant first nucleotide binding fold domain of the cystic fibrosis transmembrane regulator protein. Proc Natl Acad Sci USA 1992; 89:1539–1543.

29. Guggino WB. Outwardly rectifying chloride channels and CF: a divorce and remarriage. J Bionerg Biomembr 1993; 25:27–35.

30. Valverde MA, Díaz M, Sepúlveda FV, Gill DR, Hyde SC, Higgins CF. Volume-regulated chloride channels associated with the human multidrug-resistance P-glycoprotein. Nature 1992; 355:830–833.

31. Carter NS, Fairlamb AH. Arsenical resistant trypanosomes lack an unusual adenosine transporter. Nature 1993; 361:173–175.

32. Rosenberg H, Gerdes RG, Chegwidden K. Two systems for the uptake of phosphate in *Escherichia coli*. J Bacteriol 1977; 131:505–511.

33. Berger EA, Heppel LA. Different mechanisms of energy coupling for the shock-sensitive and shock-resistant amino acid permeases of *Escherichia coli*. J Biol Chem 1974; 249:7747–7755.

34. Rosen BP. ATP coupled solute transport systems. In: Ingraham J, Low KB, Magasanik B, Neidhardt FC, Schaechter M, Umbarger HE, eds. *Escherichia coli* and *Salmonella typhimurium*: Cellular and Molecular Biology. Washington: American Society for Microbiology, 1987:760–767.

35. Callahan R, Riordan JR. Synthetic and natural opiates interact with P-glycoprotein in multidrug-resistant cells. J Biol Chem 1993; 268:16059–16064.

36. Rosen BP, McClees JS. Active transport of calcium in inverted membrane vesicles of *Escherichia coli*. Proc Natl Acad Sci USA 1974; 71:5042–5046.

37. Marin R, Proverbio T, Proverbio F. Inside-out basolateral plasma membrane vesicles from rat kidney proximal tubular cells. Biochim Biophys Acta 1986; 858:195–201.

38. Lever JE. Active amino acid transport in plasma membrane vesicles from Simian virus 40-transformed mouse fibroblast. J Biol Chem 1977; 252:1990–1997.
39. Maloney PC, Ambudkar SV. Functional reconstitution of prokaryote and eukaryote membrane proteins. Arch Biochem Biophys 1989; 269:1–10.
40. Venkateswaran PS, Wu HC. Isolation and characterization of a phosphonomycin-resistant mutant of *Escherichia coli* K-12. J Bacteriol 1972; 110:935–944.
41. Guilfoile PG, Hutchinson CR. A bacterial analog of the *mdr* gene of mammalian tumor cells is present in the producer of daunorubicin and doxorubicin. Proc Natl Acad Sci USA 91; 88:8553–8557.
42. Rosteck PR, Reynolds PA, Hershberger CL. Homology between proteins controlling *Streptomyces fradiae* tylosin resistance and ATP-binding transport. Gene 1991; 102:27–32.
43. George AM, Levy SB. Amplifiable resistance to tetracycline, chloramphenicol, and other antibiotics in *Escherichia coli*: involvement of a non-plasmid determinant efflux of tetracycline. J Bacteriol 1983; 155:531–540.
44. Lomovskaya O, Lewis K. *emr*, an *Escherichia coli* locus for multidrug resistance. Proc Natl Acad Sci USA 1992; 89:8938–8942.
45. Neyfakh AA, Bidnenko VE, Chen LB. Efflux-mediated multidrug resistance in bacteria: similarities and dissimilarities with the mammalian system. Proc Natl Acad Sci USA 1991; 88:4781–4785.
46. Ubukata K, Ito-Yamashita N, Konno M. Cloning and expression of the *norA* gene for fluoroquinolone resistance in *Staphylococcus aureus*. Antimicrob Agents Chemother 1989; 33:1535–1539.
47. Grinius L, Dreguniene G, Goldberg EB, Liao CH, Projan SJ. A staphylococcal multidrug resistance gene product is a member of a new protein family. Plasmid 1992; 27:119–129.
48. Lewis K. Multidrug resistance pumps in bacteria: variations on a theme. Trends Biochem Sci 1994; 19:119–123.
49. Levy SB, McMurry L. Plasmid-mediated tetracycline resistance involves alternative transport systems for tetracycline. Nature 1978; 276:90–92.
50. Bell PR, Shales SW, Chopra I. Plasmid mediated tetracycline resistance in *Escherichia coli* involves in increased efflux of the antibiotic. Biochem Biophys Res Commun 1980; 93:74–81.
51. Izaki K, Arima K. Disappearance of oxytetracycline accumulation in the cells of multiple drug-resistant *Escherichia coli*. Nature 1963; 200:384–385.
52. Levy SB, Evolution and spread of tetracycline resistance determinants. J Antimicrob Chemother 1989; 241:1–3.
53. Levy SB, McMurry L. Detection of an inducible membrane protein associated with R-factor mediated tetracycline resistance. Biochem Biophys Res Commun 1974; 56:1060–1068.
54. Eckert B, Beck CF. Topology of the transposon *Tn10*-encoded tetracycline resistance protein within the inner membrane of *Escherichia coli*. J Biol Chem 1989; 264:11663–11670.
55. Rubin RA, Levy SB, Heinrickson RL, Kezdy FS. Gene duplication in the

evolution of the two complementing domains of gram-negative tetracycline efflux proteins. Gene 1990; 87:7–13.

56. Coleman DC, Chopra I, Shales SW, Hawe TGB, Foster TJ. Analysis of tetracycline resistance encoded by transposon *Tn10*: deletion mapping of tetracycline-sensitive point mutations and identification of two structural genes. J Bacteriol 1983; 153:921–929.

57. Curiale M, Levy SB. Two complementation groups mediated tetracycline resistance determined by *Tn10*. J Bacteriol 1982; 151:209–215.

58. Curiale M, McMurry LM, Levy SB. Intracistronic complementation of the tetracycline resistance membrane protein specified by *Tn10*. J Bacteriol 1984; 157:211–217.

59. Hickman R, Levy SB. Evidence that Tet protein functions as a multimer in the inner membrane of *Escherichia coli*. J Bacteriol 1988; 17:1715–1720.

60. Rubin RA, Levy SB. Interdomain hybrid Tet proteins confer tetracycline resistance only when derived from more closely related members of the *tet* gene family. J Bacteriol 1990; 172:2303–2312.

61. Yamaguchi A, Udagawa T, Sawai T. Transport of divalent cation as mediated transposon *Tn10*-encoded tetracycline resistance protein. J Biol Chem 1990; 265:4809–4813.

62. Kaneko M, Yamaguchi A, Sawai T. Energetics of tetracycline efflux encoded by *Tn10* in *Escherichia coli*. FEBS Lett 1985; 193:194–198.

63. McMurry L, Petrucci RE, Levy SB. Active efflux of tetracycline encoded by four genetically different tetracycline resistance determinants in *Escherichia coli*. Proc Natl Acad USA 1990; 77:3974–3977.

64. Hoshino T, Ikeda T, Tomizuka N, Furukawa K. Nucleotide sequence of tetracycline resistance gene of pTHT15, a thermophilic *Bacillus* plasmid: comparison with staphylococcal Tc^r controls. Gene 1985; 37:131–138.

65. Ishiwa H, Shibahara H. New shuttle vector for *Escherichia coli* and *Bacillus subtilis*. III. Nucleotide sequence analysis of tetracycline resistance gene of pAMα1 and *ori 177*. Jpn J Genet 1985; 60:485–498.

66. McMurry LM, Aronson DA, Levy SB. Susceptible *Escherichia coli* cells can actively excrete tetracyclines. Antimicrob Agents Chemother 1983; 24:544–551.

67. George AM, Levy SB. Gene in major cotransduction gap of *Escherichia coli* K-12 linkage map required for the expression of chromosomal resistance to tetracycline and other antibiotics. J Bacteriol 1983; 155:541–548.

68. Rouch DA, Cram DS, DiBerardino D, Littlejohn TG, Skurray RA. Efflux-mediated antiseptic resistance gene *qacA* from *Staphylococcus aureus*: common ancestry with tetracycline- and sugar-transport proteins. Mol Microbiol 1990; 4:2051–2062.

69. Kaatz GW, Seo SM, Ruble CA. Mechanism of fluoroquinolone resistance in *Staphylococcus aureus*. J Infect Dis 1991; 163:1080–1086.

70. Yoshida S, Kojima T, Inoue M, Mitsuhashi S. Uptake of sparfloxacin and norfloxacin by clinical isolates of *Staphylococcus aureus*. Antimicrob Agents Chemother 1991; 35:368–370.

71. Yoshida H, Bogaki M, Nakamura S, Ubukata K, Kanno M. Nucleotide

sequence and characterization of the *Staphylococcus aureus norA* gene, which confers resistance to quinolones. J Bacteriol 1990; 172:6942–6949.

72. Oshita Y, Hiramatsu K, Yokota T. A point mutation of *norA* gene is responsible for quinolone resistance in *Staphylococcus aureus*. Biochem Biophys Res Commun 1990; 172:1028–1034.

73. Neyfakh AA. The multidrug efflux transporter of *Bacillus subtilis* is a structural and functional homologue of the *Staphylococcus* NorA protein. Antimicrob Agents Chemother 1992; 36:484–485.

74. Levy SB. Active efflux for antimicrobial resistance. Antimicrob Agents Chemother 1992; 36:695–703.

75. Littlejohn TG, DiBerardino D, Messerotti LJ, Spiers SJ, Skurray RA. Structure and evolution of a family of antiseptic and disinfectant resistance genes in *Staphylococcus aureus*. Gene 1991; 101:59–66.

76. Littlejohn TG, Paulsen IT, Gillepsi MT, Tennent JM, Midgley M, Jones IG, Purewal AS, Skurray RA. Substrate specificity and energetics of antiseptic and disinfectant resistance in *Staphylococcus aureus*. FEMS Microbiol Lett 1992; 95:259–266.

77. Felmlee T, Pellett S, Lee EY, Welch RA. *Escherichia coli* hemolysin is released extracellularly without cleavage of a signal peptide. J Bacteriol 1985; 163:88–93.

78. Furukawa H, Tsay JT, Jackowski S, Takamura Y, Rock CO. Thiolactomycin resistance in *Escherichia coli* is associated with the multidrug resistance efflux pump encoded by *emrAB*. J Bacteriol 1993; 175:3723–3729.

79. Hedges RW, Baumberg S. Resistance to arsenic compounds conferred by a plasmid transmissible between strains of *Escherichia coli*. J Bacteriol 1973; 115:459–460.

80. Chen CM, Misra T, Silver S, Rosen BP. Nucleotide sequence of the structural genes for an anion pump: the plasmid-encoded arsenical resistance operon. J Biol Chem 1986; 261:15030–15038.

81. San Francisco MJD, Hope CL, Owolabi JB, Tisa LS, Rosen BP. Identification of the metalloregulatory element of the plasmid-encoded arsenical resistance operon. Nucleic Acids Res 1990; 18:619–624.

82. Wu JH, Rosen BP. Metalloregulated expression of the *ars* operon. J Biol Chem 1993; 268:52–58.

83. Wu J, Rosen BP. The *arsD* gene encodes a second *trans*-acting regulatory protein of the plasmid-encoded arsenical resistance operon. Mol Microbiol 1993; 8:615–623.

84. Mobley HLT, Rosen BP. Energetics of plasmid-mediated arsenate resistance in *Escherichia coli*. Proc Natl Acad Sci USA 1982; 79:6119–6122.

85. Rosen BP, Borbolla MG. A plasmid-encoded arsenite pump produces arsenite resistance in *Escherichia coli*. Biochem Biophys Res Commun 1984; 124:760–765.

86. Chen CM, Mobley, HLT, Rosen BP. Separate resistances to arsenate and arsenite (antimonate) encoded by the arsenical resistance operon of R-factor R773. J Bacteriol 1985; 161:758–763.

87. Ji G, Silver S. Reduction of arsenate to arsenite by the ArsC protein of the

arsenic resistance operon of the *Staphylococcus aureus* plasmid pI258. Proc Natl Acad Sci USA 1992; 89:9474–9478.

88. Oden KL, Gladysheva TB, Rosen BP. Arsenate reduction mediated by the plasmid-encoded ArsC protein is coupled to glutathione. Mol Microbiol 1994; 12:301–306.

89. Rosen BP, Weigel W, Karkaria C, Gangola P. Molecular characterization of an anion pump. The *arsA* gene product is an arsenite (antimonate)-stimulated ATPase. J Biol Chem 1988; 263:3067–3070.

90. Hsu CM, Rosen BP. Characterization of the catalytic subunit of an anion pump. J Biol Chem 1989; 264:17349–17354.

91. Karkaria CE, Chen CM, Rosen BP. Mutagenesis of a nucleotide binding site of an anion-translocating ATPase. J Biol Chem 1990; 265:7832–7836.

92. Kaur P, Rosen BP. Mutagenesis of the second putative nucleotide binding site of an anion-translocating ATPase. J Biol Chem 1992; 267:19272–19277.

93. Hsu CM, Kaur P, Karkaria, CE, Steiner RF, Rosen BP. Substrate-induced dimerization of the ArsA protein, the catalytic component of an anion-translocating ATPase. J Biol Chem 1991; 266:2327–2332.

94. Kaur P, Rosen BP. Complementation between nucleotide binding domains in an anion translocating ATPase. J Bacteriol 1993; 175:351–357.

95. Ksenzenko MY, Kessel DH, Rosen BP. Reaction of the ArsA ATPase with 2-(4′-maleimidylanilino)naphthalene-6-sulfonate. Biochemistry 1993; 32:13362–13368.

96. Kaur P, Rosen BP. In vitro assembly of an anion-stimulated ATPase from peptide fragments. J Biol Chem 1994; 269:9698–9704.

97. San Francisco MJD, Tisa LS, Rosen BP. Identification of the membrane component of the anion pump encoded by the arsenical resistance operon of R-factor R773. Mol Microbiol 1989; 3:15–21.

98. Wu JH, Tisa LS, Rosen BP. Membrane topology of the ArsB protein, the membrane component of an anion-translocating ATPase. J Biol Chem 1992; 267:12570–12576.

99. Tisa LS, Rosen BP. Molecular characterization of an anion pump: the ArsB protein is the membrane anchor for the ArsA protein. J Biol Chem 1990; 265:190–194.

100. Dey S, Dou D, Tisa LS, Rosen BP. Interaction between the catalytic and the membrane components of an anion-translocating ATPase. Arch Biochem Biophys 1994; 311:418–424.

101. Dou D, Owolabi JB, Dey S, Rosen BP. Construction of a chimeric ArsA–ArsB protein for overexpression of the oxyanion-translocating ATPase. J Biol Chem 1992; 267:25768–25775.

101a. Dey S, Dou D, Rosen BP. ATP-dependent transport in everted membrane vesicles of *Escherichia coli*. J Biol Chem 1994; 269:25442–25446.

101b. Gladysheva TB, Oden KL, Rosen BP. Properties of the arsenate reductase of plasmid R773. Biochem 1994; 33:7287–7293.

102. Rosen BP, Dey S, Dou D, Ji G, Kaur P, Ksenzenko M, Silver S, Wu J. Evolution of an ion-translocating ATPase. Ann NY Acad Sci 1992; 671:257–272.

103. Ji G, Silver S. Regulation and expression of the arsenic resistance operon from *Staphylococcus aureus* plasmid pI258. J Bacteriol 1992; 174:3684–3694.

104. Rosenstein R, Peschel P, Wieland B, Götz F. Expression and regulation of the *Staphylococcus xylosus* antimonite, arsenite and arsenite resistance operon. J Bacteriol 1992; 174:3676–3683.

104a. Dey S, Rosen BP. Dual mode of energy coupling by the oxyanion-translocating Ars B protein. J Bacteriol 1995 (in press).

105. Fojo A, Akiyama S, Gottesman MM, Pastan I. Reduced drug accumulation in multiply drug-resistant human KB carcinoma cell lines. Cancer Res 1985; 45:3002–3007.

106. Chen CJ, Chin JE, Ueda K, Clark DP, Pastan I, Gottesman, MM, Roninson IB. Internal duplication and homology with bacterial transport proteins in the *MDR1* (P-glycoprotein) gene from multidrug-resistant human cells. Cell 1986; 47:381–389.

107. Roninson IB, Chin JE, Gros P, Housman DE, Fojo A. Isolation of human *MDR* DNA sequences amplified in multidrug-resistant KB carcinoma cells. Proc Natl Acad Sci USA 1986; 83:4538–4542.

108. Hsu SI, Lothstein L, Horwitz SB. Differential overexpression of three *MDR* gene family members in multidrug-resistant J774.2 mouse cells. Evidence that distinct P-glycoprotein precursors are encoded by unique *MDR* genes. J Biol Chem 1989; 264:12053–12062.

109. Yoshimura A, Kuwazura Y, Sumizawa T, Ichikawa M, Ikeda S, Uda T, Akiyama S. Cytoplasmic orientation and two-domain structure of the multidrug transporter, P-glycoprotein, demonstrated with sequence specific antibodies. J Biol Chem 1989; 264:16282–16291.

110. Zhang JT, Ling V. Study of membrane orientation and glycosylated extracellular loops of mouse P-glycoprotein by in vitro translation. J Biol Chem 1991; 266:18224–18232.

111. Higgins CF, Hiles ID, Whalley K, Jamieson DJ. Nucleotide binding by membrane components of bacterial periplasmic binding protein-dependent transport systems. EMBO J 1985; 4:1033–1039.

112. Wilson CM, Serrano AE, Wasley A, Bogenschutz MP, Shankar AH, Wirth DF. Amplification of a gene related to mammalian *mdr* genes in drug-resistant *Plasmodium falciparum*. Science 1989; 244:1184–1186.

113. Foote SJ, Kyle DE, Marin RK, Oduola AM, Forsyth K, Kemp DJ, Coman AF. Several alleles of multidrug-resistance gene are closely linked to chloroquine resistance in *Plasmodium falciparum*. Nature 1990; 345:55–258.

114. Kuchler K, Stern RE, Thorner J. *Saccharomyces cerevisiae STE6* gene product: a novel pathway for export in eukaryotic cells. EMBO J 1989; 8:3973–3984.

115. McGrath JP, Varshavsky A. The yeast *STE6* gene encodes a homologue of the mammalian multidrug resistance P-glycoprotein. Nature 1989; 340:400–404.

116. Kamijo K, Taketani S, Yokota S, Osumi T, Hashimoto T. The 70-kDa

peroxisomal membrane protein is a member of *MDR* (P-glycoprotein)-related ATP-binding protein superfamily. J Biol Chem 1990; 265:4534–4540.

117. Berman JD. Chemotherapy for leishmaniasis: biochemical mechanisms, clinical efficacy and future strategies. Rev Infect Dis 1988; 10:560–586.

118. Croft SL, Neame KD, Homewood CA. Accumulation of [^{125}Sb]sodium stibogluconate by *Leishmania mexicana amazonensis* and *Leishmania donovani* in vitro. Comp Biochem Physiol 1981; 68C:95–98.

119. Callahan HL, Beverley SM. Heavy metal resistance: a new role for P-glycoprotein in *Leishmania*. J Biol Chem 1991; 266:18427–18430.

120. Grogl M, Martin RK, Oduola AJ, Milhous WK, Kyle DE. Characteristics of multidrug resistance in *Plasmodium* and *Leishmania*: detection of P-glycoprotein-like components. Am J Med Hyg 1991; 45:98–111.

121. Grondin K, Papadopoulou B, Oullette M. Homologous recombination between between direct repeat sequences yields P-glycoprotein containing amplicons in arsenite resistant *Leishmania*. Nucleic Acids Res 1993; 21:1895–1901.

122. Papadopoulou B, Roy G, Dey S, Rosen BP, Ouellette M. Contribution of *Leishmania* P-glycoprotein related gene *ltpgpA* to oxyanion resistance. J Biol Chem 1994; 269:11980–11986.

123. Wang Z, Rossman TG. Stable and inducible arsenite resistance in Chinese hamster cells. Toxicol Appl Pharmacol 1993; 118:80–86.

124. Lo JF, Wang HF, Tam MF, Lee TC. Glutathione *S*-transferase pi in an arsenic-resistant Chinese hamster ovary cell line. Biochem J 1992; 288:977–982.

125. Wang HF, Lee TC. Glutathione *S*-transferase facilitates the excretion of arsenic from arsenic-resistant Chinese hamster ovary cells. Biochem Biophys Res Commun 1993; 192:1093–1099.

126. Gyurasics A, Varga F, Gregus Z. Glutathione-dependent biliary excretion of arsenic. Biochem Pharmacol 1991; 42:465–468.

127. Ishikawa T. ATP-dependent glutathione π *S*–conjugate export pump. Trends Biochem Sci 192; 17:463–468.

128. Mevarech M, Rice D, Haselkorn R. Nucleotide sequence of a cyanobacterial *nifH* gene coding for nitrogenase reductase. Proc Natl Acad Sci USA 1980; 77:6476–6480.

129. de Boer PAJ, Crossley RE, Rothfield LI. A division inhibitor and a topological specificity factor encoded for by the minicell locus determine proper placement of the division septum in *Escherichia coli*. Cell 1989; 56:641–649.

130. Brusilow W. Assembly of *Escherichia coli* F_0F_1 ATPase, a large multimeric membrane-bound enzyme. Mol Microbiol 1993; 9:419–424.

131. Futai F, Noumi T, Maeda M. ATP synthase (H^+-ATPase): results by combined biochemical and molecular biological approaches. Annu Rev Biochem 1989; 58:111–136.

132. Senior AE. The proton-translocating ATPase of *Escherichia coli*. Annu Rev Biophys Biophys Chem 1990; 19:7–41.

133. Reizer J, Reizer A, Saier MH. A new subfamily of bacterial ABC-type transport systems catalyzing export of drugs and carbohydrate. Protein Sci 1992; 1:1326–1332.
134. Fath JM, Kotler R. ABC transporters: bacterial exporters. Microbiol Rev 1993; 57:995–1017.
135. Shuman HA, Panagiotidis CH. Tinkering with transporters: periplasmic binding protein-dependent maltose transport in *E. coli*. J Biomembr Bioenerg 1993; 25:613–620.
136. Kerppola RE, Ames GF. Topology of the hydrophobic membrane-bound components of the histidine periplasmic permeases. Comparison with other members of the family. J Biol Chem 1992; 267:2329–2336.
137. Saier, M.H. Computer-aided analysis of transport protein sequences: gleaning evidence concerning function, structure, biogenesis and evolution. Microbiol Rev 1994; 58:71–93.

5

β-Lactam Permeation

Karen Bush
Lederle Laboratories, Pearl River, New York

I. INTRODUCTION

A. β-Lactam Antibiotics: Structures and Physical Properties

1. Overview

β-Lactam antibiotics are broad-spectrum, potent, safe, and effective antimicrobial agents that have been used successfully for over 50 years. These agents often represent the first line of therapy for the treatment of bacterial infections. Their antimicrobial activity is based on a combination of factors, including not only the strength of interaction with the target bacterial proteins, but the ability to reach the target proteins easily. In this chapter the issue of penetration of β-lactam antibiotics will be discussed in relation to other factors of bacterial physiology that influence the fate of these molecules. This is not meant to be a comprehensive review of the literature on permeability of β-lactams through porins, as that has been covered in several excellent review articles (1–3). Nor will it cover transport of antibiotics into cytoplasmic bacterial targets, a topic covered in this book and other recent reviews (4,5). Instead, an overview of β-lactam permeation will be provided, focusing on the more recently described transport mechanisms involving some of the newer β-lactam antibiotics.

2. Structures of β-Lactam Antibiotics

All β-lactam antibiotics contain a common four-membered azetidinone ring that is capable of acylating an active-site serine residue in target proteins. Four fundamental structures found in β-lactam-containing antimicrobial agents are shown in Figure 1. These include the bicyclic penicillins, cephalosporins, and carbapenems, and the monocyclic monobactams. Structures are shown for representative antibiotics in each of these classes, including structures for many agents described in this chapter.

3. Physical Properties

Most β-lactam antimicrobial agents have relative molecular masses (M_r) in the range of 350–500 Da, although some of the more complex structures can approach sizes of 700–800 Da. These molecules differ considerably in their charges, a factor that affects their penetrability properties. The penicillin piperacillin and many cephalosporins, including cefazolin, cefoxitin, and cefotaxime, are monoanionic. Cephaloridine, imipenem, ampicillin, and the new cephalosporins, cefepime and cefpirome, exist in a zwitterionic form. Compounds with two negative and one positive charge include cefsulodin and ceftazidime. A final class of structures are dianionic and include ceftriaxone, carbenicillin, and the monobactam aztreonam. Many of these structures are shown in Figure 1.

B. Cellular Architecture: Gram-Positive and Gram-Negative Bacteria

1. Cell Wall Structure

All bacteria, with the exception of the *Archaeobacteria*, contain a peptidoglycan layer that surrounds and protects the cytoplasmic membrane (6). This peptidoglycan layer, known as the cell wall, is a network structure composed of similar building blocks, but with different cross-linking moieties among the bacteria (see Refs. 7,8). Alternate residues of β(1-4)-*N*-acetylglucosamine and *N*-acetylmuramic acid pyranoside are linked through the D-lactate of *N*-acetylmuramic acid with a tetrapeptide of the structure L-Ala-D-Glu-L-Xaa-D-Ala, for which Xaa is often a diamino acid (9). Cross-linking varies extensively, with 30–50% of the peptidoglycans cross-linked in gram-negative bacteria and bacilli, but with almost complete cross-linking in some strains of *Staphylococcus aureus* (6,10). Gram-positive bacteria contain a cell wall that is almost completely accessible to the environment, whereas gram-negative bacteria are covered by an outer membrane that acts an efficient sieve in allowing nutrients to enter the cell. In the following sections a brief description of the exterior bacterial architecture will be presented, particularly as related to permeation of β-lactam antibiotics.

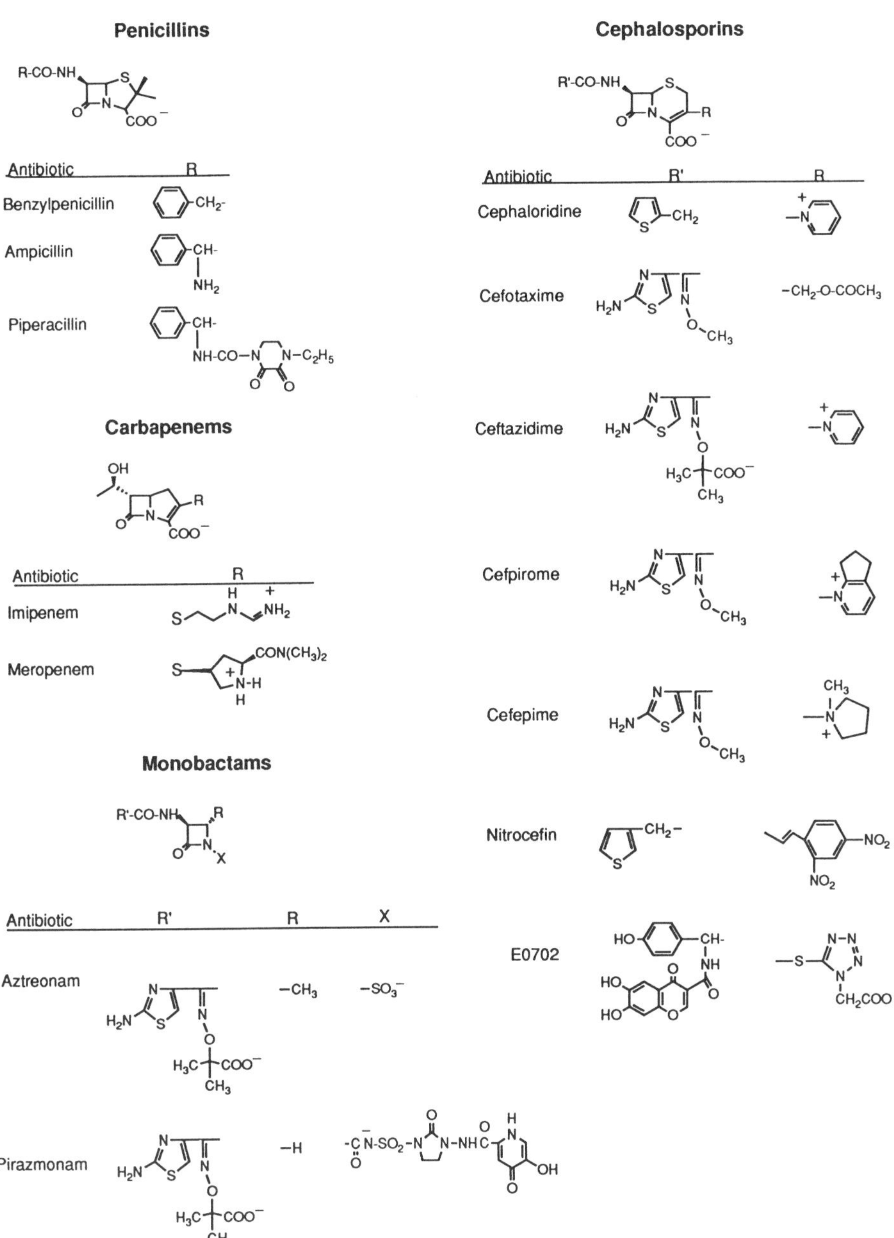

Figure 1 Structures of selected β-lactam antibiotics.

2. *Gram-Positive Bacteria*

Gram-positive bacteria are surrounded by capsular material external to the cell wall. However, the material is quite permeable and represents no significant barrier to the entry of molecules with M_r as high as 14,400, such as lysozyme. Although it is possible that electrostatic attractions or repulsions may affect the passage of antimicrobial agents through both the capsule and the cell wall, these effects are usually not considered to be significant (5).

Two major components are found in gram-positive cell walls, peptidoglycan and (lipo-)teichoic acids. A schematic representation of the cell wall is shown in Figure 2. Teichoic acids are polymers of either substituted glycerol phosphate or ribitol phosphate. They are found only in gram-positive bacteria and are major antigenic determinants on the cell surface. Peptidoglycan is the main structural component, accounting for as much as 80% of the total weight of the wall (6). The exact structure of the peptidoglycan relative to the substitutions and cross-linking of the glycan chains is quite varied and depends on the particular strain or on growth conditions. (For reviews of possible structural variations see Refs. 6,7.)

In gram-positive organisms the wall is relatively thick (11), with a high degree of cross-linking by peptide bridges between the strands of peptidoglycan. However, the walls are quite permeable and allow most large molecules to enter. In bacilli, exclusion limits as high as 60,000 have been reported (12). As a result, almost all antimicrobial agents encounter no barrier until they reach the cytoplasmic membrane. The peptidoglycan serves as a protective, but permeable, layer for the cell wall-synthesizing

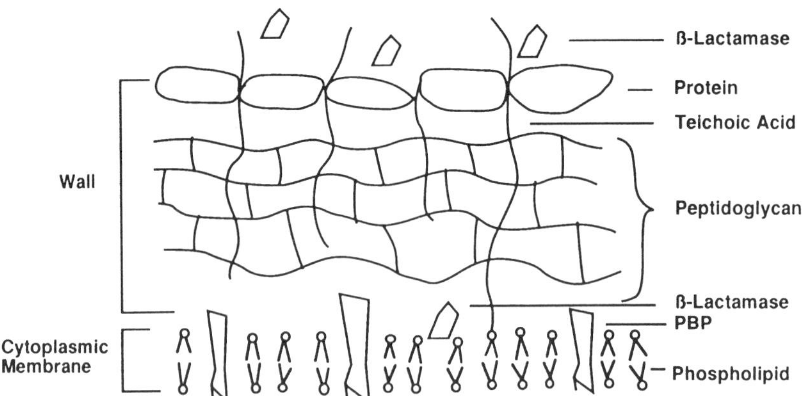

Figure 2 Structure of the cell wall of a gram-positive bacterium.

enzymes (penicillin-binding proteins; PBPs) tethered to the cytoplasmic membrane. The hydrolytic *β*-lactamases, discussed later, are often excreted into the medium, although membrane-bound forms have been identified (13,14).

Mycobacteria provide an exception to the open access found in most gram-positive bacteria. These important pathogens have a distinctive cell wall, composed of a thick peptidoglycan layer covalently linked to arabinogalactan polysaccharides that are esterified to branched, long-chain mycolic acids (15). This lipid layer provides an effective permeability barrier, similar to the outer membrane of gram-negative bacteria (16). As a result, mycobacteria are often resistant to most antibiotics (see Chap. 9).

3.   *Gram-Negative Bacteria*

A much more interesting picture of cellular architecture is provided by the gram-negative bacteria (Fig. 3). In addition to the surface-associated "enterobacterial common antigen" (17), an outer membrane structure has been added to regulate the entry of external molecules into the cell. In these organisms the peptidoglycan cell wall layer that is attached to the outer membrane is less pronounced, and the outer membrane has become the dominant feature. Several excellent review articles have been written to describe the outer membrane of gram-negative bacteria (2,3,17–20). Between the peptidoglycan layer and the cytoplasmic membrane lies the periplasmic space, which is the residence for most of the *β*-lactamases found in gram-negative bacteria. As in the gram-positive bacteria, the PBPs are attached to the cytoplasmic membrane and extend into the per-

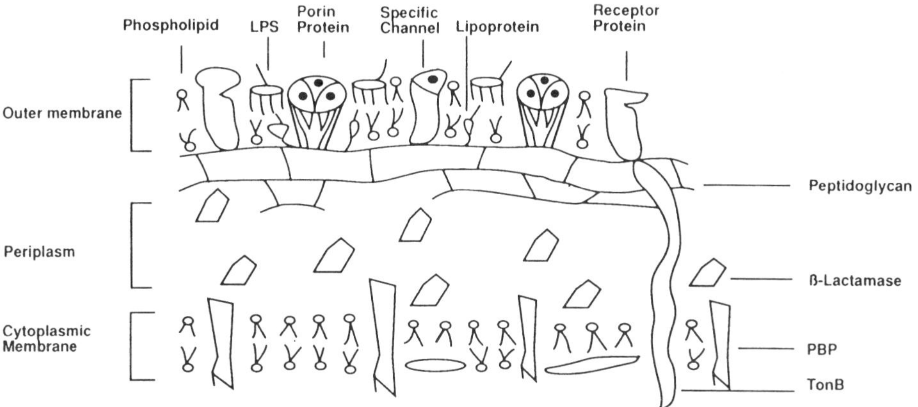

Figure 3   Structure of the cell wall of a gram-negative bacterium.

iplasm. Thus, β-lactam antibiotics need only to traverse the outer membrane to gain access to their target proteins.

The outer membrane is an asymmetrical structure, primarily composed of lipopolysaccharides (LPS), outer membrane proteins, and phospholipids. The LPS that is found on the exterior of the outer membrane exhibits considerable heterogeneity and is involved in determination of the antigenic properties of the bacteria. Phospholipids are usually segregated into the inner leaflet of the outer membrane, except in certain LPS mutants for which increased amounts of phospholipids are found on the outer leaflet (3). On the exterior surface of the outer membrane are located a variety of receptor proteins. Those involved in iron transport have been of particular interest in the development of new classes of β-lactam antibiotics.

It is the outer membrane proteins that are of greatest interest when transport of antimicrobial agents is considered. Within the outer membrane are nonspecific protein channels that act as conduits for nutrients and other small molecules that enter the cell (17). In *Escherichia coli* these porins exist as trimeric protein structures that form three separate transmembrane channels at the cell surface and merge into a single channel opening into the periplasmic space (21). Although the channels have been proposed by some researchers to exist in either an open or closed conformation through a voltage-gating mechanism, this may simply be a laboratory phenomenon, with little relevance to a clinically resistant bacterium (20). Because the porin channels provide the primary access route for β-lactam antibiotics, these proteins have been studied in great detail and their properties delineated in several of the review articles, cited previously (see also Refs. 22,23). Of special interest to readers of this book should be the recent review by Nikaido and Saier, who compared the properties of bacterial transport proteins with those of homologous proteins in eukaryotic cells (24).

A secondary uptake role has been suggested for the phospholipid bilayer of the outer membrane (25). A combination of charge and hydrophilicity may allow hydrophilic molecules to pass through this hydrophobic barrier. This mechanism may explain why antibiotics, such as ampicillin, retain a low level of antimicrobial activity in porin mutants.

C. β-Lactam Activities: Targets and Antimicrobial Activity

1. Penicillin-Binding Proteins

Penicillin-binding proteins (PBPs) are cell wall-synthesizing enzymes that are involved in the final stage of cell wall synthesis (26). Bacteria often contain multiple PBPs, several of which are essential bifunctional enzymes, with transglycosylase and transpeptidase activities (27,28). All PBPs that have yet been sequenced contain a conserved Ser-X-X-Lys motif, including the active site serine that can become acylated after interaction with a β-lactam (29–33). Penicillin has been considered as a peptide analogue for the substrate used in the final stage of cell wall synthesis (34). This proposal was based on the structural similarity of penicillin to acyl-D-alanyl-D-alanine, the terminal amino acids in the linear glycopeptide that is eventually cross-linked to form the cell wall. Other β-lactam-containing molecules may play similar roles.

The NH_2-termini of the PBPs in *E. coli* are anchored to the outer surface of the cytoplasmic membrane of the bacterial cell, such that the active sites of the enzymes are facing the periplasm (33,35,36). Cell wall synthesis that is initiated by export of precursors from the cytoplasm is completed either in the periplasm of gram-negative bacteria, or at the exterior surface of the inner membrane of gram-positive organisms. Interactions of β-lactam antibiotics with PBPs of gram-positive bacteria occur in a virtual barrier-free environment, as there is essentially free access of the antibiotic to the cell wall-synthesizing enzymes. However, access of β-lactams to PBPs in gram-negative organisms is restricted by the presence of the outer membrane. Uptake is dependent on the ease with which the antimicrobial agent can cross the outer membrane. Importantly, in both gram-negative and gram-positive organisms, transport across the cytoplasmic membrane is not required, thereby providing an advantage for the β-lactam class of antibiotics, when compared with protein or nucleic acid synthesis inhibitors that have targets in the cytoplasm.

Bacteria often produce a family of PBPs with varied capacities for binding β-lactams (37,38). In *E. coli*, four essential PBPs have been identified: PBPs 1A and 1B involved in cell elongation; PBP 2, the function of which is related to cell shape; and PBP 3, the cell wall-synthesizing enzyme responsible for septation. Monobactams and many cephalosporins have very tight binding to PBP 3 in *E. coli* (39–41), with filamentation being the initial response of the cell to β-lactams. However, there is also weaker, but significant, binding to the bifunctional PBPs 1A and 1B, eventually causing lysis of the organism. Carbapenems have very tight binding to PBP 2 in *E. coli* and other enteric bacteria (42,43). Although this interaction initially results in the formation of spherical cells, lysis subsequently occurs owing to additional binding to PBPs 1A or 1B, or both (43).

2. Antimicrobial Activity

As a group, the β-lactam antibiotics exhibit a broad spectrum of activity, with intrinsic resistance seen for only a few species of bacteria, notably

Enterococcus faecalis and mycobacteria. Most bacteria possess essential cell wall-synthesizing enzymes with high affinities for β-lactams. Interactions of a specific antibiotic with homologous wall-synthesizing enzymes in different organisms may not be easily predicted, however, resulting in a different spectrum of activity for closely related β-lactam antibiotics.

Penicillins have good antimicrobial activity against gram-positive aerobes and less activity against the gram-negative enteric bacteria. A group of semisynthetic, extended-spectrum penicillins, including piperacillin and ticarcillin, have been used to treat infections stemming from *Pseudomonas aeruginosa*; these agents also have good activity against gram-positive aerobes, and enhanced activity against enteric bacteria and anaerobes (44,45). If a β-lactam-hydrolyzing enzyme is present, most penicillins cannot be used effectively against β-lactamase-producing organisms.

Cephalosporins have been classified into "generations" of development, depending on stability to β-lactamase hydrolysis and spectrum of activity (45). The early cephalosporins had better activity against gram-positive aerobes than the later molecules, but had poor activity against the gram-negative enteric bacteria. The second- and third-generation cephalosporins exhibit improved activity against gram-negative organisms. Generally, cephalosporins are not particularly effective against *Bacteroides* spp. Monobactams have excellent targeted activity against the gram-negative enteric bacteria, but generally have no activity against gram-positive or anaerobic organisms (46). These monocyclic agents, members of the group of extended-spectrum β-lactam antibiotics, are stable to hydrolysis by many of the common chromosomally and plasmid-mediated β-lactamases.

Carbapenems, such as imipenem, meropenem, and biapenem, have the broadest range of antimicrobial activity of any of the β-lactams commercially available (47). Representatives of almost all bacteria that are susceptible to a β-lactam antibiotic can be eradicated with a carbapenem. Intrinsic resistance is seen only with those organisms that produce a carbapenem-hydrolyzing β-lactamase or a modified PBP. Currently, the occurrence of these groups of enzymes is rare (48). An exception is the methicillin-resistant staphylococci that produce a PBP with low affinity for β-lactams and are common infectious agents in some hospitals.

Antimicrobial activity of the β-lactams is dependent not only on the affinity of the target for the antibiotic, but also on the presence of the β-lactam-hydrolyzing enzymes, known as β-lactamases. As a result, combinations of β-lactams have been developed, with the purpose of protecting a labile penicillin with the addition of a β-lactamase inhibitor. Four of these combinations are now available for the treatment of β-lactamase-producing strains with intrinsic susceptibility to *β*-lactam antibiotics. Clavulanic acid has been combined with amoxicillin or ticarcillin, sulbactam is combined with ampicillin, and tazobactam has been added to piperacillin. Each of these inhibitors serves to inactivate a range of *β*-lactamases produced by a variety of bacteria (49,50).

II. MEASUREMENT OF *β*-LACTAM PERMEATION

A. Assay Techniques

Permeation of *β*-lactam antibiotics into gram-negative bacteria can be measured using a variety of analytical techniques. Two principal approaches involve either the use of intact cells, or the use of reconstituted membrane vesicles. Because the intrinsic uptake of these agents is very rapid, and only small amounts of antibiotic are measured, various tricks have been employed to obtain reliable data. The use of *β*-lactamase-mediated hydrolysis to measure a steady-state uptake of drug in intact cells is the most widely used method, but requires that the antibiotic be hydrolyzable by a well-behaved enzyme. The principal methods in the literature and their limitations are described in the following sections.

1. Radiochemical

Uptake of radiolabeled non–*β*-lactam compounds into suspended intact cells has been used to determine the molecular-sieving properties of the outer membrane (1). In this method, resuspended cells are equilibrated with the radiolabeled molecule in question, and supernatants are analyzed for radioactivity after centrifugation. It is also possible to perform these studies using cells in logarithmic growth that are treated with radioactively labeled antibiotic and then filter the cells for a more rapid determination. Uptake of ^{14}C-labeled antibiotics into intact cells has been examined using radiolabeled imipenem (51), meropenem (52), pirazmonam (53), Sch 34343, and ceftriaxone (54). For this method to work, a high specific activity of the compound is necessary because of the low permeability of some agents into resistant organisms.

In these assays, precautions must be taken to include all appropriate controls. Uninoculated broth should be incubated with the radiolabeled molecule and carried through all the subsequent separation steps as a negative control. This is especially important when a filtration step is included, as many filters can bind the radiolabeled molecule nonspecifically.

2. β-Lactamase Assays

One of the simplest assays in principle is to follow the presence, or loss, of a β-lactam spectrophotometrically. Most recently introduced cephalosporins (55) and carbapenems (56) have molar extinction coefficients greater than 5000 in the ultraviolet (UV) range for the difference spectrum observed between hydrolyzed and intact molecule. The chromogenic cephalosporin nitrocefin has a molar extinction coefficient of 14,000 at 495 nm, thereby eliminating low-level UV background absorbance in the measurements (57). Moreover, β-lactamases are highly efficient enzymes, with catalytic efficiencies approaching those for a diffusion-controlled reaction (58). Permeation of β-lactams into β-lactamase-producing organisms has been conveniently studied because of the versatility of these enzymes. It is possible to choose an organism producing a β-lactamase with a broad substrate specificity and high catalytic activity to examine the characteristics of a wide range of antibiotics. Because only a small amount of substrate (5–10 μM for cephalosporins and carbapenems) is needed to elicit a spectral response, assays based on the hydrolysis of a β-lactam are exceedingly attractive. These assays can be done in intact cells, provided all the appropriate conditions prevail (see Sec. II.B).

3. High-Performance Liquid Chromatography

High-performance liquid chromatography (HPLC) is a technique recently introduced into the β-lactam permeation arena (59). Analysis of β-lactams by HPLC has been used for many years to identify novel antibiotics and to analyze reactions after treatment of novel β-lactam molecules with β-lactamases (55,60). With the use of modern spectrophotometric detection systems, HPLC allows the intact β-lactam to be identified by both its chromatographic characteristics and its UV spectrum. Quantitation is easily accomplished from standard curves of the intact molecule. Thus, the amount of β-lactam present in a bacterial suspension can be evaluated simply by filtering the culture and analyzing the supernatant for the loss of β-lactam.

Limitations of this assay procedure include problems associated with kinetic measurements, as one cannot precisely measure when a reaction is terminated. In these assays, it is also essential to know the spectral and elution characteristics of the intact β-lactam, compared with the ring-opened molecule. Some hydrolyzed β-lactam antibiotics retain significant absorbance at the wavelength used to detect the parent β-lactam. The elution system used for analysis, therefore, must be able to separate the two components. When bacterial cultures are analyzed, it is also essential to test uninoculated broths and culture supernatants in the absence of antibiotic to determine whether there is background interference with the β-lactam-associated absorbance peaks of interest.

B. Diffusion Steady-State Model in Intact Cells

Measurement of permeability of β-lactams into intact cells was described in a classic paper by Zimmermann and Rosselet (61) and is used as the basis for permeability assays in many laboratories. A similar method was also described by Sawai et al. in 1977 (62). These methods assume that the outer membrane of gram-negative bacteria acts as a diffusion barrier to antibiotic entry into the organism. In a β-lactamase-producing organism, the kinetic properties of β-lactam hydrolysis can be used to determine the rate of entry across the outer membrane, as a consequence of two principles: first, diffusion across the outer membrane can be described by Fick's law of diffusion; and second, hydrolysis of the β-lactam antibiotic follows Michaelis–Menten kinetics. The initial studies described by Zimmermann and Rosselet were performed in *E. coli* with a broad-spectrum plasmid-mediated TEM β-lactamase in the periplasm. Sawai et al. extended these studies to *Morganella morganii* (62) and *Citrobacter freundii* (63), organisms with chromosomal cephalosporinases.

These assays assume that β-lactams reach the periplasm by passive diffusion, rather than active transport, and cross the outer membrane in a process characterized by a permeability parameter. At a given extracellular antibiotic concentration, a steady state is quickly established at which the rate of antibiotic diffusion and the rate of β-lactam hydrolysis are equal. It is also assumed that the kinetic parameters, K_m and V_{max}, are equal for cellular β-lactamase and for β-lactamase in sonicated cell suspensions. Permeability coefficients (P) can be calculated from the following equation, as modified by Nikaido (61,64):

$$V = P \times A \times (C_o - C_p) = V_{max} \times \frac{C_p}{C_p + K_m}$$

where V is the rate of β-lactam hydrolysis in intact cells; A is the area of cell surface per unit weight [132 cm^2/mg as determined for *Salmonella typhimurium* (65) and assumed to be similar for all enteric gram-negative bacteria]; C_o is the external antibiotic concentration; C_p is the steady-state periplasmic concentration of antibiotic; and K_m and V_{max} are kinetic parameters determined with β-lactamase in unclarified sonicated cell suspensions. Additional modifications of this equation have been made to account for the contribution of surface-associated β-lactamase (66).

Inhibition of β-lactamase activity has also been used to quantitate the amount of an inhibitor present in intact cells by measuring the loss of enzyme activity in the presence of an inhibitor, or a "β-lactamase-stable β-lactam," compared with an uninhibited control (67). The major problem with these assays is that few β-lactamase inhibitors are true inhibitors, but are actually poor substrates (49) and are eventually hydrolyzed. It is also important to know the stoichiometry for inhibition. For inactivators such as clavulanic acid or tazobactam, one must know the partition ratio between hydrolysis and inactivation, as these inhibitors are also hydrolyzed to some extent before a β-lactamase is inactivated (68). When this assay is used in intact cells, timing is extremely critical to be sure that a poor substrate is not hydrolyzed in the time required to extract the enzyme and measure its activity. The method has been used reasonably successfully for aztreonam, a poor substrate, with a half-life of 6.3 h for the cephalosporinase from *Enterobacter cloacae* P99 (69), and for carbapenems, cefoxitin, and cloxacillin in *E. coli*, *Ent. cloacae*, and *Citrobacter freundii* (70).

C. Reconstituted Proteoliposomes

Reconstituted membranes have been used to determine exclusion limits of specific porins or to determine rates of diffusion across the membranes. Membrane vesicles reconstituted from phospholipid, lipopolysaccharide, and porin proteins were first described by Nakae (71) and have been used extensively to study the exclusion properties of a variety of bacterial membrane proteins (72). Although the outer membrane often contains multiple porins, many studies have been carried out using outer membrane proteins from laboratory-generated strains that produce only a single porin, thereby increasing the specificity of the determination. These studies have been most frequently accomplished using strains of *E. coli* K-12 and *Sal. typhimurium* LT2 (73–75).

Early studies using a liposome efflux assay were performed by resuspending dried phospholipid and lipopolysaccharide in the presence and absence of porin proteins. This suspension was briefly sonicated in the presence of radiolabled dextran and radiolabeled substrate, equilibrated, and the vesicles filtered on Sepharose 6B. Retention of substrates was determined by calculating the ratio of substrate to dextran in the vesicle fraction and normalizing these to the ratio in vesicles not containing protein (76). Because of the time frame required to conduct these assays, even slow-diffusing molecules would have the opportunity to efflux out of the vesicles almost completely. These assays, therefore, provided a means of determining substrate specificities and exclusion limits for specific porins.

Reconstituted vesicles containing phospholipid and porin proteins can be used to determine rates of permeation by following liposome swelling. Vesicles with and without protein are suspended in 17% dextran and then diluted into an isotonic solution of test material. Liposome swelling is then measured spectrophotometrically (76), with rates measured over a 20-s period. This method can be used for a variety of molecules, although charged solutes can pose difficulties owing to the creation of membrane potential by differential diffusion of ions (3). Because of the variability in preparations of liposomes, it is important that the same batch of liposomes be used for all comparative assays in a set of data.

D. Comparison of Methods

Permeability measurements using the radiochemical method are limited by the time required to process the labeled cells. Even when cells are filtered, rather than centrifuged, full isotope equilibration is usually completed by the time the supernatant is separated from the intact cells. Nikaido et al. have calculated that the half-equilibration time across the outer membrane is less than 1 s for large molecules, such as disaccharides (64); hence, this method is not recommended for the determination of rate of uptake.

The HPLC methods are ideal for the study of β-lactam molecules that are poorly hydrolyzed by common β-lactamases (59). A major advantage is the ability to analyze low concentrations of antibiotic (e.g., 1–10 μM) that may not be accessible by standard spectrophotometric procedures. Experimental error caused by light scattering of bacterial suspensions in spectrophotometric assays is avoided in the HPLC method. However, this method presents difficulties for determining the rate of initial uptake because of the imprecision of the termination of the reaction.

Permeability measurements of reconstituted membrane vesicles have provided much of the basic information on porin specificity and sieving qualities of the outer membrane proteins. However, these results are immediately questioned because they represent an artificial situation and do not accurately reflect the natural environment of the outer membrane. The liposome efflux assay is not useful for rate measurements, but can provide estimates on the exclusion limits of specific porins. The liposome-swelling assay cannot be readily used with large cationic molecules, a disadvantage for some β-lactam antibiotics. Also, high concentrations of antibiotic (10 mM) must be used, again representing nonphysiological conditions. However, it is useful for the measurement of penetration rates for β-lactamase-stable molecules that cannot be measured using whole-cell assays.

Quantitation of permeability factors with intact cells relies heavily on the Zimmermann–Rosselet method (61), with modifications from Nikaido's laboratory to fine-tune the calculations (64,66). This method has been the most rigorously developed, primarily because of its reliance on data generated from whole-cell assays in which a dynamic steady-state process is evaluated. With the addition of the correction factors to account for surface-associated β-lactamase, this procedure should allow an accurate approximation of permeability parameters. This method, however, is limited because a β-lactam must be hydrolyzed by a periplasmic enzyme at a rate that can be measured in intact cells. Enzymes with a broad-substrate specificity are ideal for this method, although β-lactamase-stable antibiotics are difficult to evaluate, even with an HPLC finish. It was only recently that carbapenems could be studied by this assay (77,78), as these stable molecules defied analysis in intact cells.

III. UPTAKE OF β-LACTAM ANTIBIOTICS

A. Nonspecific Channels: Porins

1. *Physical Description*

Porins are hydrophilic protein channels that serve to transport nutrients across the outer membrane of gram-negative bacteria. Because they are water-filled pores, a variety of small, water-soluble materials can pass through these channels. These outer membrane proteins, generally ranging in apparent molecular size from 35 to 50 kDa, include OmpA, OmpC, OmpF, and PhoE, which are discussed in the following. These proteins are often identified on the basis of their behavior in gel electrophoresis. However, the migration of the protein bands is dependent on the method used to prepare the samples, so that care must be taken in the identification of the outer membrane proteins. For example, OmpF-like proteins run on sodium dodecyl sulfate–polyacrylamide gel electrophoresis (SDS–PAGE) at an apparent higher M_r when solubilized in SDS at low temperature, rather than high temperature (79), owing to retention of the trimeric configuration, whereas OmpA-like proteins run on SDS–PAGE at lower M_r when solubilized at low temperature because their tertiary structure has not been disrupted (80). The positions of *E. coli* OmpC and OmpF proteins are reversed, depending on whether gels are run in the presence or absence of urea. Diameters of the porins have been estimated to be 1.1 nm for the *E. coli* OmpC channel, which is only a bit smaller than the OmpF channel, with an estimated diameter of 1.2 nm (20).

In contrast with the trimeric porins OmpC and OmpF in *E. coli*, OmpA has been described as a monomeric protein that serves to maintain the integrity of the outer membrane and only recently was described as having porin activity, with diffusion rates for arabinose as much as 100-fold lower than that of OmpF (81). Although best studied in *E. coli*, a family of OmpA proteins has been identified in other gram-negative bacteria with sequence homology to the *E. coli* OmpA. Among these are Protein III in *Neisseria gonorrhoeae* (82), Omp P5 of *Haemophilus influenzae* (83), and OprF from *P. aeruginosa* (84). Large differences in pore diameters have been identified within this family, with a diameter of about 1 nm for *E. coli* OmpA, similar to that of OmpC and OmpF, but a much larger diameter of approximately 2 nm for the *P. aeruginosa* OprF (81).

Although the role of the pseudomonal OprF as a porin has been a topic of controversy (19), its role in antibiotic uptake has been strengthened by the report of an OprF-deficient, antibiotic-resistant clinical isolate (85). Evidence has been presented that minimum inhibitory concentrations (MICs) for β-lactams are increased (86) and permeability of the cephalosporin nitrocefin is decreased in an OprF mutant (87), thereby establishing the role of this protein in transport of β-lactam antibiotics. Porin activity was recently shown directly, when purified OprF was inserted into proteoliposomes and diffusion of L-arabinose was measured (88). OprF is the major porin in *P. aeruginosa* in terms of diffusion rate and size exclusion limit, and exceeds the size of *E. coli* porins. The lower permeability of *P. aeruginosa* compared with *E. coli* was attributed to the fact that only small numbers of these porins exist in the pseudomonal outer membrane.

2. Penetration Through Porins

Wild-type *E. coli* K-12, a common, well-characterized laboratory strain, produces two major outer membrane proteins that are associated with permeation of β-lactams, OmpC and OmpF. Other strains, such as *E. coli* B/r, produce only OmpF (89). In both sets of strains, loss of OmpF resulted in decreased susceptibility to many β-lactam antibiotics. For all the penicillins, cephalosporins, and the monobactam studied, the loss of OmpF resulted in diminished antimicrobial activity, particularly when accompanied by the loss of OmpC (Table 1). The loss of OmpC by itself did not affect the MICs significantly. However, even with the loss of both OmpC and OmpF, β-lactams as varied in structure as ampicillin, cefotaxime, aztreonam, and ceftazidime retained respectable antimicrobial activity, indicating that separate uptake pathways may exist for the transport of these molecules, in addition to the traditional OmpC and OmpF porins. Yamaguchi et al. have suggested that penicillins can penetrate the hydro-

Table 1 Comparison of Antimicrobial Activities of β-Lactam Antibiotics and Permeability Into Proteoliposomes From Specific Porin Mutants of *E. coli*

		MIC[a] (μg/ml)										
	Porin status	CFZ	FOX	CTX	PIP	IMP	LOR	AMP	ATM	CAR	CAZ	Ref.
E. coli strain												
B/r; CM6	F[+b]	1.0	ND[c]	ND	ND	ND	ND	0.5	ND	4.0	ND	89
HN105	F[−]	8.0	ND	ND	ND	ND	ND	4.0	ND	32	ND	89
K-12 parent	F[+], C[+]	1.0	ND	ND	ND	ND	ND	1.0	ND	8.0	ND	89
HN101	F[−], C[++]	2.0	ND	ND	ND	ND	ND	2.0	ND	128	ND	89
K-12 pop1010	F[+], C[+]	2.0	2.0	ND	ND	ND	2.0	2.0	ND	ND	ND	90
B1449	F[−], C[+]	2–4	16	ND	ND	ND	2.0	8.0	ND	ND	ND	90
B1467	F[−], C[−]	64	128	ND	ND	ND	64	16	ND	ND	ND	90
B1478	F[+], C[−]	2.0	2.0	ND	ND	ND	2.0	2.0	ND	ND	ND	90
DCO	F[+], C[+]	1.0	2.0	0.03	ND	ND	2.0	ND	0.06	ND	0.13	91
F2	F[−], C[−]	16	64	0.06	ND	ND	32	ND	0.25	ND	0.25	91
M25	F[−], C[++]	2.0	8.0	0.03	ND	ND	4.0	ND	0.25	ND	0.50	91
MC4100	F[+], C[+]	ND	1.56	0.025	0.20	0.20	ND	ND	0.05	ND	0.10	92
MH 1160 (MC4100 *ompR1*)	F[−], C[−]	ND	25	0.10	0.39	0.20	ND	ND	0.20	ND	0.20	92
Relative diffusion rate[d]	*E. coli* OmpF channel	77	46	22	<5	216	167	46	22	5	12	93
	E. coli OmpC channel	ND	ND	8	ND	280	ND	ND	12	ND	<4	93
Hydrophobicity (log P_u)[e]		−0.24	−0.02	−1.05	0.50	−1.94	2.04	0.95	ND	1.38	0.75	93
Ionic state[f]		−	−	−	−	±	±	±	− −	− −	±̲	93

Antibiotic abbreviations: CFZ, cefazolin; FOX, cefoxitin; CTX, cefotaxime; PIP, piperacillin; IMP, imipenem; LOR, cephaloridine; AMP, ampicillin; ATM, aztreonam; CAR, carbenicillin; CAZ, ceftazidime.
[a] Minimum inhibitory concentration.
[b] F, OmpF; C, OmpC; +, normal production; −, absence of Omp; + +, overproduction of Omp.
[c] Not determined.
[d] Diffusion measured in proteoliposomes with rates normalized using the diffusion rate for cephacetrile as 100.
[e] Hydrophobicity, as measured by the 1-octanol–water partition coefficient of the uncharged form of the molecule (64).
[f] Ionic state of antibiotic: −, monoanionic; ±, zwitterionic; − −, dianionic; ±̲; one positive, two negative charges

phobic phospholipid bilayer in *E. coli* mutants lacking OmpC and OmpF (25,94).

Peptide penetration is also more affected by the presence of OmpF compared with OmpC or PhoE (95). As a result of the loss of OmpF, OmpC may be overproduced to compensate (89). In some mutants deficient in both porins, PhoE, a channel that preferentially transports anions such as phosphate (64,96), is then observed (64). PhoE is also overexpressed when cells are grown in media with low phosphate concentrations (96).

Permeation of β-lactam antibiotics through *E. coli* OmpC and OmpF porins has been most thoroughly studied using specific Omp mutants in

Table 2 Comparison of Permeability Coefficients of β-Lactam Antibiotics in *E. coli* and *Ent. cloacae*

Organism	Strain	Porin status[a]	Method used for determination[b]	Permeability coefficient of cells (nm/s)						Ref.
				IMP	LOR	PIM	ROM	CTX	CAZ	
E. coli	JF701	F$^+$	PL/Dif-SS[b]	ND[c]	3570	750	643	175	95	98
	JF701	F$^+$, C$^-$	Dif-SS	ND	5260	ND	ND	ND	ND	64
	JF703	F$^-$, C$^+$	Dif-SS	ND	450	ND	ND	ND	ND	64
	LGC01	F$^+$, C$^+$	Dif-SS	14,900	1280	ND	ND	ND	ND	78
	LGC78	F$^+$, C$^-$	Dif-SS	7,100	ND	ND	ND	ND	ND	78
	LGC49	F$^-$, C$^+$	Dif-SS	6,200	ND	ND	ND	ND	ND	78
	LGC89	F$^-$, C$^-$	Dif-SS	720	ND	ND	ND	ND	ND	78
Ent. cloacae	55	F$^+$	PL/Dif-SS[b]	ND	86	15	14	5	1	99
	218R1	F$^+$	Dif-SS	ND	960	29	37	5.6	ND	59, 100
	218R2	F$^-$	Dif-SS	ND	ND	9.2	10	1.2	ND	59
Ionic state[d]				$\pm$	$\pm$	$\pm$	$\pm$	$-$	$\pm$	93, 99

Antibiotics used for comparison: IMP, imipenem; LOR, cephaloridine; PIM, cefepime; ROM, cefpirome; CTX, cefotaxime; CAZ, ceftazidime.

[a] Porin designations as in Table 1.

[b] PL, proteoliposome assay using channel porin as designated; Dif-SS, diffusion steady-state intact cell assay. Where both are designated, the intact cell permeability coefficient was determined for cephaloridine and the proteoliposome permeation rates were normalized for that value (99).

[c] Not determined.

[d] Ionic state designations as in Table 1.

isogenic backgrounds as shown in Tables 1 and 2. With both liposomes and intact cell assays, OmpF was the porin with the highest transport of β-lactam antibiotics. In liposome-swelling assays, the OmpF channel was less than 35% larger than the OmpC and OmpA channels (97). Although the channels were similar in size, penetration of penicillins and cephalosporins through OmpC was only 15–20% that for OmpF (93,97). In contrast, the rate of transport of imipenem was almost equivalent through either OmpF or OmpC in liposome-swelling assays (see Table 1; 93). As seen in Table 2 imipenem was transported through OmpC at rates almost equivalent to those observed for OmpF (78). However, smaller M_r nutrients, such as glucose, were transported through OmpC at approximately 50% the rate that for OmpF (97). OmpF was also implicated as the major β-lactam-transporting porin in *Ent. cloacae* (59), as shown by the large decrease in penetrability for the extended-spectrum cephalosporins in an F-mutant (see Table 2).

Penetration of β-lactams through OmpC and OmpF porins has been described to be more dependent on hydrophobicity and charge than on molecular size, especially for monoanionic β-lactams (93). An exclusion limit of approximately 700, which includes most β-lactam antibiotics, has been estimated to be the cutoff for the porins (71), although larger molecules, such as the dual-action cephalosporin–quinolone Ro 23-9424, also pass through the outer membrane of gram-negative organisms (101). Rates of penetration were described to be inversely dependent on the hydrophobicity of the molecule, with a tenfold increase in hydrophobicity resulting in a five- sixfold decrease in permeability for monoanionic cephalosporins (64). Negatively charged molecules, such as carbenicillin and ceftazidime, generally have slower penetration than either zwitterionic β-lactams or positively charged molecules (64,93). The fourth-generation extended-spectrum cephalosporins, cefepime and cefpirome, were transported through OmpF in both *E. coli* and *Ent. cloacae* more efficiently than the third-generation cephalosporins cefotaxime and ceftazidime (see Table 2).

Various exceptions to these generalities concerning the relation between hydrophobicity and permeability have been documented (see Table 1), particularly for those β-lactams that exist as zwitterions. For example, imipenem and cephaloridine, both zwitterionic molecules, have the highest diffusion rates of any of the antibiotics shown, but also exhibit the greatest extremes in hydrophobicity (64,102).

Relative permeability of representative cephalosporins and carbapenems into a variety of bacteria is shown in Table 3. β-Lactams appear to penetrate into *E. coli* much more easily than into other enteric gram-negative bacteria. Cephaloridine is taken up 16 times more rapidly into *E. coli* than into *Serratia marcescens* or *Ent. cloacae* and over 100 times faster than into *P. aeruginosa*. Differences in uptake of nitrocefin were

Table 3 Comparison of Permeability Coefficients of β-Lactam Antibiotics in Selected Bacteria

Organism	Strain	Permeability coefficient (nm/s)[a]				
		LOR	NIT	IMP	MER	Ref.
Escherichia coli	LGC01	1280	ND[b]	14,900	6,700	78
E. coli	C127	ND	480	ND	ND	103
Enterobacter cloacae	55	86	ND	ND	ND	99
Serratia marcescens	S6	78	ND	180	83	77
Pseudomonas aeruginosa	3-C	ND	ND	736	ND	104
P. aeruginosa	PAO4095	11	ND	ND	ND	99
P. aeruginosa	H309	ND	44[c]	ND	ND	103
P. cepacia	PC715J	ND	56[c]	ND	ND	103
Mycobacterium chelonae	PS4770	1.0	0.79	ND	ND	16

Antibiotic abbreviations: LOR, cephaloridine; NIT, nitrocefin; IMP, imipenem; MER, meropenem.
[a] Determined using the diffusion steady-state method in intact cells.
[b] Not determined.
[c] Permeability coefficient was calculated assuming a cell surface area per unit weight value of 132 cm²/mg, the value determined for *S. typhimurium* and used for other gram-negative bacteria (65).

less dramatic, although differences of eight- and tenfold were observed for *P. cepacia* and *P. aeruginosa*, respectively, compared with *E. coli.* Interestingly, transport of carbapenems was greater in *P. aeruginosa* than in *S. marcescens*, perhaps due to the *β*-lactam-selective channels present in *P. aeruginosa* (see following section). The very low rates of penetration into *Mycobacterium chelonae* for cephalosporins help to explain the poor activity of *β*-lactam antibiotics against mycobacteria.

B. *β*-Lactam Selective Channels: D2 Protein

In the mid-1980s several investigators began to report the appearance of specific resistance to imipenem in *P. aeruginosa* (51,105,106). Before this time, imipenem had been used quite effectively to treat serious infections caused by this organism. Resistance in these isolates was generally confined to imipenem (51,105,106) and was associated with the loss of an outer membrane protein in the M_r range of 45–49 kDa.

Biochemical characteristics of a heat-modifiable, outer membrane protein of 45–49 kDa are consistent with those for proteins of the D group in the outer membrane of *P. aeruginosa* (80). Initially, the missing protein in the imipenem-resistant mutants was thought to be the glucose channel-forming D1 protein (107). Later, immunoblotting techniques showed that these mutants were lacking protein D2 (also designated OprD), but produced protein D1. In proteoliposome reconstitution studies, permeation of imipenem was quite high when protein D2 was incorporated into the liposomes (104). When the L1 imipenem-hydrolyzing *β*-lactamase was introduced into isogenic pairs of *P. aeruginosa* that differed in production of the D2 protein, the penetration of imipenem, as determined by the Zimmermann–Rosselet procedure, was increased over 100-fold in the D2-producing strain, with a permeability coefficient of 736 nm/s in the strain producing D2 protein and 6 nm/s in the D2-negative strain (104). Rates of carbapenem diffusion through the D2 protein porin were approximately 2–70 times higher than those observed through other porins (108). The D2 protein also transports basic amino acids, with apparent competition between imipenem and these amino acids, as shown by elevated MICs for imipenem in the presence of the amino acids (109).

Recently, the nucleotide sequence of the protein D2 gene was determined (110). The deduced amino acid sequence lacked cysteine, was high in glycine content, and had almost equal numbers of charged amino acids scattered among the sequence. These characteristics are consistent with those previously reported for porins of gram-negative bacteria (111) and suggest an underlying structural commonality among the pore-forming channels.

C. Facilitated Uptake: Iron Transport

With the exception of lactobacilli, iron is required for bacterial membrane electron transport and as a cofactor for soluble enzymes. Free Fe^{3+} is available at very low concentrations, owing to its low solubility in the free form and its tight binding to carrier proteins, such as transferrin and lactoferrin, in mammals. As a result, bacteria have devised specific uptake systems to scavenge iron from the environment. The most important of these is the production of siderophores, molecules that specifically chelate iron in tight-binding complexes with dissociation constants of 10^{30} or higher (112). The tightly chelated iron can then be transported into cells using a set of iron-regulated outer membrane proteins (for an excellent review see Ref. 113). Pharmaceutical companies have attempted to capitalize on these uptake mechanisms by designing penicillins, cephalosporins, or monobactams that contain catechols or catechol surrogates, with the ability to chelate iron. Two excellent reviews of this area have recently been provided (114,115).

Bacterial outer membrane receptor proteins that recognize iron-complexed siderophores include at least six receptors in *E. coli*, four of which are associated with specific siderophores. These receptors include: Fiu, 83 kDa, no specific siderophore; FepA, 81 kDa, ferric enterobactin (enterochelin); FecA, 80.5 kDa, ferric citrate; FhuA, (also called TonA), 78 kDa, ferrichrome; FhuE, 76 kDa, coprogen and rhodotorulic acid; Cir, 74 kDa (see Refs. 113,116). Nikaido and Rosenberg have suggested that the Cir and Fiu proteins may serve to recapture the hydrolytic products of siderophores, such as 2,3-dihydroxybenzoic acid (98). These receptors are regulated by the amount of iron in the environment and are overproduced at low concentrations of free ferric iron.

The overriding regulator of transport of the iron-loaded siderophores across the outer membrane is the product of the *tonB* gene (118). This cytoplasmic protein, which apparently extends into the periplasm, must be functional for all the iron transport systems to be operative. Therefore, a mutation in *tonB*, resulting in a dysfunctional TonB protein, will shut down all iron transport and cause the loaded siderophores to accumulate on the cell surface. Although the smaller iron-charged siderophores, such as ferric aerobactin and ferric citrate, are small enough to enter through porins, transport of these ligands does not occur in mutants deficient in their respective receptor proteins (117).

Evidence for the role of TonB as the energy-dependent gatekeeper for the iron transport proteins has been provided specifically with the FepA receptor. Mutants of FepA, the high-affinity receptor specific for the uptake of ferric enterobactin, have been generated by deleting cell surface ligand-binding peptides of FepA (119). The resulting proteins could not bind ferric enterobactin, but the mutants producing these proteins could transport the chelated iron siderophore at high concentrations. Additional studies have shown that the FepA deletion mutant ΔRV contains FepA channels that are considerably larger than any other outer membrane porin in *E. coli* (120). High-affinity saturation kinetics were exhibited, and antibiotics such as erythromycin and bacitracin that normally do not pass through *E. coli* porins could be transported (119), indicating that the mutated FepA could function as a porin. This transport was independent of the production of TonB, in contrast with the transport of ferric enterochelin in the wild-type *E. coli*, thus confirming the role of FepA as a gated channel (119).

Numerous *β*-lactams have been designed to utilize iron uptake systems as a means of illicit entry into bacteria with low permeability for other *β*-lactam antibiotics. Among these semisynthetic analogues are catecholic ureidopenicillin, 6α-formamido penicillins, or ampicillin analogues (121–124); catechol-substituted cephalosporins (114,116,125–128); and the monobactams with catechol surrogates (46). Addition of the catechol to the cephalosporins and monobactams did nothing to enhance their activity against gram-positive organisms, but often resulted in very good gram-negative coverage, particularly for strains of *P. aeruginosa* (127,129,130). These compounds were more active when tested in low iron medium in which iron-transport proteins would be induced. At high iron concentrations, bactericidal activity was reduced at subinhibitory concentrations of antibiotics, probably due to repression of the iron receptor, or of transport proteins (125,129). Spectrophotometric studies indicated that the cephalosporins E-0702, M14659, and the monobactam pirazmonam could form complexes with iron at equimolar ratios (53,128,129), suggesting that, at low drug concentrations in the presence of excess ferric iron, a chelated antibiotic could enter through siderophore-uptake mechanisms.

Several of the iron-regulated proteins in *E. coli* are directly involved in the uptake of catechol-substituted *β*-lactams, confirming the hypothesis that an iron-chelated *β*-lactam was using a facilitated transport mechanism. In studies with iron transport-deficient mutants, the catechol cephalosporin E-0702 and the monobactam pirazmonam were shown to enter *E. coli* by the *tonB*-dependent iron-transport system (53,128). The microbiological activity of pirazmonam was also diminished by a mutation in the *cir* gene (53). Curtis et al. showed that transport of catechol-substituted cephalosporins was not only affected by mutations in the *tonB* locus, but the antibiotics had decreased microbial activity if mutations in *cir* and *fiu* were present (116). Nikaido and Rosenberg then demonstrated that the

Cir and Fiu proteins function as the receptor proteins in the transport of monomeric catechol-substituted β-lactams, including E0702 and pirazmonam (98).

Additional evidence has been presented to show that some of these molecules may also be transported by normal porin-uptake pathways. When a saturating concentration of aztreonam was mixed with pirazmonam, [^{14}C]pirazmonam uptake into *E. coli* was diminished by more than 50% (K. Bush, unpublished data). Hashizume et al. demonstrated that the catechol-substituted cephalosporins BO-1236 and BO-1341 diffused through the OmpF channel as well as through the *tonB*-dependent pathway (131). These observations would explain why antimicrobial activity is diminished, but not eliminated, when catechol-substituted molecules are tested in strains with *tonB*-dependent mutations.

IV. PERMEATION-RELATED RESISTANCE MECHANISMS

A. Outer Membrane Alterations

1. Porin Mutations

Isogenic strains of *E. coli* containing or lacking specific porins have been instrumental in establishing the specificity of transport through porins OmpF, OmpC, and OmpA. Selection of mutants with reduced susceptibilities to β-lactams because of porin deficiencies is relatively easy under laboratory conditions, as shown in at least two different laboratories by the selection of OmpF$^-$ OmpC$^-$ *E. coli* strains after overnight growth on cefoxitin (91,132). A second set of mutants was obtained in which OmpF was missing and OmpC was overexpressed, a situation similar to that reported earlier by several other groups (89,90). As shown in Table 1, this overproduction of OmpC caused a partial recovery of the antimicrobial activity of cephalosporins, such as cefoxitin and cephaloridine, but not ceftazidime or the monobactam aztreonam (91). A ceftazidime-resistant *E. coli* clinical isolate, MG32, had a very low level of OmpC, presumably contributing to its resistance to the extended-spectrum cephalosporin (133).

Porins in organisms other than *E. coli* have not been as well studied for their function and specificity. However, decreased penetration, coupled with outer membrane protein alterations, have been related to β-lactam resistance in several enteric bacteria. For example, resistance to aztreonam was associated with decreased permeability in laboratory mutants of *Ent. cloacae*, selected with extended-spectrum β-lactam antibiotics (69). A carbapenem-resistant clinical isolate of *Ent. cloacae* was shown to have not only decreased penetrability, but also to lack a major outer membrane protein of 38 kDa associated with carbapenem resistance (52). Resistance to ceftriaxone and Sch 34343 in *Ent. cloacae* was also associated with both decreased permeability and a loss of outer membrane proteins of 37–38 kDa (54). Other laboratory-generated resistant isolates of *Ent. cloacae* developed outer membrane protein mutations. Strains selected for β-lactam resistance using monobactams lost production of major outer membrane proteins with M_r of 39 kDa and 36.5 kDa (134). Carbapenem-resistant mutants of *Ent. cloacae* and *Proteus rettgeri* also lacked nonspecific porins, in contrast with the situation observed in many isolates of *P. aeruginosa* in which the specific carbapenem channel D2 protein is lacking (135).

Other studies that used laboratory-generated mutants have shown outer membrane protein alterations after selection of β-lactam-resistant organisms. This has been demonstrated in *S. marcescens* (136), *Salmonella paratyphi* A (136), *Proteus mirabilis* (132), and *Acinetobacter calcoaceticus* (137). Clinical isolates with outer membrane protein changes have also been reported for *P. cepacia* (138), *H. influenzae* (139,140), *Klebsiella pneumoniae* (141), and *S. marcescens* (142). Only in *P. cepacia*, however, was a four- to sixfold decrease in permeability associated with the loss of an oligomeric 81-kDa outer membrane protein, thereby justifying the claim that resistance in these isolates from cystic fibrosis patients was due to the loss of a porin (138). Curiously, clinical isolates of *S. marcescens*, resistant to cefotaxime and moxalactam, but susceptible to imipenem, overproduced a single outer membrane protein of either 43 or 44 kDa, perhaps a protein that is a less effective porin for the diffusion of cephalosporins than for carbapenems (142). Changes in outer membrane protein profiles in clinical isolates compared with laboratory strains are difficult to interpret, as there may be sufficient species heterogeneity among unrelated isolates to account for the observed differences.

2. Carbapenem-Specific Mutations

The discovery of the D2 protein specificity for carbapenems in *P. aeruginosa* was based on the study of imipenem-resistant clinical isolates. The MICs for penicillins, cephalosporins, and the monobactam aztreonam were never increased more than twofold when pretherapy and posttherapy imipenem-resistant isolates were compared (Table 4); in some cases MICs were decreased for these β-lactams when MICs were increased for imipenem (51,106). An unusual set of isolates was described by Quinn et al., in which three discrete populations of *P. aeruginosa* were isolated concurrently from the same patient. One was susceptible to all the β-lactams tested except carbenicillin, a second isolate was resistant to only

Table 4 Antimicrobial Activities of β-Lactam Antibiotics in Permeability Mutants of *P. aeruginosa*

P. aeruginosa source/strain	Description	Outer membrane	MIC (μg/ml) for antibiotic					Ref.
			PIP	CFS	CAZ	ATM	IMP	
Patient 1	Pretherapy		>100	>100	50	100	3.1	106
	Posttherapy	No 48-kDa protein	>100	50	25	50	25	
Patient 2	Pretherapy		6.2	1.6	1.6	3.1	6.2	106
	Posttherapy	No 48-kDa protein	6.2	1.6	1.6	3.1	25	
Patient 3	Concurrent isolate 1		6.2	3.1	0.78	3.1	1.6	106
	Concurrent isolate 2	No 45-kDa protein	3.1	1.6	0.78	1.6	12.5	
	Concurrent isolate 3		>100	25	25	25	1.6	
14179	Pretherapy		32	8	8	32	2	105
14759	Posttherapy	No 46-kDa protein	32	8	4	32	32	105
Patient 1	Pretherapy		128	ND[a]	32	ND	1	51
	Posttherapy	No 48-kDa protein	64	ND	16	ND	16	
Patient 2	Pretherapy		>256	ND	128	ND	1	51
	Posttherapy	No 49-kDa protein	>256	ND	64	ND	16	
Patient 3	Pretherapy		128	ND	16	ND	0.5	51
	Posttherapy	No 49-kDa protein	16	ND	4	ND	>64	
Patient 4	Pretherapy		4	ND	2	ND	1	51
	Posttherapy	No 49-kDa protein	8	ND	2	ND	16	
PA01			0.39	0.39	0.20	ND	0.20	109
DD-13	D2 Mutant of PA01	No D2 protein	0.78	0.39	0.39	ND	6.25	109

Antibiotic abbreviations: PIP, piperacillin; CFS, cefsulodin; CAZ, ceftazidime; ATM, aztreonam; IMP, imipenem.

[a] Not determined

imipenem, and a third was broadly resistant to all β-lactams except imipenem (106). These observations can be explained if there is an uptake system for imipenem that is separate from that used for other β-lactam antibiotics.

Resistance in these isolates was not plasmid-mediated (51), nor was it related to binding to PBPs (51,106). Hydrolysis by β-lactamases was not considered to be responsible (51,106,143), although hydrolysis at low imipenem concentrations could be a contributing factor (51). It was noted that imipenem was a less effective inducer of the group 1 cephalosporinase in resistant strains compared with induction in wild-type isolates of *P. aeruginosa* (143), suggesting a higher concentration of imipenem available for induction in the wild-type strain. When outer membrane protein profiles were compared in resistant and susceptible strains, a major outer membrane protein of an M_r range of 45–49 kDa was lacking in the resistant isolates (49,51,106). Although the exact size of the missing outer membrane protein varied according to strain, comparison of isolates from pre- and postimipenem therapy consistently exhibited the loss of a similar protein in the resistant isolates. Uptake studies with [^{14}C]imipenem showed that resistant isolates after therapy had less imipenem bound to the inner membrane protein than those isolated before therapy (51). A possible explanation for these results was decreased penetration of imipenem. However, resistance in these clinical strains was due to the loss of the D2 protein that transports only selected carbapenems within the β-lactam class of antibiotics. Selection of D2 protein mutants has recently been shown to be due to two different sets of deletion mutations in the *oprD* gene coding for the protein (144).

B. Resistance Specific to Catechol-Substituted β-Lactams

1. Resistance Caused by Mutations in Iron-Uptake Mechanisms

No catechol-substituted β-lactam antibiotic has yet been approved for clinical use, so naturally selected, resistant clinical isolates have not been identified. However, several studies have generated laboratory mutants with decreased susceptibility to the β-lactams bearing catechol or surrogate catechol substitutions. Mutation frequencies as high as 10^{-7} were reported after selection with catechol cephalosporins (116,128). *E. coli* mutants selected after growth on high concentrations of the dihydroxyisoquinolinium cephalosporin BO-1341 (126), the catechol-substituted cephalosporins from Curtis et al. (116), or E-0702 (128) have a defect in the *tonB* gene. A double *fiu cir* mutation was generated in the presence of 0.5 μg/ml GR69153 (125). Although the laboratory mutants had decreased susceptibilities, MICs were generally 6.25 μg/ml, or less, indicating a secondary uptake mechanism. Because many of these compounds appear to utilize porin uptake mechanisms in addition to the illicit transport pathway, it is likely that high-level resistance will be difficult to attain as a result of a single point mutation.

2. *Resistance Caused by Competition from the Host*

A major concern has been raised concerning the efficacy of catechol-substituted β-lactam antibiotics in mammalian systems. The binding of ferric iron to the mammalian iron-binding proteins, such as transferrin, or lactoferrin is quite tight, with binding constants of 10^{24}–10^{36} (114,145). As a result, there is little free iron left in the blood to be chelated to a foreign substance such as an antibiotic. For β-lactams to enter into bacterial cells by the iron-uptake system, the antibiotic must be chelated to iron. This occurs only if the antibiotic has a higher affinity for iron than the host transferrin or lactoferrin, or a greater affinity than the bacterially produced siderophores that may have binding constants for ferric iron as high as 10^{52} (146). It was recently demonstrated that the chelating capacity of the catechol-substituted cephalosporin M14659 was not high enough to recover the bound iron from that sequestered by transferrin, as the bactericidal activity of the antibiotic was completely inhibited in the presence of transferrin and a concentration of $FeCl_3$ capable of saturating the transferrin (129). However, Silley et al. have suggested that a low pH at the site of infection may cause transferrin to have a reduced affinity for iron, thereby providing a supply of iron at the localized site (125). In vitro studies have demonstrated that, at pH values between 5.0 and 6.0, siderophores from *P. aeruginosa* were capable of mobilizing iron from transferrin, but this did not occur at pH 7.4 (147).

C. Relationships among Permeability, β-Lactamase, and Penicillin-Binding Proteins

Three major factors determine the efficacy of a β-lactam antibiotic: penetrability, lability to hydrolysis by a β-lactamase, and affinity for the target proteins. For those β-lactams that are susceptible to hydrolysis, the combination of permeability and β-lactamase hydrolysis is most important. Because of the prevalence of β-lactamase-producing bacteria, these considerations have been explored both practically and theoretically.

In gram-negative organisms, the interplay of outer membrane permeability and hydrolysis by periplasmic β-lactamase can be evaluated quantitatively for each β-lactam antibiotic, with a composite parameter called the "target access index" (148). This index is a function of both the hydrolytic parameters V_{max} and K_m for the β-lactamase and antibiotic, and the permeability coefficient measuring entry of the antibiotic into the cell. Waley has proposed the addition of a third parameter, the rate constant for reaction of the β-lactam antibiotic with a PBP, to predict MIC values for resistant organisms (149). Another quantitative evaluation has been proposed to determine whether β-lactamase activity is sufficient to explain the antimicrobial activity of β-lactam antibiotics in gram-negative bacteria; by relating observed MICs to kinetic properties of the β-lactamase, it is possible to evaluate the relative permeability of related β-lactam antibiotics (150). In all these theoretical evaluations, it is assumed that permeability and lability to β-lactamase are highly important features in determining susceptibility to β-lactam antibiotics. It is thus no coincidence that many clinical isolates have been identified in which permeability in combination with β-lactamase production has been responsible for resistance to β-lactam antibiotics.

At one time, it was suggested that production of periplasmic β-lactamase activity directed changes in permeation of penicillins (151). However, examination of various *E. coli* mutants have shown that production of the TEM-1 β-lactamase was the sole contributing factor to penicillin resistance in these strains (152). These results were confirmed by direct measurement of permeability into *E. coli* strains with and without an R-factor that coded for the TEM β-lactamase (64).

Many studies have reported decreased permeability of β-lactam antibiotics into strains of *Ent. cloacae* that were resistant to cephalosporins (54,69,153), monobactams (69), and carbapenems (52,135). In all these strains, high-level resistance was associated with a high level of cephalosporinase expression. The role of β-lactamase production was shown by the fact that the introduction of the *ampD* gene into a hyperproducing β-lactamase strain resulted in much lower MICs for ceftazidime and carbapenems, due to the repression of cephalosporinase production (52). The enzymes produced by these *Enterobacter* strains did not efficiently hydrolyze most of the β-lactams. Hydrolysis of the carbapenems proceeded at rates of 10% or less than those for good substrates, whereas aztreonam could bind to some of these enzymes with half-lives of 2.3–6.8 h, resulting in a very slow rate of hydrolysis. In some of these strains decreased permeability was associated with the loss of outer membrane proteins with an M_r of 37 and 38 kDa (52,135).

Similar studies in *Klebsiella pneumoniae* (154), *P. rettgeri* (135), and the *Bacteroides fragilis* group (155) indicated that both β-lactamase activity and decreased permeability were associated with diminished antimicrobial activity of the β-lactam antibiotics. An important in vivo study demonstrated this interrelationship when infected rat abscesses were treated with cefoperazone and cefoperazone combined with the β-lactamase inhibitor sulbactam (154). Strains of *K. pneumoniae* were constructed to contain a TEM-2 β-lactamase, either in a wild-type background or in a strain lacking a 39-kDa outer membrane protein. As seen in Table 5, loss of the 39-kDa outer membrane protein from the low-level enzyme-producing strain increased MICs, but the antibiotics were still capable of lowering

Table 5 Efficacy of Cefoperazone (CFP) and Cefoperazone–Sulbactam (CFP–SUL) in a Rat Intra-abdominal Abscess Model

K. pneumoniae strain	β-Lactamase activity[a]	39-kDa Omp	MIC (μg/ml)		CFU ($\log_{10}$) per gram abscess[c]		
			CFP	CFP–SUL[b]	No treatment	CFP	CFP–SUL
44	0.24	+	≤0.25	≤0.25	8.5	ND[d]	4.1
44NRF	0.35	−	2	2	7.3	3.9	3.4
44NR(RP4)	87	+	>2056	64	8.4	7.8	5.2
44NRF(RP4)	49	−	>2056	256	8.2	ND	7.7

[a] Micromoles cephaloridine hydrolyzed per minute per milligram of protein
[b] CFP–SUL at a 2:1 ratio of cefoperazone to sulbactam.
[c] CFU, colony forming units.
[d] ND, not determined.
Source: Data adapted from Ref. 154.

the bacterial counts in the abscess. In the presence of high β-lactamase production, the efficacy of cefoperazone was eliminated, even when the outer membrane proteins were all present. Only when the *K. pneumoniae* expressed a high level of β-lactamase in the absence of the 39-kDa outer membrane protein was the in vivo efficacy of the β-lactamase inhibitor combination lost.

Correlations between β-lactamase production and penetrability have been made in β-lactam-resistant strains of *P. aeruginosa* (86,156,157). In these studies, the low permeability associated with *P. aeruginosa*, coupled with a feeble β-lactamase activity, were responsible for the observed resistance seen for several β-lactam antibiotics. It was estimated that a turnover number of only 0.01 s^{-1} would be sufficient to account for resistance to ceftazidime in strains producing derepressed cephalosporinase activity (86). Livermore showed that mutants of *P. aeruginosa* lacking the D2 protein required a high level of β-lactamase production to have MICs for imipenem elevated more than two- to fourfold over those observed for the wild type (157). Thus, the interplay between permeability and β-lactamase production was necessary for the full expression of resistance.

The direct influence of four different β-lactamases on susceptibility in *E. coli* strains with specific porin mutations was shown for a series of 15 β-lactam antibiotics, including cephalosporins, cephamycins, penicillins, imipenem, and aztreonam (92). The level of resistance was related to both the kind of β-lactamase and the porin mutation introduced into the host strain. Molecules that were reasonably stable to hydrolysis by the penicillinases when introduced into these strains did not show increased MICs, in contrast with piperacillin or the cephalosporins, that could be hydrolyzed by these enzymes. These results are somewhat different from the result observed in *Ent. cloacae* or *P. aeruginosa*, probably owing to the improved penetrability of these molecules into *E. coli*. The highest level of resistance was seen in strains with an effective *β*-lactamase hydrolytic activity and the loss of both OmpF and OmpC porins.

In mycobacteria, again the interplay between *β*-lactamase production and permeability has been related to low antimicrobial activity of *β*-lactam antibiotics. Although only a low level of *β*-lactamase activity is expressed (158), the permeability of *β*-lactams through the cell envelope of *M. chelonae* is also extremely low (16). Therefore, even small amounts of *β*-lactamase are sufficient to inactivate the trickle of antibiotic that approaches the PBPs, thus resulting in resistance (158).

However, in addition to the combination of permeability and *β*-lactamase, the relation between permeability and PBP binding must also be considered. In several strains of ampicillin-resistant *H. influenzae*, outer membrane protein alterations were observed in conjunction with atypical PBP profiles (139,140,159), although there appeared to be no permeability barrier to the penetration of penicillin at high antibiotic concentrations in at least one set of strains (159). Similarly, in *β*-lactam-resistant *A. calcoaceticus*, decreased permeability was not associated with changes in *β*-lactamase production, but occurred in conjunction with PBPs that had altered expression or affinity for *β*-lactam antibiotics (137).

V. CONCLUSIONS

A. Future Directions

Ideally, one would like to design novel antibiotics that can penetrate well into cells to allow efficient binding to target proteins. Aside from fairly recent attempts to synthesize catechol-substituted *β*-lactams, permeability attributes have not been addressed creatively by many antibiotic chemistry groups. Biologists are now aware of the importance of the outer membrane as a barrier to entry of molecules and are routinely testing permeability mutants of gram-negative organisms. Simply by using isogenic strains of *E. coli* or *P. aeruginosa* with different porin mutations, it is possible to determine whether decreased susceptibility to a novel molecule is due to lack of penetration, or is due to decreased binding to the target protein. If poor penetration is responsible, chemists can then design molecules with more favorable penetrability properties. For example, zwitterionic compounds are preferable as *β*-lactam agents, rather than cationic molecules that may not be transported well through porins.

Attempts to utilize facilitated transport have been quite successful in terms of microbiological activity, evidenced by the large number of potent catechol-substituted molecules synthesized. However, no successful drug candidate has yet made it to the approval stage. Because the concept is so attractive, it is likely that additional efforts will be made to design an appropriate chelating antibiotic with low toxicity. As additional specific transport mechanisms are identified, it is anticipated that ambitious drug discovery programs will attempt to incorporate specific transport characteristics into novel antimicrobial agents. Unfortunately, as described in this chapter, no single uptake mechanism may be operative, particularly across the range of gram-negative bacteria.

Computational chemists have proposed many approaches for the design of molecules that are modeled to fit into a specific conformation of a protein. These efforts become especially attractive as molecular characterization data become more available for the major bacterial proteins involved in uptake and resistance. But at least three different kinds of proteins are involved: a family of outer membrane proteins, the PBPs, and the β-lactamases. Because of the interactions among these three groups of proteins as determinants of antimicrobial activity for β-lactams, the theoretical chemist is faced with an almost impossible task. Even the most sophisticated modeling systems have not yet produced an antibiotic that can satisfy all the criteria needed for optimal efficacy. Perhaps Frere et al. were correct in describing structure–activity relations in the β-lactam family as "an impossible dream" (160).

B. Summary

Permeation of β-lactam antibiotics into bacteria is one of the most critical factors that can affect their microbiological activity. Ultimately, the affinity of the killing target protein for the antibiotic and the presence of an effective inactivating enzyme will determine whether a novel molecule exhibits antimicrobial activity. For β-lactams, good penetration through the outer membrane of gram-negative bacteria is essential for activity, and this can occur through a variety of pathways. Traditionally, in *E. coli* it has been assumed that uptake of β-lactams proceeded primarily through the OmpF porins, with lesser, but significant transport through the OmpC porin. In organisms such as *P. aeruginosa*, carbapenem-selective channels have now been identified that transport only one class of β-lactam. The illicit transport systems provided by the iron-uptake receptors represent yet another form of uptake mechanism.

Mutations in OmpF, OmpC, and related enterobacterial outer membrane proteins are quite common, resulting in diminished microbiological activity for many *β*-lactam antibiotics. Nevertheless, it is rare that a transportable molecule cannot trickle into a bacterial cell, even in the presence of porin mutations. Evidence is accumulating that nonporin antibiotic-uptake systems exist, particularly in mutants, or in organisms, such as *P. aeruginosa*, that have inefficient porin-mediated uptake pathways (2). Additional porin activities continue to be described for proteins such as OmpA. Mutations in the iron receptor proteins may result in porin proteins that are capable of the nonspecific uptake of a variety of molecules. It is but a matter of time before various other redundant systems are identified, as the transport of nutrients from the environment is an essential feature in the life of a bacterial cell. Fortunately, for us, *β*-lactam antibiotics are small enough to be able to slip through the outer membrane using a variety of pathways designed for nutrient uptake. But, because of the evolutionary versatility exhibited by bacteria, it is inevitable that these organisms will devise alternative mechanisms to elude the perils posed by their antagonistic environment.

REFERENCES

1. Nikaido H. Transport through the outer membrane of bacteria. Methods Enzymol 1986; 125:265–278.
2. Hancock REW, Bell A. Antibiotic uptake into gram-negative bacteria. Eur J Clin Microbiol Infect Dis 1988; 7:713–720.
3. Nikaido H, Vaara M. Molecular basis of bacterial outer membrane permeability. Microbiol Rev 1985; 49:1–32.
4. Georgopapadakou NH. Antibiotic permeation through the bacterial outer membrane. J Chemother 1990; 2:275–279.
5. Livermore DM. Antibiotic uptake and transport by bacteria. Scand J Infect Dis (Suppl.) 1991; 74:15–22.
6. Ward JB. Biosynthesis of peptidoglycan: points of attack by wall inhibitors. In: Tipper DJ, ed. Antibiotic Inhibitors of Bacterial Cell Wall Synthesis. Vol 127. Oxford: Pergamon Press, 1985:1–43.
7. Strominger JL. Penicillin-sensitive enzymatic reactions in bacterial cell wall synthesis. Harvey Lect 1969; 64:179–213.
8. Ghuysen J-M, Frere J-M, Joris B, et al. Inhibition of enzymes involved in bacterial cell wall synthesis. In: Sandler M, Smith HJ, eds. Design of Enzyme Inhibitors as Drugs. Oxford: Oxford University Press, 1989:523–572.
9. Ghuysen J-M. Use of bacteriolytic enzymes in determination of wall structure and their role in cell metabolism. Bacteriol Rev 1968; 32:425–464.
10. Tipper DJ, Berman MF. Structures of the cell wall peptidoglycan of *Staphylococcus epidermidis* Texas 26 and *Staphylococcus aureus* Copenhagen. Chain length and average sequence of cross-bridge peptides. Biochemistry 1969; 8:2183–2192.
11. Ghuysen JM. The bacterial DD-carboxypeptidase-transpeptidase enzyme

system. In: Brown WE, ed. E. R. Squibb Lectures on Chemistry of Microbial Products. Tokyo: University of Tokyo Press, 1977.

12. Scherrer P, Gerhardt P. Molecular sieving by the *Bacillus megaterium* cell wall and protoplast. J Bacteriol 1971; 107:718–735.

13. Nielsen JBK, Lampen JO. β-Lactamase III of *Bacillus cereus* 569: membrane lipoprotein and secreted protein. Biochemistry 1983; 22:4652–4656.

14. Connolly AK, Waley SG. Characterization of the membrane β-lactamase in *Bacillus cereus* 569/H/9. Biochemistry 1983; 22:4647–4651.

15. Trias J, Jarlier V, Benz R. Porins in the cell wall of mycobacteria. Science 1992; 258:1479–1481.

16. Jarlier V, Nikaido H. Permeability barrier to hydrophilic solutes in *Mycobacterium chelonei*. J Bacteriol 1990; 172:1418–1423.

17. Nikaido H, Nakae T. The outer membrane of gram-negative bacteria. Adv Microb Physiol 1979; 20:163–250.

18. Lugtenberg B, Alphen LV. Molecular architecture and functioning of the outer membrane of *Escherichia coli* and other gram-negative bacteria. Biochim Biophys Acta 1983; 737:51–115.

19. Hancock REW, Siehnel R, Martin N. Outer membrane proteins of *Pseudomonas*. Mol Microbiol 1990; 4:1069–1075.

20. Nikaido H. Porins and specific channels of bacterial outer membranes. Mol Microbiol 1992; 6:435–442.

21. Engel A, Massalski A, Schindler H, Dorset DL, Rosenbusch JP. Porin channel triplets merge into single outlets in *Escherichia coli* membranes. Nature 1985; 317:643–645.

22. Rosenbusch JP. Structural and functional properties of porin channel in *E. coli* outer membranes. Experientia 1990; 46:167–173.

23. Benz R, Bauer K. Permeation of hydrophilic molecules through the outer membrane of gram-negative bacteria. Eur J Biochem 1988; 176:1–19.

24. Nikaido H, Saier MH. Jr. Transport proteins in bacteria: common themes in their design. Science 1992; 258:936–942.

25. Yamaguchi A, Hiruma R, Sawai T. Phospholipid bilayer permeability of β-lactam antibiotics. J Antibiot 1982; 35:1692–1699.

26. Spratt BG. Properties of the penicillin-binding proteins of *Escherichia coli* K12. Eur J Biochem 1977; 72:341–352.

27. Frere J-M, Joris B. Penicillin-sensitive enzymes in peptidoglycan biosynthesis. CRC Crit Rev Microbiol 1985; 11:299–396.

28. Spratt BG. Penicillin-binding proteins and the future of β-lactam antibiotics. J Gen Microbiol 1983; 129:1247–1260.

29. Buchanan CE, Ling M-L. Isolation and sequence analysis of *dacB*, which encodes a sporulation-specific penicillin-binding protein in *Bacillus subtilis*. J Bacteriol 1992; 174:1717–1725.

30. Dowson CG, Hutchison A, Spratt BG. Extensive re-modeling of the transpeptidase domain of penicillin-binding protein 2B of a penicillin-resistant South African isolate of *Streptococcus pneumoniae*. Mol Microbiol 1989; 3:95–102.

31. Popham DL, Setlow P. Cloning, nucleotide sequence, and regulation of the *Bacillus subtilis pbpE* operon, which codes for penicillin-binding protein 4* and an apparent amino acid racemase. J Bacteriol 1993; 175:2917–2925.

32. Song MD, Wachi M, Doi M, Ishino F, Matsuhashi M. Evolution of an inducible penicillin-target protein in methicillin-resistant *Staphylococcus aureus* by gene fusion. FEBS Lett 1987; 221:167–171.

33. Spratt BG, Cromie KD. Penicillin-binding proteins of gram-negative bacteria. Rev Infect Dis 1988; 10:699–711.

34. Tipper DJ, Strominger JL. Mechanism of action of penicillins: a proposal based on their structural similarity to acyl-D-alanyl-D-alanine. Proc Natl Acad Sci USA 1965; 54:1133–1141.

35. Pratt JM, Jackson ME, Holland IB. The C-terminus of penicillin-binding protein 5 is essential for localization to the *E. coli* inner membrane. EMBO J 1986; 5:2399–2405.

36. Edelman A, Bowler L, Broome-Smith JK, Spratt BG. Use of a *β*-lactamase fusion vector to investigate the organization of penicillin-binding protein 1B in the cytoplasmic membrane of *Escherichia coli*. Mol Microbiol 1987; 1:101–106.

37. Georgopapadakou NH, Liu FY. Penicillin-binding proteins in bacteria. Antimicrob Agents Chemother 1980; 18:148–157.

38. Georgopapadakou NH. Penicillin-binding proteins and bacterial resistance to *β*-lactams. Antimicrob Agents Chemother 1993; 37:2045–2053.

39. Curtis N, Orr D, Ross GW, Boulton MG. Affinities of penicillins and cephalosporins for the penicillin-binding proteins of *Escherichia coli* K-12 and their antibacterial activity. Antimicrob Agents Chemother 1979; 16:533–539.

40. Bush K, Liu FY, Smith SA. Interactions of monobactams with bacterial enzymes. Society for Industrial Microbiology, 1987; 153–164. (Pierce G, ed. Developments in Industrial Microbiology. Vol 27, suppl. 1).

41. Georgopapadakou NH, Smith SA, Cimarusti CM, Sykes RB. Binding of monobactams to penicillin-binding proteins of *Escherichia coli* and *Staphylococcus aureus*: relation to antibacterial activity. Antimicrob Agents Chemother 1983; 23:98–104.

42. Ubukata K, Hikida M, Yoshida M, et al. In vitro activity of LJC10,627, a new carbapenem antibiotic with high stability to dehydropeptidase I. Antimicrob Agents Chemother 1990; 34:994–1000.

43. Spratt BG, Jobanputra V, Zimmermann W. Binding of thienamycin and clavulanic acid to the penicillin-binding proteins of *Escherichia coli* K-12. Antimicrob Agents Chemother 1977; 12:406–409.

44. Fu KP, Neu HC. Piperacillin, a new penicillin active against many bacteria resistant to other penicillins. Antimicrob Agents Chemother 1978; 13:358–367.

45. Turck M. Clinical application of the newer *β*-lactam antibiotics. J Antimicrob Chemother 1988; 22 (suppl A):45–62.

46. Sykes RB, Koster WH, Bonner DP. The new monobactams: chemistry and biology. J Clin Pharmacol 1988; 28:113–119.

47. Birnbaum J, Kahan FM, Kropp H, MacDonald JS. Carbapenems, a new class of beta-lactam antibiotics. Am J Med 1985; 78 (suppl 6A):3–21.

48. Payne DJ. Metallo-β-lactamases—a new therapeutic challenge. J Med Microbiol 1993; 39:93–99.

49. Bush K. β-lactamase inhibitors from laboratory to clinic. Clin Microbiol Rev 1988; 1:109–123.

50. Knowles JR. Penicillin resistance: the chemistry of β-lactamase inhibition. Accounts Chem Res 1985; 18:97–104.

51. Lynch MJ, Drusano GL, Mobley HLT. Emergence of resistance to imipenem in *Pseudomonas aeruginosa*. Antimicrob Agents Chemother 1987; 31:1892–1896.

52. Lee EH, Nicolas MH, Kitzis MD, Pialoux G, Collatz E, Gutmann L. Association of two resistance mechanisms in a high-level imipenem-resistant clinical isolate of *Enterobacter cloacae*. Antimicrob Agents Chemother 1991; 35:1093–1098.

53. Bush K, Tanaka SK, Ohringer S, Bonner DP. Mode of action studies: pirazmonam in *Escherichia coli* and *Pseudomonas aeruginosa*. Intersci Conf Antimicrob Agents Chemother 1987; 27:abstr 1218.

54. Marchou B, Bellido F, Charnas R, Lucain C, Pechere J-C. Contribution of β-lactamase hydrolysis and outer membrane permeability to ceftriaxone resistance in *Enterobacter cloacae*. Antimicrob Agents Chemother 1987; 31:1589–1595.

55. Bush K, Freudenberger JS, Sykes RB. Interaction of azthreonam and related monobactams with β-lactamases from gram-negative bacteria. Antimicrob Agents Chemother 1982; 22:414–420.

56. Monks J, Waley SG. Imipenem as substrate and inhibitor of β-lactamases. Biochem J 1988; 253:323–328.

57. O'Callaghan C, Morris A, Kirby SM, Shingler AH. Novel method for detection of β-lactamases by using a chromogenic cephalosporin substrate. Antimicrob Agents Chemother 1972; 1:283–288.

58. Fisher JF, Knowles JR. Bacterial resistance to β-lactams: the β-lactamases. Annu Rep Med Chem 1978; 13:239–248.

59. Bellido F, Pechere J-C, Hancock RW. Novel method for measurement of outer membrane permeability to new β-lactams in intact *Enterobacter cloacae* cells. Antimicrob Agents Chemother 1991; 35:68–72.

60. Wells JS, Trejo WH, Principe PA, Sykes RB. Obafluorin, a novel β-lactone produced by *Pseudomonas fluorescens*. Taxonomy, fermentation and biological properties. J Antibiot 1984; 37:802–803.

61. Zimmermann W, Rosselet A. Function of outer membrane of *Escherichia coli* as a permeability barrier to beta-lactam antibiotics. Antimicrob Agents Chemother 1977; 12:368–372.

62. Sawai T, Matsuba K, Yamagishi S. A method for measuring the outer membrane-permeability of β-lactam antibiotics in gram-negative bacteria. J Antibiot 1977; 30:1134–1136.

63. Sawai T, Matsuba K, Tamura A, Yamagishi S. The bacterial outer-membrane permeability of β-lactam antibiotics. J Antibiot 1979; 32:59–65.

64. Nikaido H, Rosenberg EY, Foulds J. Porin channels in *Escherichia coli*: studies with β-lactams in intact cells. J Bacteriol 1983; 153:232–240.

65. Smit J, Kamio Y, Nikaido H. Outer membrane of *Salmonella typhimurium*: chemical analysis and freeze-fracture studies with lipopolysaccharide mutants. J Bacteriol 1975; 124:942–958.

66. Liu W, Nikaido H. Contribution of the cell-surface-associated enzyme in the Zimmerman–Rosslet assay of outer membrane permeability to β-lactam antibiotics. Antimicrob Agents Chemother 1991; 35:177–179.

67. Kojo H, Shigi Y, Nishida M. A novel method for evaluating the outer membrane permeability to β-lactamase-stable β-lactam antibiotics. J Antibiot 1980; 33:310–316.

68. Bush K, Macalintal C, Rasmussen BA, Lee VJ, Yang Y. Kinetic interactions of tazobactam with β-lactamases from all major structural classes. Antimicrob Agents Chemother 1993; 37:851–858.

69. Bush K, Tanaka SK, Bonner DP, Sykes RB. Resistance caused by decreased penetration of β-lactam antibiotics into *Enterobacter cloacae*. Antimicrob Agents Chemother 1985; 27:555–560.

70. Hashizume T, Yamaguchi A, Sawai T. Outer membrane permeability of imipenem in comparison with other β-lactam antibiotics. J Antibiot 1986; 39:153–156.

71. Nakae T. Outer membrane of *Salmonella*. Isolation of protein complex that produces transmembrane channels. J Biol Chem 1976; 251:2176–2178.

72. Nikaido H. Proteins forming large channels from bacterial and mitochondrial outer membranes: porins and phage lambda receptor protein. Methods Enzymol 1983; 97:85–100.

73. Nurminen M, Lounatmaa K, Sarvas M, Makela PH, Nakae T. Bacteriophage-resistant mutants of *Salmonella typhimurium* deficient in two major outer membrane proteins. J Bacteriol 1976; 127:941–955.

74. Hall MN, Silhavy TJ. The *ompB* locus and the regulation of the major outer membrane porin proteins of *Escherichia coli* K12. J Mol Biol 1981; 146:23–43.

75. Chai T-J, Foulds J. Two bacteriophages which utilize a new *Escherichia coli* major outer membrane protein as part of their receptor. J Bacteriol 1978; 135:164–170.

76. Luckey M, Nikaido H. Specificity of diffusion channels produced by λ-phage receptor protein of *Escherichia coli*. Proc Natl Acad Sci USA 1980; 77:167–171.

77. Yang Y, Bhachech N, Macalintal C, Weiss W, Bush K. Characterization of the carbapenem biapenem (L627): permeability, and interactions with penicillin-sensitive proteins. Intersci Conf Antimicrob Agents Chemother 1992; 32:abstr 143.

78. Cornaglia G, Guan L, Fontana R, Satta G. Diffusion of meropenem and imipenem through the outer membrane of *Escherichia coli* K-12 and correlation with their antibacterial activities. Antimicrob Agents Chemother 1992; 36:1902–1908.

79. Hancock REW, Poole K, Benz B. Outer membrane protein P of *Pseudomo-*

nas aeruginosa: regulation by phosphate deficiency and formation of small anion-specific channels in lipid bilayer membranes. J Bacteriol 1982; 150:730–738.

80. Hancock REW, Carey AM. Outer membrane of *Pseudomonas aeruginosa*: heat- and 2-mercaptoethanol-modifiable proteins. J Bacteriol 1979; 140:902–910.

81. Sugawara E, Nikaido H. Pore-forming activity of OmpA protein of *Escherichia coli*. J Biol Chem 1992; 267:2507–2511.

82. Blake MS, Wetzler LM, Gotschlich EC, Rice PA. Protein III: structure, function and genetics. Clin Microbiol Rev 1989; 2:S60–S63.

83. Munson RS, Grass S, West R. Molecular cloning and sequence of the gene for outer membrane protein P5 of *Haemophilus influenzae*. Infect Immun 1993; 61:4017–4020.

84. Woodruff WA, Hancock REW. *Pseudomonas aeruginosa* outer membrane protein F: structural role and relationship to the *Escherichia coli* OmpA protein. J Bacteriol 1989; 171:3304–3309.

85. Piddock LJV. Quinolone/ureidopenicillin cross-resistance. Lancet 1987; 2:907.

86. Hancock REW, Woodruff WA. Roles of porins and β-lactamase in β-lactam resistance of *Pseudomonas aeruginosa*. Rev Infect Dis 1988; 10:770–775.

87. Nicas TI, Hancock REW. *Pseudomonas aeruginosa* outer membrane permeability: isolation of a porin protein F-deficient mutant. J Bacteriol 1983; 153:281–285.

88. Nikaido H, Nikaido K, Harayama S. Identification and characterization of porins in *Pseudomonas aeruginosa*. J Biol Chem 1991; 266:770–779.

89. Harder KJ, Nikaido H, Matsuhashi M. Mutants of *Escherichia coli* that are resistant to certain beta-lactam compounds lack the ompF porin. Antimicrob Agents Chemother 1981; 20:549–552.

90. Jaffe A, Chabbert YA, Semonic O. Role of porin proteins OmpF and OmpC in the permeation of β-lactams. Antimicrob Agents Chemother 1982; 22:942–948.

91. Curtis NAC, Eisenstadt R, Turner KA, White AJ. Porin-mediated cephalosporin resistance in *Escherichia coli* K-12. J Antimicrob Chemother 1985; 15:642–644.

92. Hiraoka M, Okamoto R, Inoue M, Mitsuhashi S. Effects of β-lactamases and *omp* mutation on susceptibility to β-lactam antibiotics in *Escherichia coli*. Antimicrob Agents Chemother 1989; 33:382–386.

93. Yoshimura F, Nikaido H. Diffusion of β-lactam antibiotics through the porin channels of *Escherichia coli* K-12. Antimicrob Agents Chemother 1985; 27:84–92.

94. Yamaguchi A, Tomiyama N, Hiruma R, Sawai T. Difference in pathway of *Escherichia coli* outer membrane permeation between penicillins and cephalosporins. FEBS Lett 1985; 181:143–148.

95. Alves RA, Gleaves JT, Payne JW. The role of outer membrane proteins in peptide uptake by *Escherichia coli*. FEMS Microbiol Lett 1985; 27:333–338.

96. Tommassen J, Lugtenberg B. Localization of *phoE*, the structural gene for outer membrane protein in *Escherichia coli* K-12. J Bacteriol 1981; 147:118–123.

97. Nikaido H, Rosenberg EY. Porin channels in *Escherichia coli*: studies with liposomes reconstituted from purified proteins. J Bacteriol 1983; 153:241–252.

98. Nikaido H, Rosenberg EY. Cir and Fiu proteins in the outer membrane of *Escherichia coli* catalyze transport of monomeric catechols: study with β-lactam antibiotics containing catechol and analogous groups. J Bacteriol 1990; 172:1361–1367.

99. Nikaido H, Liu W, Rosenberg EY. Outer membrane permeability and β-lactamase stability of dipolar ionic cephalosporins containing methoxyimino substituents. Antimicrob Agents Chemother 1990; 34:337–342.

100. Hancock REW, Bellido F. Factors involved in the enhanced efficacy against gram-negative bacteria of fourth generation cephalosporins. J Antimicrob Chemother 1992; 29 (suppl A):1–6.

101. Georgopapadakou NH, Bertasso A, Chan KK, et al. Mode of action of the dual-action cephalosporin Ro 23-9424. Antimicrob Agents Chemother 1989; 33:1067–1071.

102. Nikaido H. Role of permeability barriers in resistance to β-lactam antibiotics. In: Tipper DJ, ed. Antibiotic Inhibitors of Bacterial Cell Wall Biosynthesis. International Encyclopedia of Pharmacology and Therapeutics. Vol. 127. Oxford: Pergamon Press, 1985:203–239.

103. Parr TR Jr, Moore RA, Moore LV, Hancock REW. Role of porins in intrinsic antibiotic resistance of *Pseudomonas cepacia*. Antimicrob Agents Chemother 1987; 31:121–123.

104. Trias J, Nikaido H. Outer membrane protein D2 catalyzes facilitated diffusion of carbapenems and penems through the outer membrane of *Pseudomonas aeruginosa*. Antimicrob Agents Chemother 1990; 34:52–57.

105. Buscher KH, Cullmann W, Dick W, Wendt S, Opferkuch W. Imipenem resistance in *Pseudomonas aeruginosa* is due to diminished expression of outer membrane proteins. J Infect Dis 1987; 156:681–684.

106. Quinn JP, Dudek EJ, DiVincenzo CA, Lucks DA, Lerner SA. Emergence of resistance to imipenem during therapy for *Pseudomonas aeruginosa* infections. J Infect Dis 1986; 154:289–294.

107. Trias J, Rosenberg EY, Nikaido H. Specificity of the glucose channel formed by protein D1 of *Pseudomonas aeruginosa*. Biochim Biophys Acta 1988; 938:493–496.

108. Satake S, Yoshihara E, Nakae T. Diffusion of β-lactam antibiotics through liposome membranes reconstituted from purified porins of the outer membrane of *Pseudomonas aeruginosa*. Antimicrob Agents Chemother 1990; 34:685–690.

109. Fukuoka T, Masuda N, Takenouchi T, Sekine N, Iijima M, Ohya S. Increase in susceptibility of *Pseudomonas aeruginosa* to carbapenem antibiotics in low-amino-acid media. Antimicrob Agents Chemother 1991; 35:529–532.

110. Yoneyama H, Yoshihara E, Nakae T. Nucleotide sequence of the protein D2 gene of *Pseudomonas aeruginosa*. Antimicrob Agents Chemother 1992; 36:1791–1793.

111. Gerbl-Rieger S, Peters J, Kellermann J, Lottspeich F, Baumeister W. Nucleotide and derived amino acid sequences of the major porin of *Comamonas acidovorans* and comparison of porin primary structures. J Bacteriol 1991; 173:2196–2205.

112. Nielands JB. Microbial iron compounds. Annu Rev Biochem 1981; 50:715–731.

113. Harris AM. Catechol-substituted cephalosporins. Curr Opin Invest Drugs 1993; 2:109–118.

114. Miller MJ, Malouin F. Microbial iron chelators as drug delivery agents: the rational design and synthesis of siderophore–drug conjugates. Accounts Chem Res 1993; 26:241–249.

115. Nielands JB. Microbial envelope proteins related to iron. Annu Rev Microbiol 1982; 36:285–309.

116. Curtis NAC, Eisenstadt RL, East SJ, Cornford RJ, Walker LA, White AJ. Iron-regulated outer membrane proteins of *Escherichia coli* K-12 and mechanism of action of catechol-substituted cephalosporins. Antimicrob Agents Chemother 1988; 32:1879–1886.

117. Braun V. The unusual features of the iron transport systems of *Escherichia coli*. Trends Biol Sci 1985; 75–78.

118. Frost GE, Rosenberg H. Relationship between the *tonB* locus and iron transport in *Escherichia coli*. J Bacteriol 1975; 124:704–712.

119. Rutz JM, Liu J, Lyons JA, et al. Formation of a gated channel by a ligand-specific transport protein in the bacterial outer membrane. Science 1992; 258:471–475.

120. Liu J, Rutz JM, Feix JB, Klebba PE. Permeability properties of a large gated channel within the ferric enterobactin receptor, FepA. Proc Natl Acad Sci USA 1993; 90:10653–10657.

121. Basker MJ, Edmondson RA, Knott SJ, Ponsford RJ, Slocombe B, White SJ. In vitro antibacterial properties of BRL 36650, a novel 6α-substituted penicillin. Antimicrob Agents Chemother 1984; 26:734–740.

122. Basker MJ, Frydrych CH, Harrington FP, Milner PH. Antibacterial activity of catecholic piperacillin analogues. J Antibiot 1989; 42:1328–1329.

123. Best DJ, Burton G, Davies DT, et al. Structure–activity relationships of some arylglycine analogues and catechol isosteres of BRL 36650, a 6α-formamido penicillin. J Antibiot 1990; 43:574–577.

124. Ohi N, Aoki B, Shinozaki T, et al. Semisynthetic β-lactam antibiotics. I. Synthesis and antibacterial activity of new ureidopenicillin derivatives having catechol moieties. J Antibiot 1986; 39:230–241.

125. Silley P, Griffiths JW, Monsey D, Harris AM. Mode of action of GR69153, a novel catechol-substituted cephalosporin, and its interaction with the *tonB*-dependent iron transport system. Antimicrob Agents Chemother 1990; 34:1806–1808.

126. Sanada M, Hashizume T, Matsuda K, Nakagawa S, Tanaka N. Mode of

action of BO-1341: transport pathway through the outer membrane of *Escherichia coli*. Drugs Exp Clin Res 1988; 14:397–402.

127. Weissberger BA, Abruzzo GK, Fromtling RA, et al. L-658,310, a new injectable cephalosporin. I. In vitro antibacterial properties. J Antibiot 1989; 42:795–806.

128. Watanabe N-A, Nagasu T, Katsu K, Kitoh K. E-0702, a new cephalosporin, is incorporated into *Escherichia coli* cells via the *tonB*-dependent iron transport system. Antimicrob Agents Chemother 1987; 31:497–504.

129. Mochizuki H, Yamada H, Oikawa Y, et al. Bactericidal activity of M14659 enhanced in low-iron environments. Antimicrob Agents Chemother 1988; 32:1648–1654.

130. Iwamatsu K, Atsumi K, Sakagami K, et al. A new antipseudomonal cephalosporin CP6162 and its congeners. J Antibiot 1990; 43:1450–1463.

131. Hashizume T, Sanada M, Nakagawa S, Tanaka N. Comparison of transport pathways of catechol-substituted cephalosporins, BO-1236 and BO-1341, through the outer membrane of *Escherichia coli*. J Antibiot 1990; 43:1617–1620.

132. Sawai T, Hiruma R, Kawana N, Kaneko M, Taniyasu F, Inami A. Outer membrane permeation of β-lactam antibiotics in *Escherichia coli*, *Proteus mirabilis*, and *Enterobacter cloacae*. Antimicrob Agents Chemother 1982; 22:585–592.

133. Bakken JS, Sanders CC, Thomson KS. Selective ceftazidime resistance in *Escherichia coli*: association with changes in outer membrane protein. J Infect Dis 1987; 155:1220–1225.

134. Aggeler R, Then RF, Ghosh R. Reduced expression of outer-membrane proteins in β-lactam-resistant mutants of *Enterobacter cloacae*. J Gen Microbiol 1987; 133:3383–3392.

135. Raimondi A, Traverso A, Nikaido H. Imipenem- and meropenem-resistant mutants of *Enterobacter cloacae* and *Proteus rettgeri* lack porins. Antimicrob Agents Chemother 1991; 35:1174–1180.

136. Dang P, Gutmann L, Quentin C, Williamson R, Collatz E. Some properties of *Serratia marcescens*, *Salmonella paratyphi* A, and *Enterobacter cloacae* with non–enzyme-dependent multiple resistance to β-lactam antibiotics, aminoglycosides, and quinolones. Rev Infect Dis 1988; 10:899–904.

137. Obara M, Nakae T. Mechanisms of resistance to β-lactam antibiotics in *Acinetobacter calcoaceticus*. J Antimicrob Chemother 1991; 28:791–800.

138. Aronoff SC. Outer membrane permeability in *Pseudomonas cepacia*: diminished porin content in a β-lactam-resistant mutant and in resistant cystic fibrosis isolates. Antimicrob Agents Chemother 1988; 32:1636–1639.

139. Mendelman PM, Chaffin DO, Stull TL, Rubens CE, Mack KD, Smith AL. Characterization of non–β-lactamase-mediated ampicillin resistance in *Haemophilus influenzae*. Antimicrob Agents Chemother 1984; 26:235–244.

140. Reid AJ, Simpson IN, Harper PB, Amyes SGB. Ampicillin resistance in *Haemophilus influenzae*: identification of resistance mechanisms. J Antimicrob Chemother 1987; 20:645–656.

141. Pangon B, Bizet C, Buré A, et al. In vivo selection of a cephamycin-resis-

tant, porin-deficient mutant of *Klebsiella pneumoniae* producing a TEM-3 β-lactamase. J Infect Dis 1989; 159:1005–1006.

142. Hashizume T, Sanada M, Nakagawa S, Tanaka N. Alteration in expression of *Serratia marcescens* porins associated with decreased outer membrane permeability. J Antimicrob Chemother 1993; 31:21–28.

143. Buscher K-H, Cullmann W, Dick W, Opferkuch W. Imipenem resistance in *Pseudomonas aeruginosa* resulting from diminished expression of an outer membrane protein. Antimicrob Agents Chemother 1987; 31:703–708.

144. Yoneyama H, Nakae T. Mechanism of efficient elimination of protein D2 in outer membrane resistance of imipenem-resistant *Pseudomonas aeruginosa*. Antimicrob Agents Chemother 1993; 37:2385–2390.

145. Finkelstein RA, Sciortino CV, McIntosh MA. Role of iron in microbe–host interactions. Rev Infect Dis 1983; 5:S759–S777.

146. Raymond K, Carrano CJ. Coordination chemistry and microbial iron transport. Accounts Chem Res 1979; 12:183–190.

147. Sriyosachati S, Cox CD. Siderophore-mediated iron acquisition from transferrin by *Pseudomonas aeruginosa*. Infect Immun 1986; 52:885–891.

148. Nikaido H, Normark S. Sensitivity of *Escherichia coli* to various β-lactams is determined by the interplay of outer membrane permeability and degradation by periplasmic β-lactamases: a quantitative predictive treatment. Mol Microbiol 1987; 1:29–36.

149. Waley SG. An explicit model for bacterial resistance: application to β-lactam antibiotics. Microbiol Sci 1987; 4:143–146.

150. Frere J-M. Quantitative relationship between sensitivity to β-lactam antibiotics and β-lactamase production in gram-negative bacteria-I. Steady state treatment. Biochem Pharmacol 1989; 38:1415–1426.

151. Yamamoto T, Yokota T. beta-Lactamase-directed barrier for penicillins of *Escherichia coli* carrying R plasmids. Antimicrob Agents Chemother 1977; 11:936–940.

152. Crowlesmith I, Howe TGB. Characterization of β-lactamase-deficient (*bla*) mutants of the R plasmid R1 in *Escherichia coli* K-12 and comparison with similar mutants of RP1. Antimicrob Agents Chemother 1980; 18:667–674.

153. Vu H, Nikaido H. Role of β-lactam hydrolysis in the mechanism of resistance of a β-lactamase-constitutive *Enterobacter cloacae* strain to expanded-spectrum β-lactams. Antimicrob Agents Chemother 1985; 27:393–398.

154. Rice LB, Carias LL, Etter L, Shlaes DM. Resistance to cefoperazone–sulbactam in *Klebsiella pneumoniae*: evidence for enhanced resistance resulting from the coexistence of two different resistance mechanisms. Antimicrob Agents Chemother 1993; 37:1061–1064.

155. Malouin F, Lamothe F. The role of β-lactamase and the permeability barrier on the activity of cephalosporins against members of the *Bacteroides fragilis* group. Can J Microbiol 1987; 33:262–266.

156. Bayer AS, Peters J, Parr TR Jr, Chan L, Hancock REW. Role of β-lactamase in in vivo development of ceftazidime resistance in an experimental

Pseudomonas aeruginosa endocarditis model. Antimicrob Agents Chemother 1987; 31:253–258.

157. Livermore DM. Interplay of impermeability and chromosomal β-lactamase in imipenem-resistant *Pseudomonas aeruginosa*. Antimicrob Agents Chemother 1992; 36:2046–2048.

158. Jarlier V, Gutmann L, Nikaido H. Interplay of cell wall barrier and β-lactamase activity determines high resistance to β-lactam antibiotics in *Mycobacterium chelonae*. Antimicrob Agents Chemother 1991; 35:1937–1939.

159. Parr TR Jr, Bryan LE. Mechanism of resistance of an ampicillin-resistant, β-lactamase-negative clinical isolate of *Haemophilus influenzae* type b to β-lactam antibiotics. Antimicrob Agents Chemother 1984; 25:747–753.

160. Frere J-M, Joris B, Varetto L, Crine M. Structure–activity relationships in the β-lactam family: an impossible dream. Biochem Pharmacol 1988; 37:125–137.

6

Aminoglycoside Transport

Michael H. Miller
Albany Medical College, Albany, New York

I. INTRODUCTION

The aminoglycosides—aminocycletols bactericidal antibiotics with broad-spectrum activity against facultative and aerobic gram-positive and gram-negative pathogens and *Mycobacterium tuberculosis*. Most aminoglycosides are naturally occurring compounds and contain amino sugars linked by a glycosidic linkage to another amino sugar or a cyclic alcohol. They are hydrophilic molecules, of molecular weights from 467 to 587, which are bases at physiological pH ($pK_b \geq 8$). Aminoglycosides are subdivided into two major classes on the basis of the aminocycletol moiety. The streptidine subclass contains a central nonaminohexose sugar and a terminal aminocycletol; streptomycin is the only clinically important antibiotic of this subclass (Fig. 1A). The 2-deoxystreptamine subclass (see Fig. 1B) includes three families: the neomycin, kanamycin, and gentamicin families. Each is characterized by a central 2-deoxystreptamine ring attached by glycosidic linkages to amino sugars.

Since the introduction of streptomycin in 1944, intensive research has focused on the mechanism(s) of aminoglycoside action (28). However, as yet, there is no completely satisfactory model of how the pleiotropic effects of these compounds lead to loss of cell viability. Bacterial inhibition and killing involves noncovalent binding to one or more sites on the bacte-

"

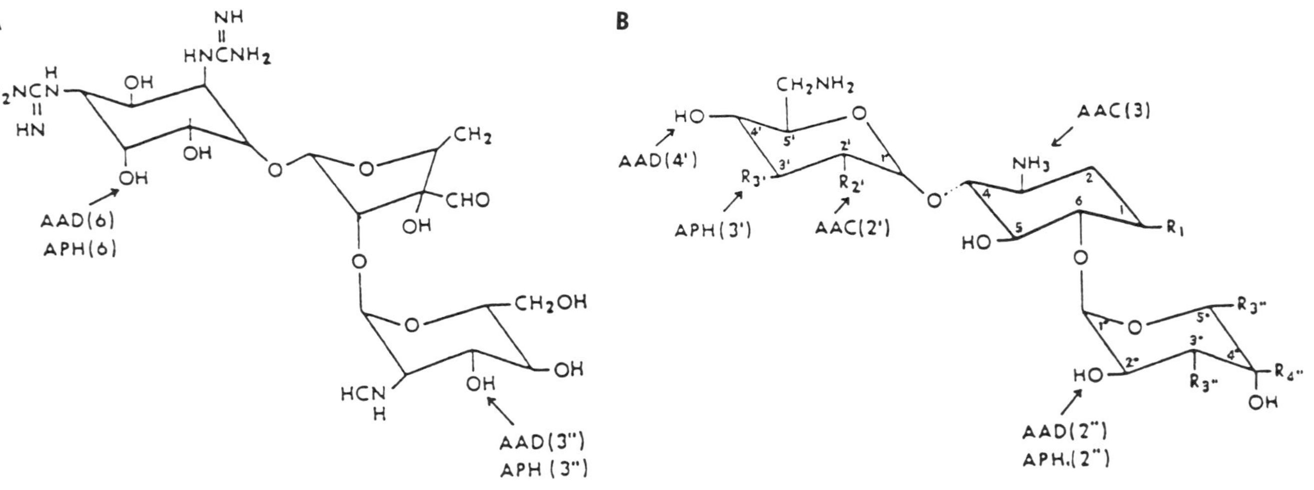

Agent	R_1	R_2	R_3'	R_4'	R_3''	R_4''	R_5''
Kanamycin	NH_2	—	OH^*	OH^*	NH_2	—	CH_2OH
Tobramycin	NH_2	NH_2^*	—	OH^*	NH_2	—	CH_2OH
Gentamicin	NH_2	NH_2^*	—	—	$NHCH_3$	$—CH_3$	—
Amikacin	$NH—C—C—CH_2—CH_2—NH_2$	$—OH$	$—OH$	$—OH^*$	$—NH_2$	—	CH_2OH

aAsterisk (*) indicates a site of enzymatic modification.

Figure 1 Structures of (A) streptomycin and (B) 2-deoxystreptamine subclass. The latter includes most common aminogly-cosides.

rial ribosome, thereby causing misreading and initiation blockade. Aminoglycoside uptake is also recognized as a key factor (14,28,42,92).

Most uptake studies have been done using either the streptidine, streptomycin, or the 2-deoxystreptamines, gentamicin or tobramycin. Although there are similarities in the uptake of each aminoglycoside, there may be differences in the uptake of compounds from different subclasses that have not, as yet, been fully evaluated (13,66). Nevertheless, in this chapter the assumption is made that general uptake mechanisms are similar for the streptidine and the 2-deoxystreptamine subclasses in *Escherichia coli*, *Pseudomonas aeruginosa*, *Staphylococcus aureus*, and *Bacillus subtilis* cells and membrane vesicles.

Alterations in uptake are observed in resistant strains. However, depending on the mechanism of resistance, decreased uptake in these strains may or may not be the only cause for resistance. Physiological conditions present at the site of infection may also decrease the activity of aminoglycosides in situ; for example, decreased aminoglycoside uptake is associated with a decreased external pH (pH$_o$), redox potential, or rate of growth. Physiological resistance is particularly important to the clinical resistance of aminoglycosides. Resistance is also associated with mutations that affect ribosomal binding or components of the membrane energization complex (14,42,92), and with aminoglycoside-modifying enzymes. Resistance can be absolute or relative. Absolute resistance is associated with the inability of aminoglycosides to kill bacteria at clinically achievable concentrations and is due to either ribosomal mutations for streptomycin or plasmid-mediated NH$_2$-acetylation, or OH-phosphorylation or adenylation of specific side chains for both aminoglycoside subclasses (see Fig. 1). Relative resistance involves an increase in minimum inhibitory concentration (MIC) values, but these are still lower than clinically achievable aminoglycoside concentrations in the serum of patients. Nevertheless, relatively resistant strains may also cause therapeutic failures, since aminoglycoside concentrations in infected tissue are often less than those in the serum, and drug activity in tissues is diminished. Relative resistance may be caused by one or more mutations that decrease drug transport. Similar to ribosomal mutations for streptomycin or mutations of the membrane energization complex, aminoglycoside-modifying enzymes decrease drug transport (29,61). Thus, both microbial and physiological resistance are associated with decreased transport.

The primary site of action for aminoglycosides is the bacterial ribosome. Therefore, these compounds must traverse one (gram-positive bacteria) or two (gram-negative bacteria) cell envelope barriers before binding to the lethal target. Since aminoglycosides are charged, hydrophilic bases, they do not cross lipid membranes, such as those in mammalian cells or artificial phospholipid bilayers. As a result, uptake across lipid bilayers in bacteria necessitates either a transporter or a leak pathway. Although no aminoglycoside transporter has been identified, all energy-dependent transporters in bacteria are membrane proteins or protein complexes. In gram-negative bacteria, aminoglycosides must first traverse the outer membrane, the outer leaflet of which contains lipopolysaccharide. The inner leaflet of the outer membrane and both leaflets of the cytoplasmic membrane contain phospholipids. However, a significant proportion of both the outer and the cytoplasmic membranes is made up of proteins. Entry across the outer membrane may occur by self-promoted pathways (42,82,92) or porin protein channels (97); entry through the inner membrane occurs by specific or nonspecific transporters.

In general, most reviews refer to aminoglycoside *uptake*, rather than *transport*. This is due to uncertainty about the specificity and saturability of aminoglycoside uptake when compared with other bacterial transport systems (92). The ability of the highly charged aminoglycosides to traverse the cytoplasmic membrane, in conjunction with the fact that uptake is energy-dependent, gated, and sulfhydryl reagent-sensitive, suggests transport through a translocator protein. However, no transport protein has been rigorously sought or identified. Moreover, even though uptake is both energy-dependent and gated, the presence of an intracellular sink in bacterial cytoplasm makes it impossible to determine whether uptake occurs against a concentration gradient in cells. Energy regulation of aminoglycoside uptake could occur by the opening of a voltage-gated channel (facilitated diffusion), or by a carrier or "permease" (active transport). Therefore, we will use the terms energy-dependent and transporter when referring to the bioenergetics and nature of the uptake system, respectively.

II. MEASUREMENT OF AMINOGLYCOSIDE UPTAKE AND ENERGY QUANTITATION

Aminoglycoside uptake has been characterized in aerobic (*P. aeurginosa*), facultative (*E. coli*), and anaerobic (*Bacteroides fragilis*) gram-negative bacteria, and in anaerobic (*Clostridium perfringens*) and facultative gram-positive (*S. aureus, Bacillus megaterium, B. subtilis, Enterococcus faecalis, Streptococcus* spp.) bacteria. In *E. coli* and *S. aureus*, uptake has been determined under both aerobic and anaerobic growth conditions (13,64). Uptake has also been measured in spheroplasts of *E. coli* and right-side-out membrane vesicles of *E. coli* and *Pseudomonas putida*, prepared according to standard methods (48,49), and in *E. coli* vesicles containing the components of protein synthesis (14).

Studies in bacteria have generally employed log-phase cells in nutrient broth or minimal medium, with glucose or succinate as the carbon source. Since cations decrease aminoglycoside activity, media should not be supplemented with cations such as Ca^{2+} or Mg^{2+}. When performing aminoglycoside-uptake studies, careful attention to the phase and rate of bacterial growth is important; growth rate correlates with the rate of aminoglycoside uptake (78). Stationary-phase cells are resistant to aminoglycosides, and the magnitude of the cytoplasmic membrane electrical potential ($\Delta\psi$) decreases as cells go from log- to stationary-phase growth (51). However, growth rate itself has no effect on the magnitude of $\Delta\psi$ (51). Since uptake is often measured over minutes, it is not generally necessary to buffer media, and it appears that certain buffers themselves may inhibit uptake. However, since external pH has a dramatic effect on aminoglycoside uptake, it is important to adjust the pH of an unbuffered medium and carefully monitor pH changes when uptake is to be measured over a prolonged period. The regulation of pH is particularly important when measuring uptake under anaerobic conditions and with streptococci (72).

Since there are limitations to the study of uptake processes in whole cells, many investigators have attempted to characterize the kinetics and bioenergetics of uptake in membrane vesicles. Uptake studies in vesicles have several advantages over those in cells. In susceptible bacteria, transport of antibiotics takes place simultaneously with cell death or alterations in physiological activity, including inhibition of protein synthesis (28), decreased rates of growth (78), increased membrane permeability (27,28), and decreased membrane potential (57). Each perturbation alters the aminoglycoside-uptake process. In cells, the presence of an intracellular sink makes it difficult to determine if uptake is occurring against a concentration gradient. Although studies in membrane vesicles are important for understanding the biochemistry and biophysics of uptake, any comprehensive model of action must also consider the plethora of membrane and cytoplasmic perturbations that occur in whole-cell systems.

Initial attempts to study aminoglycoside uptake in right-side-out vesicles of *E. coli* were unsuccessful (14,83,93). To date, all attempts to develop an aminoglycoside-competent transport system in vesicles have used variations of methods originally described by Kaback (48,49). Bryan modified Kaback's methods and prepared *E. coli* vesicles with ribosomal fractions using methods initially described by Modolell (74). After a 20-min lag, uptake was seen in vesicles provided with an energy source and ribosomal fractions. Uptake did not occur in vesicles treated with KCN, or when a potential of -125 mV was generated with valinomycin in vesicles preloaded with K^+ (14). This potential was associated with uptake in whole-cell systems. Subsequent studies by Thomson, using right-side-out membrane vesicles of *P. putida* (93), showed streptomycin uptake in vesicles energized with ascorbic acid and phenazine methosulfate (ASC–PMS). Uptake was blocked by carbonylcyanide-*m*-chlorophenylhydrozone (CCCP). Dalhoff (23) demonstrated uptake of unlabeled aminoglycosides in *E. coli* vesicles. However, the methods used to energize vesicles and the sensitivity and reproducibility of the uptake system were not described in detail, and measurements of membrane potential were not performed. Recent studies by Leviton et al. have demonstrated uptake in *E. coli* membrane vesicles prepared by using a variation of Kaback's method in which vesicles were prepared in potassium 2-(*N*-morpholino)ethanesulfonic (MES) buffer, rather than potassium phosphate buffer (57). Although the inhibitory effects of cations on aminoglycoside uptake is well described (9,42), anions (including phosphate) also inhibit aminoglycoside uptake.

Aminoglycoside-uptake studies have generally used radiolabeled streptomycin, gentamicin, or tobramycin. The lack of commercial availability of one or more of these compounds has presented problems in the past; at present, none are available. However, methods for the preparations of radiolabeled streptomycin and gentamicin suitable for transport studies have been described (1,67). Uptake studies in bacteria generally use log-phase cells to which radiolabeled aminoglycosides are added. One- to five-milliliter samples are quenched with a salt solution. Samples are then filtered through a glass fiber, cellulose nitrate, or polycarbonate bacterial filters. Filters are pretreated with high concentrations of unlabeled aminoglycosides to help prevent ionic binding. Binding to filters varies; we prefer Whatman glass fiber filters. Filters are then counted in a liquid scintillation counter. An alternative system, with unlabeled aminoglycosides, has been used in both cells and membrane vesicles. Kanamycin uptake in *B. subtilis* has been measured by centrifuging and washing cells, then lysing cells with lysozyme. In these studies, intracellular drug content was measured by a disk-diffusion microbiological assay (91). Alternatively, changes in drug concentrations in the supernatant have been used to estimate uptake in *E. coli* cells and membrane vesicle preparations (23). These techniques are less sensitive than those that use radiolabeled compounds.

Generally, uptake per unit time is measured and expressed per unit cell mass, using a preestablished relation between turbidity and protein or dry weight. The absence of lysis or changes of cell morphology of aminoglycoside-treated cells makes turbidimetric determination of cell mass the method of choice. Uptake is linear when expressed per absorbance unit, despite that many cells exposed to aminoglycosides are unable to form colonies at 24 h (the functional definition of cell death). Uptake should not be expressed per unit viable bacteria because, even in the absence of an increase in cell-associated drug, killing itself will suggest uptake when none exists.

Many studies have characterized the bioenergetics of aminoglycoside uptake. It is important to review some of the potential pitfalls of measuring $\Delta\psi$, ΔpH, and ATP. The electrochemical gradient of protons (or proton motive force; $\Delta\mu_{H^+}$) consists of an electrical potential ($\Delta\psi$) and a chemical gradient of protons (ΔpH). The magnitude of each can be determined in cells and vesicles by measuring the steady-state distribution of radiolabeled lipophilic cations, such as tetraphenylphosphonium bromide (TTP^+) or acetylsalicyclic acid, respectively. All procedures require separation of cells or vesicles from the reaction mixture. This can be done by a variety of methods; membrane filtration provides a simple form of separation that can be used for the determination of kinetic rate constants. Flow dialysis is another useful method, particularly in membrane vesicles, since it is both sensitive and reproducible and permits various manipulations during the course of the same experiment. However, since equilibration within the flow–dialysis apparatus is slow, only steady-state concentrations can be determined. Adequate oxygenation is necessary whatever method is used. Centrifugation through oil has also been used to separate cells from supernatant (51).

Adenosine triphosphate and $\Delta\mu_{H^+}$ are interconvertible by the H^+-ATPase complex. It is important to note that manipulations that decrease $\Delta\mu_{H^+}$ also cause a fall in intracellular ATP levels. However, ATP levels can be maintained even with a fall in $\Delta\mu_{H^+}$ by using strains with $\Delta uncBC$ mutations. This class of mutants contains a deletion of the genes encoding the H^+-ATPase complex. As a result, the mutants cannot hydrolyze ATP in response to a collapse of $\Delta\mu_{H^+}$. The ATP content in cells can be conveniently measured with the luciferin–luciferase assay (33).

The outer membrane in gram-negative bacteria acts as a barrier for TPP^+ as well as many chemicals and ionophores. Although ethylene diaminetetraacetic acid (EDTA) treatment permits TPP^+ to access the cell interior, EDTA itself alters aminoglycoside uptake by both specific and nonspecific effects (39).

III. KINETICS AND BIOENERGETICS OF UPTAKE IN BACTERIAL CELLS AND CYTOPLASMIC MEMBRANE VESICLES

The discussion of aminoglycoside uptake will consider translocation across the outermost portions of the cell envelope (polysaccharide capsules, the outer membrane of gram-negative bacteria, and the peptidoglycan layer). The phases of uptake across the cytoplasmic membrane and the bioenergetics and biochemical parameters that regulate uptake will also be considered.

Aminoglycoside uptake across the cytoplasmic membrane in *E. coli* and *S. aureus* can be divided into three phases: an initial phase of nonspecific binding, followed by two energy-dependent phases (Fig. 2). The duration and rate of the first energy-dependent phase (EDP I) is concentration-dependent, and no killing occurs during this phase (9,12,14,69). The second, and more rapid, phase of uptake (EDP II) requires ribosomal binding and is associated with killing (9,12,14,29,60,69). In the absence of a ribosomal sink (e.g., in strains with *rpsL* mutations, or in certain strains with aminoglycoside-modifying enzymes), only EDP I uptake kinetics occur (9,10,29). During early EDP II, rapid uptake is directly proportional to killing (33,63). However, despite continued drug uptake, after the first few minutes, there is little additional killing, despite continued uptake.

The bioenergetics regulating uptake will be considered in detail in the next section. Aminoglycoside uptake is generally dependent on membrane potential. For a given aminoglycoside concentration there is a critical threshold (gate) for uptake. Once this gate is exceeded, for several minutes uptake is proportional to $\Delta\psi$. When membrane potential is dissipated with protonophores, uptake may also be regulated by ATP.

A. Effects of Chemicals and Metabolic Inhibition on Aminoglycoside Uptake

1. Carbonylcyanide-m-chlorophenylhydrozone and Dinitrophenol

Chemicals that inhibit energy generation or maintenance (protonophores), membrane proteins (sulfhydryl reagents), membrane fluidity (anesthetics), or microbial respiration (respiratory poisons) provided early evidence that aminoglycoside uptake was energy-dependent (4,5,9). However, it was often difficult with these chemicals to distinguish between specific and nonspecific effects on uptake. The $\Delta\mu_{H^+}$ is the proximate driving force for many active transport processes and is involved in the oxidative generation of ATP. Early studies showed that the protonophore CCCP (and dinitrophenol; DNP) blocked streptomycin uptake (5). Although protonophores collapsed $\Delta\mu_{H^+}$ and blocked aminoglycoside uptake, the specificity of these experiments was uncertain. For example, early studies with protonophores were done in *E. coli* cells. In cells, high concentrations were required to dissipate $\Delta\mu_{H^+}$, owing to the outer membrane barrier (5). Treatment with CCCP not only dissipates $\Delta\mu_{H^+}$, but also causes a fall in ATP concentration. The effects of chemicals on membrane bioener-

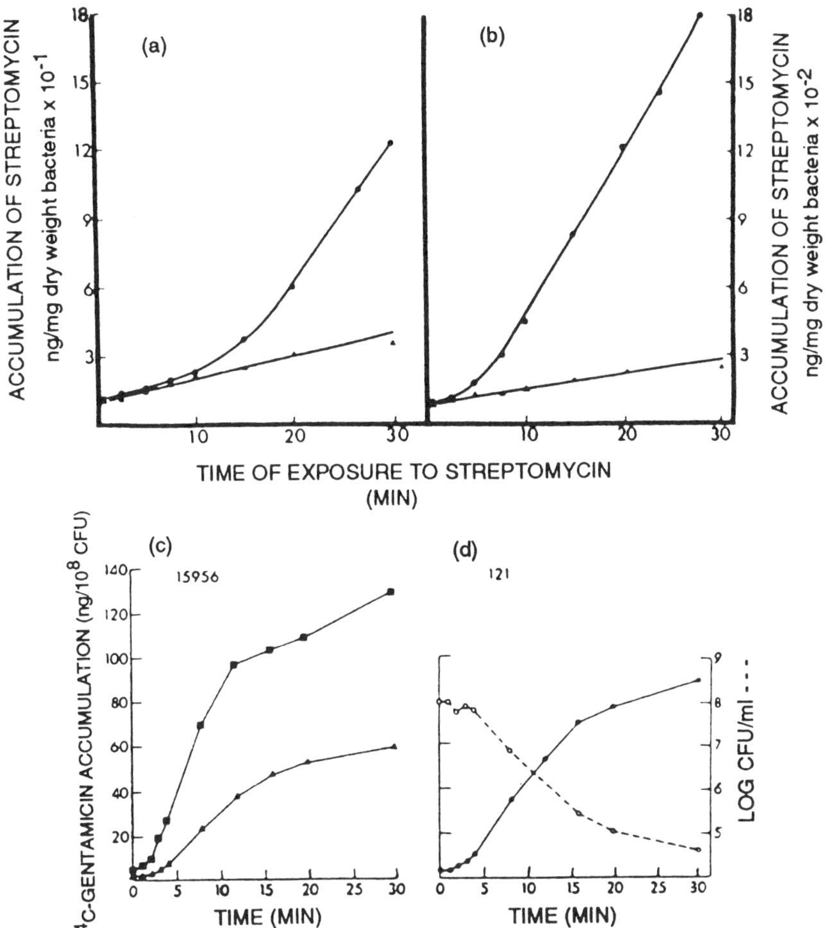

Figure 2 Aminoglycoside accumulation in *E. coli* and *S. aureus*. (a,b) Streptomycin accumulation in an *E. coli* K-12 strain (●) and a *rspL* mutant (▲) at (a) 10 μg/ml and (b) 50 μg/ml streptomycin. (c,d) Gentamicin accumulation kinetics in (c) *S. aureus* 15956 at 0.5 μg/ml (▲) and 1.0 μg/ml (■) gentamicin, and in (d) *S. aureus* 121 at 0.5 μg/ml gentamicin, showing the association between drug accumulation (●, solid line) and killing (○, broken line).

getics or cell growth were not determined in these early studies. Moreover, at high concentrations, CCCP acts as a sulfhydryl reagent (50). Sulfhydryl reagents, themselves, block aminoglycoside uptake (5,9,57). Inhibitors of metabolism used to study aminoglycoside uptake are listed in Table 1.

2. *Toluene*

The effects of toluene have also been prominently featured in models of aminoglycoside uptake. Early studies in cells have shown that aminoglycoside uptake is irreversible; aminoglycoside efflux does not occur following the addition of the protonophores CCCP or DNP (5,28,84). However, Andry and Bockrath (5) showed that the addition of 2% toluene to streptomycin-preloaded cells was associated with rapid streptomycin efflux. These studies suggested that uptake occurred against a concentration gradient. The addition of toluene to *E. coli* during EDP II causes a rapid efflux of the aminoglycosides streptomycin and tobramycin. However, toluene also causes cellular lysis, with a lysis half-life of approximately 30 min (57). Therefore, efflux from preloaded cells might be due to loss of the aminoglycosides that are bound to a cytoplasmic sink. This effect, rather than actively transported drug moving down a concentration gradient, may explain toluene-induced efflux in cells.

In contrast, when 2% toluene was added to *E. coli* before EDP II, Anand and Davis (4) showed a virtually instantaneous stimulation of streptomycin influx. These studies suggested that toluene-induced membrane damage bypassed the aminoglycoside membrane uptake system (4,28).

B. Mutations That Affect Uptake

The effects of mutations in *E. coli*, *B. subtilis* and, to a lesser extent, *S. aureus* have helped characterize aminoglycoside uptake. Several of these mutations, along with their effects on uptake, are listed in Table 2. Most

Table 1 Effects of Different Reagents and Conditions on Aminoglycoside Uptake in Wild-Type *E. coli*

Challenge	Concentration (mM)	Relative uptake
None		+ + + + +
Ice bath		0
Dinitrophenol	2.0	0
KCN	0.5	0
KAsO$_4$	10.0	+
NEM	1.0	+ +
NaF	5.0	+ + +

Source: After Ref. 5.

Table 2 Mutations That Affect Uptake in Bacteria

Organism	Category	Genotype	Phenotype	Effect on uptake
E. coli	H^+-ATPase	*uncA*	H^+-ATPase-	Increased
		uncB	F_0 gate	Decreased
	Cytochrome/respiration		8-Aminolevulinate	Decreased
		ubi	Ubiquinone	Decreased
		hemA	Cytochrome	Decreased
		ubiD	Ubiquinone	Decreased
	30S Ribosome	*rpsL*	30S-Binding mutant	EDPII decreased
B. subtilis	Cytochrome/respiration	*aroD*	Menaquinones	Decreased
		strC	Cytochrome aa_3	Decreased
S. aureus	H^+-ATPase		F_0 leak	Decreased
	Cytochrome/respiration		Respiratory	Decreased
			Quinone	Decreased
			Hemin	Decreased
P. aeruginosa	Cytochrome/respiration		Cytochrome *c552*/ nitrate reductase	Decreased
			Cytochrome *d*	Decreased

mutations fall into three classes: mutants with alterations in the H^+-ATPase complex, mutants with alterations in the membrane energization complex (i.e., cytochromes and/or respiration) and mutations that affect global regulatory mechanisms (catabolite repression and stringent regulation). These mutations may not be mutually exclusive, since both classes may effect the cytoplasmic membrane energy state. On the other hand, there is evidence that the cytoplasmic membrane energy state and the components of respiration may independently regulate uptake (13,66).

Mutants of the H^+-ATPase complex may affect the F_1 or F_0 portion of the membrane protein complex. Aminoglycosides themselves select for one class of mutants; those for which the F_0 channel has become leaky to protons. Those mutants selected with aminoglycosides uncouple proton flux from ATP synthesis and active transport (68). In *E. coli*, F_0 mutants show both relative resistance to, and decreased uptake of, aminoglycosides. The proton leak is blocked by the carbodimide N,N'-dicyclohexylcarbodiimide (DCCD) in both *E. coli* and *S. aureus*. Several incompletely characterized mutants of *S. aureus* show aminoglycoside resistance and decreased aminoglycoside uptake that normalizes after the addition of DCCD. However, since in *S. aureus* wild-type cells, DCCD increases the magnitude of $\Delta\mu_{H^+}$ (33), it is uncertain whether these mutants have an alteration in F_0. Although F_1 mutations with altered ATPase activity also show the uncoupled phenotype, they maintain the electrochemical proton gradient and show increased aminoglycoside uptake (10).

A second class of uptake-deficient mutants has been identified. These mutants have alterations in respiratory function involving cytochromes or respiratory quinones. Mutations causing defective cytochromes have been identified in *E. coli* (*hemA*), *B. subtilis* (*strC*) and *P. aeruginosa*. In most of these mutants, the magnitude of the membrane potential was not compared with that in wild-type strains. An exception is an *S. aureus* mutant that showed both normalization of aminoglycoside uptake and an increase in the membrane potential with the addition of menadione (17). Importantly, a cytochrome-deficient mutation of *B. subtilis* (*strC*) caused decreased uptake, despite a membrane potential similar to that of the wild-type parent. These studies suggest that the components of the respiratory system may have functions, other than energy transduction, that regulate aminoglycoside uptake (9,66). Both Bryan and Taber have suggested that a membrane energization complex may be important in the generation and maintenance of $\Delta\psi$ and may also function as part of the transport system itself (13,14,92). Several additional uptake-deficient mutants with alterations in respiratory quinones have been identified in gram-negative (ubiquinone) and gram-positive (menaquinone) bacteria (12,69,92).

Additional mutants with decreased aminoglycoside uptake include an incompletely characterized mutant of *E. coli* that shows defective coupling of $\Delta\mu_{H^+}$ and transport of a variety of substrates. This mutant shows normal electron transport, ATP levels, and $\Delta\mu_{H^+}$. Mutations of *E. coli* and *S. aureus* with decreased ribosomal binding of streptomycin (*rpsL*) also cause decreased uptake (9,98). Parenthetically, there have been no studies that rigorously characterize all mutations that decrease aminoglycoside activity in *E. coli*. The most comprehensive study selected for mutants by using drug concentrations just above the MIC (94). However, in this study, all slow-growing strains were discarded. Importantly, most of the transport-deficient mutants of in *S. aureus* occurred in strains that were slow growing (69). Mutants with alterations in global regulation included catabolite repression and stringent regulation. As reviewed by Hancock (42,43), adenylate cyclase-deficient (*cya*) and cAMP receptor protein-deficient mutations cause increased resistance and decrease uptake of aminoglycosides. The addition of glucose has the same effects. The addition of cAMP to strains with *cya* mutations restores susceptibility and aminoglycoside uptake. Mutations affecting the outer membrane of *P. aeruginosa* are discussed in Chapter 10.

C. Effects of Antibiotics on Uptake

1. Inhibitors of Protein Synthesis

Chloramphenicol, which inhibits protein synthesis by blocking covalent linkage of the nascent protein strand to the AA-transfer RNA, blocks aminoglycoside uptake in *E. coli* and *S. aureus* when added before or concomitant with aminoglycosides. However, the addition of chloramphenicol after the rapid phase of uptake has begun, has little or no effect on further uptake (28,57). These studies suggest that active protein synthesis is necessary for the induction of uptake, but is not necessary during EDP II. The mechanism by which chloramphenicol exerts its inhibitory effects is unknown.

Puromycin, which also inhibits protein synthesis, has an effect on uptake different from that of chloramphenicol (47). At low, but still inhibitory concentrations, it stimulates, rather than inhibits, streptomycin uptake in *E. coli* when added simultaneously with aminoglycosides, whereas at higher concentrations, it inhibits aminoglycoside uptake (47). The mechanisms of the dose-related, disparate effects of puromycin are unclear. It has been suggested that the stimulatory effect of puromycin might be analogous to the aminoglycoside effect associated with EDP II. That is, both puromycin and aminoglycosides cause a premature termination of the nascent protein chain that increases the number of runoff ribosomes (47), thought to be the putative cytoplasmic sink (14). On the other hand, the inhibitory effects may be due to the nascent proteins before they reach a length sufficient to form nonspecific channels (28). Interestingly, puromycin-induced, increased streptomycin uptake occurs not only in susceptible cells, but in *rpsL* as well (47).

2. Cell Wall-Active Antibiotics

Combination therapy with antibiotics that act on cell envelope and aminoglycosides has been used in the treatment of serious infections with both gram-positive and gram-negative bacteria. Several early studies showed that the addition of a β-lactam, vancomycin, or detergents before or concomitant with aminoglycosides caused bactericidal synergism in vitro and increased survival in certain infections in humans when compared with monotherapy. Initial studies by Plotz and Davis in *E. coli* showed that the addition of penicillin to low concentrations of streptomycin was associated with a stimulation of streptomycin uptake (87). Several years later, using *Enterococcus faecalis*, Moellering and colleagues showed that cell wall agents induced the uptake of otherwise sublethal concentrations of streptomycin and caused bactericidal synergy (75). Although many subsequent studies have shown bactericidal synergy between β-lactams and aminoglycosides in other pathogenic bacteria, in most instances, the assumption that the mechanism of β-lactam–aminoglycoside synergism is due to induction of aminoglycoside uptake has not been confirmed experimentally.

The precise mechanism by which β-lactams cause a breach in the cell envelope, thereby facilitating aminoglycoside uptake, is not completely understood. Gram-positive bacteria differ from gram-negatives both in the absence of an outer membrane and the presence of a multilayered peptidoglycan envelope (Fig. 3). The cell envelope of gram-positive bacteria does not act as a barrier to molecules larger than aminoglycosides. Therefore, it is unclear how an alteration of peptidoglycan structure would facilitate aminoglycoside uptake. When the stimulatory effects of several β-lactams on aminoglycoside uptake were examined in *Staphylococcus aureus*, *Enterococcus faecalis*, *Streptococcus mitis*, and *Streptococcus sanguis*, important differences were observed (72,98). Although aminoglycoside uptake and bactericidal synergy were noted in both staphylococci and enterococci, neither was seen with the viridans streptococci *S. mitis*

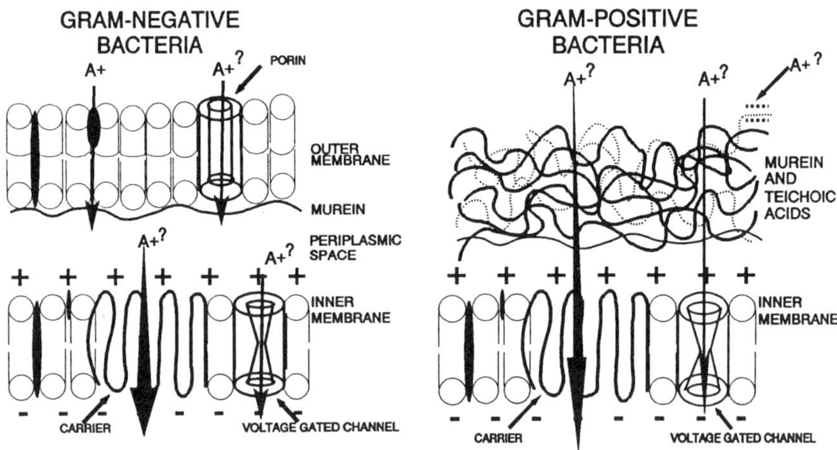

Figure 3 Putative routes of aminoglycoside uptake across the outer and inner membranes of gram-negative and gram-positive bacteria. Uptake across the outer membrane in *P. aeruginosa* occurs through self-generated pathways, whereas in enterobacteria it may also involve porins. The nature of the translocation across the cytoplasmic membrane is speculative, although the transporter(s) are likely proteins. The proton export, which occurs during respiration or anaerobically, creates a polarity across the inner membrane ($\Delta\psi$), which is interior negative and alkaline. Membrane potential, in turn, regulates uptake by either opening a voltage-gated channel or driving active uptake across a transmembrane carrier by a uniport mechanism. Although respiratory quinones are involved in the generation of $\Delta\psi$, they also may form part of the translocation machinery itself. In gram-positive bacteria, there is no outer membrane barrier. However, phosphate groups of the teichoic acids may bind some aminoglycoside molecules, limiting access to the cytoplasmic membrane translocation apparatus. Uptake across the inner membrane appears to be similar to that in gram-negative bacilli.

or *S. sanguis* II (72). The *S. mitis* strains show rapid killing after the addition of penicillin, whereas those of *S.* sanguis II are tolerant to β-lactam antibiotics. Other laboratories have suggested that β-lactam-induced aminoglycoside uptake in viridans streptococci is strain-specific (96). However, these studies measured cell mass, using direct protein measurement. Penicillin causes lysis of viridans streptococci, but not enterococci, releasing protein into the supernatant. As a result, the correlation between protein and cell mass is lost in washed cells (M. Miller, unpublished observations). Therefore, studies suggesting that penicillin stimulates aminoglycoside uptake in viridans streptococci are difficult to interpret.

In contrast, in time–kill studies with *S. aureus* (98) and *E. faecalis* (72,75), β-lactam induction of facilitated streptomycin uptake and synergy was observed. In abbreviated time–kill uptake studies in *S. aureus*, this effect was seen only when otherwise subinhibitory concentrations of aminoglycosides and β-lactam concentrations that were above the MIC were used (98).

We have proposed a model to explain why β-lactams stimulate aminoglycoside uptake in *S. aureus* and *E. faecalis*, but not *S. mitis* or *S. sanguis* (72). Tomasz has shown that penicillin causes the rapid release of teichoic acid in gram-positive bacteria (54). We believe that anionic teichoic acids in *S. aureus* and *E. faecalis* bind low concentration of aminoglycosides (98). Important differences in murein chemistry are found in different gram-positive cocci (98). In contrast with most gram-positive cocci, streptococci and staphylococci are relatively resistant to high salt concentrations. In addition, they are the only gram-positive organisms that grow on a modified MacConkey's medium containing detergents and high salt concentrations (30). Our model suggests that differences in cell envelope teichoic acids cause genus-specific differences in barrier function for cations (98). Penicillin-induced disruption of the multilayered cell wall allows aminoglycosides to access the cytoplasmic membrane and cell interior (98).

The outer membrane of gram-negative bacilli, a known barrier to the uptake of aminoglycosides, is covalently linked (through lipoprotein) to the cell wall. Therefore, facilitated aminoglycoside uptake caused by disruption of this barrier by cell wall-active agents such as β-lactams appears to be a reasonable explanation for synergy. On the other hand, β-lactams that bind to different penicillin-binding proteins (PBPs) cause marked differences in the extent of peptidoglycan degradation and lysis (see Chap. 5). It is possible that β-lactams with different PBP affinities might differ in the extent of β-lactam-induced aminoglycoside uptake (71).

3. Other Antibiotics

Another potential method to increase aminoglycoside uptake and associated bactericidal effects is to combine antibiotic ionophores with
aminoglycosides. Like streptomycin, the antibiotic ionophore nigericin
is a fermentation product of *Streptomyces*. Nigericin, developed as an
anticoccidiostat antibiotic for animals, was never investigated in humans
because of its toxicity and lack of bactericidal effects. It increases the
membrane potential of the cytoplasmic membrane and stimulates the uptake of an otherwise subinhibitory aminoglycoside, causing bactericidal
synergism in vitro under a variety of experimental conditions (60,63,64).

D. Effects of Growth Rates, pH, and Redox Potential

Aminoglycoside uptake is decreased at low pH, when bacteria are growing
slowly, and when facultative bacteria are grown in an anaerobic environment. These in vitro conditions often mimic in vivo conditions at sites of
infection in humans.

1. Growth Rate

In *E. coli* and *Bacillus megaterium* grown in chemostat culture under
phosphate-limiting conditions, the relative rates of aminoglycoside uptake
are proportional to the rates of growth. Although uptake does not require
protein or DNA synthesis, the rates of uptake appear tightly linked to the
rate of RNA synthesis (79). Studies by Kasket demonstrated that the
magnitude of $\Delta\psi$ is not altered by growth rate. Therefore, growth-associated regulation of aminoglycoside uptake appears to be independent of
energy. The observation that rates of uptake in ubi^+ and ubi^- were independent of respiration suggests that growth-associated regulation of aminoglycoside uptake is not mediated by a membrane energization complex
involving quinones.

Growth rate itself appears to regulate uptake independently of other
factors. Even though the mechanism of this regulation is unknown, it has
been suggested that growth may enhance an intracellular sink that occurs
when the number of active ribosomes involved in protein synthesis is
maximal (79). Another possible mechanism of growth regulation involves
global regulation and the stringent response. Amino acid-starved auxotrophs of *E. coli* show decreased aminoglycoside uptake. Under the same
experimental conditions strains with rel^- mutations show normal uptake,
suggesting that growth rate-associated regulation of aminoglycoside uptake might be associated with the stringent response. Interestingly, aminoglycosides themselves depress the stringent response (79).

2. Effect of pH

That aminoglycosides are less active at an acidic pH has been known for many years (31). It was thought initially that enhanced activity of aminoglycosides was associated with pH-dependent partitioning, uncharged drug traversing the hydrophobic membrane barrier of gram-negative bacteria under alkaline conditions. Although this hypothesis no longer explains the effects of pH on uptake, pH partitioning may still play a role when external pH values are greater than 7.5. Once it was recognized that many charged substrates are actively transported by membrane carriers in response to the electrochemical proton gradient, another mechanism of pH regulation was suggested (13,24,63,69). Although a detailed description of the bioenergetics of uptake will be given in the section on energy transduction, to understand pH regulation one must review the chemiosmotic theory of Mitchell (63,73) as it relates to transport. According to this hypothesis, proton exclusion during respiration or ATP hydrolysis leads to the generation of a transmembrane electrochemical gradient of hydrogen ions ($\Delta \mu_{H^+}$) that is the immediate driving force for many biological processes. The proton electrochemical gradient is composed of electrical and chemical components, according to the relationship:

$$\Delta \mu_{H^+} = \Delta \psi - Z \Delta \text{pH}$$

in which $\Delta \psi$ represents the electrical potential across the plasma membrane and ΔpH the transmembrane difference in H^+ concentration (Z is a constant, equal to 58.8 at room temperature). For transport, the chemiosmotic hypothesis predicts that transport is driven by $\Delta \psi$ (interior negative) for cationic substrates. Importantly, external pH affects the relative contribution of $\Delta \psi$ and ΔpH on $\Delta \mu_{H^+}$ (38,51,89). At an acidic pH, the chemical gradient of protons is large, since the internal pH is tightly maintained at 7.5–7.8. This is associated with a compensatory decrease in $\Delta \psi$, which maintains $\Delta \mu_{H^+}$ (see foregoing equation) at a constant level over a range of pHs. The partitioning of $\Delta \psi$ and ΔpH over a pH range from 5 to 7.5 was employed in early studies with *S. aureus* to demonstrate a relation between $\Delta \psi$ and both aminoglycoside uptake and killing. There was a linear correlation between early gentamicin uptake and killing and $\Delta \psi$ (63). When uptake rates were extrapolated to the abscissa ($\Delta \psi$), it appeared that a potential of approximately (-75 mV) was required to initiate uptake. These studies and those of Damper and colleagues (24) suggested that aminoglycoside uptake was gated. Once this threshold of $\Delta \psi$ was exceeded, initial uptake and killing were both proportional to membrane potential (63). Parenthetically, the threshold of -75 mV was later shown to be low owing to the measurement of $\Delta \psi$ in stationary-phase bacteria.

Uptake was measured in log-phase cells (63) and, as mentioned, $\Delta\psi$ decreases as a function of the phase (51), but not rate, of growth (77,79).

3. Effect of Anaerobic Growth

Decreased aminoglycoside uptake is observed when facultative bacteria, such as *E. coli* or *S. aureus*, are incubated under anaerobic conditions (13,64). Studies by Bryan in *E. coli* showed that, when terminal electron acceptors other than oxygen (nitrate and fumarate) were used, aminoglycoside uptake was less than that under aerobic growth conditions. Streptomycin uptake was also absent in the strict anaerobes *Clostridium perfringens* and *Bacterioides fragilis* (11). However, when *B. fragilis* was grown in the presence of respiratory chain precursors (menadione and hemin), aminoglycoside uptake was observed (11). Since $\Delta\psi$ was not measured in these studies, it was uncertain whether decreased uptake was associated with a fall in membrane potential, respiration, or both. Since the decreased uptake under anaerobic conditions may have been due to the effect that anaerobiosis has on the membrane energy state, we examined this hypothesis in *S. aureus*. In that organism, at pH 6.5 and under anaerobic conditions, membrane potential was approximately 75% of that seen aerobically. This potential was less than the threshold necessary to induce aminoglycoside uptake (11).

IV. UPTAKE ACROSS THE OUTER MEMBRANE

In considering uptake across the cell envelope we will consider the potential barriers for both gram-negative and gram-positive bacteria, ionic binding to capsular polysaccharides, and peptidoglycan (see Fig. 3).

A. Ionic Surface Binding

1. Gram-Negative Bacteria

Capsular polysaccharides present in both gram-negative and gram-positive bacteria present a negatively charged, hydrophilic barrier to aminoglycoside entry (see Fig. 3). Although the significance of this outermost barrier has not been carefully studied, it is generally thought to be small when compared with the membrane barriers of gram-negative bacilli.

2. Gram-Positive Bacteria

The gram-positive cell envelope does not generally impede substrate access to cells. Nevertheless, we believe that ionic binding to teichoic acids in the envelope of certain gram-positive bacteria may be an important barrier to aminoglycoside uptake (98). The peptidoglycan of gram-positive bacteria, unlike that of gram-negatives, is a multilayered structure consisting of murein, which is covalently linked to negatively charged teichoic acids. In addition, lipoteichoic acids extend from the cytoplasmic membrane through the peptidoglycan layer. Both cell wall and lipoteichoic acids bind streptomycin (56). In *Streptomyces* spp., an aminoglycoside-producing organism, drug yields are increased by washing cells with salts. Cations, such as Mg^{2+}, other aminoglycosides, and spermidine, all displace aminoglycosides ionically bound to teichoic acids. This possible barrier effect has been incorporated into a model of β-lactam–aminoglycoside synergy in gram-positive bacteria (98).

B. Uptake Across the Gram-Negative Outer Membrane

Uptake of a variety of antibiotics across the outer membrane of gram-negative bacteria has been extensively studied in cells and proteoliposomes of *E. coli* and *P. aeruginosa* (9,11–14). In general, two potential routes of entry occur: entry by leak or self-generated pathways, and diffusion through water-filled porin channels. Although most hydrophilic compounds traverse the outer membrane through porins, aminoglycosides may be an exception.

Liposome-swelling studies with *E. coli*, using reconstituted proteoliposomes, suggested that aminoglycosides traversed the outer membrane through porin channels (97). However, this method of measuring uptake may not be specific or quantitative for ions, particularly cations, which create Donnan potentials, inducing complex buffer and other counterion movement. As a result, the route of passage of aminoglycosides through the outer membrane of enteric bacteria is uncertain. More extensive studies have been performed in *P. aeruginosa*, a genus that shows higher intrinsic resistance to aminoglycosides than enteric bacteria. In this organism, porins do not represent a major entry pathway; rather, as shown by a number of indirect observations, aminoglycosides traverse the outer membrane by a self-promoted pathway in which lipopolysaccharide–Mg^{2+} cross-bridging is breached by aminoglycosides and other polycations (42,76,82).

C. Uptake Across the Cytoplasmic Membrane

Uptake across the cytoplasmic membrane includes an initial, energy-independent, ionic binding and two subsequent, energy-dependent phases termed EDP I and EDP II (9). Ionic binding occurs at both the outer and cytoplasmic membranes (9,57).

1. Ionic Binding

When aminoglycosides are added to whole cells, a virtually instantaneous binding occurs; there is a concentration-dependent association between the aminoglycoside added and the extent of this initial binding. The early phase of "uptake" has been best characterized in whole-cell preparations of gram-negative bacilli. Since aminoglycosides bind to cells with increased barrier function, it is thought that aminoglycosides bind to the outer membrane. Cations diminish initial binding, suggesting that early "uptake" represents anionic binding to constituents of the cell envelope. This early-binding phase is not associated with changes in cell growth or viability. Instantaneous binding also occurs in right-side-out vesicles and, like that in whole cells, is not inhibited by protonophores or maleimides. In membrane vesicles, binding represents approximately 25% of membrane-associated drug and is also virtually instantaneous.

2. Energy-Dependent Phase I

Following the initial energy-independent phase of uptake, there is an energy-dependent phase I (EDP I), which requires both energy and cell growth. Early studies suggested that both the duration and rate of EDPI was proportional to drug concentrations; this initial energy-dependent phase of uptake is not associated with killing. As a result, in whole-cell preparations, it was difficult to distinguish between true uptake or ionic binding to growing cells. It has been suggested that EDP I represents transport throughout a cytoplasmic membrane carrier or carriers (14,69), or uptake by a leak pathway (28). Studies in membrane vesicles have recently shown that no uptake occurs in the absence of energy and that the requirements in EDP I are identical with those ascribed to both EDP I and EDP II in cells (57).

Both the duration and rate of EDP I are dependent on the concentration of aminoglycoside used (9,39; see Fig. 2). EDP I is not associated with either cell death or inhibition of protein synthesis. In *E. coli* with an *rpsL* mutations, or strains with streptomycin-modifying enzymes, EDP I, but not EDP II, is observed for streptomycin (9). Since in vitro studies demonstrate that both enzymatically modified aminoglycosides and native streptomycin show decreased binding to ribosomes from wild-type and strains with *rspL* mutations, respectively (25,26), it appears that EDP I represent uptake across the cytoplasmic membrane in the absence of ribosomal binding. However, EDP I has variously been characterized as a specific uptake, mediated by a membrane energization complex (14) or uptake through nonspecific channels (28).

It has also been postulated that EDP I is an artifact caused by continued cell growth in association with ionic binding to the cell surface (84). However, several experiments in whole cells suggest that EDP I is not an artifact. Both slope and duration of EDP I in *E. coli* and *S. aureus* are dependent on drug concentration; nonspecific binding would not cause these effects. Recent studies in *E. coli* membrane vesicles have also shed additional light on uptake in the absence of ribosomal binding (57); that is, EDP I-type uptake. Studies in whole-cell preparations of *E. coli* and *S. aureus* suggested that aminoglycoside uptake in a medium buffered with potassium phosphate was less than that in an unbuffered medium at the same pH (M. Miller, unpublished data). As a result, we prepared vesicles using potassium 2-(*N*-morpholino)ethanesulfonic acid (MES) buffer, rather than potassium phosphate. Aminoglycoside uptake was measured at 37°C using radiolabeled tobramycin at a concentration of 200 μg/ml. Vesicles were energized with ASC and PMS to ensure a maximal electrochemical potential (65). Although tobramycin accumulation was measured over 10–12 min (Fig. 4), uptake reached a peak at 3–5 min. To measure vesicle-associated aminoglycoside in the absence of $\Delta\psi$, energized vesicles were exposed to the protonophore CCCP, or treated with the ionophore valinomycin, which decreases $\Delta\psi$ and increases ΔpH (see later). Surface binding in the absence of $\Delta\psi$ was also shown by measuring vesicle-associated tobramycin in the absence of electron donors. As with cells, the initial surface binding of aminoglycosides to unenergized vesicles or to vesicles that are initially energized with ASC–PMS and then deenergized with either CCCP or valinomycin was virtually instantaneous. In vesicles, but not in cells (9,12–14,41,69), binding represents up to 25% of vesicle-associated tobramycin.

Studies with the *N*-ethylmaleimide (NEM) were also performed to characterize the effect of sulfhydryl reagents on aminoglycoside uptake (57). The NEM had no effect on energy-independent binding, but blocked subsequent uptake (see Fig. 4). In vesicles, the relatively lipophilic maleimide NEM blocked not only tobramycin uptake but also the uptake of lactose, melibiose, and proline. Studies by Kaback have shown that this blockade is due to inactivation of carrier proteins, rather than the ability of vesicles to generate $\Delta\mu_{H^+}$ (21). Studies with sulfhydryl reagents have been confirmed in whole-cell preparations of *E. coli* and *S. aureus*; both NEM and the more hydrophilic glutathione maleimide blocked tobramycin uptake at concentrations that did not alter cell growth (M. Miller, unpublished data), suggesting that the aminoglycoside transporter is a protein with accessible sulfhydryl groups on the external face of the cytoplasmic membrane.

Studies using membrane vesicles of *P. putida* (93) have shown aminoglycoside uptake kinetics similar to that in our *E. coli* vesicle preparations. When *P. putida* vesicles were energized with ASC–PMS, streptomycin

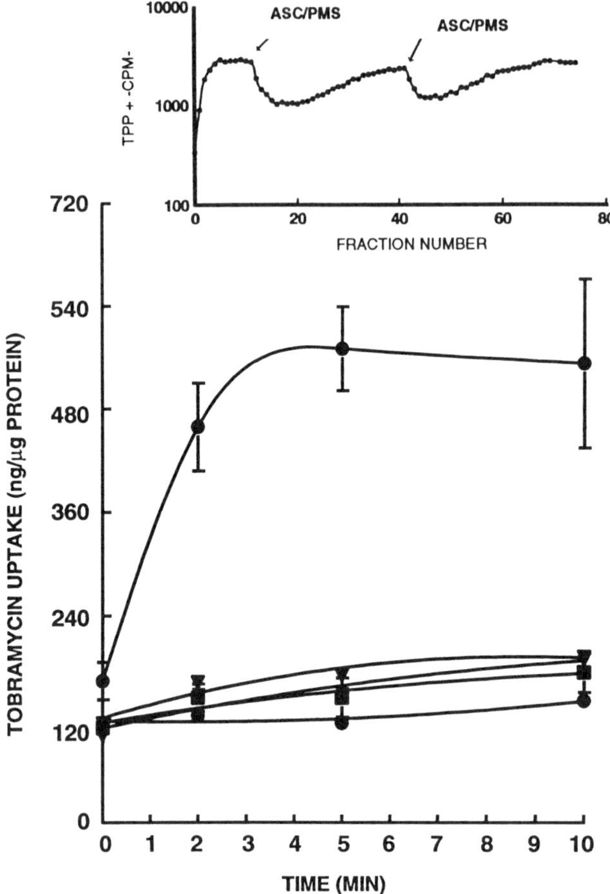

Figure 4 Tobramycin uptake in *E. coli* membrane vesicles energized with 20 mM (○) and 0.1 mM ASC–PMS (●). Also shown is the uptake in vesicles energized with ASC–PMS and then treated with 20 µM CCCP (△) or 0.05 mM NEM before the addition of 200 µg/ml tobramycin (▲). Uptake in unenergized vesicles is also shown for comparison (●).

uptake was noted which, similar to that in *E. coli*, was blocked by CCCP. In *P. putida* the concentration of streptomycin inside cells was approximately double that in the medium.

3. Energy-Dependent Phase II

The third phase of aminoglycoside uptake that is seen with susceptible strains of *E. coli* and *S. aureus* is called EDP II. Unlike EDP I, this phase is associated with protein synthesis inhibition and cell death (see Fig. 2). Uptake during EDP II is more rapid than that during EDP I, but is also concentration-dependent and regulated by $\Delta\psi$. For streptomycin, EDP II does not occur in *E. coli* with *rpsL* mutations or strains with streptomycin-modifying enzymes. However, under certain conditions, EDP II kinetics are observed in the absence of cell death. Puromycin, which at low concentrations increases the number of runoff ribosomes, is associated with accelerated uptake, much like that seen during EDP II. Moreover, gentamicin dose–response studies in isogenic, gentamicin-susceptible and resistant strains of *S. aureus* also showed a dissociation between EDP II kinetics and killing (61). These studies examined aminoglycoside uptake, killing, and changes in optical density in clinical isolates with AAC (6′) and APH (2″) activity (Fig. 5). Like previous studies with streptomycin in *E. coli* with aminoglycoside-modifying enzymes (29), at low concentrations of gentamicin, uptake was less than that in susceptible strains. However, at higher, but still subinhibitory concentrations, uptake was at least comparable with that in a susceptible strain that showed EDP II kinetics. These studies demonstrate that the dissociation between uptake and killing is not limited to a single bacterial species or aminoglycoside. Finally, although there was no killing in the strain with aminoglycoside-modifying activity, at high concentrations there was a decrease in cell growth, as measured turbidimetrically in both the resistant and susceptible strains. This suggested that at higher drug concentrations, modified deoxystreptamines may bind to nonlethal ribosomal targets, inducing an increase in the intracellular sink, which results in enhanced uptake, in the absence of killing.

IV. ENERGETICS OF UPTAKE

Although studies examining the effects of external pH on cells suggested that the rate of aminoglycoside uptake was regulated by membrane potential and was gated, these studies were inconclusive. To better demonstrate the association of $\Delta\psi$ with uptake, membrane potential was manipulated at a fixed external pH with carbodiimides and ionophores, and drug activity or uptake studies were performed in cells and membrane vesicles (57).

It has been proposed that the bioenergetics of aminoglycoside uptake (13,24,69,73) were consistent with the chemiosmotic theory. Accordingly, electrical potential was necessary for the uptake of cationic aminoglycosides (63,69). Furthermore, it appeared that physiological resistance (low pH or anaerobiosis) could be understood using this model, since these and other in situ conditions decrease aminoglycoside uptake and membrane potential (14,33,63,69).

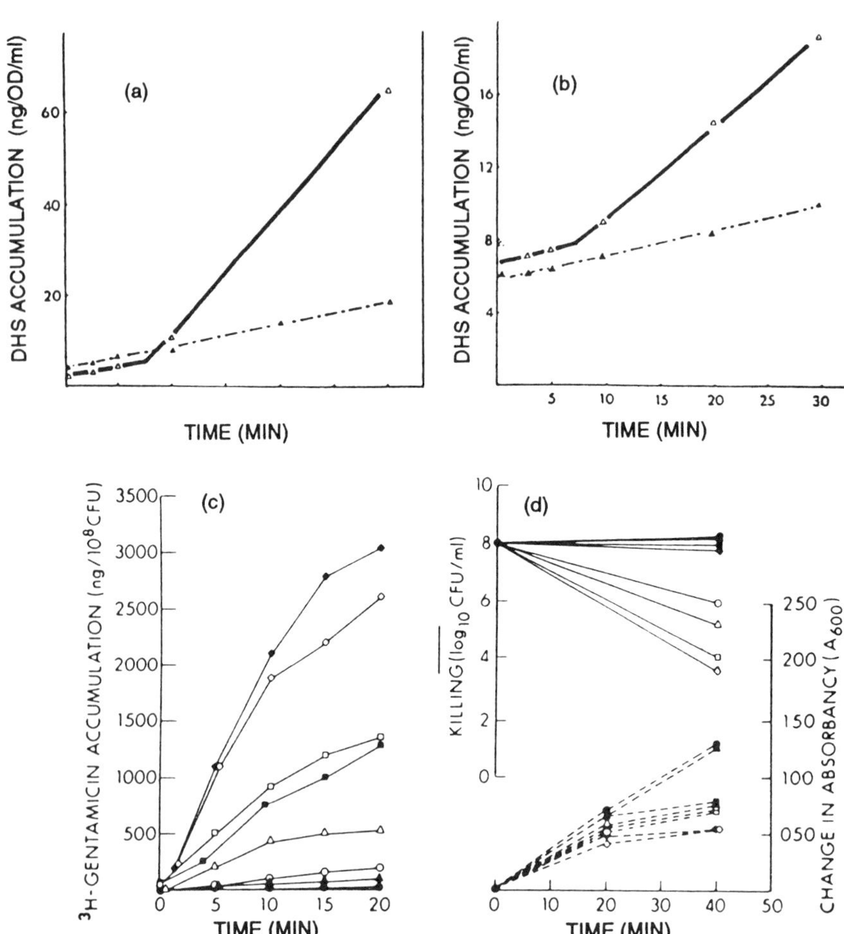

Figure 5 (a) Accumulation of 0.5 μg/ml of dihydrostreptomycin by *E. coli* strains ML308.225 (△—△) and ML308.227 with plasmid-mediated, streptomycin-modifying enzyme activity (▲–▲–▲); (b) uptake in spheroplasts of the same strains. (c) Dose–response relation between external gentamicin concentration and [³H]gentamicin uptake in gentamicin-resistant *S. aureus* strain LM 36 (MIC, 125 μg/ml) at 1.0 (●), 2.5 (▲), 5.0 (■), and 10 (◆) μg/ml of gentamicin. Data for gentamicin-susceptible LM 361 (MIC, 0.4 μg/ml) at the same gentamicin concentrations are also shown (open symbols). (d) Growth rate as a function of absorbance (dashed lines) and viability (solid lines) for the two strains. Gentamicin concentrations (and symbols) as in c.

A. Studies in Cells Treated with Ionophores

Initial uptake studies in *S. aureus* showing that aminoglycoside uptake was dependent on membrane potential used the ionophores nigerin and valinomycin. To ensure that the effects of ambient pH were caused by the changes in the magnitude of $\Delta\psi$, the effects of ionophores on uptake and killing were tested at a constant external pH. The ionophore nigericin catalyzes the transmembrane, electrically neutral exchange of H^+ for K^+, thereby collapsing ΔpH, with a compensatory increase in $\Delta\psi$. Valinomycin has the opposite effect: it increases membrane permeability to K^+ and, in the presence of external K^+, causes $\Delta\psi$ to fall. At pH_o 5.0, where $\Delta\psi$ is relatively low and aminoglycoside uptake and killing were negligible, nigericin increased $\Delta\psi$ at the expense of ΔpH, causing an increase in aminoglycoside uptake and initiation of killing (Fig. 6A). Conversely, valinomycin at a more alkaline pH abolished aminoglycoside uptake and killing in conjunction with a fall in $\Delta\psi$ (see Fig. 6B). Nigericin also induced aminoglycoside uptake in cells grown under anaerobic conditions, during which $\Delta\psi$ was below the critical threshold (64).

Attempts to demonstrate a nigericin dose-dependent association between uptake and $\Delta\psi$ at a fixed external pH were equivocal. There was a correlation between nigericin concentration, uptake, and $\Delta\psi$; however, these studies gave quantitatively unsatisfactory results, in part, owing to the growth-inhibiting and lethal effects of nigericin.

B. Studies with *N,N'*-Dicyclohexylcarbodiimide

To circumvent the problems with nigericin, and to demonstrate dose-dependent association between uptake and $\Delta\psi$, at a fixed external pH, and measure the critical threshold required for the induction of uptake, dose–response studies with N,N'-dicyclohexylcarbodiimide (DCCD) were performed. The carbodiimide DCCD is a highly reactive carboxyl reagent that binds to the F_0 channel of the proton-translocating adenosine triphosphatase (H^+-ATPase) complex, rendering it impermeable to protons. In *S. aureus*, DCCD increased the magnitude of $\Delta\psi$ without inhibiting cell growth (33). Cells exposed to increasing concentrations of DCCD showed a concentration-dependent increase in $\Delta\psi$, with no measurable effect on ΔpH at external pH ranging from 5.0 to 7.5 (33). There was no uptake at pH 5.0 (Fig. 7), for which $\Delta\psi = -140$ mV. However, raising the magnitude of $\Delta\psi$ with DCCD induced drug uptake in a DCCD concentration-dependent manner. At pH 6.0, where $\Delta\psi$ exceeds the critical threshold, uptake occurs in the absence of DCCD. However, uptake was further enhanced in a DCCD concentration-dependent manner. In other experiments, gentamicin uptake (10 × MIC) was studied in log-phase

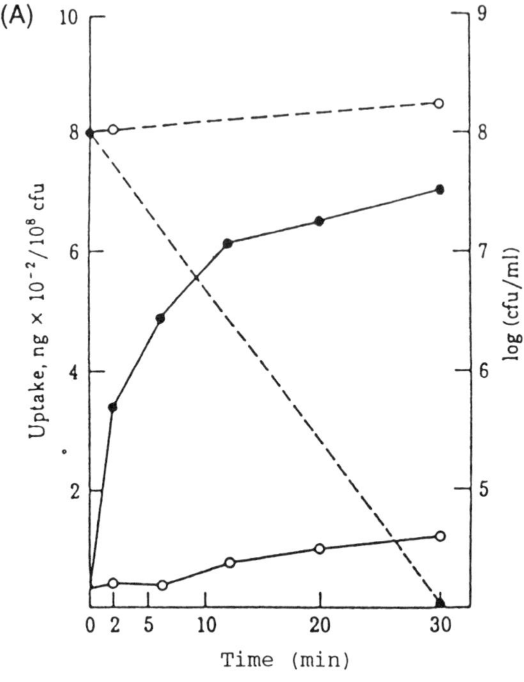

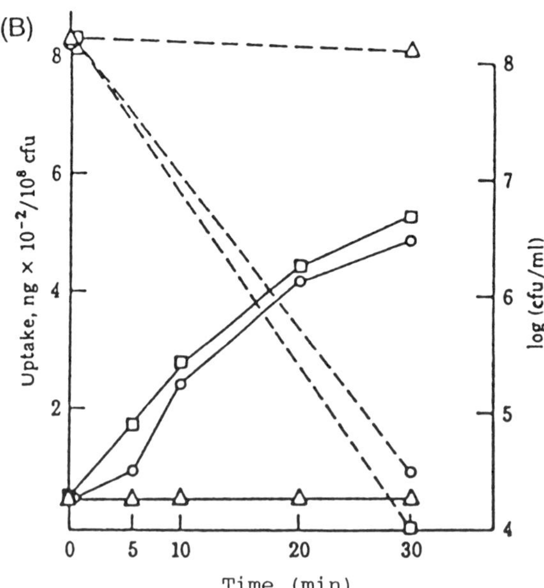

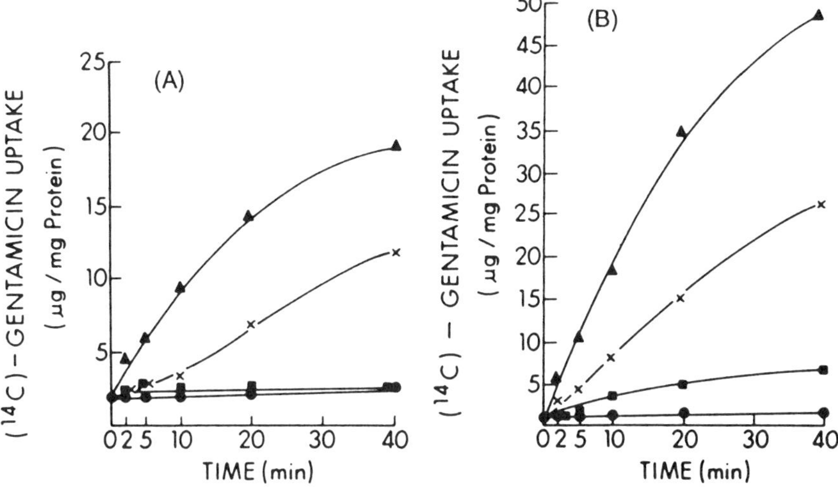

Figure 7 Effect of DCCD on gentamicin uptake in *S. aureus* at (A) pH 5.0 and (B) 6.0. At each pH, baseline uptake values were established in the presence (●) or absence (■) of chloramphenicol. DCCD at 40 μM (×) or 100 μM (▲) was added to log-phase cultures 15 min before time zero.

cells under identical conditions. At both pH 5.0 and 6.0, early killing was proportional to uptake.

These studies suggested that the initiation of uptake requires a critical threshold, and that above this threshold, drug uptake was directly proportional to $\Delta\psi$. The observation that aminoglycoside uptake is dependent on $\Delta\psi$ and is gated has been independently shown by several investigators, using a variety of bacterial strains, including *E. coli*, *B. subtilis*, and *S. aureus* (14,24,34,40). However, the magnitude of the gate is dependent on aminoglycoside concentration. Studies by Bryan with *B. subtilis* showed that the critical threshold necessary for the initiation of streptomycin uptake was dependent on the concentration of streptomycin used (9). In these studies, $\Delta\psi$ was regulated by varying the external K^+ concentra-

---

Figure 6 (A) [^{3}H]Gentamicin uptake (●, ○; solid lines) and killing (●, ○; broken lines) in *S. aureus* 86 W at pH 5.0 in the presence (open symbols) and absence (closed symbols) of 0.05 μM nigericin. (B) Gentamicin uptake (solid lines) and killing (broken lines) in nutrient broth, pH 6.8, in the presence of gentamicin (□), gentamicin plus 2 μM valinomycin (○), gentamicin plus valinomycin plus 50–100 μM KCl (△).

tion. Confirmatory studies with *S. aureus* by Mandel (60) and Eisenberg (33) also showed that increasing the magnitude of $\Delta\psi$ lowered the concentration of gentamicin at which uptake occurred. In this instance the magnitude of $\Delta\psi$ was increased by DCCD or media alkalization. Both groups of investigators showed that, after several minutes of incubation, increasing electrical potential (14,70) did not further enhance aminoglycoside uptake.

C. Tobramycin Uptake in Membrane Vesicles

Tobramycin uptake in vesicles energized with D-lactate was compared with that in vesicles energized with ASC–PMS to determine whether or not aminoglycoside uptake in vesicles, similar to that in cells (14,24,63), was gated. There was no uptake in D-lactate-energized vesicles ($\Delta\psi$ = −95 mV). The addition of nigericin did not stimulate uptake, despite an increase in $\Delta\psi$ to −110 mV (57). These studies suggest that tobramycin uptake in *E. coli* membrane vesicles is gated at between −110 and −120 mV. This value is remarkably similar to that in *E. coli* cells, for which the gate has been estimated at between −107 and −125 mV (14).

Since studies with ionophores demonstrated that uptake in cells was regulated by $\Delta\psi$, rather than $\Delta\mu_{H^+}$ (14,33,63), uptake studies were repeated in membrane vesicles treated with ionophores. Previous studies in *E. coli* cells and right-side-out vesicles have shown that at pH 6.6 and an external K^+ of 100 mM, $\Delta\psi$ can be increased or decreased with the ionophores nigericin and valinomycin, respectively (35,88). The disparate effects of these ionophores on $\Delta\psi$ demonstrate that aminoglycoside uptake is regulated by $\Delta\psi$ and not by ΔpH or $\Delta\mu_{H^+}$ (38). As in whole-cell systems (60,63), nigericin addition to vesicles energized with ASC–PMS increased tobramycin uptake, and valinomycin decreased it (57).

Earlier studies on aminoglycoside uptake in *P. putida* (93) demonstrated kinetics similar to those in *E. coli* vesicle preparations. Moreover, in both *E. coli* and vesicles energized with ASC–PMS, aminoglycoside uptake was blocked by CCCP and intracellular concentrations (C_i) were approximately twofold higher than extracellular concentrations (C_o).

The effect of CCCP and 1% toluene in vesicles that were either energized with ASC–PMS and then preloaded with tobramycin for 10 min, or exposed to tobramycin in the absence of electron donors, was also examined. Treatment with CCCP dissipates both $\Delta\psi$ and ΔpH and causes efflux of substrates that have been actively transported. The addition of CCCP was not associated with efflux of preaccumulated tobramycin (Fig. 8), but caused complete efflux of preaccumulated proline (not shown). Addition

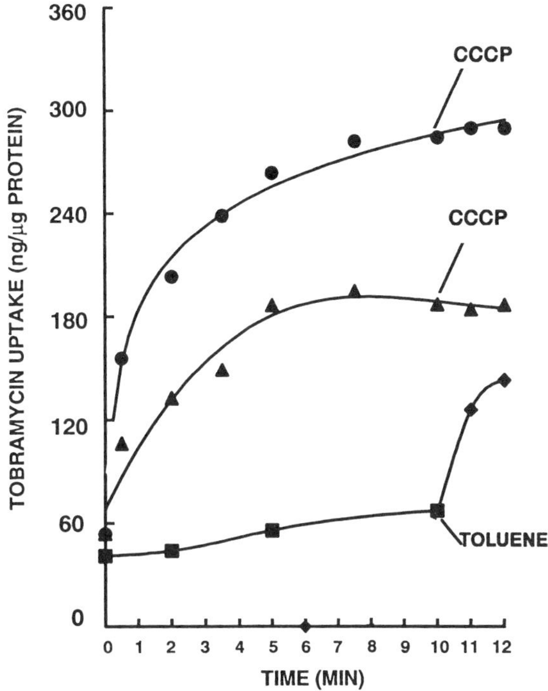

Figure 8 Tobramycin uptake in cytoplasmic membrane vesicles derived from *E. coli* ML308-225. Toluene (1%) was added to unenergized vesicles at 10 min (■). Alternatively, vesicles were energized with 20 mM ASC–0.1 mM PMS in the absence (▲) or presence (●) of 0.4 mM nigericin at 0 min, then treated with 20 mM CCCP at 10 min.

of CCCP did not cause tobramycin to efflux from vesicles exposed to 0.4 μM nigericin, for which the tobramycin C_i/C_o was 2.83.

To confirm that following energization with ASC–PMS, aminoglycoside concentrations inside vesicles did not reach thermodynamic equilibrium with $\Delta\psi$, toluene was also added following 10-min preloading with tobramycin. Toluene addition was not associated with aminoglycoside efflux in preloaded vesicles, confirming C_i/C_o ratios, with or without nigericin, of approximately 2.8 and 1.1, respectively. Moreover, in both vesicles (M. Miller, unpublished data) and cells treated with toluene (4,28), there was an initial stimulation or uptake, suggesting a bypass of the putative membrane carrier.

D. Additional Studies in Cells Further Characterizing the Bioenergetics of Aminoglycoside Uptake

Physiological substrates can be actively transported into bacteria in response to ATP or membrane potential (36,49). Several substrates have independent uptake systems that can be driven by either $\Delta\mu_{H^+}$ or ATP. Although uptake driven by ATP- and $\Delta\mu_{H^+}$-associated systems require plasma membrane carriers (36,49), ATP uptake requires periplasmic-binding proteins (36). Since it is difficult to manipulate or measure membrane energy in the presence of an intact outer membrane, strains carrying *acrA* mutations were used to determine whether ATP might also be able to regulate aminoglycoside uptake. Initial studies suggested that these mutants are defective in outer membrane barrier function (22), but more recent work suggests that they are unable to actively export a variety of preaccumulated cytoplasmic substrates, owing to an inactivation of a multidrug efflux complex (59). Manipulation of membrane energy with ionophores and the determination of $\Delta\psi$ with TPP^+ is possible in *acrA* mutants (39,53). Concentrations of CCCP equal to or less than 8 mM abolish $\Delta\psi$ (39). We confirmed studies by Kinoshita showing that, after a lag of several hours, there is a resumption of growth in *E. coli acrA* strains exposed to CCCP (39,65). Growth was arbitrarily separated into five phases [note that these phases of growth are not related to phases of aminoglycoside uptake (e.g., EDP I and EDP II)]. Phase I represents growth before CCCP addition, and phase II is the brief period after CCCP addition when there is no decrease in replication, as determined turbidimetrically. During phase III, cell replication ceases, resuming after several hours at increasing rates (phase IV), until phase V is reached. During phase V the doubling time was identical with that in phase I (no CCCP) cells.

To ensure that neither CCCP nor TPP^+ were lost from the system or rendered nonfunctional owing to a new barrier effect, we compared the uptake of substrates driven by ion motive gradients or ATP, measured flagellar motion (which is $\Delta\psi$-dependent) by phase-contrast microscopy, and compared TPP^+ uptake in phase V cells washed and resuspended in buffer with or without CCCP (39). However, since the publication of this manuscript, several pumps that actively export cations (59) or CCCP (58) have been described. Nevertheless, the observation that, in phase V cells, uptake of proline ($\Delta\psi$ driven in K^+ buffer), but not methionine (ATP driven) was absent, in conjunction with the lack of flagellar motion, suggested that membrane potential was low or absent. Moreover, the maintenance for 20 min of TPP^+ C_i/C_0 ratios of more than 100 in phase V cells resuspended in buffer, and ratios of unity in CCCP-treated phase V cells, further suggests that the apparent absence of $\Delta\psi$ was not due to an efflux pump.

Studies in phase V cells showed that both cell growth and aminoglycoside uptake was associated with the restoration of intracellular ATP levels. As shown in Figure 9, aminoglycoside uptake during phase I (for which ATP = 6.6 nM/mg protein and $\Delta\psi$ = -179 mV) and phase V (for which $\Delta\mu_{H^+}$ = 0 and ATP = 6.7 nM/mg protein) were comparable.

Whereas earlier studies suggested that, during phase I, membrane potential regulated uptake without the contribution of ATP, it was important to establish that ATP played no role. Recent studies examining transport membrane vesicles suggest that both $\Delta\mu_{H^+}$ and ATP are important (18–20). Moreover, since many manipulations that decrease $\Delta\mu_{H^+}$ also decrease ATP, the importance of each cannot be determined unless the two are uncoupled. To do this we constructed a mutant of CL2 (*E. coli acrA rpsL*) that was deleted for the entire *unc* operon ($\Delta uncBC$) by using sequential transduction with P1vir (39). Previous studies have shown that strains with *uncA* mutations maintain intracellular ATP content in the presence of protonophores (5). We confirmed this by exposing log-phase CL2 *acrA uncBC* mutants to 16 μM CCCP and measuring ATP levels (data not shown). Tobramycin uptake studies in CCCP-treated, *uncBC acrA* mutants in phase I, II, and V are shown in Figure 10. Uptake occurred in phase I and V cells and was absent in phase II cells, despite the maintenance of ATP. Moreover, killing kinetics were similar to that seen in *unc*$^+$ cells (see Fig. 4). In phase I cells, 1 mM sodium arsenate decreased ATP by 90%, but had no effect on the rate of killing (data not shown). These data, in conjunction with earlier studies, strongly suggest that ATP has no role in phase I uptake.

E. Effects of Aminoglycosides on Membrane Potential in Susceptible *acrA* Mutants of *E. coli*

Recent models of the aminoglycoside uptake have focused both on the effects that aminoglycosides themselves may have on membrane potential and the nature of the carrier system(s) (6,14,15,28,84). Previous studies, using a variety of methods to measure the effects of aminoglycoside on $\Delta\psi$, are contradictory (14,15,84). It has also been suggested that the calculation of $\Delta\psi$ from TPP$^+$ uptake may be inaccurate in *E. coli* treated with aminoglycosides (34). However, in recent studies, streptomycin did not alter TPP$^+$ uptake in a high level streptomycin-resistant mutant of *E. coli* (AS-1 *rpsL*) (57). Moreover, $\Delta\psi$ fell from -168 to -135 mV in cells

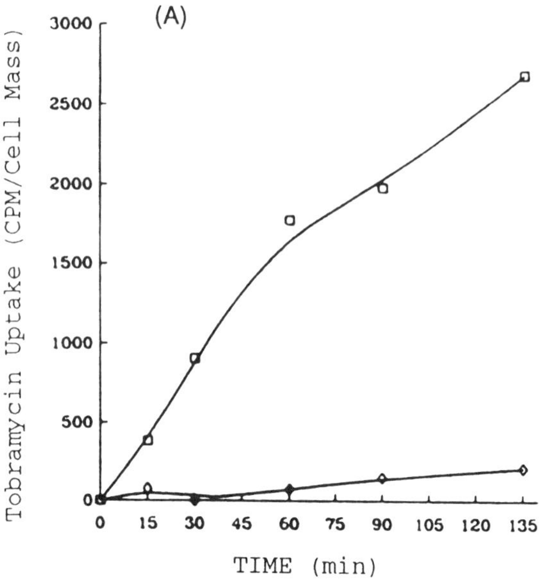

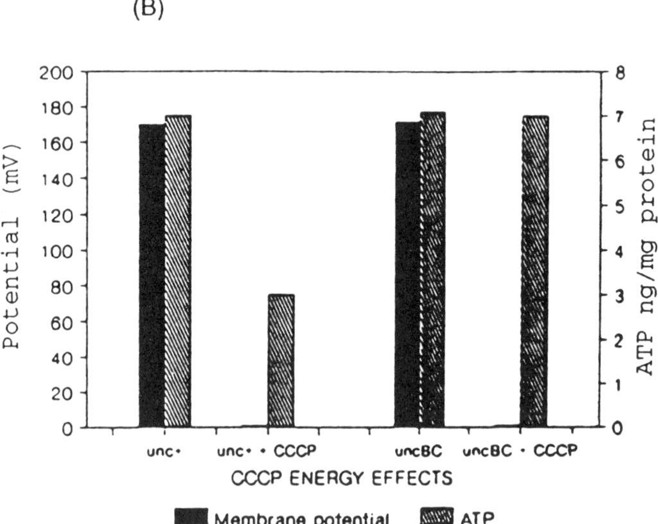

Figure 9 (A) [³H]Tobramycin uptake in *E. coli acrA Δ uncBC* strain HF2 in Luria broth containing 100 mM Tris HCl, pH 7.5, before (phase I, □) and after (phase II, ◇) the addition of 8 μM CCCP. Tobramycin (8 × MIC) was added at time zero, CCCP 5 min before the addition of tobramycin. (B) Effects of CCCP on

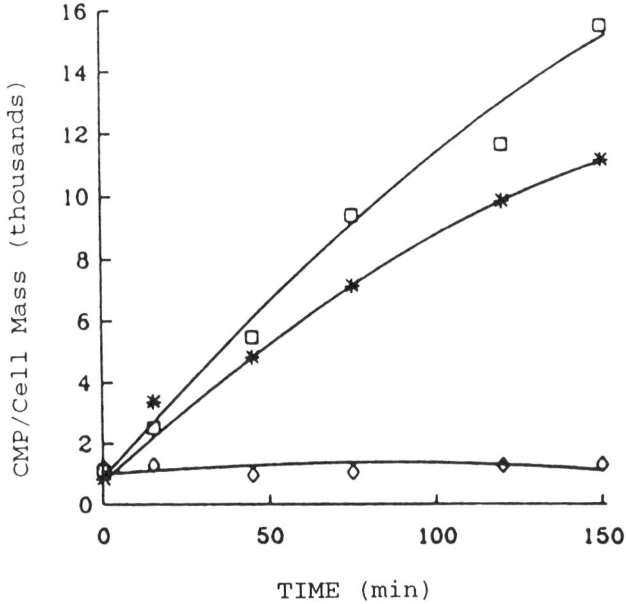

Figure 10 [^{3}H]Tobramycin uptake in *E. coli acrA* CL2 during phases I (□), II (◇), and V (∗) in Luria broth containing Tris HCl, pH 7.5. Tobramycin (16 × MIC) was added to all cells at time zero, and [^{3}H]tobramycin uptake assays were performed at 37°C. CCCP (16 μM) was added to phase II cells 5 min before the addition of tobramycin.

treated with 0–25 μg/ml tobramycin (57). Higher concentrations of tobramycin did not associate with a further decrease in potential.

There have been no systematic efforts to identify the aminoglycoside transporter or transporters. Nevertheless, several models have been proposed based on bacterial transport systems, or on biochemical and bioenergetic observations describing aminoglycoside uptake in cells and membrane vesicles (6,14,15,28,84). For natural substrates, protein carriers are integral to all known energy-driven transport systems or chan-

---

membrane potential and ATP levels in *acrA unc*+ strain CL2 and *acrA ΔuncBC* strain HF2. Membrane potential and ATP levels were measured before and 15 min after the addition of 16 μM CCCP to logarithmic-phase cells in M9 minimal medium plus 0.5% glucose, pH 7.5. Membrane potential was determined by equilibrium distribution of [^{3}H]TPP+, and ATP levels by the luciferin–luciferase assay.

nels. Studies in vesicles suggest that aminoglycosides do not diffuse across the cytoplasmic membrane by a leak pathway. Therefore, it is hard to envision a mechanism of energy-dependent uptake without a protein carrier. In cells and membrane vesicles, sulfhydryl reagents inhibit transport of natural substrates with known protein carriers by inactivating the carriers (21). Sulfhydryl reagents demonstrate varying degrees of membrane penetration and inhibit transport without decreasing respiration or membrane energization (21). Models suggesting that the aminoglycoside transport system is atypical may not be warranted, since these models are often based on conflicting experimental systems (28,84).

VI. MODELS OF UPTAKE AND THEIR RELATION TO MECHANISM OF ACTION OF AMINOGLYCOSIDES

Several models describing the potential mechanisms of the induction of EDP II that involve membrane carriers will be discussed. Data suggesting that the aminoglycoside transporter is a voltage-gated channel will be outlined, and the merits and shortcomings of each model will be considered.

A. Models of EDPII and Their Relation with Aminoglycoside-Induced Lethality

The most elegant and comprehensive model has been proposed by Bryan: Uptake across the cytoplasmic membrane occurs when aminoglycosides bind to a respiratory quinone or a series of transporters linked to quinones (14). Reduction in response to intramembranous electron transport produces a negatively charged aminoglycoside transporter. When the membrane potential reaches a critical threshold, aminoglycosides are actively accumulated across the membrane in response to $\Delta\psi$. Initial cytoplasmic binding involves polysomes as the binding sink (14), and binding to ribosomes induces a perturbation of the ribosomal cycle that accelerates the rate of uptake to the ribosomal sink. Ribosomal effects, presumably involving alteration in protein synthesis, are associated with an eventual loss of cytoplasmic membrane integrity and, thereby, loss of permeability control. The loss of the ribosomal sink in *rpsL* mutants or strains with aminoglycoside-modifying enzymes is associated with the absence of EDP II uptake.

Several models addressing the events leading to EDP II or to cell death have recently been proposed (6,15,28). Although the observation that aminoglycoside uptake is irreversible has been known for years (5,28), the mechanism of aminoglycoside trapping is unknown (28). These new models attempt to explain irreversible uptake, which is assumed to be a critical event leading to cell death. These models are partly based on the seminal studies of Bryan (9,11–14) and Davis (3,4,27), and each represents a modification or expansion of Bryan's model.

A unifying hypothesis to explain how the pleiotropic effects of aminoglycosides cause cell death has recently been proposed by Davis (28). This hypothesis suggests that aminoglycoside-initiated misreading of mRNA results in altered proteins that are inserted into to the cytoplasmic membrane, forming nonspecific channels. These channels are thought to facilitate the uptake or efflux of a variety of substrates, including aminoglycosides themselves (EDP II). Four key factors are identified in this model: (1) misreading, (2) secondary membrane damage, (3) energy-dependent irreversible uptake, and (4) initiation blockade. Uptake before misreading is thought to occur through a leak pathway (28). According to this hypothesis, inhibition of protein synthesis prevents the initial formation of channels, blocking uptake, but has no effect on rapid uptake once it has commenced. Both observations are consistent with the early and late effects of chloramphenicol on aminoglycoside uptake (5,28,60). However, this hypothesis assumes that initial aminoglycoside uptake occurs through a leak pathway or uptake during EDP II occurs by a transporter that differs from that during EDP I. Recent studies with membrane vesicles made from cells not exposed to aminoglycosides suggest that the aminoglycoside uptake bioenergetics are identical with those in whole-cell systems during EDP I and early and late EDP II (57). These observations cannot be reconciled with a leak pathway.

Busse and colleagues have recently proposed a model (6,15) that is similar to that championed by Davis. Both models suggest that aminoglycoside-induced misreading of base pairs during mRNA translation is associated with the formation of nonspecific channels capable of transporting aminoglycosides into cells. From studies in *E. coli*, Busse hypothesized that these transient channels cause intracellular trapping of aminoglycosides (6,15). As with Davis's hypothesis, voltage-gated uptake during late EDP II and by vesicles is difficult to reconcile with uptake by many nonspecific channels. On the other hand, the well-documented loss of cytoplasmic membrane integrity (28) and the fall in membrane potential may, as suggested by both models, be due to the insertion of misread proteins into the cytoplasmic membrane (6,15,27,28) that form nonspecific channels.

B. Is the Aminoglycoside Transporter a Carrier or Channel?

Until the aminoglycoside transporter (or transporters) has been identified and reconstituted, its nature will remain speculative. We have recently proposed a mechanism of aminoglycoside trapping in which an aminoglycoside-associated decrease in the magnitude of $\Delta \psi$ prevents efflux through voltage-gated channels (57). This hypothesis represents a modification of earlier model in which aminoglycoside uptake was linked to $\Delta \psi$ according to chemiosmotic theory (14,55,92). The older model suggested that aminoglycosides were actively transported through a membrane carrier by a uniport mechanism. However, both voltage-dependent carriers and channels are proteins that traverse the cytoplasmic membrane (2,85), and the observation that aminoglycoside uptake by vesicles is voltage-gated suggests that the transporter has properties of a channel. Translocation by channels differs from that by carriers, in that the former is bidirectional, orders of magnitude more rapid, and not saturable at low substrate concentrations and nonconcentrative (95).

In addition to gating, other characteristics of aminoglycoside uptake are also difficult to reconcile with the chemiosmotic model, but are consistent with transport through channels. These include the inability to saturate the carrier at low substrate concentrations; uptake and killing kinetics proportional to $\Delta \psi$ for 2–4 min (33,63), uptake being dependent on aminoglycoside concentration, and the irreversibility of uptake.

In general, carriers are saturated at lower substrate concentrations than are channels. Although the determination of K_t values for antibiotics in susceptible bacteria is fraught with technical problems (i.e., cells may be inhibited or killed during the antibiotic uptake process), studies by Bryan with *E. coli rpsL* showed that uptake was saturable at high streptomycin concentrations (9). Moreover, the K_t for streptomycin in membrane vesicles of *Pseudomonas putida* was 15 mM (93), and no known substrates show competitive inhibition of aminoglycoside uptake. Thus, streptomycin uptake is saturable in vesicles and cells, it occurs at high K_t values, consistent with transport by channels.

The early proportionality between membrane potential and both killing and uptake has been interpreted according to the chemiosmotic model. However, uptake by voltage-gated channels offers an alternative explanation. Voltage-gated channels do not "open" or "close" at a given potential (16,44). Rather, at the single-channel level, gating transitions are stochastic. Even though the number of open channels per unit membrane fluctuates spontaneously, the likelihood of being in an open configuration varies over a narrow range of membrane potential (16,44). To understand the alteration of the apparent magnitude of the gate by external aminoglycoside concentration, it is also important that following the initiation of uptake, aminoglycosides themselves stimulate a series of events (EDP II). This autostimulation greatly increases aminoglycoside uptake and is necessary for lethal activity (14,68).

That transport through channels is bidirectional suggests a mechanism for irreversible aminoglycoside uptake. Although studies examining the effect of aminoglycosides on $\Delta\psi$ have been contradictory (6,14,15,41), recent data suggest that aminoglycosides decrease $\Delta\psi$. Previous studies have also shown that, after several minutes, the addition of either gentamicin (14) or streptomycin (41) to *E. coli* cells was associated with a fall in the magnitude of $\Delta\psi$ by 20–30 mV, which is comparable with that seen when *E. coli* cells are exposed to tobramycin. We propose that at a lower magnitude of $\Delta\psi$, sufficient uptake occurs at high aminoglycoside concentrations to initiate EDP II, despite fewer channels being in the open configuration (57). An increase in the magnitude of $\Delta\psi$ would open more channels so that otherwise subinhibitory concentrations of aminoglycosides initiate EDP II and killing.

This model may also explain why uptake and killing are proportional to membrane potential for only a brief period. Since the percentage of channels in the open configuration is a function of the magnitude of $\Delta\psi$, it follows that, at a fixed external aminoglycoside concentration, the initial rate of aminoglycoside uptake is proportional to $\Delta\psi$. However, the internal and external aminoglycoside concentrations rapidly reach equilibrium, and the apparent relation between the magnitude of $\Delta\psi$ and the rate of uptake would cease.

Finally, we propose an alternative model to explain aminoglycoside-induced killing. Aminoglycosides themselves decrease the magnitude of $\Delta\psi$. Since transport through channels is bidirectional, the closure of the voltage-gated channels would cause irreversible "trapping" of intracellular aminoglycosides. This hypothesis might also explain why the aminoglycosides are bactericidal, whereas other inhibitors of protein synthesis that do not alter $\Delta\psi$ or enter by voltage-gated channels are bacteriostatic. The failure of tobramycin efflux after the addition of CCCP is consistent with this model.

VII. CONCLUSIONS AND FUTURE DIRECTIONS

Aminoglycosides continue to have a prominent role in the therapy of life-threatening bacterial infections. New approaches to the more effective use of existing aminoglycosides and the development of new agents in this class require a better understanding of their mechanism(s) of action. Although we do not understand how aminoglycosides kill bacteria, both transport and trapping appear to be necessary for killing; both microbial and physiological resistance is often associated with impaired uptake (9,12–14,29,60,62,64). Recent data characterizing the pharmacodynamics of aminoglycosides have demonstrated that bacterial killing correlates with clinically relevant concentrations and that inhibition persists after drug removal (35). Although these observations have already brought about a change in the way aminoglycosides are administered, an understanding of aminoglycoside pharmacodynamics at the cellular level is rudimentary (7). Additional data characterizing the unique mechanisms of translocation (uptake and efflux) may also be important in understanding aminoglycoside pharmacodynamics. Aminoglycosides continue to be first-line agents in the treatment of the reemerging pathogens *Mycobacterium tuberculosis* and the enterococci. They are used in the treatment of multidrug-resistant tuberculosis strains; in patients who cannot tolerate oral medications, or as part of short course regimens. The mechanism of aminoglycoside resistance in multidrug-resistant *M. tuberculosis* strains has not been rigorously studied. Since mutations do not cause high-level resistance to the 2-deoxystreptamines in other bacteria, and no plasmids or aminoglycoside-modifying enzymes have been reported in *M. tuberculosis*, decreased transport may play an important role in resistance. The increasing prevalence of aminoglycoside-modifying enzymes in enterococci has been associated with an inability to treat some patients (80). Difference in aminoglycoside uptake in gram-positive and gram-negative bacteria of streptidine and 2-deoxystreptamines aminoglycosides (61; M. Miller, unpublished data) may be particularly important to pursue as it relates to these pathogens.

Areas of future research of aminoglycoside transport can be divided into those of which the primary focus is mechanistic, and those of which primary focus is therapeutic. However, this division is artificial, since a better understanding of aminoglycoside translocation (uptake and efflux) will enhance our knowledge of their mechanisms of action and resistance and will be important in drug design. Whereas uptake across the outer membrane of *P. aeruginosa* has been extensively characterized (42,76,82), little is known about uptake in facultative gram-negative bacilli. Models of EDP II, the aminoglycoside-induced rapid phase of uptake, implicate either nonspecific channels or alterations in the ribosomal binding (6,15,28,92). Interestingly, other antibiotics that inhibit protein synthesis have disparate effects of uptake, and the reasons for these important differences are unclear (5,85). Although translocation across the cytoplasmic membrane requires one or more protein transporters, a direct role of respiratory quinones in membrane energization complex has also been hypothesized (14). Descriptive studies of aminoglycoside uptake have suggested that the translocation machinery is a cytoplasmic membrane carrier or channel. However, neither construct fits all experimental data or better-characterized models of translocation in bacteria or higher organisms.

Even though bioenergetic studies have clearly involved membrane potential as the proximate regulator of uptake, under unusual circumstances, uptake may also require ATP (39). Studies implicating ATP need to be repeated in light of recent data suggesting a confounding role of efflux pumps (58,59). The identification and reconstitution of aminoglycoside carrier(s) are important not only in understanding how these drugs work, but such studies may also serve as models for transport in bacteria and eukaryotic cells.

It is generally assumed that the highly lipophilic aminoglycosides do not penetrate into mammalian cells. Indeed, aminoglycosides are used as an in vitro experimental tool to distinguish between intra- and extracellular bacteria. However, several studies suggest that some uptake into eukaryotic cells does occur. The inactivity of aminoglycosides within mammalian cells may be a function of the local microenvironment and trafficking, rather than that of simply poor penetration. Moreover, the clinical benefit of aminoglycosides in animal models of mycobacterial infections also suggests an eukaryotic, intracellular site of action. The penetration of aminoglycosides into eukaryotic cells can be increased by using liposomal preparations (90). Intracellular *Salmonella* are killed by liposomal preparations of aminoglycosides. Although there are many alternatives for the therapy of typhoid fever, the liposomal formulation may be useful in the therapy of other intracellular pathogens, such as mycobacteria, for which there are few therapeutic alternatives (see Chap. 9).

REFERENCES

1. Abad JP, Amils R. Synthesis of active nitroguaiacol ether derivatives of streptomycin. Antimicrob Agents Chemother 1990; 34:1908–1914.
2. Ames GF, Lecar H. ATP-dependent bacterial transporters and cystic fibrosis: analogy between channels and transporters. FASEB J 1992; 6:2660–2666.
3. Anand N, Davis B. Effect of streptomycin on *Escherichia coli*. Nature 1960; 4705:22–23.
4. Anand N, Davis BD, Armitage AK. Uptake of streptomycin in *Escherichia coli*. Nature 1960; 186:22–24.
5. Andry K, Bockrath RC. Dihydrostreptomycin accumulation in *E. coli*. Nature 1974; 251:534–536.
6. Bakker EP. Aminoglycoside and aminocyclitol antibiotics: hygromycin B is an atypical bactericidal compound that exerts effects on cells of *Escherichia coli* characteristic for bacteriostatic aminocyclitols. J Gen Microbiol 1992; 138:563–569.
7. Barmada S, Kohlhepp S, Leggett J, Dworkin R, Gilbert D. Correlation of tobramycin induced inhibition of protein synthesis with postantibiotic effect in *Escherichia coli*. Antimicrob Agents Chemother 1993; 37:2678–83.

8. Bermudez LE, Yau Yong AO, Lin JP, Cogger J, Young LS. Treatment of disseminated *Mycobacterium avium* complex infection of beige mice with liposome encapsulated aminoglycosides. J Infect Dis 1990; 161:1262–8.

9. Bryan LE, Van Den Elzen HM. Streptomycin accumulation in susceptible and resistant strains of *Escherichia coli* and *Pseudomonas aeruginosa*. Antimicrob Agents Chemother 1976; 9:928–938.

10. Bryan LE, Van Den Elzen HM. Effects of membrane-energy mutations and cations on streptomycin and gentamicin accumulation by bacteria: a model for entry of streptomycin and gentamicin in susceptible and resistant bacteria. Antimicrob Agents Chemother 1977; 12 163-177.

11. Bryan LE, Kowand SK, Van Den Elzen HM. Mechanism of aminoglycoside antibiotic resistance in anaerobic bacteria: *Clostridium perfringens* and *Bacteroides fragilis*. Antimicrob Agents Chemother 1979; 15:7–13.

12. Bryan LE, Van Den Elzen HM. Effects of membrane-energy mutations and actions on streptomycin and gentamicin accumulation by bacteria: a model for entry of streptomycin in susceptible and resistant bacteria. Antimicrob Agents Chemother 1979; 12:163–177.

13. Bryan LE, Kwan S. Mechanisms of aminoglycoside resistance of anaerobic bacteria and facultative bacteria grown anaerobically. J Antimicrob Chemother 1981; 8 (suppl D):1–8.

14. Bryan LE, Kwan S. Roles of ribosomal binding, membrane potential, and electron transport in bacterial uptake of streptomycin and gentamicin. Antimicrob Agents Chemother 1983; 23:835–845.

15. Busse HJ, Wostmann C, Bakker E. The bactericidal action of streptomycin: membrane permeabilization caused by the insertion of mistranslated proteins into the cytoplasmic membrane of *Escherichia coli* and subsequent caging of the antibiotic inside the cells due to degradation of these proteins. J Gen Microbiol 1992; 138:551–561.

16. Catterall W. Structure and function of voltage-sensitive ion channels. Science 1988; 242:50–61.

17. Chambers HF, Miller MH. Emergence of resistance to cephalothin and gentamicin during combination therapy for methicillin-resistant *Staphylococcus aureus* endocarditis in rabbits. J Infect Dis 1987; 155:581–585.

18. Chen L, Tai PC. ATP is essential for protein translocation into *E. coli* membrane* vesicles. Proc Natl Acad Sci USA 1985; 82:4384–4388.

19. Chen L, Tai PC. Roles of H^+-ATPase and proton motive force in ATP-dependent protein translocation in vitro. J Bacteriol 1986; 167:389–392.

20. Chen L, Tai PC. Effects of nucleotides on ATP-dependent protein translocation into *Escherichia coli* membrane vesicles. J Bacteriol 1986; 168:828–832.

21. Cohn DE, Kaczorowski GJ, Kaback HR. Effects of the proton electrochemical gradient on maleimide inactivation of active transport in *Escherichia coli* membrane vesicles. Biochemistry 1981; 20:3308–3313.

22. Coleman WG Jr, Leive L. Two mutations which affect the barrier function of the *Escherichia coli* K-12 outer membrane. J Bacteriol 1979; 139:899–910.

23. Dalhoff A. Aminoglycoside accumulation by membrane vesicles of *Esche-*

richia coli and *Streptococcus faecalis*. Zentrabl Bakt Mikrobiol Hyg 1983; 254:333–342.

24. Damper PD, Epstein W. Role of the membrane potential in bacterial resistance to aminoglycoside antibiotics. Antimicrob Agents Chemother 1981; 20:803–808.

25. Davis J. Bacterial resistance to aminoglycoside antibiotics. J Infect Dis 1971; 124 (suppl):7–10.

26. Davis J, Kagan SA. What is the mechanism of plasmid-determined resistance to aminoglycoside antibiotics? In: Drews J, Hogenau G, eds. R-Factors: Their Properties and Possible Control. Topics in Infectious Diseases, vol 2. New York: Springer-Verlag, 1977:207–219.

27. Davis BD, Chen L, Tai PC. Misread protein creates membrane channels: an essential step in the bactericidal action of aminoglycosides. Proc Natl Acad Sci USA 1986; 83:6164–6168.

28. Davis B. Mechanism of bacterial action of aminoglycosides. Microbiol Rev 1987; 51:341–350.

29. Dickie P, Bryan LE, Pickard MA. Effect of enzymatic adenylylation on dihydrostreptomycin accumulation in *Escherichia coli* carrying an R-factor: model explaining aminoglycoside resistance by inactivating mechanisms. Antimicrob Agents Chemother 1978; 14:569–580.

30. Difco Laboratories, Inc. Dehydrated culture media and reagents for microbiology. In: Difco Manual, 10th ed. Detroit: Difco Laboratories, 1984.

31. Donovick R, Bayan AP, Canales P, Pansy F. The influence of certain substances on the activity of streptomycin. III. Differential effects of various electrolytes on the action of streptomycin. J Bacteriol 1948; 56:125–37.

32. Drusano GL. The role of pharmacokinetics in the outcome of infections. Antimicrob Agents Chemother 1988; 32:289–297.

33. Eisenberg ES, Mandel LJ, Kaback HR, Miller MH. Quantitative association between electrical potential across the cytoplasmic membrane and early gentamicin uptake and killing in *Staphylococcus aureus*. J Bacteriol 1984; 157:863–867.

34. Emling F, Holtje JV. Autostimulation of dihydrostreptomycin uptake in *Bacillus subtilis*. J Gen Microbiol 1987; 133:3495–3504.

35. Felle H, Porter JS, Slayman CL, Kaback HR. Quantitative measurements of membrane potential in *Escherichia coli*. Biochemistry 1980; 19:3585–3590.

36. Ferro-Luzzi Ames G. Structure and mechanism of bacterial periplasmic transport systems. J Bioenerg Biomembr 1988; 20:1–18.

37. Frace AM, Gargus JJ. Molecular biology of membrane transport proteins. Curr Top Membr 1991; 39:3–36.

38. Friedberg I, Kaback HR. Electrochemical proton gradient in *Micrococcus lysodeikticus* cells and membrane vesicles. J Bacteriol 1980; 142:651–8.

39. Fraimow HS, Greenman JB, Leviton IM, et al. Tobramycin uptake in *Escherichia coli* is driven by either electrical potential or ATP. J Bacteriol 1991; 173:2800–2808.

40. Gilman S, Saunders VA. Accumulation of gentamicin by *Staphylococcus aureus*: the role of the transmembrane electrical potential. J Antimicrob Chemother 1986; 17:37–44.

41. Goss SR, Spicer AB, Nichols WW. Bioenergetics of dihydrostreptomycin transport by *Escherichia coli*. FEBS Lett 1988; 228:245–248.

42. Hancock REW. Aminoglycoside uptake and mode of action—with special reference to streptomycin and gentamicin. J Antimicrob Chemother 1981; 8:249–276, 429–445.

43. Hancock REW, Nikaido H. Resistance to antibacterial agents acting on cell membranes. In: Bryan LE, ed. Antimicrobial Drug Resistance. New York: Academic Press, 1984:147–171.

44. Hille B. Ionic Channels of Excitable Membranes. Sunderland, MA: Sinauer Associates, 1992.

45. Hoch DH, Finkelstein A. Gating of large toxin channels by pH. Ann NY Acad Sci 1985; 456:33–35.

46. Holtje JV. Streptomycin uptake via an inducible polyamine transport system in *Escherichia coli*. Eur J Biochem 1978; 86:345–351.

47. Hurwitz C, Braun CB, Rosano CL. Role of ribosome recycling in uptake of dihydrostreptomycin by sensitive and resistant *Escherichia coli*. Biochim Biophys Acta 1981; 652:168–176.

48. Kaback HR. Bacterial membranes. Methods Enzymol 1971; 22:99–120.

49. Kaback HR. Transport across isolated bacterial cytoplasmic membranes. Biochim Biophys Acta 1972; 265:367–416.

50. Kaback HR, Reeves JP, Short SA, Lombardi FJ. Mechanisms of active transport in isolated bacterial membrane vesicles. The mechanism of action of carbonylcyanide *m*-chlorophenylyhydrazone. Arch Biochem Biophys 1974; 160:215–22.

51. Kashket ER. Effects of aerobiosis and nitrogen source on the proton motive force in growing *Escherichia coli* and *Klebsiella pneumoniae* cells. J Bacteriol 1981; 146:377–384.

52. Kashiwagi K, Kobayashi H, Igarashi K. Apparently unidirectional polyamine transport by proton motive force in polyamine-deficient *Escherichia coli*. J Bacteriol 1986; 165:972–977.

53. Kinoshita N, Unemoto T, Kobayashi H. Proton motive force is not obligatory for growth of *Escherichia coli*. J Bacteriol 1984; 160:1074–1077.

54. Kitano K, Tomasz A. Triggering of autolytic cell wall degradation in *Escherichia coli* by beta-lactam antibiotics. Antimicrob Agents Chemother 1979; 16:838–848.

55. Konings WN, Otto R, Ten Brink B. Relation between the proton motive force and solute transport in bacteria. Biochem Soc Trans 1984; 12:152–154.

56. Kusser W, Zimmer K, Fiedler F. Characteristics of the binding of aminoglycoside antibiotics to teichoic acids. Eur J Biochem 1985; 151:601–605.

57. Leviton IM, Fraimow HS, Carrasco N, Miller MH. Tobramycin uptake in *Escherichia coli* membrane vesicles. Antimicrob Agents Chemother 1995; 39:467–475.

58. Lomovskaya O, Lewis K. *emr*, an *Escherichia* coli locus for multidrug resistance. Proc Natl Acad Sci USA 1992; 89:8938–42.

59. Ma D, Cook DN, Alberti M, Pon NG, Nikaido H, Hearst JE. Molecular cloning and characterization of *acrA* and *acrE* genes of *Escherichia coli*. J Bacteriol 1993; 175:6299–313.

60. Mandel LJ, Eisenberg ES, Simkin NJ, Miller MH. Effect of *NN'*-dicyclohexyl-carbodiimide and nigericin on *Staphylococcus aureus* susceptibility to gentamicin. Antimicrob Agents Chemother 1983; 24:440–442.

61. Mandel LJ, Murphy E, Steigbigel NH, Miller MH. Gentamicin uptake in *Staphylococcus aureus* possessing plasmid-encoded, aminoglycoside-modifying enzymes. Antimicrob Agents Chemother 1984; 26:563–569.

62. Manoil C, Beckwith J. *TnphoA*: a transposon prove for protein export signals. Proc Natl Acad Sci USA 1985; 82:8129–8133.

63. Mates SM, Eisenberg ES, Mandel LJ, Patel L, Kaback HR, Miller MH. Membrane potential and gentamicin uptake in *Staphylococcus aureus*. Proc Natl Acad Sci USA 1982; 79:6693–6697.

64. Mates SM, Patel L, Kaback HR, Miller MH. Membrane potential in anaerobically growing *Staphylococcus aureus* and its relationship to gentamicin uptake. Antimicrob Agents Chemother 1983; 23:526–530.

65. Matsushita K, Kaback HR. D-Lactate oxidation and generation of the proton electrochemical gradient in membrane vesicles from *Escherichia coli* GR19N and in proteoliposomes reconstituted with purified D-lactate dehydrogenase and cytochrome oxidase. Biochemistry 1986; 25:2321–2327.

66. McEnroe AS, Taber HW. Correlation between cytochrome aa_3 concentrations and streptomycin accumulation in *Bacillus subtilis*. Antimicrob Agents Chemother 1984; 26:507–512.

67. Merlin TL, Davis GE, Anderson WL, Moyzis RK, Griffith JK. Aminoglycoside uptake increased by *tet* gene expression. Antimicrob Agents Chemother 1989; 33:1549–52.

68. Miller MH, Wexler MA, Steigbigel NH. Single and combination antibiotic therapy of *Staphylococcus aureus* experimental endocarditis: emergence of gentamicin resistant mutants. Antimicrob Agents Chemother 1978; 14:336–343.

69. Miller MH, Edberg SC, Mandel LJ, Behar CF, Steigbigel NH. Gentamicin uptake in wild-type and aminoglycoside-resistant small colony mutants of *Staphylococcus aureus*. Antimicrob Agents Chemother 1980; 18:722–729.

70. Miller MH, Mandel LJ, Mates SM, Simkin NJ, Kaback HR. Effect of specific alterations of membrane energization on gentamicin accumulation and killing in sensitive *S. aureus*. *Intersci Conf Antimicrob Agents Chemother* 1981; 21:507 Abstr.

71. Miller MH. Mechanisms of β-lactam/aminoglycoside potentiation in *P. aeruginosa* and *E. coli*. Clin Res 1986; 34:526A.

72. Miller MH, El-Sokkary MA, Feinstein SA, Lowy FD. Penicillin-induced effects on streptomycin uptake and early bactericidal activity differ in viridans group and enterococcal streptococci. Antimicrob Agents Chemother 1986; 30:763–768.

73. Mitchell P. Chemiosmotic Coupling and Energy Transduction. Bodmin, UK: Glynn Research, 1968.

74. Modolell J. The S-30 system from *E. coli*. In: Last JA, Laskin AI, eds. Protein Biosynthesis in Bacterial Systems. New York: Marcel Dekker, 1971:1–5.

75. Moellering RC Jr, Weinberg AN. Studies on antibiotic synergism against enterococci. II. Effect of various antibiotics on the uptake of C_{14}-labelled streptomycin by enterococci. J Clin Invest 1971; 50:2580–2584.

76. Moore RA, Hancock REW. Involvement of outer membrane of *Pseudomonas cepacia* in aminoglycoside and polymyxin resistance. Antimicrob Agents Chemother 1986; 30:923–926.

77. Muir ME, Hanwell DR, Wallace BJ. Characterization of a respiratory mutant of *Escherichia coli* with reduced uptake of aminoglycoside antibiotics. Biochim Biophys Acta 1981; 638:234–241.

78. Muir ME, Van Heswyck RS, Wallace BJ. Effect of growth rate on streptomycin accumulation by *Escherichia coli* and *Bacillus megaterium*. J Gen Microbiol 1984; 130:2015–2022.

79. Muir ME, Ballesteros M, Wallace BJ. Respiration rate, growth rate and the accumulation of streptomycin in *Escherichia coli*. J Gen Microbiol 1985; 131:2573–79.

80. Murray B. New aspects of antimicrobial resistance and resulting therapeutic dilemas. J Infect Dis 1991; 163:1184–1194.

81. Newman MJ, Foster DL, Wilson TH. Purification and reconstitution of functional lactose carrier from *Escherichia coli*. J Biol Chem 1981; 256:11804–11808.

82. Nicas TI, Hancock RE. Alteration of susceptibility to EDTA, polymyxin B and gentamicin in *Pseudomonas aeruginosa* by divalent cation regulation of outer membrane protein HI. J Gen Microbiol 1983; 129:509–517.

83. Nichols WW, Young SN. Respiration-dependent uptake of dihydrostreptomycin by *Escherichia coli*. J Biochem 1985; 228:505–512.

84. Nichols WW. On the mechanism of translocation of dihydrostreptomycin across the bacterial cytoplasmic membrane. Biochim Biophys Acta 1987; 895:11–23.

85. Nikaido H, Saier MH Jr. Transport proteins in bacteria: common themes in their design. Science 1992; 258:936–942.

86. Nunoki K, Florio V, Catterall W. Activation of purified calcium channels by stoichiometric protein phosphorylation. Proc Natl Acad Sci USA 1989; 86:6816–6820.

87. Plotz PH, Davis BD. Synergism between streptomycin and penicillin: a proposed mechanism. Science 1962; 135:1067–1068.

88. Ramos S, Schuldiner S, Kaback HR. The electrochemical gradient of protons and its relationship to active transport in *Escherichia coli* membrane vesicles. Proc Natl Acad Sci USA 1976; 73:1892–1896.

89. Ramos S, Kaback HR. pH dependent changes in proton:substrate stoichiometries during active transport in *Escherichia coli* membrane vesicles. Biochemistry 1977; 16:4270–5.

90. Swenson CE, Stewart KA, Hammett JL, Fitzsimmons WE, Ginsberg RS. Pharmacokinetics and in vivo activity of liposome-encapsulated gentamicin. Antimicrob Agents Chemother 1990; 34:235–40.

91. Taber HW, Halfenger GM. Multiple aminoglycoside-resistent mutants of *Bacillus substilis*, deficient in accumulation of kanamycin. Antimicrob Agents Chemother 1976; 9:251–259.

92. Taber HW, Mueller JP, Miller PF, Arrow AS. Bacterial uptake of aminoglycoside antibiotics. Microbiol Rev 1987; 51:439–457.

93. Thomson TB, Crider BP, Eagon RG. The kinetics of dihydrostreptomycin uptake in *Pseudomonas putida* membrane vesicles: absence of inhibition by cations. J Antimicrob Chemother 1985; 16:157–163.

94. Thorbjarnardottir SH, Magnusdottir RA, Eggertsson G. Mutations determining generalized resistance to aminoglycoside antibiotics in *Escherichia coli*. Mol Gen Genet 1978; 161:89–98.

95. Wilson DB. Cellular transport mechanisms. Annu Rev Biochem 1978; 47:933–960.

96. Yee Y, Farber B, Mates S. Mechanism of penicillin streptomycin synergy for clinical isolates of viridans streptococci. J Infect Dis. 1986; 154:531–4.

97. Yoneyama H, Nakae T. Small diffusion pore in the outer membrane of *Pseudomonas aeruginosa*. Eur J Biochem 1986; 157:33–38.

98. Zenilman JM, Miller MH, Mandel LJ. In vitro studies simultaneously examining effect of oxacillin on uptake of radiolabeled streptomycin and on associated bacterial lethality in *Staphylococcus aureus*. Antimicrob Agents Chemother 1986; 30:877–882.

7

Tetracycline Uptake and Efflux in Bacteria

Ian Chopra
SmithKline Beecham Pharmaceuticals, Surrey, England

I. INTRODUCTION

A. Perspective

The tetracyclines are a group of antibiotics that were discovered at Lederle Laboratories in 1948, with the isolation of chlortetracycline from *Streptomyces aureofaciens* (1). Subsequently, other tetracyclines were identified, either as naturally occurring molecules, or as products of semisynthetic approaches (1,2). Several of the tetracyclines have been developed for the therapy of human or veterinary bacterial infections (Table 1), and these have been referred to as first- (1948–1957) and second-generation (1965–1972) tetracyclines (3). The therapeutic usefulness of the tetracyclines arises from their relative safety and their broad-spectrum profile; that is, they exhibit activity against most gram-positive and gram-negative bacteria (including obligate anaerobes), chlamydiae, mycoplasmas, rickettsiae, and protozoan parasites (3).

Since the bacterial ribosome is the target of those tetracyclines used clinically (see Sec. I.B), it is clear that to reach their intracellular target they must cross one or two membranes, depending on whether the organism is gram-positive or gram-negative. These aspects will be considered in more detail in subsequent sections. Removal of tetracyclines from the

Table 1 Principal Tetracyclines Used for the Therapy of Infectious Diseases

Chemical name	Generic name	Trade name	Year of discovery
7-Chlorotetracycline	Chlortetracycline	Aureomycin	1948
5-Hydroxytetracycline	Oxytetracycline	Terramycin	1948
Tetracycline	Tetracycline	Achromycin	1953
6-Demethyl-7-chlorotetracycline	Demethylchlorotetracycline	Declomycin	1957
6-Methylene-5-hydroxytetracycline	Methacycline	Rondomycin	1965
6-Deoxy-5-hydroxytetracycline	Doxycycline	Vibramycin	1967
7-Dimethylamino-6-demethyl-6-deoxy tetracycline	Minocycline	Minocin	1972

cytoplasm is an important mechanism of resistance to this class of antibiotics (3,4). Hence, this chapter also considers the molecular mechanisms by which tetracyclines leave the cytoplasm through efflux across the bacterial cytoplasmic membrane.

B. Tetracycline Targets

Studies conducted in intact bacteria during the 1950s and early 1960s established that several tetracyclines were primarily inhibitors of bacterial protein synthesis (4). Subsequent work has confirmed this, and it is now established that those tetracyclines listed in Table 1 are indeed inhibitors of bacterial protein synthesis (3). Inhibition of protein synthesis results from disruption of codon–anticodon association between tRNA and mRNA, thereby preventing binding of aminoacyl-tRNA to the ribosomal acceptor (A) site (3). This is mediated by binding of drug to a single site on the 30S ribosomal subunit (3). Nevertheless, interaction of these tetracyclines with the 30S ribosomal subunit is reversible, since these agents are bacteriostatic (3,8; Table 2).

Recently a second class of tetracycline analogues has been identified, the primary target of which is not the bacterial ribosome (3,5–8; see Table 2). These agents do not have an intracellular target site and appear to inhibit bacterial growth by nonspecific disruption of cytoplasmic membrane integrity, leading to a bactericidal response. They are also toxic to mammalian cells. Since these molecules do not enter the bacterial cytoplasm, discussion of their transport into and out of the cell is clearly

Table 2 Structure–Activity Relationships Within the Tetracycline Series

Analog	Structure	MIC(μg ml) for *E.coli* [a]	Type of inhibition		Ribosome as primary target
			Bacteriostatic	Bactericidal	
Tetracycline	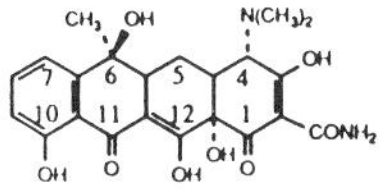	0.5	+		+
Chlortetracycline	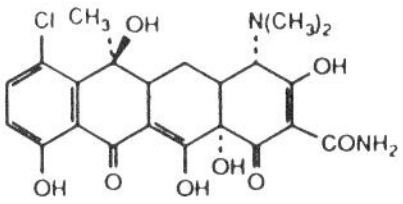	0.25	+		+
Minocycline	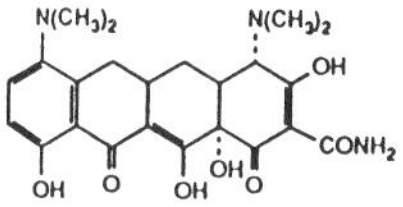	0.25	+		+
Doxycycline	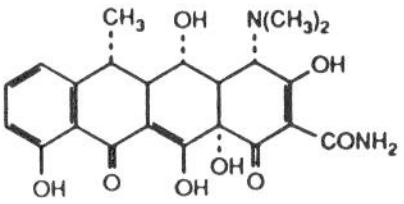	0.25	+		+
Anhydrotetracycline	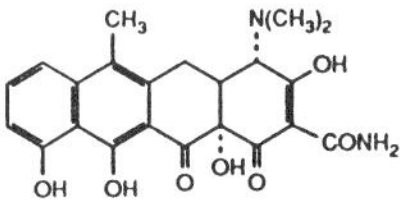	2.0		+	−
Anhydrochlortetracycline	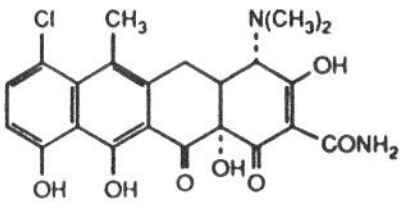	4.0		+	−
6-Thiatetracycline	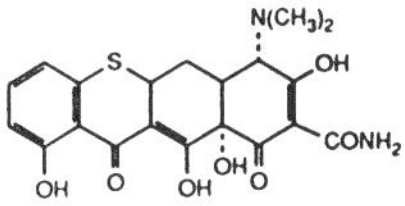	0.5		+	−
Chelocardin	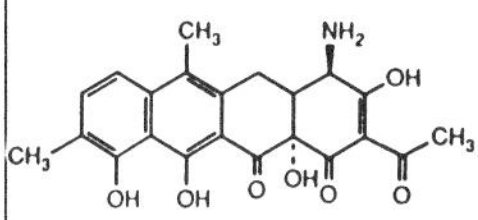	0.5		+	−
4-Epi-anhydrochlortetracycline	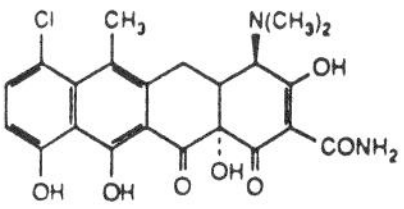	8.0		+	−

[a] *E.coli* k12 MC 4100 grown in M63 minimal medium

irrelevant. Accordingly, the so-called atypical tetracyclines, which have no potential as chemotherapeutic agents (3,8), will not be considered further in this chapter.

C. Dissociation Schemes for Tetracyclines

To consider tetracycline uptake and efflux processes (see Secs. III and IV) an overview of the protonation, and chelation behavior of tetracyclines is necessary. The tetracyclines are acids that can ionize in aqueous solution, and dissociation schemes are available for tetracycline (T), oxytetracycline (ϕ), and minocycline (M) (Fig. 1; Table 3). Tetracycline has three protonation sites (4,9) with pK values of 3.3, 7.7, and 9.7 (see Table 3) that are assigned to the tricarbonylmethane group (C-1 through C-3 region; see Table 2), the phenolic β-diketone system (C-10 through C-12 region; see Table 2), and the dimethylamino group (C-4 substituent; see Table 2). Oxytetracycline and minocycline also possess these protonation sites, but minocycline contains an additional titratable group with a pK value of 5.0, representing the dimethylamino group substituted at the C-7 position of the molecule (see Table 2).

At neutral pH the forms TH_2, TH^-, ϕH_2, and ϕH^- are preponderant for tetracycline and oxytetracycline, whereas for minocycline, MH_2 is the

$$(a) \quad TH_3^+ \underset{K_1}{\rightleftharpoons} (H^+) + TH_2 \underset{K_2}{\rightleftharpoons} (H^+) + TH^- \overset{K_3}{\underset{K_S}{\rightleftharpoons}} \begin{matrix} (H^+) + T^{2-} \\ + Mg^{2+} \\ (THMg)^+ \end{matrix}$$

$$(b) \quad \phi H_3^+ \underset{K_1}{\rightleftharpoons} (H^+) + \phi H_2 \underset{K_2}{\rightleftharpoons} (H^+) + \phi H^- \overset{K_3}{\underset{K_S}{\rightleftharpoons}} \begin{matrix} (H^+) + \phi^{2-} \\ + Mg^{2+} \\ (\phi HMg)^+ \end{matrix}$$

$$(c) \quad MH_4^{2+} \underset{K_1}{\rightleftharpoons} (H^+) + MH_3^+ \underset{K_1'}{\rightleftharpoons} (H^+) + MH_2 \underset{K_2}{\rightleftharpoons} (H^+) + MH^- \overset{K_3}{\underset{K_S}{\rightleftharpoons}} \begin{matrix} (H^+) + M^{2-} \\ + Mg^{2+} \\ (MHMg)^+ \end{matrix}$$

Figure 1 Dissociation schemes for (a) tetracycline hydrochloride, (b) oxytetracycline hydrochloride, and (c) minocycline hydrochloride. (From Ref. 4.)

Table 3 Ionization Constants (K_1, K_1', K_2, K_3) of Tetracycline, Oxytetracycline, and Minocycline Hydrochloride and Stability Constants (K_s) of Complexes with Magnesium

Antibiotic	pK_1	pK_1'	pK_2	pK_3	pK_s
Tetracycline	3.3		7.7	9.7	4.16–4.29
Oxytetracycline	3.3		7.3	9.1	3.80–3.96
Minocycline	2.8	5.0	7.8	9.5	ND[a]

[a]ND, not determined; but minocycline does form magnesium chelates.
Source: Ref. 4.

major species (4,10). The TH^-, ϕH^-, and MH^- anions chelate divalent cations, including magnesium (see Table 3). However, tetracycline–metal chelates are less soluble than the free antibiotics (10).

II. MEASUREMENT OF TETRACYCLINE TRANSPORT

Tetracycline transport has been studied in whole cells, and in right-side-out and everted membrane vesicles (4,11). Whole-cell and vesicle systems allow kinetic studies of transport, but membrane vesicles are more suitable than whole cells for establishing the energy requirements for transport (11). Everted vesicles are the most appropriate system for studying tetracycline efflux systems located in the cytoplasmic membrane (11). Three experimental approaches have been applied to measure tetracyclines: one uses fluorescence spectroscopy, the second uses conversion of tetracyclines to their chromogenic anhydro- analogues, and the third uses radioactively labeled tetracyclines. All three methods have been applied to whole cells (e.g., see Refs. 4, 11–19), but only radioactively labeled tetracyclines have been applied to studies utilizing membrane vesicles (e.g., see Refs. 4,11,19–21).

Measurement of tetracycline transport by fluorescence spectroscopy depends on fluorescence enhancement of the antibiotic as it enters the cell. The method has been used in uptake studies of a number of tetracycline analogues (12). Typically, bacteria are harvested from midexponential-phase cultures (approximately 5×10^8 organisms per milliliter) and resuspended (5×10^9 organisms per milliliter) in phosphate- or Tris-based buffers containing a carbon source (glucose or glycerol). Tetracycline is added, and fluorescence enhancement is measured at 520 nm following excitation at 400 nm (12–15). Although the method can provide a qualitative estimate of tetracycline uptake into bacteria, it is neither applicable to kinetic studies, nor to studies concerning the pH-dependence of transport (4,14).

Conversion of tetracyclines to their chromogenic anhydro analogues provides a reliable method for the determination of absolute amounts of tetracyclines accumulated by whole cells. In this method, bacteria exposed to tetracyclines are harvested by centrifugation, and the cell-bound antibiotic is quantitatively converted to the anhydro analogue by heating in the presence of concentrated hydrochloric acid. The quantity of anhydrotetracycline in the sample is then determined spectrophotometrically (13–17).

The use of radioactively labeled tetracyclines for studies of tetracycline transport in whole cells and vesicles has been widely reported (e.g., see Refs. 4,11,18–21). Typically, uptake of antibiotic is started by addition of radioactive tetracycline to a cell or vesicle suspension, followed by removal of samples and rapid filtration through membrane filters. Radioactivity retained on the filters is quantified by scintillation spectroscopy. Radioactive uptake methods in conjunction with everted membrane vesicle systems have been particularly useful in defining the nature of energy coupling for tetracycline efflux, identification of magnesium as a cofactor, and establishing that the transport process (efflux) is saturable (4,11,19,20) (Table 4).

Table 4 Properties of Tetracycline Influx and Efflux Systems in Membrane Vesicles from *Pseudomonas putida* (19) and *Escherichia coli* (20,21)

	Kinetic constants		Optima for influx/efflux	
Transport system	K_m (μM)	V_{max} (nmol/min/mg protein)	pH	[Mg^{2+}] (mM)
Pseudomonas putida influx	2,500	50	NE	NE
Escherichia coli influx	ND	ND	6.9	1
P. putida, TetA(A)-mediated efflux	2.0–3.5	0.15	NE	NE
E. coli TetA(B)-mediated efflux	6	0.1–1	7.7	3–10

ND, not determinable; NE, not established.
Source: Ref. 4.

III.   TETRACYCLINE UPTAKE PROCESSES

A.   The Gram-Negative Outer Membrane

1.   Introduction

The structure and organization of the gram-negative outer membrane have been extensively reviewed in recent years (22–24), and readers are referred to these articles for detailed accounts of outer-membrane composition and architecture. In terms of charge distribution across the outer membrane, a Donnan equilibrium exists across the membrane (negative charge inside) (25).

By analogy with other antibiotics and solutes (24,26), we can predict that hydrophobicity will also be a major determinant of the uptake of tetracyclines across the outer membrane. That is, hydrophobic analogues will diffuse more slowly across the outer membrane, reflecting the relative impermeability of the membrane to hydrophobic molecules, owing to the presence of lipopolysaccharides in the outer leaflet of the bilayer. Experimental data indicate that the hydrophobicity of tetracyclines is, indeed, a determinant of outer-membrane permeability; there is good correlation between hydrophobicity and susceptibility of *Escherichia coli* to a series of tetracycline analogues, the more hydrophobic members being less effective antibacterial agents (Fig. 2). The relation between hydrophobicity and outer membrane uptake has also been confirmed by methods that are not based on the growth inhibitory properties of tetracyclines. Chopra and Hacker (27) assessed uptake of tetracyclines into a strain of *E. coli* carrying a *tetA–lacZ* translational fusion, in which expression of β-galactosidase is controlled by the pSC101 *tetR* repressor gene. The ability of tetracycline analogues to induce β-galactosidase synthesis was correlated with their hydrophobicity, such that hydrophobic analogues were relatively poor enzyme inducers (27). Therefore, the data obtained using the translational fusion system are in accord with the susceptibility–hydrophobicity relation presented in Figure 2.

By further analogy with other antibiotics and solutes, we would expect hydrophilic tetracyclines (e.g., tetracycline) to diffuse through the hydrophilic transmembrane protein (porin) channels and relatively hydrophobic tetracyclines (e.g., minocycline) to diffuse through the lipopolysaccharide-rich regions of the outer membrane. These assertions are supported by experimental data that are discussed in the following sections.

2.   Porin-Dependent Uptake Pathway

Porin-deficient mutants of *E. coli* become more resistant to tetracycline, supporting the contention that diffusion of the antibiotic occurs through porin channels (3,4,28). Furthermore, since strains with *ompF* mutations

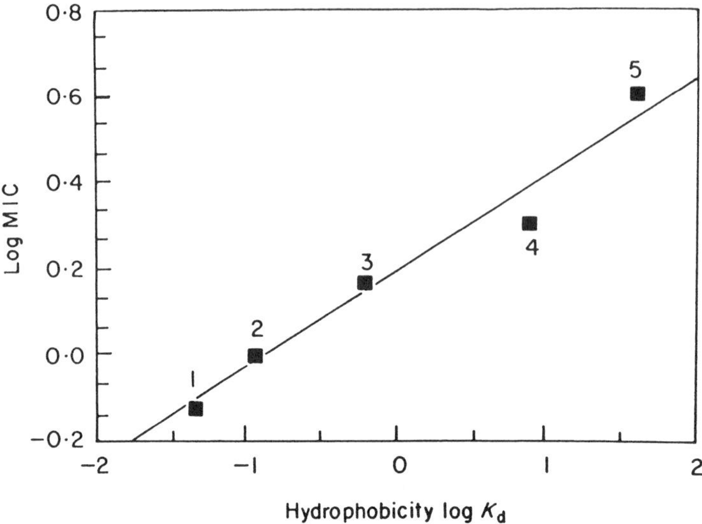

Figure 2 Relation between the antimicrobial activity of tetracyclines and their hydrophobicity. The graph is a plot of the logarithm of the chloroform/buffer distribution constant at pH 7.0 (log K_d) versus the logarithm of the minimum inhibitory concentration (MIC) against wild-type *E. coli* K-12, for a series of tetracycline analogues. 1, tetracycline; 2, methacycline; 3, doxycycline; 4, 6-demethyl-6-deoxytetracycline; 5, minocycline. (From Ref. 3.)

are more resistant than those with *ompC* mutations, tetracycline appears to have a preference for porins formed by the OmpF protein (3,4,28). The Donnan equilibrium across the outer membrane favors the diffusion of positively charged species through porin channels. Therefore, binding of magnesium to the TH^- anion (see Fig. 1) will lead to the formation of a cationic chelate of tetracycline that will be able to cross the outer membrane in response to the Donnan equilibrium, resulting in uphill concentration of the antibiotic in the periplasm (4,9). The concept that tetracycline crosses the outer membrane as a cationic chelate of magnesium is consistent with utilization of OmpF pores for uptake, since these channels are cation-selective (29).

3. Lipid Bilayer-Dependent Uptake Pathway

As noted in Section III.A.1, hydrophobicity–activity relations imply that the influx of hydrophobic tetracycline analogues, such as minocycline, occurs through the lipid bilayer regions of the outer membrane. Nikaido and Thanassi (9) recently proposed that minocycline does, indeed, penetrate the lipid-rich regions of the outer membrane. These authors suggest that, in contrast with tetracycline, the permeating species (i.e., minocycline) is not charged, does not respond to the Donnan potential, and accordingly, is not concentrated in the periplasm. This is consistent with the decreased efficacy of hydrophobic tetracycline analogues against gram-negative bacteria (9) (see Fig. 2).

Experimental evidence supporting the view that minocycline diffuses through the lipid-rich region of the outer membrane has been obtained. This is summarized as follows:

1. The susceptibility of porin-deficient mutants of *E. coli* to minocycline is unaltered (28), consistent with the view that the porin pathway does not operate for minocycline uptake.
2. The susceptibility of deep-rough lipopolysaccharide mutants of *E. coli* to minocycline is enhanced (30), consistent with penetration of drug through the lipid region.
3. Polymyxin B nonapeptide (PMBN), a probe that enhances permeability by the lipid-dependent pathway (24), enhances β-galactosidase induction by minocycline in an *E. coli* strain containing a *tetA–lacZ* fusion (27).

B. The Cytoplasmic Membrane

1. Lack of Evidence for Carrier-Mediated Transport

It has been known for many years that uptake of tetracycline and its accumulation within bacteria are energy-dependent processes (3,4). A simple explanation for these phenomena would be an active, carrier-mediated transport system for uptake across the cytoplasmic membrane (4). If uptake is mediated by a specific transporter, it is expected that saturation kinetics for tetracycline uptake would be observed. Failure to demonstrate saturation kinetics has been consistently reported both in gram-negative and gram-positive bacteria, and infinitely high K_m values have been obtained (3,4,9,19,21,31–33; see Table 4). The absence of a carrier-mediated uptake system for tetracyclines explains why it has not been possible to isolate chromosomal mutants resistant to high levels of tetracycline (32). Furthermore, attempts to identify putative transport systems through the use of mutants deficient in known uptake mechanisms have also failed to provide evidence for carrier-mediated transport of tetracyclines across the bacterial cytoplasmic membrane (30,34). These observations are consistent with other experimental findings that demonstrate that tetracycline diffuses through the phospholipid bilayers of liposomes (35).

2. Biochemical Basis for Uptake of Tetracyclines

Nikaido and Thanassi (9) have recently presented strong arguments supporting the uptake of uncharged tetracycline species across the bacterial cytoplasmic membrane. The apparent energy-dependent accumulation of tetracycline, therefore, simply appears to represent distribution of the uncharged species across the membrane in response to the pH gradient component of the proton motive force (9,36). Since the cytoplasmic pH (approximately 7.8) is higher than the external pH (approximately 6.1), Yamaguchi et al. (36) propose that the uncharged tetracycline species will dissociate into anion and proton after entering the cell. Furthermore, this dissociation may be facilitated by the formation of magnesium–tetracycline chelates, resulting in intracellular accumulation of tetracyclines (36). A model for the uptake of tetracycline across the cytoplasmic membrane and its accumulation in bacteria, based on the foregoing discussion, is presented in Figure 3.

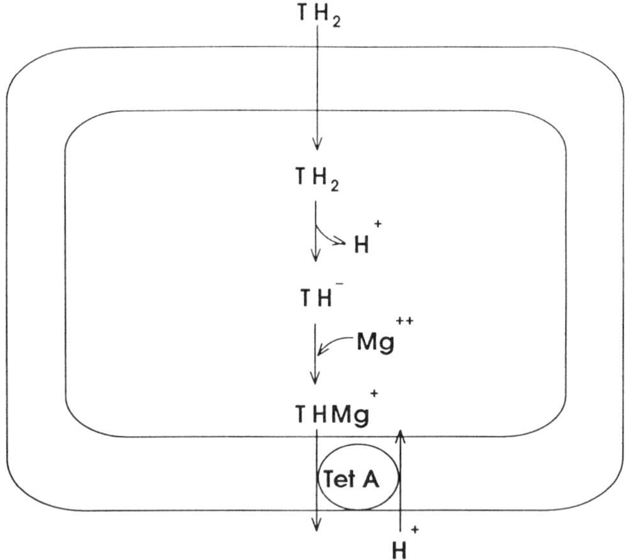

Figure 3 Proposed mechanism for tetracycline uptake and efflux across the bacterial cytoplasmic membrane. Abbreviations: Mg^{2+}, divalent magnesium cation; TH_2 and TH^-, protonated and deprotonated tetracycline, respectively, $THMg^+$, magnesium–tetracycline chelate complex; TetA, proton-coupled tetracycline antiporter. (Based on Ref. 36.)

IV. EFFLUX OF TETRACYCLINES

A. Mechanism of Efflux: Biochemical and Energetic Considerations

Efflux of tetracyclines from the bacterial cytoplasm constitutes a clinically important mechanism of resistance to this class of antibiotic (3,4,11,37). The process is saturable, is magnesium-dependent (see Table 4), and is mediated by distinct membrane-located carrier (efflux) proteins (see Sec. IV.B.1) encoded by genes that are frequently located in transposable elements and plasmids (3,4).

The energetic basis of efflux has been established only for tetracycline, but it is assumed to apply in general to any tetracycline that is a substrate for an efflux protein. Efflux of tetracycline is driven by the proton motive force and involves an electrically neutral proton–tetracycline antiport system, with exchange of a monocationic (probably magnesium)–tetracycline chelate complex for a proton (3,38) (see Fig. 3). These observations are consistent with the presence of magnesium–tetracycline chelates formed during the uptake of tetracyclines into the cell (see Sec. III.B.2).

Evidence supporting the energetic basis of efflux just described is as follows. Dependence on the electrochemical proton gradient is suggested by stimulation of tetracycline uptake into everted vesicles following incubation with substrates for electron transport, such as lactate, NADH, or phenazine methosulfate–sodium ascorbate (PMS–ASC) (11,19,20,38). Inhibition of lactate, NADH, or PMS–ASC stimulated uptake of tetracycline into everted vesicles by agents that inhibit or destroy the electrochemical proton gradient [e.g., 2,4,-dinitrophenol (DNP) and carbonylcyanide-m-chlorophenylhydrazone (CCCP)] is also consistent with dependence of efflux on the electrochemical proton gradient (11,19,20,38). The relative contribution of the electrical ($\Delta\psi$) and proton (ΔpH) gradients to efflux have been established by using valinomycin (which dissipates the membrane potential, $\Delta\psi$) and nigericin (which dissipates the chemical gradient of protons, ΔpH). The NADH-induced transport of tetracycline into everted vesicles was inhibited by nigericin, but not by valinomycin, indicating that efflux is driven by the proton gradient across the membrane (38). Furthermore, transport studies using artificially imposed pH (ΔpH) and electrical gradients ($\Delta\psi$) indicated that ΔpH alone can drive efflux, suggesting an electrically neutral antiport system of protons and a cationic form of tetracycline (38). In addition to the coupling of protons (antiport) to efflux, some efflux proteins are also able to use potassium ions in exchange for tetracycline (39–41).

B. Efflux Proteins

1. *Properties and Substrate Profiles*

Eight genetic determinants (TetA through TetF, TetK, and TetL) have
been described in bacteria that encode tetracycline efflux proteins
(3,4,11,20). Nomenclature for the genes and proteins mediating efflux is
as follows: the structural gene in each determinant that encodes the efflux
protein is designated *tetA* and the corresponding protein TetA (42). The
genes and products of particular Tet determinants are identified in paren-
thesis after the symbols [i.e., the gene encoding the efflux protein in the
TetB determinant is designated *tetA(B)* and the efflux protein itself as
TetA(B) (42)].

Total nucleotide sequences are available for the *tetA(A)*, *tetA(B)*,
tetA(C), *tetA(D)*, *tetA(K)*, and *tetA(L)* genes (43–49). The deduced amino
sequences of the proteins encoded by these genes indicate a set of hydrophobic proteins, ranging in size from 459 amino acids for *tetA(K)* [pre-
dicted relative molecular mass (M_r) 50.7 kDa] to 394 amino acids for
tetA(D) (predicted M_r 41.1 kDa).

By comparing the deduced amino acid sequences of a variety of membrane transport proteins, Griffith et al. (49) have identified four families
within the large class of transporters. The TetA(A), TetA(B), TetA(C),
and TetA(D) proteins are all members of the second (II) family, which
also includes other transport proteins, such as Bmr and NorA, which
mediate efflux of drugs (11,37). Within this group of tetracycline transporters, the pairs that are most closely related are TetA(A)–TetA(C) and Tet-
A(B)–TetA(D) (46). The TetA(K) and TetA(L) proteins are members of
the third (III) family, which also contains other transporters believed to
mediate efflux of antibiotics and antiseptics in microorganisms.

Attempts to deduce the substrate specificities of different efflux proteins have been made by considering the level of protection they confer
against various tetracyclines. From this approach it was concluded that
TetA(B) recognized (and removed) both first- and second-generation tetracyclines (see Table 1), whereas others, for example, TetA(A), TetA(C),
TetA(D), TetA(K), and TetA(L), provide poor protection against (i.e., do
not recognize) second-generation analogues, in particular, minocycline
(see Sec. IV.B.3 for discussion).

The limitations of the foregoing approach toward identification of substrate specificities have been discussed by Guay and Rothstein (50) and
relate principally to the use of nonisogenic strains and systems not permitting comparable expression of *tetA* genes. The substrate specificities of
the TetA(B), TetA(C), and TetA(K) proteins have now been investigated
by the cloning of their structural genes into an isogenic background and

adjusting their level of expression to provide equivalent resistance to tetracycline. The ability of each efflux system to confer protection against other tetracyclines was then determined with these "normalized" expression systems (50). In contrast with previous conclusions, TetA(B) and TetA(C) conferred very similar levels of resistance to a variety of tetracycline analogues (50). However, TetA(K) does differ from TetA(B) and TetA(C) in not conferring high-level resistance to the second-generation analogues minocycline and doxycycline (50). These analogues, in contrast with those recognized by TetA(K), lack a hydroxyl substituent at the 6 position (see Table 2). Therefore, TetA(K) may be unable to recognize or transport (efflux) analogues lacking a hydroxyl substituent at this position (50).

2. *Topographical Organization of Efflux Proteins*

The deduced primary amino acid sequences of various tetracycline efflux proteins have been used to predict the secondary structure of the proteins (3,39,46,49,51). With the exception of the TetA(K) protein, each efflux protein was predicted to have an even number of membrane-spanning α-helices [14 for TetA(L), 12 for the remainder].

The *tetA(K)* gene was originally sequenced by Khan and Novick (52). Hydropathy analysis of the derived primary amino acid sequence suggested, in contrast with the Tet efflux proteins described earlier, the presence of an odd number (i.e., 13 α-helical, membrane-spanning regions; 52). Although an odd number of membrane-spanning regions might occur, most transport proteins, including other Tet proteins, possess an even number of α-helices (39,49). Recently, however, the *tetA(K)* nucleotide sequence has been reexamined, revealing several earlier sequencing errors (47). Examination of the corrected sequence shows that TetA(K) is likely to contain 14 transmembrane regions (47).

The topographical organization of TetA(B) has been probed using biochemical techniques, and it was found that the NH_2-terminus of the protein is located on the cytoplasmic side of the membrane (51). By extrapolation from the studies with TetA(B), models for the organization of the other closely related proteins TetA(A), TetA(C), and TetA(D) can be deduced (46,53). Figure 4 illustrates the proposed secondary structure of TetA(C), showing the location of the NH_2- and COOH-termini.

3. *Functional Domains*

A complete understanding of the functional domains within tetracycline efflux proteins will ultimately depend on elucidation of their three-dimensional structure at the atomic level. This will require purification, crystallization, and x-ray diffraction analysis of the proteins (39). These are challenging objectives for which the first step will be availability of stable,

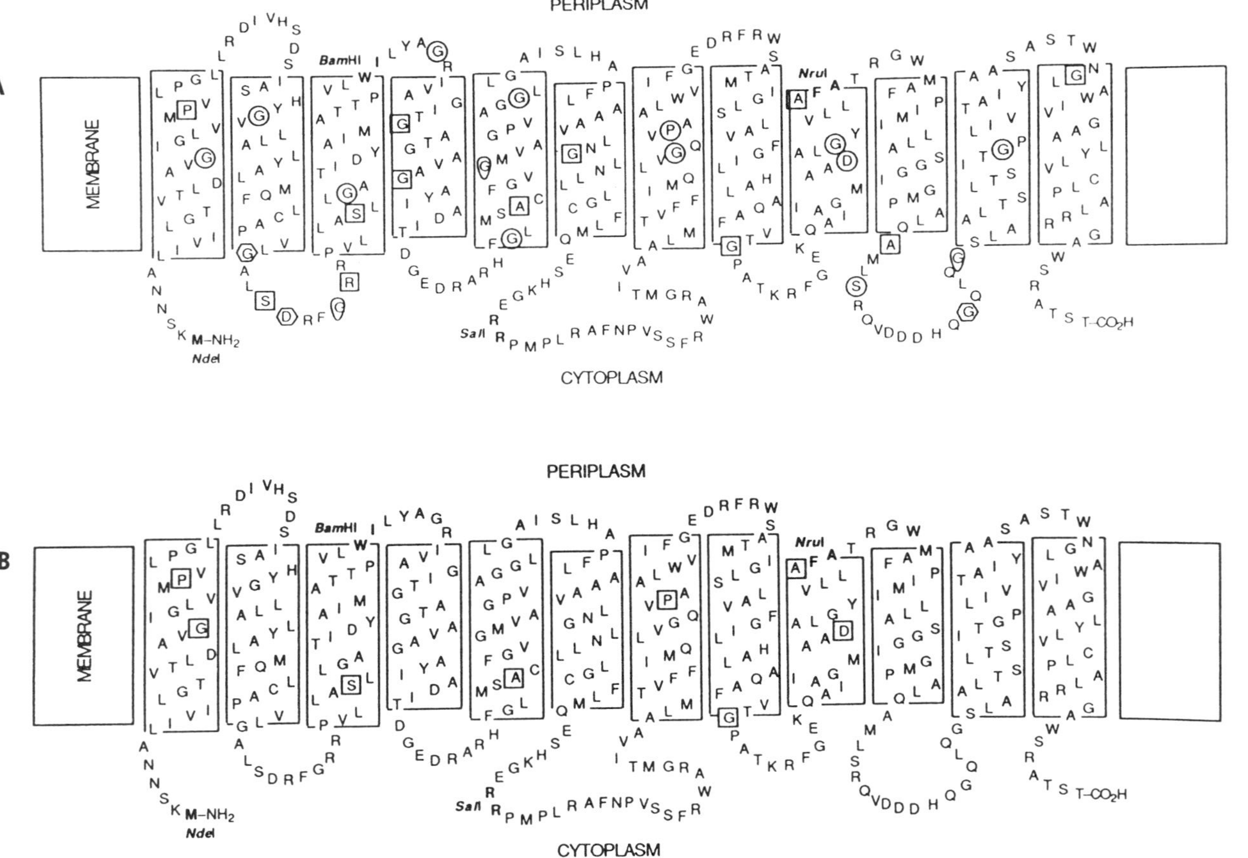

undenatured proteins in sufficient quantities for analytical purposes. Although some progress has been made toward purification of the proteins (54), the requirements for x-ray diffraction analysis have not yet been achieved and would seem to be distant objectives (39).

In the absence of tertiary structure analysis, functional domains in the Tet efflux proteins can be predicted only by comparison of sequence data among transporters and by mutagenesis specifically directed toward the *tet* genes. These studies are described in the following.

Yamaguchi et al. (56) have suggested that the following functional domains are necessary for a proton-coupled antiporter system: (1) a substrate-binding site fluctuating between high- and low-affinity states; (2) at least two gating regions, one on the cytoplasmic face and the other on the periplasmic face, which open and close in response to affinity changes at the binding site; and (3) a proton transfer site, the protonation–deprotonation of which affects the affinity of the binding site and probably the opening and closing of the gates.

The most detailed attempts to identify functional domains within Tet proteins have been applied to the TetA(B) and TetA(C) proteins. The two-dimensional topology (see Fig. 4) of the TetA(C) efflux protein (396 residues) will serve as a reference protein for the following discussion. On the basis of overall sequence comparisons between different transporters, Griffith et al. (49) suggest that substrate (i.e., tetracycline) specificity is determined primarily by sequence motifs located in the COOH-terminal halves of the efflux proteins. This hypothesis is based on the general observation that the COOH-terminal halves of transporters that recognize structurally dissimilar substrates are less conserved than the NH_2-terminal halves (49). In contrast, the relative homology among the NH_2-terminal halves of a variety of proton-dependent transporters suggests that the NH_2-terminal halves of the Tet proteins are probably important for proton-coupled efflux (49). These suggestions do not preclude interaction at the tertiary level between NH_2- and COOH-terminal regions of the protein.

Yamaguchi and co-workers have conducted a series of experiments involving site-directed mutagenesis within the *tetA(B)* gene designed to

---

Figure 4 Model of the two-dimensional topology of the TetA(C) efflux protein and the location of hydroxylamine-induced missense mutations that abolish activity of the protein. (A) All amino acid alterations; (B) location in the membrane-spanning regions of those amino acid alterations that abolish efflux activity without the introduction of a charged residue. The number of independent occasions on which a specific codon was altered is indicated by the following symbols: □, one; ○, two; ⟨⟩, three; ⟨⟩, four. (From Ref. 58.)

explore functional domains within the TetA(B) transporter (55–57). The region defined by the sequence GXXSDRFGRR facing the cytoplasm between the second and third transmembrane regions [residues 62–71 in TetA(B); residues 64–73 in TetA(C); see Fig. 4] is highly homologous among transporters in families I, II, and IV (49) with the SD (Ser-Asp) dipeptide absolutely conserved in all tetracycline transporters (3). Conversion of Asp-66 in TetA(B) to Asn-66 completely abolishes tetracycline efflux, and replacement of Ser-65 with Cys-65 renders the mutant protein susceptible to attack by sulfydryl agents, such as *N*-ethylmaleimide, which completely inhibit transport activity, even in the presence of tetracycline (55). These residues are also important in the activity of the TetA(C) protein because hydroxylamine-induced missense mutations abolishing resistance arise at these sites (58) (Fig. 4, residues 67/68). The importance of the region GXXSDRFGRR in the function of TetA proteins is further confirmed by the observation that several other residues in this region, in addition to the SD dipeptide, are the sites of missense mutations abolishing resistance by TetA(C) (58; see Fig. 4). Since the loop region GXXSDRFGRR is highly cationic, whereas the transported (effluxed) substrate is probably a magnesium–tetracycline chelate (see Fig. 3), it is unlikely that this region of TetA proteins would be able to form a stable binding site for the substrate, owing to electrical repulsion (3,55). Indeed, it has been suggested that this region may comprise the cytoplasmically orientated gate for tetracycline release, opening in conjunction with proton translocation (3,55).

Histidine residues are known to be important components of charge–relay systems involved in the protonation–deprotonation cycle of several proton-translocating membrane proteins (see Ref. 56). Since the histidine-specific reagent diethyl pyrocarbonate inhibits the activity of TetA(B), Yamaguchi et al. (56) have proposed that one or more histidine residues plays a role in proton transfer within the TetA(B) efflux protein. The only conserved histidine residue in TetA proteins is located in transmembrane region 8 [residue 257 in TetA(B), residue 259 in TetA(C); see Fig. 4]. Although there is no other charged residue in helix 8, a negatively charged residue, aspartic acid, occurs at a similar position in the adjacent transmembrane domain that comprises helix 9 [residue 285 in TetA(B), residue 287 in TetA(C)] (see Fig. 4). Replacement of His-257 by glutamic acid or aspartic acid in TetA(B) produced mutants that mediated downhill efflux of tetracycline, without proton translocation, and with decreased affinity for the substrate, thereby confirming a role for this histidine residue in the charge–relay process (56). Furthermore, when Asp-285 in TetA(B) is replaced by asparagine, lysine, or glutamic acid, tetracycline–proton antiport activity is lost (57). A role for Asp-285/287 in expression of tetracycline resistance is also supported by the results of missense mutagenesis in *tetA(C)* (58; see Fig. 4).

Missense mutations causing loss of tetracycline resistance in TetA(C) have been identified at many sites not discussed in the foregoing (58) (see Fig. 4). Undoubtedly, loss of function could result from radical structural changes, arising, for example, from substitution of a charged residue within a membrane-spanning α-helix (58). However, even when such mutants are accounted for, it is evident that several mutations that do not introduce charge into transmembrane regions, nevertheless, abolish expression of resistance (58) (see Fig. 4). The precise role of the residues affected remains to be established.

V. CONCLUSIONS AND FUTURE DIRECTIONS

A. Comparison with Other Antibiotic Transport Systems

How do the mechanisms for transport of tetracyclines in bacteria compare with those employed by other antibiotics? Passage of agents across the gram-negative outer membrane can occur by (1) self-promoted uptake, during which the antibiotics (e.g., aminoglycosides) displace divalent cations from lipopolysaccharide; (2) facilitated diffusion using outer membrane receptor proteins normally involved in iron transport (e.g., albomycin, catecholic β-lactams); or (3) passive diffusion through porin channels or lipid bilayer regions (e.g., noncatecholic β-lactams, quinolones) (9,59,60). As discussed in this chapter, the mechanisms of tetracycline uptake across the outer membrane fall into category 3.

Transport of antibiotics across the cytoplasmic membrane can be mediated by the following processes: (1) carrier-mediated transport, energized by the proton motive force (e.g., cycloserine, fosfomycin); (2) carrier-mediated group translocation (e.g., streptozocin); or (3) distribution in response to the pH gradient that exists across the cytoplasmic membrane (e.g., quinolones) (9,59,60). As discussed in this chapter, tetracycline uptake across the cytoplasmic membrane conforms to mechanism 3.

The relation of Tet efflux proteins to other membrane transporters has already been discussed in the context of the four families identified by Griffith et al. (49). Table 5 specifically compares the Tet transporters with other systems that mediate antibiotic efflux in bacteria. The substrates transported (effluxed), the nature of energy coupling for transport, and

Table 5 Microbial Antibiotic Efflux Systems

Gene	Substrates transported	Energy source	Transporter family	Ref.
msrA	Macrolides	ATP	Unknown	11,37,61
tet	Tetracyclines	PMF	II and III	3,4,11,37,49
bmr	Rhodamine (Rh)	PMF	II	11,37,49
	Ethidium bromide (Eb)			
	Chloramphenicol (Cm)			
	Puromycin (Pur)			
	Fluoroquinolones (Fq)			
norA	Rh, Eb, Cm, Pur, Fq	PMF	II	11,37,49

assignment (where known) to the transporter families defined by Griffith et al. (49) are indicated.

B. The Influence of Transport on Drug Design

Improved understanding of the mechanism of tetracycline efflux leads to the possibility of (1) designing novel tetracycline analogues that are not recognized by Tet transporters, and (2) discovering or designing Tet efflux pump inhibitors that might be combined with existing tetracycline drugs to overcome resistance.

Rational drug design approaches in both areas probably will ultimately depend on definition of the tertiary structure of the Tet transporters and identification of the key residues involved in the recognition of tetracyclines and their active efflux. However, even though the three-dimensional structure of a TetA protein is not yet available, there are promising indications, discussed in the following, that both foregoing objectives 1 and 2 are achievable.

It has already been noted that TetA(K) is unable to recognize or transport the second-generation analogues minocycline or doxycycline (see Sec. IV.B.1). Furthermore, new *N,N*-dimethylglycylamido derivatives of minocycline and 6-demethyl-6-deoxytetracycline, the so-called glycylcyclines (Fig. 5), have recently been reported that are active against organisms expressing *tetA*, *tetB*, *tetC*, *tetD*, and *tetK* determinants (62). These observations imply that the Tet transporters fail to recognize the glycylcyclines.

Relative to efflux pump inhibitors, Nelson et al. (63) recently described a series of tetracycline analogues that inhibit TetA(B)-mediated efflux of tetracyclines. The inhibitors comprise a series of 13-(alkylthio) and 13-

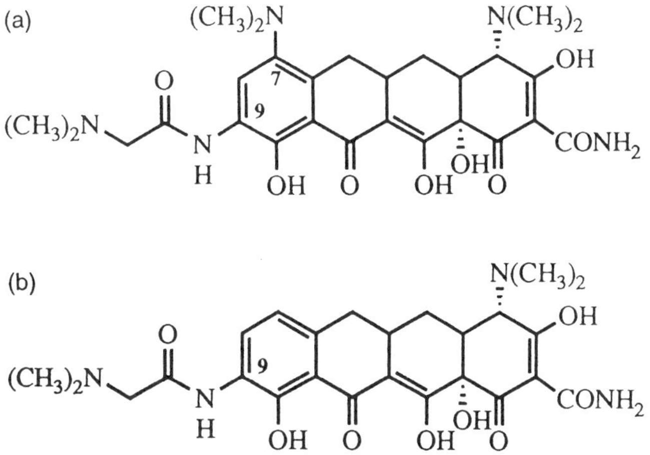

Figure 5 Structure of (a) *N,N*-dimethylglycylamido-minocycline and (b) *N,N*,dimethylglycylamido-6-deoxytetracycline.

(arylthio) derivatives of 5-hydroxy-6-deoxytetracycline. The most active members exhibited IC_{50} values of 0.3 μM against the TetA(B) efflux pump in everted *E. coli* membrane vesicles, but the antibacterial properties of these inhibitors against resistant strains in combination with other tetracyclines has not yet been reported (63). Finally, sensitive screening assays for the detection of inhibitors of tetracycline efflux pumps have recently been described (64). Such systems offer the prospect of discovering efflux pump inhibitors from chemical compound libraries or natural product sources.

REFERENCES

1. Mitscher LA. The Chemistry of the Tetracycline Antibiotics. New York: Marcel Dekker, 1978.
2. Rogalski W. Chemical modification of the tetracyclines. In Hlavka JJ, Boothe JH, eds. The Tetracyclines. Handbook of Experimental Pharmacology, Vol. 78. Berlin: Springer-Verlag, 1985:179–316.
3. Chopra I, Hawkey PM, Hinton M. Tetracyclines, molecular and clinical aspects. J Antimicrob Chemother 1992; 29:245–277.
4. Chopra I. Mode of action of the tetracyclines and the nature of bacterial resistance to them. In Hlavka JJ, Boothe JH, eds. The Tetracyclines. Handbook of Experimental Pharmacology, Vol. 78. Berlin: Springer-Verlag, 1985:317–392.
5. Rasmussen B, Noller HF, Daubresse G, Oliva B, Misulovin Z, Rothstein

     DM, Ellestad GA, Gluzman Y, Tally FP, Chopra I. Molecular basis of tetracycline action: identification of analogs whose primary target is not the bacterial ribosome. Antimicrob Agents Chemother 1991; 35:2306–2311.

6. Oliva B, Chopra I. *tet* determinants provide poor protection against some tetracyclines: further evidence for division of tetracyclines into two classes. Antimicrob Agents Chemother 1992; 36:876–878.

7. Oliva B, Gordon G, McNicholas P, Ellestad G, Chopra I. Evidence that tetracycline analogs whose primary target is not the bacterial ribosome cause lysis of *Escherichia coli*. Antimicrob Agents Chemother 1992; 36:913–919.

8. Chopra I. Tetracycline analogs whose primary target is not the bacterial ribosome. Antimicrob Agents Chemother 1994; 38:637–640.

9. Nikaido H, Thanassi DG. Penetration of lipophilic agents with multiple protonation sites into bacterial cells: tetracyclines and fluoroquinolones as examples. Antimicrob Agents Chemother 1993; 37:1393–1399.

10. Barringer WC, Shultz W, Sieger GM, Nash RA. Minocycline hydrochloride and its relationship to other tetracycline antibiotics. Am J Pharm 1974; 146:179–191.

11. Levy SB. Active efflux mechanisms for antimicrobial resistance. Antimicrob Agents Chemother 1992; 36:695–703.

12. Samra Z, Krausz-Steinmetz J, Sompolinsky D. Transport of tetracyclines through the bacterial cell membrane assayed by fluorescence: a study with susceptible and resistant strains of *Staphylococcus aureus* and *Escherichia coli*. Microbios 1979; 21:7–21.

13. Shales SW, Chopra I, Ball PR. Evidence for more than one mechanism of plasmid-determined tetracycline resistance in *Escherichia coli*. J Gen Microbiol 1980; 121:221–229.

14. Smith MCM, Chopra I. Limitations of a fluorescence assay for studies on tetracycline transport into *Escherichia coli*. Antimicrob Agents Chemother 1983; 23:175–178.

15. Sumita Y, Shishido K. Regulation of tetracycline accumulation in *Bacillus subtilis* bearing *B. subtilis* plasmid pNS1981. FEMS Microbiol Lett 1985; 30:403–406.

16. Smith MCM, Chopra I. Energetics of tetracycline transport into *Escherichia coli*. Antimicrob Agents Chemother 1984; 25:446–449.

17. Mortimer PGS, Piddock LJV. The accumulation of five antibacterial agents in porin-deficient mutants of *Escherichia coli*. J Antimicrob Chemother 1993; 32:195–213.

18. Del Bene VE, Rogers M. Comparison of tetracycline and minocycline transport in *Escherichia coli*. Antimicrob Agents Chemother 1975; 7:801–806.

19. Hedstrom RC, Crider BP, Eagon RG. Comparison of kinetics of active tetracycline uptake and active tetracycline efflux in sensitive and plasmid RP4-containing *Pseudomonas putida*. J Bacteriol 1982; 152:255–259.

20. McMurry LM, Petrucci RE, Levy SB. Active efflux of tetracycline encoded by four genetically different tetracycline resistance determinants in *Escherichia coli*. Proc Natl Acad Sci USA 1980; 77:3974–3977.

21. McMurry LM, Cullinane JC, Petrucci RE, Levy SB. Active uptake of tetracycline by membrane vesicles from susceptible *Escherichia coli*. Antimicrob Agents Chemother 1981; 20:307–313.

22. Nikaido H, Nakae T. The outer membrane of gram negative bacteria. Adv Microb Physiol 1979; 20:163–250.

23. Osborn MJ, Wu HCP. Proteins of the outer membrane of gram negative bacteria. Annu Rev Microbiol 1980; 34:369–422.

24. Nikaido H, Vaara M. Molecular basis of bacterial outer membrane permeability. Microbiol Rev 1985; 49:1–32.

25. Stock JB, Rauch B, Roseman S. Periplasmic space in *Salmonella typhimurium* and *Escherichia coli*. J Biol Chem 1977; 252:7850–7861.

26. Nikaido H. Role of permeability barriers in resistance to beta-lactam antibiotics. Pharmacol Ther 1985; 27:197–231.

27. Chopra I, Hacker K. Uptake of minocycline by *Escherichia coli*. J Antimicrob Chemother 1992; 29:19–25.

28. Chopra I, Eccles SJ. Diffusion of tetracycline across the outer membrane of *Escherichia coli* K-12: involvement of protein Ia. Biochem Biophys Res Commun 1978; 83:550–557.

29. Hancock REW. Role of porins in outer membrane permeability. J Bacteriol 1987; 169:929–933.

30. Ball PR, Chopra I, Eccles SJ. Accumulation of tetracyclines by *Escherichia coli* K-12. Biochem Biophys Res Commun 1977; 77:1500–1507.

31. McMurry L, Levy SB. Two transport systems for tetracycline in sensitive *Escherichia coli*: critical role for an initial rapid uptake system insensitive to energy inhibitors. Antimicrob Agents Chemother 1978; 14:210–219.

32. Argast M, Beck C.F. Tetracycline uptake by susceptible *Escherichia coli* cells. Arch Microbiol 1985; 141:260–265.

33. Chopra I, Ismail S, Oliva B. Lack of evidence for a saturable tetracycline transport system in *Staphylococcus aureus*. Antimicrob Agents Chemother 1991; 35:2643–2644.

34. Chopra I, Ismail S. Uptake of tetracycline by *Escherichia coli* is not mediated by the sodium dependent glutamate transport system. J Antimicrob Chemother 1990; 26:722–724.

35. Argast M, Beck C.F. Tetracycline diffusion through phospholipid bilayers and binding to phospholipids. Antimicrob Agents Chemother 1984; 26:263–265.

36. Yamaguchi A, Ohmori H, Kaneko-Ohdera MJ, Nomura T, Sawai T. ΔpH-dependent accumulation of tetracycline in *Escherichia coli*. Antimicrob Agents Chemother 1991; 35:53–56.

37. Chopra I. Efflux-based antibiotic resistance mechanisms: the evidence for increasing prevalence. J Antimicrob Chemother 1992; 30:737–744.

38. Kaneko M, Yamaguchi A, Sawai T. Energetics of tetracycline efflux system encoded by *Tn10* in *Escherichia coli*. FEBS Lett 1985; 193:194–198.

39. Henderson PJF, Maiden MCJ. Homologous sugar transport proteins in *Escherichia coli* and their relatives in both prokaryotes and eukaryotes. Philos Trans R Soc Lond B 1990; 326:391–410.

40. Dosch DC, Salvacion FF, Epstein W. Tetracycline resistance element of pBR322 mediates potassium transport. J Bacteriol 1984; 160:1188–1190.
41. Guay GG, Tuckman M, McNicholas P, Rothstein DM. The *tet(K)* gene from *Staphylococcus aureus* mediates the transport of potassium in *Escherichia coli*. J Bacteriol 1993; 175:4927–4929.
42. Levy SB, McMurry LM, Burdett V, Courvalin P, Hillen W, Roberts MC, Taylor DE. Nomenclature for tetracycline resistance determinants. Antimicrob Agents Chemother 1989; 33:1373–1374.
43. Waters SH, Rogowsky P, Grinsted J, Altenbuchner J, Schmitt R. The tetracycline resistance determinants of *RP1* and *Tn1721*: nucleotide sequence analysis. Nucleic Acids Res 1983; 11:6089–6105.
44. Hillen W, Schollmeier K. Nucleotide sequence of the *Tn10* encoded tetracycline resistance gene. Nucleic Acids Res 1983; 11:525–539.
45. Peden KWC. Revised sequence of the tetracycline-resistance gene of pBR322. Gene 1983; 22:277–280.
46. Varela MF, Griffith JK. Nucleotide and deduced protein sequences of the class D tetracycline resistance determinant: relationship to other antimicrobial transport proteins. Antimicrob Agents Chemother 1993; 37:1253–1258.
47. Guay GG, Khan SA, Rothstein DM. The *tet(K)* gene of plasmid pT181 of *Staphylococcus aureus* encodes an efflux protein that contains 14 transmembrane helices. Plasmid 1993; 30:163–166.
48. Hoshino T, Ikeda T, Tomizuka N, Furukawa K. Nucleotide sequence of the tetracycline resistance gene of pTHT15, a thermophilic *Bacillus* plasmid: comparison with staphylococcal tetracycline-resistant controls. Gene 1985; 37:131–138.
49. Griffith JK, Baker ME, Rouch OA, Page MGP, Skurray RA, Paulsen IT, Chater KF, Baldwin SA, Henderson PJF. Membrane transport proteins: implications of sequence comparisons. Curr Opin Cell Biol 1992; 4:684–695.
50. Guay GG, Rothstein DM. Expression of the *tetK* gene from *Staphylococcus aureus* in *Escherichia coli*: comparison of substrate specificities of TetA(B), TetA(C), and TetK efflux proteins. Antimicrob Agents Chemother 1993; 37:191–198.
51. Eckert B, Beck CF. Topology of the transposon *Tn10*-encoded tetracycline resistance protein within the inner membrane of *Escherichia coli*. J Biol Chem 1989; 264:11663–11670.
52. Khan SA, Novick RP. Complete sequence of pT181, a tetracycline resistance plasmid from *Staphylococcus aureus*. Plasmid 1983; 10:251–259.
53. Sheridan RP, Chopra I. Origin of tetracycline efflux proteins: conclusions from nucleotide sequence analysis. Mol Microbiol 1991; 5:895–900.
54. Hickman RK, McMurry LM, Levy SB. Overproduction and purification of the *Tn10*-specified inner membrane tetracycline resistance protein Tet using fusions to β-galactosidase. Mol Microbiol 1990; 4:1241–1251.
55. Yamaguchi A, Ono N, Akasaka T, Noumi T, Sawai T. Metal–tetracycline H$^+$ antiporter of *Escherichia coli* encoded by a transposon, *Tn10*. The role of the conserved dipeptide, Ser^{65}–Asp^{66}, in tetracycline transport. J Biol Chem 1990; 265:15525–15530.

56. Yamaguchi A, Adachi K, Akasaka T, Ono N, Sawai T. Metal–tetracycline H$^+$ antiporter of *Escherichia coli* encoded by a transposon, *Tn10*. Histidine 257 plays an essential role in H$^+$ translocation. J Biol Chem 1991; 266:6045–6051.

57. Yamaguchi A, Akasaka T, Ono N, Someya Y, Nakatani M, Sawai T. Metal–tetracycline H$^+$ antiporter of *Escherichia coli* encoded by a transposon, *Tn10*. Roles of the aspartyl residues located in the putative transmembrane helices. J Biol Chem 1992; 267:7490–7498.

58. McNicholas P, Chopra I, Rothstein DM. Genetic analysis of the *tetA*(*C*) gene on plasmid pBR322. J Bacteriol 1992; 174:7926–7933.

59. Chopra I. Molecular mechanisms involved in the transport of antibiotics into bacteria. Parasitology 1988; 96:S25–S44.

60. Chopra I. Transport of antibiotics into bacteria. Annu Rep Med Chem 1989; 24:139–146.

61. Ross JI, Eady EA, Cove JH, Cunliffe WJ, Baumberg S, Wooton JC. Inducible erythromycin resistance in staphylococci is encoded by a member of the ATP-binding transport super-gene family. Mol Microbiol 1990; 4:1207–1214.

62. Testa RA, Petersen PJ, Jacobus NV, Sum P-E, Lee VJ, Tally FP. In vitro and in vivo antibacterial activities of the glycylcyclines, a new class of semi-synthetic tetracyclines. Antimicrob Agents Chemother 1993; 37:2270–2277.

63. Nelson ML, Park BH, Andrews JS, Georgian VA, Thomas RC, Levy SB. Inhibition of the tetracycline efflux antiport protein by 13-thio-substituted 5-hydroxy-6-deoxytetracyclines. J Med Chem 1993; 36:370–377.

64. Rothstein DM, McGlynn M, Bernan V, McGarhen J, Zaccardi J, Cekleniak N, Bertrand KP. Detection of tetracyclines and efflux pump inhibitors. Antimicrob Agents Chemother 1993; 37:1624–1629.

8
Quinolone Uptake and Efflux

Nafsika H. Georgopapadakou
Roche Research Center, Nutley, New Jersey

I. INTRODUCTION

A. Perspective and Definitions

Quinolones are totally synthetic antibiotics, as opposed to β-lactams (Chap. 5), aminoglycosides (Chap. 6), and tetracyclines (Chap. 7), which are natural or semisynthetic products. They have low eukaryotic toxicity and broad-spectrum, bactericidal activity. Early compounds, such as nalidixic acid, which was discovered in the early 1960s from a synthetic precursor of the antimalarial chloroquine (1), have a 1,8-naphthyridine nucleus (Fig. 1). Later compounds, such as norfloxacin, ciprofloxacin, fleroxacin, sparfloxacin, and the 1-aryl quinolones, have a quinolone nucleus with a fluorine substituent at C-6 and a heterocyclic ring, usually piperazine or pyrrolidine, at C-7 (Fig. 1 and 2). In some quinolones, such as ofloxacin and T-3761, there is also a 1,8-bridge giving rise to a third ring fused to the quinolone nucleus. Recent variations on the quinolone nucleus, the 2,3-isothiazoloquinolones, benzonaphthyridines, and fused tricyclic quinolones, will not be discussed since so far they have not reached the clinic because of poor antibacterial activity or host toxicity.

The early history of quinolones [reviewed by Albrecht (2)] was unremarkable; nalidixic acid was an antibiotic active against gram-negative aerobes and used exclusively in urinary tract infections since its achiev-

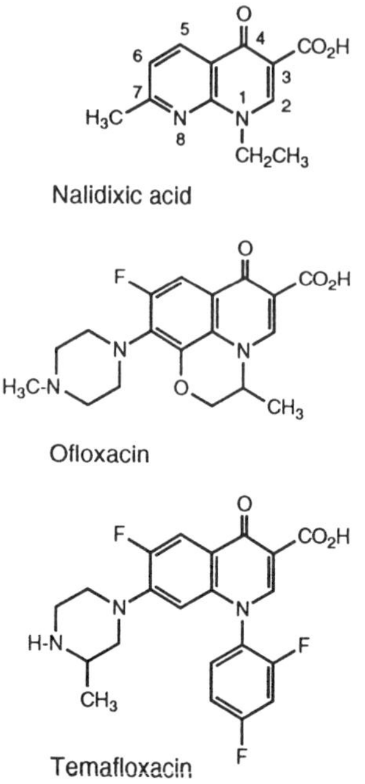

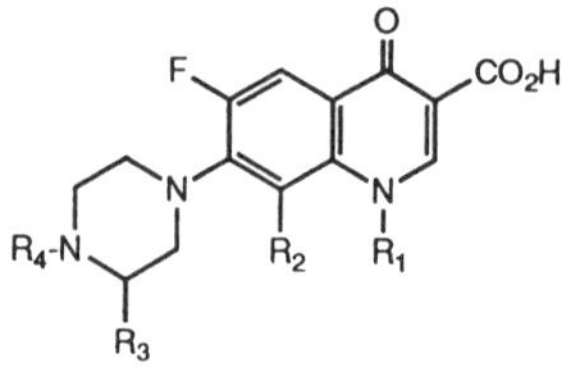

	R_1	R_2	R_3	R_4
Ciprofloxacin	◁	-H	-H	-H
Fleroxacin	$-CH_2CH_2F$	-F	-H	$-CH_3$
Lomefloxacin	$-CH_2CH_2F$	-F	$-CH_3$	-H
Norfloxacin	$-CH_2CH_3$	-H	-H	-H
Pefloxacin	$-CH_2CH_3$	-H	-H	$-CH_3$

Figure 1 Structures of quinolones in clinical use. The 1-aryl quinolone temafloxacin was withdrawn because of adverse effects.

able serum concentration was below that needed to inhibit most systemic pathogens (3). Oxolinic acid (quinoline nucleus), cinoxacin (cinnoline nucleus), and pipemidic acid (pyridopyrimidine nucleus), which were introduced in the 1970s, had only modest improvements in activity; in addition, oxolinic acid and cinoxacin had central nervous system effects. However, with the introduction of the fluorine substituent at C-6 of the quinolone nucleus in the early 1980s, compounds emerged that had greatly increased antibacterial potency (up to 1000-fold) and spectrum and possessed favorable pharmacokinetics permitting both oral and parenteral administration. Several such compounds are currently in clinical use, the most prominent being ciprofloxacin, with worldwide sales of over a billion dollars in 1993. Antibacterial activity of quinolones includes less common, difficult-to-treat pathogens such as *Mycobacterium tuberculosis*, *Legionella* species, and even rickettsiae. Compounds with improved gram-positive and anaerobe activity, such as sparfloxacin and clinafloxacin (Fig. 2), are under development.

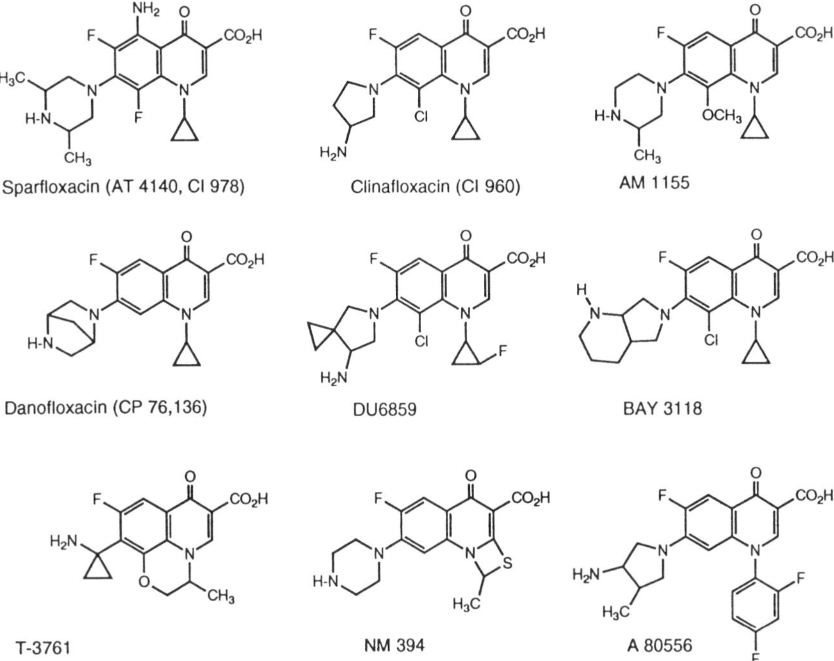

Figure 2 Structures of quinolones in development.

The intense research activity on quinolones during the past decade has given rise to an enormous number of compounds, patents, and publications. There are several excellent reviews (4–12) and monographs (13–17), which cover the spectrum of quinolone activity, mechanism of action, resistance, pharmacokinetics, clinical uses, and toxicity. An important factor in the antimicrobial activity of quinolones is their ability to enter bacterial and mammalian cells and achieve high intracellular levels. This review focuses on bacterial quinolone transport and its contribution to the mechanism of action and resistance.

B. Quinolone Targets

1. DNA Gyrase

The action of nalidixic acid was shown to be bactericidal and to result from inhibition of bacterial DNA biosynthesis soon after its discovery (18,19). Its molecular target, DNA gyrase, was discovered over a decade

decade later (20). The mechanism of inhibition of DNA gyrase by both nalidixic acid and novobiocin, an antibacterial discovered in the 1950s, was elucidated shortly thereafter (21,22). DNA gyrase is a tetrameric protein of two 97-kDa subunits (A subunits) and two 90-kDa subunits (B subunits), encoded by the genes *gyrA* and *gyrB*, respectively (reviewed in Refs. 23–25). It is a unique and essential bacterial enzyme, which introduces negative supercoils into closed circular, double-stranded DNA, thereby leading to strand separation necessary for replication and transcription. In addition, it has swivel action, thereby relieving the torsional tension generated by replication and transcription. All gyrase-catalyzed reactions involve the introduction of a double-strand break in the DNA with a four-base stagger between the break sites, strand passage, and religation. The transient double-strand break is bridged by two phosphodiester bonds to Tyr residues [Tyr-122 in *Escherichia coli* (26)] in the two A subunits of the enzyme and the 5′-ends of the two DNA strands. The B subunit is the site of DNA-dependent ATP hydrolysis and inhibition by novobiocin. Both A and B subunits are required for all enzyme activities.

Quinolones act by immediately, selectively, and reversibly forming a complex with DNA gyrase on DNA (reviewed recently in Ref. 27). They trap the reaction intermediate in which the gyrase has broken the phosphodiester backbone of DNA (cleavage complex). According to a model, hydrogen bonding of quinolones to the unpaired bases of the staggered DNA is involved (28). However, direct interaction with DNA gyrase complexed with DNA now seems more likely (29). The interaction with gyrase involves the N-terminal region of the A subunit, particularly residues 67–106 (quinolone resistance-determining region, QRDR; Ref. 30) and the quinolone nucleus; the C-7 substituent can vary with little effect on inhibitory activity. The overall result is blockage of chromosome replication and introduction of intracellular DNA lesions (31), which in turn trigger the SOS response (32) and ultimately lead to cell death. The mechanism of bacterial killing is still incompletely understood (33). The SOS response may not be involved, since mutations affecting several proteins in the SOS response *increase* susceptibility to quinolones. Time-kill studies have shown that quinolones are rapidly bactericidal for a wide range of bacteria at minimal inhibitory concentrations (MICs) (34). In *E. coli*, quinolones cause filamentation, distinguishable from cephalosporin-induced filamentation by the additional effects on nucleoid segregation (35). The induction of filamentation and nucleoid segregation is shared by agents that cleave DNA, such as mitomycin C, and is part of the SOS response. Quinolones differ in their physiological effects from coumarins, another class of DNA gyrase-acting drugs, which simply inhibit enzyme activity

(36). Protein synthesis is required for the bactericidal effect of quinolones; chloramphenicol and rifampicin generally antagonize quinolone action (37). Quinolones themselves may act antagonistically at high concentrations, an effect described as paradoxical (38). However, the newer, more potent quinolones can kill bacteria in stationary phase in the presence of inhibitors of protein synthesis (39).

2. *Topoisomerase IV*

Quinolones also inhibit *E. coli* topoisomerase IV, a tetrameric enzyme homologous to DNA gyrase (A subunit, 75 kDA; B subunit, 70 kDa) (40), but at much higher concentrations (41). Topoisomerase IV is mechanistically similar to DNA gyrase: it introduces transient double-strand breaks on DNA (type II topoisomerase) (40,42). However, topoisomerase IV has a discrete cellular function; it is involved in decatenation, i.e., the resolution of interlinked circular daughter chromosomes following replication (42–44). Topoisomerase IV may be the quinolone target in *Staphylococcus aureus* (45) and in cases of DNA gyrase–associated quinolone resistance, although the latter has not yet been shown.

C. Quinolone Resistance

Anaerobic pathogens, such as *Bacteroides*, *Clostridium*, and other anaerobic cocci and bacilli, are intrinsically resistant to quinolones currently in use at clinically achievable tissue or fluid levels. In addition, several important gram-positive pathogens, such as methicillin-resistant *S. aureus* (MRSA), enterococci, and hemolytic streptococci, are also resistant. Of the gram-negative aerobic bacteria, *Pseudomonas aeruginosa* and enterobacteria are becoming increasingly resistant (see Chap. 1). There is incomplete cross-resistance between quinolones (46–48).

In contrast to β-lactam and aminoglycoside resistance, quinolone resistance is exclusively chromosomal (49–51). Indeed, quinolones have been reported to promote *loss* of plasmids and to inhibit transfer of R-factor-mediated resistance through their effects on DNA gyrase activity (52,53). Quinolone resistance mechanisms are commonly associated with (a) decreased outer-membrane permeation through altered porins; (b) increased efflux through cytoplasmic membrane; and (c) decreased sensitivity of DNA gyrase, particularly the A subunit. There is no reported quinolone modification by bacteria.

Serial exposure of bacteria to increasing concentrations of a quinolone results in stepwise increase in resistance to the quinolone exposed and to other quinolones (54). Resistance appears to result from reduced inhibition of DNA gyrase, increased efflux, and, in gram-negative bacteria, loss of outer-membrane proteins, particularly the OmpF porin (55–59). The major form of quinolone resistance is altered DNA gyrase; decreased quinolone accumulation is associated with low-level, pleiotropic resistance. High-level resistance is associated exclusively with changes in DNA gyrase, particularly in the narrow region between Ala-67 and Gln-106 of the A subunit. Spontaneous, single-step resistance to quinolones occurs at a relatively low frequency ($<10^{-9}$) in the laboratory. However, studies with several clinical isolates have shown that high-level, DNA gyrase–associated, quinolone resistance can occur in a single step (60). A combination of decreased permeability and DNA gyrase changes has been seen in experimental endocarditis with *P. aeruginosa* (61), experimental peritonitis with *Enterobacter cloacae* (62), and other infection models.

II. MEASUREMENT OF QUINOLONE TRANSPORT

A. Protonation Schemes for Quinolones

To understand quinolone uptake and efflux, the protonation and chelation behavior of quinolones must be briefly considered. Like tetracyclines (see Chap. 7), quinolones are acids that can ionize in aqueous solution; a general protonation scheme is shown in Figure 3 (63). Most quinolones have two protonation sites, on the carboxylate (pK ~6) of the nucleus and on the amine (pK ~8.8) of the 7-substituent. At neutral pH, the zwitterionic and uncharged forms, evident in the microscopic but not macroscopic protonation scheme of Figure 3, predominate. It is the uncharged form that diffuses through the cytoplasmic membrane (64). The zwitterionic form can chelate divalent cations, such as calcium and magnesium, which has implications for transport through the outer membrane (65). The importance of the two species in the overall uptake depends on which of the two steps is rate-limiting.

B. Transport Assays

Quinolone transport has been studied in whole cells, protoplasts, and everted vesicles, the latter being the most appropriate for studying quinolone efflux. Cells or vesicles are separated from the external medium by filtration or centrifugation. Filtration can be on glass fiber, cellulose nitrate, or polycarbonate filters and is especially convenient with radiolabeled quinolones (66). Centrifugation can be direct, through silicone oil (67–69), or may involve aqueous two-phase systems [polyethylene glycol (PEG)/dextran, PEG/salts] (70). In the silicone oil method, after incuba-

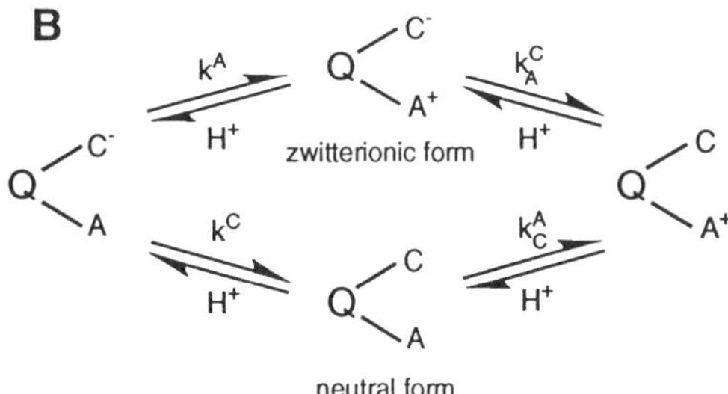

Figure 3 Protonation scheme for quinolones. Shown are macroscopic (upper panel) and microscopic (lower panel) protonation forms and their dissociation constants for three quinolones. (A) The amino group of the piperazine; (B) the carboxylate group of the quinolone nucleus. (Data from Ref. 63.)

tion of a cell suspension with quinolones, a 0.5-ml sample is placed onto 0.5 ml ice-cold silicone oil ($d = 1.04$) in a 1.5-ml Eppendorf tube. The tubes are centrifuged, frozen, cut in the middle of the oil layer, and quinolone concentration is determined in the pellet.

Quinolone concentration is determined by three types of assays: spectrophotometric [based on absorbance (71) or fluorescence (72)], radiometric (73), and microbiological (55). Typically, bacteria are grown to midlog phase and incubated with 1–10 μg/ml quinolone. Samples are removed at different times, and cell-associated quinolone is determined. The different assays generate comparable data (74). The fluorimetric assay, which exploits the natural fluorescence of the quinolone nucleus, is the most versa-

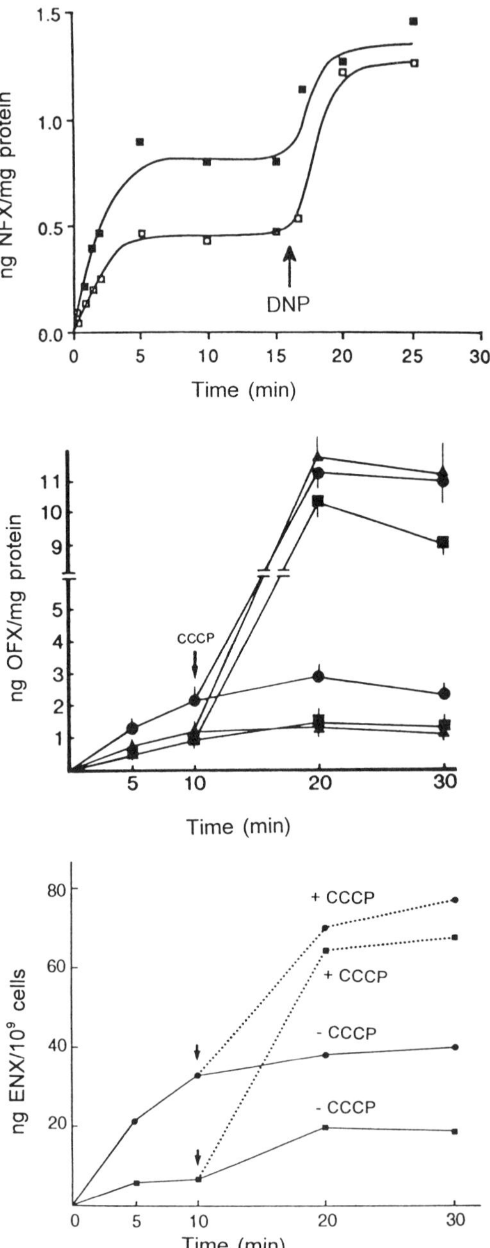

Figure 4 Quinolone accumulation in *E. coli*, *P. aeruginosa*, and *S. aureus*. Upper panel: *E. coli* strains AG100 (■) and LM218 (□). Middle panel: *P. aeruginosa*

tile and convenient assay for measuring quinolone accumulation in bacteria. It has thus been adopted by many workers in the field. For fleroxacin, the excitation and emission maxima are at 282 nm and 442 nm, respectively (72); other quinolones have similar spectra (75). Fluorescence is maximal at pH 3.0, linear at 1–100 ng/ml fleroxacin, and quenched by acetone or boiling the cells. With a cell suspension of ~40 mg/ml (OD_{660} = 20), quinolone accumulation can be measured at 1 μg/ml external concentration. Although this is higher than quinolone MICs for most bacteria, it is still lower than therapeutically achievable serum concentrations of quinolones, which range between 2 and 8 mg/ml depending on the quinolone.

In its early version, the fluorimetric assay involved incubating cells with quinolone at 37°C for 10 min, diluting and washing cells with buffer at room temperature, treating cells with glycine hydrochloride at pH 3.0 to release the quinolone, and measuring the released quinolone fluorimetrically. Under these conditions, blocking energy production by the uncouplers 2,4-dinitrophenol (DNP) and carbonyl cyanide m-chlorophenylhydrazone (CCCP) did not affect quinolone accumulation (65). In a later version (76), cells were not diluted with buffer after incubation with quinolone, but were washed immediately at 4°C. Under these conditions, DNP (0.25 mM) and CCCP (2 mM) increased quinolone accumulation, particularly in quinolone-resistant mutants (Fig. 4). A direct correlation was obtained between hydrophobicity, measured by the log of the octanol/pH 7.2 buffer distribution, and the intracellular accumulation of 11 quinolones in *S. aureus*, while *P. aeruginosa* and *E. coli* gave an inverse correlation (69).

In determining quinolone accumulation, different investigators have used different cell parameters and thus results from different laboratories are often difficult to compare. To help the reader with the primary literature, correlations between the different cell parameters and optical density are shown in Table 1 for three major pathogens.

C. Transport in Cells, Spheroplasts, and Vesicles

Most studies have focused on *E. coli* (55,65,73,77); other enterobacteria, *P. aeruginosa*, and *S. aureus* have been examined to a lesser extent. In

---

strains KG1079 (●), TN501 (■), and TN508 (▲). Lower panel: *S. aureus* SA113 (●) and SA113(pTUS20) (■). Quinolones (final concentrations: norfloxacin, 0.125 μM; enoxacin, 10 μg/ml; ofloxacin, 10 μg/ml) were added at time zero. Energy poisons (final concentrations: DNP, 2 mM; CCCP, 0.1 mM) were added at the time indicated by the arrows. (From Refs. 76, 88, and 101, with permission.)

Table 1 Cell Parameters in Different Bacteria at an OD_{660} of 1

| | | Concn. (mg/ml) | | | Intracellular |
| | | Cells | Cells | | vol |
Organism	CFU/ml	(wet wt)	(dry wt)	Protein	(% wet wt)
E. coli					
ATCC 25922	9×10^8	3.0 ± 0.1	0.44 ± 0.02	0.24 ± 0.04	55
JF568	ND	2.5 ± 0.1	0.41 ± 0.01	0.21 ± 0.04	ND
P. aeruginosa	8×10^8	2.7 ± 0.2	0.42 ± 0.02	0.16 ± 0.01	ND
PAO1					
S. aureus ATCC	5×10^8	1.5 ± 0.1	0.30 ± 0.02	0.18 ± 0.02	52
29213					

ND, not determined.
Source: McCaffrey et al. (75).

all bacteria studied, quinolones are taken up rapidly, reaching a plateau within 2 min. At 10 μg/ml external concentration (27–45 μM depending on the quinolone), the steady-state concentration ranges from 50 to 300 ng quinolone/mg dry weight of cells, corresponding to a two- to 12-fold quinolone accumulation. Uptake is nonsaturable in *E. coli*, *P. aeruginosa*, and *S. aureus* (67,73,75,77,78) and is affected by both temperature (73,79) and pH (77–79). Spheroplasts have about half of the steady-state concentration seen in whole cells (77).

Starting with the pioneering studies of Rosen and McClees 20 years ago (Ref. 80; see also Chap. 4), energy-dependent efflux has been measured in inside-out (everted) vesicles, where it appears as energy-dependent uptake. The energy requirement is defined by the energy sources and inhibitors. Thus, quinolone efflux (measured as accumulation in everted vesicles) is stimulated by glucose or lactose and is inhibited by cyanide, which blocks electron transport, or DNP and CCCP, which depolarize the energized membrane (81). Further, it is saturable with a K_m of 0.2 mM.

III. QUINOLONE UPTAKE

A. Gram-Negative Outer Membrane

The outer membrane, the distinguishing feature of gram-negative bacteria, envelopes and is covalently linked to peptidoglycan. Structurally, it is a protein-rich, asymmetrical lipid bilayer containing phospholipids in the inner leaflet and lipopolysaccharides (LPS) of different saccharide chain lengths in the outer leaflet, which interact with one another via Mg^{2+}-

Table 2 Quinolone Uptake in Different Bacteria

Organism	Quinolone	Ext. concn. (μg/ml)	Steady-state uptake	Method	Ref.
E. coli					
K12 J53	CFX	0.15	0.004 μg/mg dry wt. cells	Radio. assay	78
K12 JF568	CFX	10	0.28 μg/mg dry wt. cells	Fluor. assay	75
ATCC 25922	CFX	10	0.28 μg/mg dry wt. cells	Fluor. assay	75
K16	CFX	16	0.35 μg/mg dry wt. cells	Radio. assay	79
SA 1306	ENX	5	0.3 μg/mg dry wt. cells	Radio. assay	73
K12 JF568	FLX	10	0.13 μg/mg dry wt. cells	Fluor. assay	75
ATCC 25922	FLX	10	0.09 μg/mg dry wt. cells	Fluor. assay	75
KL16	LFX	10	0.06 μg/mg dry wt. cells	Fluor. assay	114
AG100	NFX	0.125	0.5 ng/mg protein	Radio. assay	81
CS109	NFX	1	0.15 μg/mg dry wt. cells	uv assay	71
KP05124	NFX	2	0.5 μg/mg dry wt. cells	Radio. assay	68
CS109	NFX	10	0.4 μg/mg dry wt. cells	Bioassay	55
KL16	NFX	10	0.25 μg/mg dry wt. cells	Bioassay	55
Q1	NFX	10	0.012 μg/mg cells	Fluor. assay	115
K12 JF568	NFX	10	0.23 μg/mg dry wt. cells	Fluor. assay	75
ATCC 25922	NFX	10	0.21 μg/mg dry wt. cells	Fluor. assay	75
K12 JF568	OFX	10	0.12 μg/mg dry wt. cells	Fluor. assay	75
ATCC 25922	OFX	10	0.10 μg/mg dry wt. cells	Fluor. assay	75
K12 JF568	PFX	10	0.17 μg/mg dry wt. cells	Fluor. assay	75
ATCC 25922	PFX	10	0.14 μg/ml dry wt. cells	Fluor. assay	75
P. vulgaris					
08602	OFX	10	0.006 μg/mg dry wt. cells	Fluor. assay	99
P. aeruginosa					
PAO503	CFX	0.15	0.006 μg/mg dry wt. cells	Radio. assay	78
PAO2	CFX	10	0.04 μg/mg dry wt. cells	Bioassay	67
PAO1	CFX	10	0.10 μg/mg dry wt. cells	Fluor. assay	95
PAO1	FLX	10	0.06 μg/mg dry wt. cells	Fluor. assay	75
PAO1	NFX	10	0.10 μg/mg dry wt. cells	Fluor. assay	75
PAO1	OFX	10	0.06 μg/ml dry wt. cells	Fluor. assay	75
KG1079	OFX	10	0.002 ng/mg protein	Fluor. assay	99
PAO1	PFX	10	0.10 μg/ml dry wt. cells	Fluor. assay	75
S. aureus					
ATCC 29213	CFX	10	0.14 μg/mg dry wt. cells	Fluor. assay	75
SA113	ENX	10	0.04 ng/10^9 cells	Radio. assay	101
ATCC 29213	FLX	10	0.14 μg/mg dry wt. cells	Fluor. assay	75
NCTC 8532	LFX	10	0.09 μg/mg dry wt. cells	Fluor. assay	114
ATCC 29213	NFX	10	0.19 μg/mg dry wt. cells	Fluor. assay	75
MS16008	NFX	10	0.5 μg/mg dry wt. cells	Bioassay	110

(continued)

Table 2 (*Continued*)

Organism	Quinolone	Ext. concn. (μg/ml)	Steady-state uptake	Method	Ref.
534	NFX	16	0.015 ng/mg protein	Radio. assay	102
ATCC 29213	OFX	10	0.19 μg/ml dry wt. cells	Fluor. assay	75
ATCC 29213	PFX	10	0.24 μg/ml dry wt. cells	Fluor. assay	75
MS16008	SFX	10	0.5 μg/ml dry wt. cells	Bioassay	110
SA113	SFX	10	0.015 ng/10^9 cells	Radio. assay	101

CFX, ciprofloxacin; ENX, enoxacin; FLX, fleroxacin; LFX, lomefloxacin; NFX, norfloxacin; OFX, ofloxacin; PFX, pefloxacin; SFX, sparfloxacin.

salt bridges as well as outer-membrane proteins (82–84). Functionally, it is a molecular sieve with water-filled channels, formed by 35- to 45-kDa proteins (porins), through which nonspecific transport of small molecules occurs. It thus protects the bacterial cell from such damaging agents as antibiotics, bile salts, and mammalian hydrolytic enzymes (85).

In *E. coli* K12 outer membrane there are two porins, OmpC and OmpF, which trimerize and form channels of 11- and 12-A diameter, respectively, with an exclusion limit of 600–800 Da (86). The two porins are reciprocally regulated at the transcriptional level (87). High osmolarity (300 mosm) and high temperature (37°C), conditions that prevail in the body, favor OmpC production, and thus the narrower channel, at the expense of OmpF. Like β-lactams (see Chap. 5), quinolones cross the outer membrane of *Enterobacteria* predominantly through the porin pathway. Laboratory *OmpF*, *marA*, and *OmpR* mutants of *E. coli* and *Salmonella typhimurium* that have decreased expression of OmpF show a two- to fourfold decrease in susceptibility to quinolones and a concomitant decrease in quinolone uptake and steady-state concentration (55,56,73,88). Conversely, *E. coli* mutants with decreased OmpC have no change in susceptibility or uptake (57). Most important, quinolone-resistant clinical isolates lack OmpF (55,77,89), suggesting that this pathway may be clinically relevant despite the expected suppression of OmpF in favor of OmpC under conditions that prevail in the body. There may be some additional factor mediating quinolone uptake, since *marA* strains have a lower initial rate of uptake and steady-state concentration of norfloxacin than *ompF* strains (88). In addition, there may be "self-promoted" quinolone entry through lipid patches in the outer membrane resulting from the removal of LPS-bound magnesium and destabilization of the outer membrane by quinolones (65). Accordingly, magnesium and calcium ions decrease uptake, a situation reminiscent of that with tetracyclines (see Chap. 7). The non-porin pathway may be particularly important for hydrophobic quinolones, such as tosufloxacin (90), in bacteria whose permeability is relatively poor, such as *P. aeruginosa*, or in bacteria whose loose LPS exposes hydrophobic membrane domains, such as *Hemophilus influenzae*.

Quinolones probably use the porin pathway in *Enterobacteria* in general (91), although direct evidence, such as studies with porin mutants, is lacking. In *P. aeruginosa*, on the other hand, they probably use the 45-kDa D2 protein which has been implicated in the transport of imipenem (92) (see Chap. 5). In this organism, the other outer-membrane proteins and lipopolysaccharide may also play a role (67,93–96) and the self-promoted pathway may be operating.

In *H. influenzae*, whose porin channel has an exclusion limit similar to that of *E. coli*, quinolones probably also use the porin pathway though they may use additional nonporin pathways. This organism has a loose LPS structure and is uniquely, for a gram-negative bacterium, susceptible to some hydrophobic antibiotics such as the newer macrolides (see Chap. 1).

Since newer quinolones are active against the important anaerobe *Bacteroides fragilis*, their transport in that organism would be of interest. *B. fragilis* porins have not yet been characterized, though its pores appear to have an exclusion limit similar to that of *P. aeruginosa* (97).

B. Bacterial Cytoplasmic Membrane

The cytoplasmic membrane is the next barrier encountered by quinolones on their way to the target; the peptidoglycan does not pose a barrier for small molecules. This membrane is a conventional phospholipid bilayer, which allows diffusion of hydrophobic antibiotics such as novobiocin and erythromycin (hence their gram-positive activity). Accordingly, there is a decrease in the MICs of quinolones against *S. aureus* with increasing quinolone hydrophobicity, defined as partitioning between *n*-octanol and pH 7.2 phosphate buffer (partition coefficient range: 0.046–4.4). Quinolones probably cross the cytoplasmic membrane uncharged (64) and their apparent concentrative uptake may be in response to Donnan potential. The cytoplasmic pH, ~7.8, is higher than the external pH, ~6.1 (98), and the quinolone species becomes zwitterionic upon entering the cell (see Sec. II.A).

IV. QUINOLONE EFFLUX

Although early experiments showed no effect of DNP and CCCP on quinolone accumulation (65,73,76,78), starting with the work of Cohen et al.

(81), energy-dependent efflux has been shown in *E. coli* (75,81), *Proteus vulgaris* (99), *P. aeruginosa* (76), and *S. aureus* (100–102) (Fig. 4). The gene encoding this system, *norA*, has been identified and cloned (101,103). Interestingly, *norA* is associated with an eight- to 64-fold increase in resistance to hydrophilic quinolones but only twofold resistance to hydrophobic quinolones (73). *NorA* codes for a highly hydrophobic protein that contains 12 putative transmembrane segments (104,105) and has significant sequence homology to the tetracycline efflux transporters (Tet proteins) of gram-negative bacteria (see Chap. 7). *NorA* preferentially mediates efflux of hydrophilic quinolones and does not provide resistance to tetracyclines (106).

V. CONCLUSIONS AND FUTURE DIRECTIONS

The understanding of quinolone transport has progressed rapidly at both cellular and molecular levels. As discussed in this chapter, quinolone accumulation is the net result of both uptake and efflux (Fig. 5). Uptake

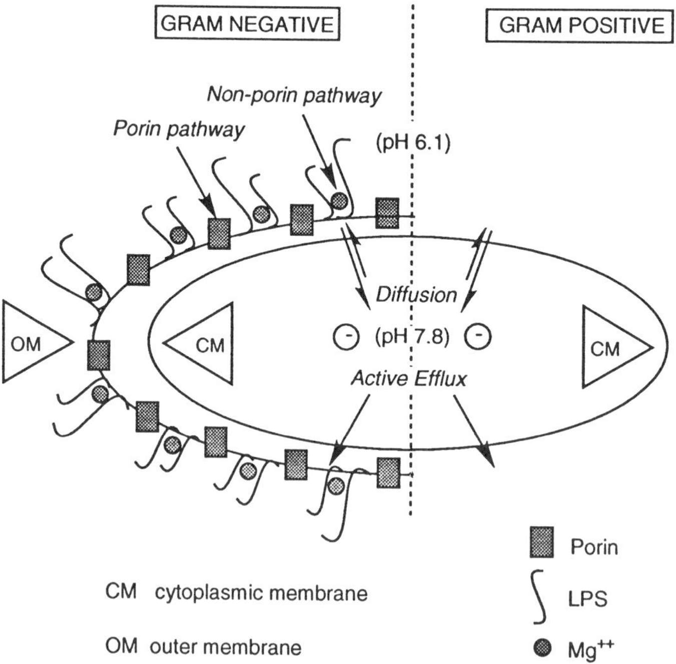

Figure 5 Quinolone transport in gram-negative and gram-positive bacteria.

across the outer membrane involves passive diffusion through porin channels or lipid bilayer regions; uptake across the cytoplasmic membrane involves distribution of the quinolone in response to the pH gradient that exists across the cytoplasmic membrane. Efflux occurs across the cytoplasmic membrane, is energy-dependent, and involves a membrane-spanning protein, NorA.

Transport may be a less important factor in resistance to quinolones than β-lactams, aminoglycosides, or tetracyclines, at least in aerobic bacteria. This may due to the fact that, contrary to β-lactams and aminoglycosides, quinolones are not degraded and, contrary to tetracyclines, they are rapidly bactericidal. However, transport may be a more important factor in quinolone resistance of anaerobes, such as *B. fragilis*, where quinolones may not be bactericidal (38).

Like antiparasitic antimonials (Chap. 14) and antitumor antifolates (Chap. 16), decreased quinolone accumulation appears to accompany low levels of resistance and may precede alterations in DNA gyrase. Thus, decreased accumulation may be the first line of defense in bacteria, parasites, and tumor cells presented with a cytotoxic compound.

Issues, both theoretical and experimental, persist. For example, outer-membrane changes associated with quinolone resistance almost always occur with alterations in DNA gyrase, which could lead to alterations in DNA supercoiling and thereby altered gene expression. It is therefore possible that some outer-membrane alterations may be the result, rather than the cause, of quinolone resistance.

Most of the quinolone transport studies have been carried out at quinolone concentrations that far exceed MICs. Some physiological subtleties may be lost under these conditions. It is recalled that the physiologically important interactions of β-lactamases and broad-spectrum cephalosporins occur at low cephalosporin concentrations (thus the importance of catalytic efficiency; see Chap. 5). If a specific transport system for the uptake of quinolones exists, it will most likely operate at low quinolone concentrations (see also imipenem transport in *P. aeruginosa*; Chap. 5).

The contribution of quinolone accumulation to resistance is often inferred from negative $gyrA^+$ plasmid complementation experiments (107,108). However, these may be falsely negative if the plasmid is unstable in the organism being studied (109).

A final caveat has to do with time scale of the quinolone transport studies and the cell manipulations involved. As was recently pointed out (64), quinolone leakage most likely occurs during the cell washings that precede quinolone determination and may affect reliability of data.

Nevertheless, mechanistic studies have started to produce valuable insights into this important factor of quinolone action and resistance and may have considerable impact on the design, development, and utility of new quinolones. For example, there is evidence for cross-resistance between quinolones and imipenem in *P. aeruginosa* following quinolone, but not imipenem, treatment, and that hydrophobic quinolones, like sparfloxacin (110), are effluxed less readily. The role of efflux (reviewed in Ref. 111) may be particularly important in the relative resistance of this organism to many antibacterial agents, including quinolones (112), and may occur across both cytoplasmic and outer membranes (113).

ACKNOWLEDGMENTS

I thank Drs. John Chapman, John Pace, and Mildred Rivera for their contributions; Lisa Cummings, Anne Bertasso, and Catherine McCaffrey for their excellent technical assistance; and Roche management for being supportive of the work carried out in my laboratory.

REFERENCES

1. Lesher GY, Forelich ED, Gruet MD, Bailey JH, Brundage RP. 1,8-Naphthyridine derivatives. A new class of chemotherapeutic agents. J Med Pharm Chem 1962; 5:1063–1068.
2. Albrecht R. Development of antibacterial agents of the nalidixic acid type. Prog Drug Res 1977; 21:9–104.
3. Ronald AR, Turck M, Petersdorf RG. A critical evaluation of nalidixic acid in urinary tract infections. N Engl J Med 1966; 275:1081–1089.
4. Chu, DTW, Fernandes PB. Recent developments in the field of quinolone antibacterial agents. Adv Drug Res 1991; 21:39–144.
5. Bryan LE, Bedard J. Impermeability to quinolones in gram-positive and gram-negative bacteria. Eur J Clin Microbiol 1991; 10:232–239.
6. Piddock LJV. Mechanism of quinolone uptake into bacterial cells. J Antimicrob Chemother 1991; 27:399–403.
7. Piddock LJV. New quinolones and gram-positive bacteria. Antimicrob Agents Chemother 1994; 38:163–169.
8. Piddock LJV. Resistance to quinolones and fluoroquinolones. In: Bryan LE, ed. Microbial Resistance to Drugs. Handbook of Experimental Pharmacology, Vol 91. Berlin: Springer-Verlag, 1989:169–192.
9. Maxwell A. The molecular basis of quinolone action. J Antimicrob Chemother 1992; 30:409–416.
10. Hooper DC, Wolfson JS. Fluoroquinolone antimicrobial agents. N Engl J Med 1991; 324:384–394.
11. Neu HC. Clinical utility of DNA gyrase inhibitors. Pharmacol Ther 1989; 41:207–221.
12. Neu HC. Quinolone antimicrobial agents. Annu Rev Med 1992; 43:465–486.
13. Andreole V, ed. The Quinolones. New York: Academic Press, 1988.

14. Wolfson JS, Hooper DC, eds. Quinolone Antimicrobial Agents. Washington, DC: American Society for Microbiology, 1989.
15. Fernandes PB, ed. International Telesymposium on Quinolones. Barcelona: JR Prous, 1989.
16. Siporin C, Heifetz CL, Domagala JM, eds. The New Generation of Quinolones. New York: Marcel Dekker, 1990.
17. Hooper DC, Wolfson JS, eds. Quinolone Antimicrobial Agents, 2nd ed. Washington, DC: American Society for Microbiology, 1993.
18. Goss WA, Deitz WH, Cook TM. Mechanism of action of nalidixic acid on *Escherichia coli*. J Bacteriol 1964; 88:1112–1118.
19. Deitz WH, Cook TM, Gross WA. Mechanism of action of nalidixic acid on *Escherichia coli*. III. Conditions required for lethality. J Bacteriol 1966; 91:768–773.
20. Gellert M, Mizuuchi K, O'Dea MH, Nash HA. DNA gyrase: an enzyme that introduces superhelical turns into DNA. Proc Natl Acad Sci USA 1976; 73:3872–3876.
21. Gellert M, Mizuuchi K, O'Dea MH, Itoh T, Tomizawa JI. Nalidixic acid resistance: a second character involved in DNA gyrase activity. Proc Natl Acad Sci USA 1977; 74:4772–4776.
22. Sugino A, Peebles CL, Kreuzer KN, Cozzarelli NR. Mechanism of action of nalidixic acid: purification of *Escherichia coli nalA* gene product and its relationship to DNA gyrase and a novel nicking-closing enzyme. Proc Natl Acad Sci USA 1977; 74:4767–4771.
23. Reece RJ, Maxwell A. DNA gyrase: structure and function. Crit Rev Biochem Mol Biol 1991; 26:335–375.
24. Wang JC. DNA topoisomerases. Annu Rev Biochem 1985; 54:665–697.
25. Gellert M. DNA topoisomerases. Annu Rev Biochem 1981; 50:879–910.
26. Horowitz DS, Wang JC. Mapping of the active site tyrosine of *Escherichia coli* DNA gyrase. J Biol Chem 1987; 262:5339–5344.
27. Hooper DC, Wolfson JS. Mechanisms of quinolone action and bacterial killing. In: Hooper DC, Wolfson JS, eds. Quinolone Antibacterial Agents. Washington, DC: American Society for Microbiology, 1993:53–75.
28. Shen LL, Mitscher LA, Sharma PN, O'Donnell TJ, Chu DWT, Cooper CS, Rosen T, Pernet AG. Mechanism of inhibition of DNA gyrase by quinolone antibacterials: a cooperative drug-DNA binding model. Biochemistry 1989; 28:3886–3894.
29. Yoshida H, Nakamura M, Bogaki M, Ito H, Kojima T, Hattori H, Nakamura S. Mechanism of action of quinolones against *Escherichia coli* DNA gyrase. Antimicrob Agents Chemother 1993; 37:839–845.
30. Yoshida H, Bogaki M, Nakamura M, Nakamura S. Quinolone-resistance-determining region in the DNA gyrase *gyrA* gene of *Escherichia coli*. Antimicrob Agents Chemother 1990; 34:1271–1272.
31. Kreuzer KN, Cozzarelli NR. *Escherichia coli* mutants thermosensitive for deoxyribonucleic acid gyrase subunit A: effects of DNA replication, transcription, and bacteriophage growth. J Bacteriol 1979; 140:424–435.

32. Walker G. Mutagenesis and inducible responses to deoxyribonucleic acid damage in *Escherichia coli*. Microbiol Rev 1984; 48:60–93.

33. Drlica K, Coughlin S, Gennaro ML. Mode of action of quinolones: biochemical aspects. In: Siporin C, Heifetz CL, Domagala JM, eds. The New Generation of Quinolones. New York: Marcel Dekker, 1990:45–62.

34. Sonstein SA. Mode of action of quinolones: antibacterial aspects. In: Siporin C, Heifetz CL, Domagala JM, eds. The New Generalization of Quinolones. New York: Marcel Dekker, 1990:63–78.

35. Georgopapadakou NH, Bertasso A. Effects of quinolones on nucleoid segregation in *Escherichia coli*. Antimicrob Agents Chemother 1991; 35:2645–2648.

36. Engle EC, Manes SH, Drlica K. Differential effects of antibiotics inhibiting gyrase. J Bacteriol 1982; 149:92–98.

37. Smith JT. Awakening the slumbering potential of the quinolones. Pharm J 1989; 15:299–305.

38. Lewin CS, Morrissey I, Smith JT. The mode of action of quinolones: the paradox in activity of low and high concentrations and activity in the anaerobic environments. Eur J Clin Microbiol Infect Dis 1991; 10:240–248.

39. Zeiler H. Evaluation of the in vitro bactericidal action of ciprofloxacin on cells of *Escherichia coli* in the logarithmic and stationary phases of growth. Antimicrob Agents Chemother 1985; 28:524–527.

40. Kato J, Suzuki H, Ikeda H. Purification and characterization of DNA topoisomerase IV in *Escherichia coli*. J Biol Chem 1992; 267:25676–25684.

41. Hoshino K, Kitamura A, Morrissey I, Sato K, Kato J-I, Ikeda H. Comparison of inhibition of *Escherichia coli* topoisomerase IV by quinolones with DNA gyrase inhibition. Antimicrob Agents Chemother 1994; 38:2623–2627.

42. Kato J, Nishimura Y, Imamura R, Niki H, Hiraga S, Suzuki H. New topoisomerase essential for chromosome segregation in *Escherichia coli*. Cell 1990; 63:393–404.

43. Adams DE, Shekhtman EM, Zechiedrich EL, Schmid M, Cozzarelli NR. The role of topoisomerase IV in partitioning bacterial replicons and the structure of catenated intermediates in DNA replication. Cell 1992; 71:277–288.

44. Peng H, Marians KJ. Decatenation activity of topoisomerase IV during *oriC* and pBR322 DNA replication in vitro. Proc Natl Acad Sci USA 1993; 90:8571–8575.

45. Ferrero L, Cameron B, Manse B, Lagneaux D, Crouzet J, Famechon A, Blanche F. Cloning and primary structure of *Staphylococcus aureus* DNA topoisomerase IV: a primary target of fluoroquinolones. Mol Microbiol 1994; 13:641–653.

46. Barry AL, Jones RN. Cross resistance among cinoxacin, ciprofloxacin, DJ-6783, enoxacin, nalidixic acid, norfloxacin and oxolinic acid after in vitro selection of resistant populations. Antimicrob Agents Chemother 1984; 25:775–777.

47. Traub WH. Incomplete cross-resistance of nalidixic acid and pipemidic

acid–resistant variants of *Serratia marcescens* against ciprofloxacin, enoxacin, and norfloxacin. Chemotherapy 1985; 31:34–39.

48. Thomson KS, Sanders C. Dissociated resistance among fluoroquinolones. Antimicrob Agents Chemother 1994; 38:2095–2100.

49. Burman LG. Apparent absence of transferable resistance to nalidixic acid in pathogenic gram-negative bacteria. J Antimicrob Chemother 1977; 3:509–516.

50. Smith JT. Mutational resistance to 4-quinolone antibacterial agents. Eur J Clin Microbiol 1984; 3:347–350.

51. Courvalin P. Plasmid-mediated 4-quinolone resistance: a real or apparent absence? Antimicrob Agents Chemother 1990; 34:681–684.

52. Hirai K, Irikura T, Iyobe S, et al. Inhibition of conjugal transfer of R-plasmids by norfloxacin in *Pseudomonas aeruginosa*. Chemotherapy 1984; 32:471–476.

53. Michel-Briand Y, Uccelli V, Laporte JM et al. Elimination of plasmids from *Enterobacteriaceae* by 4-quinolone derivatives. J Antimicrob Chemother 1986; 18:667–674.

54. Hooper DC, Wolfson JS. Mechanisms of bacterial resistance to quinolones. In: Hooper DC, Wolfson JS, eds. Quinolone Antibacterial Agents. Washington, DC: American Society for Microbiology, 1993:97–118.

55. Hirai K, Aoyama H, Suzue S, Irikura T, Iyobe S, Mitsuhashi S. Isolation and characterization of norfloxacin-resistant mutants of *Escherichia coli* K-12. Antimicrob Agents Chemother 1986; 30:248–253.

56. Hirai K, Aoyama H, Irikura T, Iyobe S, Mitsuhashi S. Differences in susceptibility to quinolones of outer membrane mutants of *Salmonella typhimurium* and *Escherichia coli*. Antimicrob Agents Chemother 1986; 29:535–538.

57. Chapman JS, Bertasso A, Georgopapadakou NH. Fleroxacin resistance in *Escherichia coli*. Antimicrob Agents Chemother 1989; 33:239–241.

58. Masecar BL, Celesk RA, Robillard NJ. Analysis of acquired ciprofloxacin resistance in a clinical strain of *Pseudomonas aeruginosa*. Antimicrob Agents Chemother 1990; 34:281–286.

59. Watanabe M, Inoue M, Mitsuhashi S. In vitro activity of amifloxacin against outer membrane mutants of the family *Enterobacteriaceae* and frequency of spontaneous resistance. Antimicrob Agents Chemother 1989; 33:1837–1840.

60. Gootz TD, Martin BA. Characterization of high-level quinolone resistance in *Campylobacter jejuni*. Antimicrob Agents Chemother 1991; 35:840–845.

61. Chamberland S, Bayer AS, Schollaardt T, Wong SA, Bryan LE. Characterization of mechanisms of quinolone resistance in *Pseudomonas aeruginosa* strains isolated in vitro and in vivo during experimental endocarditis. Antimicrob Agents Chemother 1989; 33:624–634.

62. Lucain C, Regamey P, Bellido F, Pechere J.-C. Resistance emerging after pefloxacin therapy of experimental *Enterobacter cloacae* peritonitis. Antimicrob Agents Chemother 1989; 33:937–943.

63. Takacs-Novak K, Noszal B, Hermecz I, Kereszturi G, Podanyi B, Szasz G. Protonation equilibria of quinolone antibacterials. J Pharm Sci 1990; 79:1023–1028.

64. Nikaido H, Thanassi DG. Penetration of lipophilic agents with multiple protonation sites into bacterial cells: tetracyclines and fluoroquinolones as examples. Antimicrob Agents Chemother 1993; 37:1393–1399.

65. Chapman JS, Georgopapadakou NH. Routes of quinolone permeation in *Escherichia coli*. Antimicrob Agents Chemother 1988; 32:438–442.

66. Kaatz GW, Seo SM, Ruble CA. Mechanisms of fluoroquinolone resistance in *Staphylococcus aureus*. J Infect Dis 1991; 163:1080–1086.

67. Celesk RA, Robillard NJ. Factors influencing the accumulation of ciprofloxacin in *Pseudomonas aeruginosa*. Antimicrob Agents Chemother 1989; 33:1921–1926.

68. Valisena S, Palumbo M, Parolin C, Palu G, Meloni GA. Relevance of ionic effects on norfloxacin uptake by *Escherichia coli*. Biochem Pharmacol 1990; 40:431–436.

69. Bazile S, Moreau N, Bouzard D, Essiz M. Relationships among antibacterial activity, inhibition of DNA gyrase, and intracellular accumulation of 11 fluoroquinolones. Antimicrob Agents Chemother 1992; 36:2622–2627.

70. Moreau N, Lacroix P, Fournel L. Antibiotic uptake by bacteria as measured by partition in polymer aqueous phase systems. Anal Biochem 1984; 141:94–100.

71. Kotera Y, Watanabe M, Yoshida S, Inoue M, Mitsuhashi S. Factors influencing the uptake of norfloxacin by *Escherichia coli*. J Antimicrob Chemother 1991; 27:733–739.

72. Chapman JS, Georgopapadakou NH. A fluorometric assay for quinolone uptake by bacterial cells. Antimicrob Agents Chemother 1989; 33:27–29.

73. Bedard J, Wong S, Bryan LE. Accumulation of enoxacin by *Escherichia coli* and *Bacillus subtilis*. Antimicrob Agents Chemother 1987; 31:1348–1354.

74. Mortimer PGS, Piddock LJV. A comparison of methods used for measuring the accumulation of quinolones by *Enterobacteriaceae*, *Pseudomonas aeruginosa* and *Staphylococcus aureus*. J Antimicrob Chemother 1991; 28:639–653.

75. McCaffrey C, Bertasso A, Pace J, Georgopapadakou NH. Quinolone accumulation in *Escherichia coli*, *Pseudomonas aeruginosa*, and *Staphylococcus aureus*. Antimicrob Agents Chemother 1992; 1601–1605.

76. Lei Y, Sato K, Nakae T. Ofloxacin-resistant *Pseudomonas aeruginosa* mutants with elevated drug extrusion across the inner membrane. Biochem Biophys Res Commun 1991; 178:1043–1048.

77. Hooper DC, Wolfson JS, Souza KS, Ng EY, McHugh GL, Swartz MN. Mechanisms of quinolone resistance in *Escherichia coli*: characterization of *nfxB* and *cfxB*, two mutant resistance loci decreasing norfloxacin accumulation. Antimicrob Agents Chemother 1989; 33:283–290.

78. Bedard J, Chamberland S, Wong S, Schollaardt T, Bryan LE. Contribution of permeability and sensitivity to inhibition of DNA synthesis in determining

susceptibility of ciprofloxacin for *Escherichia coli*, *Pseudomonas aeruginosa* and *Alcaligenes faecalis*. Antimicrob Agents Chemother 1989; 33:1457–1464.

79. Diver JM, Piddock LJV, Wise R. The accumulation of five quinolone antibacterial agents by *Escherichia coli*. J Antimicrob Chemother 1990; 25:319–333.

80. Rosen BP, McClees. Active transport of calcium in inverted membrane vesicles of *Escherichia coli*. Proc Natl Acad Sci USA 1974; 71:5042–5046.

81. Cohen SP, Hooper DC, Wolfson JS, Souza KS, McMurry LM, Levy SB. Endogenous active efflux of norfloxacin in susceptible *Escherichia coli*. Antimicrob Agents Chemother 1988; 32:1187–1191.

82. Nikaido H, Vaara M. Molecular basis of bacterial outer membrane permeability. Microbiol Rev 1985; 49:1–32.

83. Lugtemberg B, Van Alpen L. Molecular architecture and functioning to the outer membrane porin proteins of *Escherichia coli* and other gram-negative bacteria. Biochim Biophys Acta 1983; 737:51–115.

84. Georgopapadakou NH. Antibiotic permeation through the bacterial outer membrane. J Chemother 1990; 2:275–279.

85. Nikaido H. Prevention of drug access to bacterial targets: permeability barrier and active efflux. Science 1994; 264:382–388

86. Benz R. Porins from bacterial and mitochondrial outer membranes. CRC Crit Rev Biochem 1985; 19:145–190.

87. Hall MN, Silhavy TJ. The *ompB* locus and the regulation of the major outer membrane porin proteins of *Escherichia coli* K12. J Mol Biol 1979; 146:23–43.

88. Cohen SP, McMurry LM, Hooper DC, Wolfson JS, Levy SB. Cross-resistance to fluoroquinolones in multiple antibiotic resistant (Mar) *Escherichia coli* selected by tetracycline or chloramphenicol: decreased drug accumulation associated with membrane changes in addition to OmpF reduction. Antimicrob Agents Chemother 1989; 33:1318–1325.

89. Aoyama H, Sato K, Kato T, Hirai K. Norfloxacin resistance in a clinical isolate of *Escherichia coli*. Antimicrob Agents Chemother 1987; 31:1640–1641.

90. Mitsuyama J-I, Itoh Y, Takahata M, Okamoto S, Yasuda T. In vitro antibacterial activities of tosufloxacin against and uptake of tosufloxacin by outer membrane mutants of *Escherichia coli*, *Proteus mirabilis*, and *Salmonella typhimurium*. Antimicrob Agents Chemother 1992; 36; 2030–2036.

91. Dechene M, Leying H, Cullman W. Role of the outer membrane for quinolone resistance in enterobacteria. Chemotherapy 1990; 36:13–23.

92. Yamano Y, Nishikawa T, Komatsu Y. Outer-membrane proteins responsible for the penetration of β-lactams and quinolones in *Pseudomonas aeruginosa*. J Antimicrob Chemother 1990; 26:175–184.

93. Daikos GL, Lolans VT, Jackson GG. Alterations in the outer membrane proteins of *Pseudomonas aeruginosa* associated with selective resistance to quinolones. Antimicrob Agents Chemother 1988; 32:785–787.

94. Fukuda H, Hosaka M, Hirai K, Iyobe S. New norfloxacin resistance genc

in *Pseudomonas aeruginosa* PAO. Antimicrob Agents Chemother 1990; 34:1757–1761.

95. Hirai K, Suzue S, Irikura T, Iyobe S, Mitsuhashi S. Mutations producing resistance to norfloxacin in *Pseudomonas aeruginosa*. Antimicrob Agents Chemother 1987; 31:582–586.

96. Yoshida T, Muratani T, Iyobe S, Mitsuhashi S. Mechanisms of high-level resistance to quinolones in urinary tract isolates of *Pseudomonas aeruginosa*. Antimicrob Agents Chemother 1994; 38:1466–1469.

97. Kobayashi Y, Akatsuka A, Nakae T. Electron microscopic visualization of the outer membrane permeability of *Bacteroides fragilis*. FEMS Microbiol Lett 1987; 48:325–329.

98. Kashket ER. Stoichiometry of the H^+-ATPase of growing and resting *Escherichia coli*. Biochemistry 1981; 21:5534–5538.

99. Ishii H, Sato K, Hoshino K, Sato M, Yamaguchi A, Sawaii T, Osada Y. Active efflux of ofloxacin by a highly quinolone-resistant strain of *Proteus vulgaris*. J Antimicrob Chemother 1991; 28:827–836.

100. Nakanishi N, Yoshida S, Wakebe H, Inoue M, Yamaguchi T, Mitsuhashi S. Mechanism of clinical resistance to fluoroquinolones in *Staphylococcus aureus*. Antimicrob Agents Chemother 1991; 35:2562–2567.

101. Yoshida H, Bogaki M, Nakamura S, Ubukata K, Konno M. Nucleotide sequence and characterization of the *Staphylococcus aureus norA* gene, which confers resistance to quinolones. J Bacteriol 1990; 172:6942–6949.

102. Cundy KV, Fasching CE, Willard KE, Peterson LR. Uptake of ^{3}H-norfloxacin in methicillin-resistant *Staphylococcus aureus*. J Antimicrob Chemother 1991; 28:491–497.

103. Ubukata K, Itoh-Yamashita N, Konno M. Cloning and expression of the norA gene for fluoroquinolone resistance in *Staphylococcus aureus*. Antimicrob Agents Chemother 1989; 33:1535–1539.

104. Neyfakh AA, Bidnenko VE, Chen LB. Efflux-mediated multidrug resistance in bacteria: similarities and dissimilarities with mammalian system. Proc Natl Acad Sci USA 1991; 88:4781–4785.

105. Neyfakh AA, Borsch CM, Kaatz GW. Fluoroquinolone resistance protein NorA of *Staphylococcus aureus* is a multidrug efflux transporter. Antimicrob Agents Chemother 1993; 37:128–129.

106. Kaatz GW, Seo SM, Ruble CA. Efflux-mediated fluoroquinolone resistance in *Staphylococcus aureus*. Antimicrob Agents Chemother 1993; 37:1086–1094.

107. Hashmi ZS, Smith JMB. Quinolone resistance in *Pseudomonas aeruginosa*. J Antimicrob Chemother 1994; 33:881–883.

108. Yoshida T, Muratani T, Iyobe S, Mitsuhashi S. Mechanisms of high-level resistance to quinolones in urinary tract isolates of *Psuedomonas aeruginosa*. Antimicrob Agents Chemother 1994; 38:1466–1469.

109. Soussy CJ, Wolfson JS, Ng EY, Hooper DC. Limitations of plasmid complementation test for determination of quinolone resistance due to changes in the gyrase A protein and identification of conditional quinolone resistance locus. Antimicrob Agents Chemother 1993; 37:2588–2592.

110. Yoshida H, Kojima T, Inoue M, Mitsuhashi S. Uptake of sparfloxacin and norfloxacin by clinical isolates of *Staphylococcus aureus*. Antimicrob Agents Chemother 1991; 35:368–370.
111. Levy SB. Active efflux mechanisms for antimicrobial resistance. Antimicrob Agents Chemother 1992; 36:695–703.
112. Li X-Z, Livermore DM, Nikaido H. Role of efflux pumps in intrinsic resistance of *Pseudomonas aeruginosa*: resistance to tetracycline, chloramphenicol, and norfloxacin. Antimicrob Agents Chemother 1994; 38:1732–1741.
113. Poole K. Bacterial multidrug resistance—emphasis on efflux mechanisms and *Pseudomonas aeruginosa*. J Antimicrob Agents Chemother 1994; 34:453–456.
114. Piddock LJV, Hall MC, Wise R. Mechanism of action of lomefloxacin. Antimicrob Agents Chemother 1990; 34:1088–1093.
115. Moniot-Ville N, Guibert J, Moreau N, Acar JF, Collatz E, Gutmann L. Mechanisms of quinolone resistance in a clinical isolate of *Escherichia coli* highly resistant to fluoroquinolones but susceptible to nalidixic acid. Antimicrob Agents Chemother 1991; 35:519–523.

9

Antibiotic Transport in Mycobacteria

Joaquim Trias
Universitat de Barcelona, Barcelona, Spain

I. INTRODUCTION

Mycobacteria are gram-positive organisms that are the causative agents of tuberculosis, leprosy, and some of the most frequent systemic bacterial infections in patients with acquired immunodeficiency syndrome (AIDS). According to the World Health Organization (WHO), over a billion people are infected with *Mycobacterium tuberculosis*, the agent of tuberculosis, with approximately 10 million of new cases yearly worldwide (1). Leprosy, caused by *M. leprae*, is still a major problem in Asia and Africa, where the leprosy patients are estimated to total 10 million (2). New, emerging mycobacteria that are associated with immunosuppression are isolated more frequently in patients with AIDS, and disseminated infections by *M. avium-intracellulare* complex may occur in all AIDS patients who do not die of other causes (3).

Mycobacteria are naturally resistant to a wide variety of antimicrobial agents. The first antibiotic to be effective against *M. tuberculosis* was streptomycin, developed in 1944. The major breakthrough in the therapy of mycobacterial infections came when isoniazid, effective in the treatment of tuberculosis, and rifampin were developed. Nevertheless, the treatment of mycobacterial infections is still far from satisfactory because (a) there are very few effective antibiotics active against mycobacterial infections, (b) there is no good therapy for the treatment of AIDS-associated *M. avium-intracellulare* infections, and (c) the number of drug-resistant strains is increasing.

The main cause for the natural resistance of mycobacteria to antibiotics is the structure of the cell envelope. Mycobacteria have a large amount of lipids that act as an efficient permeability barrier. To be effective, an antimycobacterial agent has to overcome this barrier and reach the target in the cell. In addition, antibiotics must reach the intracellular mycobacteria present in the infected host. Thus, an ideal drug or combination of drugs should permeate quickly through both the mycobacterial cell wall and the cytoplasmic and phagosomal membranes of the mammalian cell.

New effective antimycobacterial agents are needed to treat infections caused by atypical mycobacteria and multidrug-resistant mycobacteria and to shorten the duration of treatment and, consequently, improve therapy.

II. BIOLOGY OF CLINICALLY IMPORTANT MYCOBACTERIA

Several mycobacterial species are pathogenic and, until the emergence of AIDS, they were traditionally placed in three main groups: (a) mycobacteria associated with leprosy, with only one human pathogen, *M. leprae*; (b) mycobacteria associated with tuberculosis, mainly *M. tuberculosis* and *M. bovis*; and (c) nontuberculosis mycobacteria associated with a variety of rare diseases (1,2,4). With the emergence of AIDS in the 1980s, the number of immunocompromised patients and associated infections, such as those caused by *M. tuberculosis* and *M. avium-intracellulare* complex, increased (1,3,5,6). Other mycobacterial species are also isolated from AIDS patients with some frequency.

A general feature of mycobacterial disease is that mycobacteria are intracellular parasites (1–3). They can multiply in the macrophage and other cell types and thereby escape the immune system. The intracellular population is more difficult to reach with antibiotics, and this limits the number of antimycobacterials that can be effectively used to treat the infection.

A. Clinically Important Mycobacteria

1. *Leprosy*

Leprosy remains a common disease in the developing world and is still found in Southern Europe and the United States. It is caused by *M. leprae*, which is an obligate intracellular parasite that can survive and multiply in macrophages, Schwann cells, and the perineural cells of the nerve bundle. The treatment of leprosy is based on the use of dapsone, clofazimine, rifampin, and a thioamide, and can take several years. Drug susceptibility in leprosy is difficult to monitor because *M. leprae* is not culturable. Most of the resistant strains have been attributed to poor compliance to drug therapy (2).

2. *Tuberculosis*

Tuberculosis is still a major disease worldwide and is increasing in some developed countries. Most of the infections are caused by *M. tuberculosis*. Tuberculosis caused by *M. bovis* is decreasing because of better control of food and cattle. The AIDS epidemic and the increase of homelessness have marked the resurgence of tuberculosis in the United States and other countries (1). *Mycobacterium tuberculosis* and the other mycobacteria associated with tuberculosis can survive and multiply in the macrophage.

The therapy of tuberculosis is based on the use of two drugs, isoniazid and rifampin, to which a third and sometimes a fourth drug may be added. The choice of the third drug depends on the patient tolerance and the progression of the disease. The therapy of tuberculosis is long relative to the therapy of other infections; the short-term course takes 6 months and a long one takes 2 years. The emergence of multidrug-resistant strains has been associated with poor patient compliance to the drug therapy (1). Resistant strains have been isolated ever since isoniazid and rifampin were used, although outbreaks of multidrug-resistant tuberculosis have been extremely rare. Recently, several outbreaks with multidrug-resistant organisms have been reported, and these are usually associated with immunocompromised patients (7,8).

3. *Mycobacterial Infections Associated with AIDS*

Outbreaks of tuberculosis are common in the early stages of AIDS (5), and the incidence of systemic mycobacterial infections increases at late stages of human immunodeficiency virus (HIV) infection (3,6). The most common systemic mycobacterial disease associated with AIDS is caused by *M. avium-intracellulare* complex in North America, Western Europe, Australia, and Japan, and by *M. tuberculosis* in Africa, Latin America, and the Caribbean (3,5,6); infections by other mycobacteria are less frequent. In the nonimmunocompromised host, infections by *M. avium-intracellulare* complex are rare. Bacterial strains of the *M. avium-intracellulare* complex can survive and grow in the macrophage; they are naturally resistant to almost all antibiotics (3), and therapy is still a problem. Infected patients are usually treated with a combination of clofazimine, rifampin, a quinolone, and an aminoglycoside (5,6).

4. *Pathogenesis*

A key feature in the pathogenesis of mycobacteria is their entry and survival in mammalian cells. Mycobacteria bind to macrophages through complement receptors (9,10) or through a 30-kDa fibronectin receptor (11,12). After phagocytosis by the macrophage, they resist the bactericidal action of the phagolysosome fusion and reside in a vacuole defective in acidification (13,14). These vacuoles acquire some lysosomal enzymes, but lack the proton-ATPase responsible for their acidification (15). The mycobacterial cell wall plays an important role in modulating the vacuole environment (16–18). Therefore, to be effective, antimycobacterial agents must reach the vacuoles of macrophages where the bacterium survives. Otherwise, the population that remains in macrophages will be a reservoir for future infections.

B. Antibiotic Targets

Mycobacteria are naturally resistant to a large number of antibiotics, although most of their antibiotic targets examined are sensitive. For example, mycobacteria have several penicillin-binding proteins with high affinity for β-lactams (19,20). Their DNA gyrase is fully sensitive to many quinolones, in good agreement with the high susceptibility of mycobacteria to these compounds (21). Their ribosomes are also susceptible to the action of aminoglycosides (22,23) and rifampins (24). Thus, it should theoretically be possible to use these drugs if they could permeate faster through the cell wall of mycobacteria.

C. Composition and Properties of the Mycobacterial Cell Wall

1. *Composition and Structure of the Cell Wall*

The cell wall of mycobacteria is unique among gram-positive bacteria. In addition to a typical type IV, thick peptidoglycan layer found in gram-positive bacteria (25–27), the mycobacterial cell wall contains polysaccharides (galactans and arabinans), lipopolysaccharides, lipids (such as mycolic acids or glycolipids), and proteins. They form a unique structure that is responsible for some of the more relevant properties of mycobacteria (Fig. 1).

2. *The Core Structure of the Cell Wall*

The core structure of the mycobacterial cell wall consists of a macromolecule formed by the peptidoglycan, covalently linked to arabinogalactan polysaccharides to which mycolic acids are esterified. The peptidoglycan

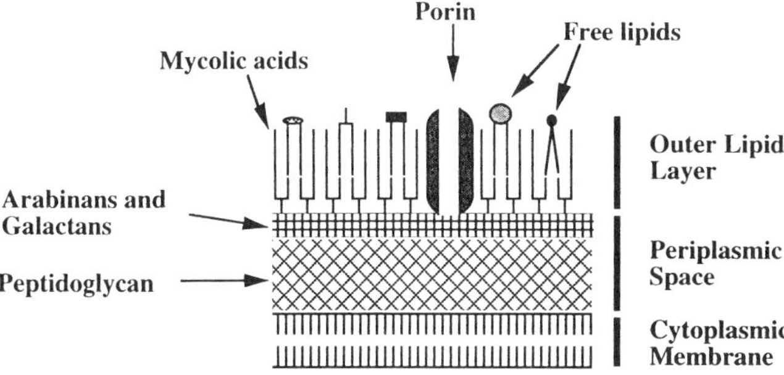

Figure 1   Hypothetical structure of the cell wall of mycobacteria.

is linked to galactans by a disaccharide phosphate composed of rhamnose and N-acetylglucosamine. The latter is linked to the peptidoglycan by a phosphodiester bridge to a murein residue of the peptidoglycan, and the former is linked to a galactose residue (25). The galactans are homopolysaccharides formed by D-galactosyl residues in the furanose form. They are composed of 30 residues of galactose, with alternating residues of 5- and 6-linked β-D-galactose (28). The arabinans are the other main homopolysaccaride found in the cell wall, and approximately two arabinans are linked to a galactan. The arabinan homopolysaccharide is formed of 5-linked α-D-arabinose residues and is branched at 3,5-linked arabinose units. The arabinan ends form one of the most characteristic structures of the cell wall of mycobacteria: the pentasaccharide where the mycolic acids are esterified (25). Mycolic acids are long, branched, unsaturated fatty acids, unique to mycobacteria and some related organisms. They are esterified to the arabinan residues of the peptidylarabinogalactan molecules and are the backbone of the permeability barrier of the cell wall of mycobacteria. Their structure and chemical composition vary from species to species (25–27; Fig. 2).

Other molecules found in the cell wall, but not covalently linked to the mycobacterial cell wall core structure, include lipopolysaccharides, free lipids, and proteins (24–26,29).

Lipoarabinomannans are major component lipopolysaccharides of the mycobacterial cell wall that are present in all species of the genus. They consist of a backbone of mannan (1–6) D-mannose, with the reducing end composed of phosphatidylinositol and esterified to palmitoyl and tuberculostearoyl residues (30–33). Attached to the mannan backbone are residues of arabinans responsible for the antigenic nature of the lipoarabinomannan (33), which is exposed to the surface where it has a main role in

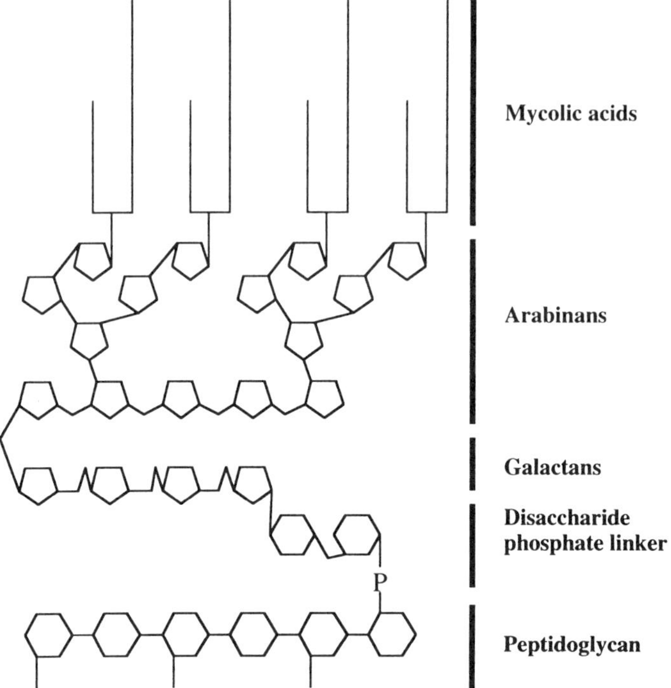

Figure 2 Core structure of the mycobacterial cell wall.

the pathogenicity of *M. tuberculosis* (17). The anchorage site of lipoarabinomannans is uncertain, although their exposure outside of the cell suggests that they are probably anchored to the outer lipid layer of the cell wall (34–36); however, there are some claims that it may be anchored in the cytoplasmic membrane (31,32). Other short-chained or medium-chained lipids are also present in the cell wall. They are in the lipid layer in close contact with the mycolate backbone, forming a membrane structure (29,37).

Proteins are also found in the cell wall. Some recognize cellular receptors and play a key role in the phagocytosis of mycobacteria by the macrophage (9–12). Others have pore-forming properties and participate in the diffusion of hydrophilic compounds through the cell wall. Only one porin has yet been identified in the mycobacterial cell wall (38,39). The channel formed by the porin is wide, has negative point charges, and, consequently, positively charged molecules can diffuse faster. It is voltage-gated and is present in low numbers in the cell envelope (38,39). There are also iron receptors in the cell wall that are induced under iron starvation conditions and suggest the presence of specific channels (40).

Despite the good knowledge of the chemical composition of the myco-bacterial cell wall and the many structural studies by electron microscopy, the physical structure of the cell wall is not well understood. Recently, from X-ray diffraction of the cell wall of *M. chelonae*, the first evidence was presented that the cell wall lipids are organized in a membrane fashion (37), thus explaining the permeability properties of the mycobacterial cell wall.

3. Properties of the Cell Wall

It has been traditionally assumed that the mycobacterial cell wall plays an important role in the natural resistance and susceptibility to antibiotics. It is well known that the addition of detergents or inhibitors of the synthe-sis of cell wall components to the medium substantially lowers the minimal inhibitory concentration (MIC) of antimycobacterial drugs (41–43). Pre-sumably, detergents permeabilize the cell envelope and help the diffusion of antimycobacterial agents, thereby lowering their MICs.

Only recently have the permeability properties of the mycobacterial cell wall been studied in the fast-growing species *M. chelonae* and *M. smegmatis* (44; J. Trias, unpublished results). The permeability of the cell wall of mycobacteria to small hydrophilic molecules is among the lowest in prokaryotes (44–47). The permeability coefficients to β-lactams are 10–100 times lower in *M. chelonae* than in *Pseudomonas aeruginosa* (45), a gram-negative bacterium that has one of the lowest permeabilities to small hydrophilic compounds among gram-negative bacteria (Table 1). Permeability is thus the main factor to explain the natural resistance of mycobacteria to antibiotics (20).

Table 1 Cell Wall or Outer Membrane Permeability Coefficients to β-Lactams in *M. chelonae*, *M. smegmatis*, *P. aeruginosa*, and *Escherichia coli*

	Permeability coefficient (10^{-8} cm/s)			
β-Lactam	*M. chelonae*	*M. smegmatis*	*P. aeruginosa*	*E. coli*
Cephaloridine	10	100	130	52,600
Cephapirin	4.1	NA[a]	NA	19,400
Cephacetrile	1.8	NA	75	4,000
Cephalothin	2.7	10	NA	NA
Nitrocefin	7.9	NA	60	740

[a] NA, data not available.
Source: Refs. 44–47; Trias J, unpublished observations.

III. MEASUREMENT OF DRUG TRANSPORT

Most antimycobacterial drugs—as do antibacterial drugs in general—have their targets in the cytoplasm or in the cytoplasmic membrane inside the cell wall. To reach their targets, drugs must cross the lipid layer of the cell wall, diffuse through the periplasm, and in some cases, cross the cytoplasmic membrane.

The natural low permeability of mycobacteria to a wide range of antibiotics is the main factor responsible for their natural resistance to antibiotics. Therefore, it is essential to understand and explore the pathways operating in the cell wall that could be used for entry of potential new antibiotics and to understand the mechanism of action of the antimycobacterial agents that are currently in use.

A. Measurement of Drug Transport Through the Cell Envelope

The measurement of drug transport in mycobacteria is similar to the methods used for studying drug transport in other bacteria (48). The similarity is closer to the gram-negative, than to the gram-positive, bacteria because of the additional lipid layer in mycobacteria. There are also some features unique to mycobacteria. The high lipid content of the outer shell of the mycobacterial cell wall makes some measurements difficult to perform when intact cells are used. Mycobacteria tend to aggregate, owing to the hydrophobicity of their cell surface. This is a major problem when measuring drug uptake or diffusion. Cells must be in suspension so that we can assume, when performing the experiments, that we are measuring the uptake of a single cell and not a cell aggregate. The problem of cell aggregation can make uptake experiments or intact-cell experiments difficult to perform. Special care has to be taken when choosing the strains and the culture medium. Since the production of surface lipids is dependent on the strain and media, a medium that will produce a minimal or negligible aggregation has to be chosen. Trypticase soy agar (Difco) has yielded good results with fast-growing mycobacteria, but other minimal media specific for growth of mycobacteria or other rich media that include glycerol have not yielded good results (J. Trias, unpublished results).

Media that include detergents in their composition should be avoided. Detergents, such as Triton X-100 or Tween, interact with the lipid layer of the cell wall. When performing intact-cell experiments or uptake experiments the presence of detergents should be avoided completely because they can modify the permeability properties of the cell wall. The addition of detergent in the medium can overcome the aggregation problem, but it interferes with the structure and composition of membranes, thereby making transport measurements difficult to analyze.

When studying the transport of a drug, we often have to calculate the concentration of the drug in the periplasmic space. This concentration can be calculated by using the several published methods applied to calculate the concentration in the periplasm of a gram-negative bacterium (49). Similarly, in mycobacteria we can define a periplasmic space that occupies the space between the cytoplasmic membrane and the outer lipid layer. We find in this space the peptidoglycan, the galactans, and the arabinans (see Fig. 1), and drug-modifying enzymes, such as β-lactamases. The volume of the mycobacterial periplasmic space relative to the cell has not yet been measured.

B. Measurement of Drug Transport Through the Cytoplasmic Membrane

To measure transport and establish transport kinetics of the cytoplasmic membrane, it is important to obtain viable spheroplasts. Most of the techniques applied to obtain spheroplasts in gram-positive bacteria cannot be applied in mycobacteria because of the presence of the lipid layer. Several methods published in recent years for mycobacteria use glycine and lysozyme (50–52). Glycine (20%) is apparently effective in helping the lysozyme reach the peptidoglycan and to spheroplast the cells (50).

C. Measurement of Drug Transport in *Mycobacterium leprae*

No data are available on drug transport in *M. leprae*. The measurement of transport in noncultivable mycobacteria requires the use of indirect methods that are usually unavailable in most laboratories.

IV. TRANSPORT OF ESTABLISHED ANTIMYCOBACTERIAL AGENTS

Most of the research on the uptake of antimycobacterial drugs was published in the 1970s and was developed with fast-growing and slow-growing mycobacteria (other than *M. leprae*, which is not culturable in artificial media or tissue cultures). Unfortunately, most published experiments have been performed with detergents that permeabilize the cell wall lipid layer. This invalidates some of the results, because transport kinetics change, and some enzymes leak out of the periplasm. The knowledge of the permeation and transport of antibiotics into the mycobacterial cell is extremely poor, and the number of papers dealing validly with uptake or permeability is very low. This section will review the transport of antimycobacterial agents into the cell.

Antimycobacterial agents first have to permeate through the cell wall. Basically, diffusion through the cell wall can take place through the porin channel (39,40) and through the lipid layer (44). The porin channel present in the cell wall of mycobacteria has point negative charges and allows the facilitated diffusion of hydrophilic compounds that have a net positive charge (39). Neutral compounds can also diffuse, as can negatively charged ones, but at a lower rate. Overall, the permeability to hydrophilic compounds is very low, and small compounds permeate more rapidly. Among the antibiotics that are hydrophilic and active against mycobacterial cells, isoniazid and aminoglycosides have the physicochemical properties that allow them to use the porin pathway: they are hydrophilic and have positive charges. Aminoglycosides may interact also with other cell envelope structures and enter the cell by a self-promoted uptake (53,54). Some of the quinolones are also hydrophilic and could use the porin pathway. Although negatively charged, they are usually chelated with Mg^{2+} (55). The presence of Mg^{2+} could help them diffuse through the porin channel by forming bridges with the negative charges present in or around the channel (39).

The other major antimycobacterial agents, rifampins, macrolides, hydrophobic tetracyclines, ethionamide, and clofazimine, are hydrophobic molecules and permeate mainly through the lipid layer.

A. Isoniazid

Isoniazid is the hydrazide of isonicotinic acid. Its mechanism of action involves its conversion to an active compound by catalase (56) and subsequent inhibition of an early step in the synthesis of mycolic acids (57). The presence of catalase is necessary for the susceptibility of *M. tuberculosis* to isoniazid (56,57). The drug is accumulated by the mycobacterial cell and can reach 50 times the extracellular concentration (58). The accumulation process is oxygen-dependent and indicates the use of energy. However, neither system for transport through the cytoplasmic membrane nor through the lipid layer has been identified. Isoniazid is a very small hydrophilic molecule and could use the porin pathway to cross the lipid layer.

The *M. avium-intracellulare* complex organisms are resistant to the action of isoniazid. Rastogi and co-workers (59) postulated that isoniazid could not cross the cell wall, and that was the main reason for the natural resistance. To increase the cell wall permeability to isoniazid, a palmitoyl tail was added to the isoniazid molecule: *M. avium-intracellulare* showed increased susceptibility to this molecule. It is likely that the increase in permeation came from the detergent properties of the new molecule. Palmitoyl isoniazid has the structure of a detergent, which would allow permeation through the lipid layer instead of the porin pathway.

B. Rifampins

Rifampin and isoniazid are the mainstays of the treatment of tuberculosis and other mycobacterial diseases. *Mycobacterium tuberculosis* is usually susceptible to this antibiotic, and most of the resistant strains have mutations in the β-subunit of the RNA polymerase (24). Impaired permeability to rifampin is the main cause for the natural resistance to this antibiotic in some *M. intracellulare* and *M. avium* strains that have sensitive RNA polymerase (60). Rifampin uptake studies in *M. avium* showed the uptake to be low (60,61) and, in *M. intracellulare*, the addition of a detergent, Tween 80, sensitized resistant strains (62). Thus, permeabilizing the cell wall helps the diffusion of rifampin (60–62). The large size and the hydrophobicity of rifampin suggest that the main pathway for crossing the cell envelope is diffusion through the lipid layer.

C. Aminoglycosides

Streptomycin was the first antibiotic effective against mycobacteria. Its uptake, studied in *M. tuberculosis*, involves two steps: the first is presumably a binding step at the cell wall, whereas the second is active transport through the cytoplasmic membrane (54). Aminoglycosides may thus follow the "self-promoted" uptake also seen in gram-negative bacteria (53).

The permeability barrier of the cell wall has not been measured, but there is some evidence that it is high. A large difference exists in inactivation of aminoglycosides between intact and broken cells (63), and spheroplasts are more sensitive to aminoglycosides than are intact cells (53). Similar findings were obtained in "opaque" mutants in *M. intracellulare* (64). The MIC for streptomycin was decreased by a factor of 10 when detergents were added to the medium (62,64).

D. D-Cycloserine

D-Cycloserine is used as a second-line drug in the treatment of tuberculosis and other mycobacterial diseases. Most of the resistance is attributed to the increased expression of the target enzyme D-alanyl-D-alanine synthetase. Transport of D-cycloserine through the cytoplasmic membrane can take place using the alanine-glycine-D-serine uptake system. In addition, being a small hydrophilic molecule, D-cycloserine could diffuse through the porin pathway. Uptake experiments performed with a pair of isogenic susceptible and resistant strains of *M. tuberculosis* showed no differences of transport between them (65).

E. β-Lactams

The permeability of β-lactam antibiotics has been measured in fast-growing mycobacteria, *M. chelonae* and *M. smegmatis* (20,44; J. Trias, unpublished results). The permeability coefficients for β-lactams are low (see Table 1). Permeability to imipenem and cefoxitin has not been measured; these antibiotics are not hydrolyzed by the mycobacterial β-lactamase, and their hydrophilicity and small size allows them to permeate across the mycobacterial cell wall by the porin pathway.

F. Quinolones

Susceptibility of mycobacteria to quinolones has received considerable attention, because this family of antimicrobial agents has in vitro and vivo activity against mycobacteria, including *M. tuberculosis*, *M. avium-intracellulare*, *M. leprae*, and fast-growing mycobacteria. The good activity of quinolones can be attributed to a combination of transport and gyrase sensitivity. The mycobacterial gyrase is inhibited by quinolones, and mutations in *gyrA* lead to resistance to quinolones in mycobacteria (21). The way quinolones permeate into the mycobacterial cell is unknown; they could cross through the lipid layer, or take a hydrophilic pathway. When uncharged, quinolones are lipophilic and could diffuse through the lipid layer (66). Quinolones can also diffuse through porin channels when they are charged or chelated with divalent cations such as Mg^{2+} or Ca^{2+} (55,66).

G. Macrolides and Tetracyclines

Macrolides that show good antimycobacterial activity, clarithromycin and azithromycin, and a tetracycline that is active against mycobacteria, minocycline, are large hydrophobic molecules. How they cross the cell wall is unknown, but presumably, they can diffuse through the lipid layer.

H. Clofazimine and Other Antimycobacterial Agents

Clofazimine is rapidly taken up by cells (61). By virtue of its high hydrophobicity, it likely permeates through the lipid layer of the cell envelope. The transport of other antimycobacterial agents has not been studied, and there are no data on their diffusion through the cell envelope (Fig. 3).

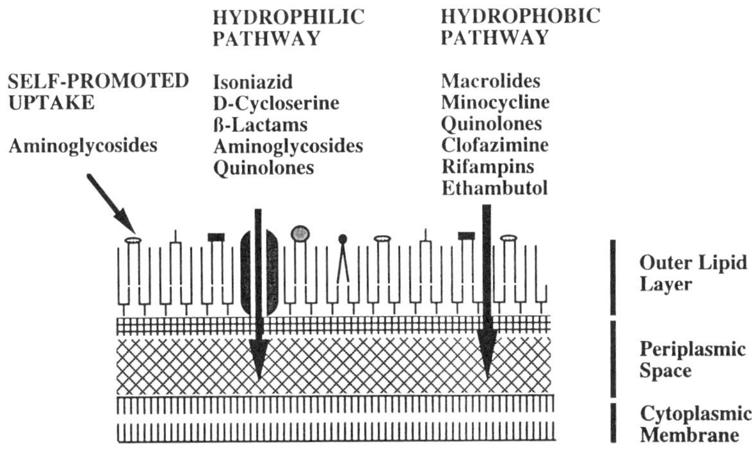

Figure 3   Pathways for antibiotic diffusion through the mycobacterial cell wall.

V. AGENTS THAT INCREASE DRUG TRANSPORT

A. Ethambutol

The mode of action of ethambutol is not completely understood, and its primary target remains unknown. The addition of ethambutol to intact mycobacterial cells inhibits glucose metabolism (67). This could have a direct effect on the cell wall structure by inhibiting the synthesis of the arabinans present in the cell wall (42,67–69). In combination with other antibiotics, ethambutol acts synergistically and potentiates them (69–72).

B. Detergents

Detergents have a synergistic effect, similar to ethambutol, lowering the MICs of antibiotics in mycobacteria. They can permeabilize the mycobacterial cell wall by releasing some of its components to the external medium. Isoniazid palmitoyl derivatives should be included here, as their action reflects the combined effects of the detergent and isoniazid moieties (59).

VI. CONCLUSIONS AND FUTURE DIRECTIONS

Mycobacterial diseases are very difficult to treat because mycobacteria are naturally resistant to a wide variety of chemotherapeutic agents. Drugs belonging to well-known antimicrobial families and showing good activity against mycobacteria are being developed (Table 2). A major effort to discover and develop new drugs that can overcome the high resistance of mycobacteria to antibiotics is needed. The main factor for the high resistance is the low permeability of the cell wall. A good antibiotic, or group of antibiotics, should reach the target in the mycobacterial cell and should be effective against both intracellular and extracellular bacteria.

Rational drug design should take into account these two factors. The ways that drugs reach their targets in the mycobacterial cell have to be explored. Basically, a drug can cross the cell wall by diffusing through the lipid layer or through a hydrophilic channel. However, some of the most effective drugs against mycobacteria are highly hydrophobic, reflecting both diffusion through the lipid layer of the cell wall and active uptake by macrophages. Recently developed hydrophobic drugs, such as sparfloxacin, clarithromycin, azithromycin, or minocycline, are active against mycobacteria (73–75). The porin channel present in mycobacteria could also be used by small hydrophilic antibiotics, although the permeability to hydrophilic compounds in mycobacteria remains poor. Imipenem and isoniazid, both small and hydrophilic, are a good example of this class of antimycobacterial agents. A third unexplored pathway would be the use of specific channels. There are some good indications that these channels exist in mycobacteria: (a) mycobacteria grown under iron-deficiency conditions induce the synthesis of siderophores, mycobactins, and iron receptors in the cell wall; and (b) the growth of mycobacteria under phosphate starvation conditions also induces the synthesis of new proteins in the cell wall. These channels could be used by new, rationally designed drugs to more efficiently reach their target in the cell.

Table 2 Promising Antimycobacterial Agents

Antimicrobial class	Examples
β-Lactams	Imipenem
Tetracyclines	Doxycycline
	Minocycline
Quinolones	Ciprofloxacin
	Ofloxacin
	Sparfloxacin
Macrolides	Clarithromycin
	Azithromycin

The cell wall itself is an area with attractive possibilities for new targets: it is involved in the pathogenesis of mycobacteria, plays a main role in resistance to antibiotics, and is a structure unique to mycobacteria and related organisms. Drugs that inhibit the synthesis of cell wall components increase the susceptibility of mycobacteria to antimicrobial compounds (14,67–72), presumably by increasing the cell wall permeability. However, the contributions of specific cell wall components to the overall barrier function, especially during drug resistance, must be defined. As cell wall biosynthesis becomes better known, the enzymes involved in the regulation and synthesis of the cell wall will become natural targets for antibiotics.

REFERENCES

1. Bloom BR, Murray CJL. Tuberculosis: commentary on a reemergent killer. Science 1992; 257:1055–1064.
2. Hastings RC, Gillis TP, Krahenbuhl JL, Franzblau SG. Leprosy. Clin Microbiol Rev 1988; 1:330–348.
3. Inderlied CB, Kemper CA, Bermudez LEM. The *Mycobacterium avium* complex. Clin Microbiol Rev 1993; 6:266–310.
4. Wolinsky E. Nontuberculous mycobacteria and associated diseases. Am Rev Respir Dis 1979; 119:107–109.
5. Barnes PF, Bloch AB, Davidson PT, Snider DE. Tuberculosis in patients with human immunodeficiency virus infection. N Engl J Med 1991; 324:1644–1650.
6. Horsburgh CR. *Mycobacterium avium* complex infection in the acquired immunodeficiency syndrome. N Engl J Med 1991; 324:1332–1338.
7. Small PM, Shafer RW, Hopewell PC, Samiir PS, Murphy MJ, Desmond E, Sierra MF, Schoolnik GK. Exogenous reinfection with multidrug-resistant *Mycobacterium tuberculosis* in patients with advanced HIV infection. N Engl J Med 1993; 328:1137–1144.
8. Frieden TR, Sterling T, Pablos-Mendez A, Kilburn JO, Cauthen GM, Dooley SW. The emergence of drug-resistant tuberculosis in New York City. N Engl J Med 1993; 328:521–526.
9. Schlesinger LS, Bellinger-Kawahara CG, Payne NR, Horwitz MA. Phagocytosis of *Mycobacterium tuberculosis* is mediated by human monocyte complement receptors and complement component C3. J Immunol 1990; 144:2771–2780.
10. Schlesinger LS, Horwitz MA. Phagocytosis of leprosy bacilli is mediated by complement receptors CR1 and CR3 on human monocytes and complement C3 in serum. J Clin Invest 1990; 85:1304–1314.
11. Roecklein JA, Swartz RP, Yeager Y. Nonopsonic uptake of *Mycobacterium avium* complex. J Lab Clin Med 1992; 119:772–781.
12. Bermudez LM, Young LS, Enkel H. Interaction of *Mycobacterium avium*

complex with human macrophages: roles of membrane receptors and serum proteins. Infect Immun 1991; 59:1697–1702.

13. Armstrong JA, Hart PD. Response of cultured macrophages to *Mycobacterium tuberculosis*, with observations on fusion lysosomes with phagosomes. J Exp Med 1971; 134:713–740.

14. McDonough KA, Kress Y, Bloom BR. Pathogenesis of tuberculosis: interaction of *Mycobacterium tuberculosis* with macrophages. Infect Immun 1993; 61:2763–2773.

15. Sturgill-Koszycki S, Schlesinger PH, Chakraborty P, Haddix PL, Collins HL, Fok AK, Allen RD, Gluck SL, Heuser J, Russell DG. Lack of acidification in *Mycobacterium* phagosomes produced by exclusion of vesicular proton-ATPase. Science 1994; 263:678–681.

16. Chan J, Fujiwara T, Brennan P, McNeil M, Turco SJ, Sibille JC, Snapper M, Aisen P, Bloom BR. Microbial glycolipids: possible virulence factors that scavenge oxygen radicals. Proc Natl Acad Sci USA 1989; 86:2453–2457.

17. Chan J, Fan X, Hunter SW, Brennan PJ, Bloom BR. Lipoarabinomannan, a possible virulence factor involved in persistence of *Mycobacterium tuberculosis* within macrophages. Infect Immun 1991; 59:1755–1761.

18. Frechel C, Ryper A, Rastogi N, David H. The electron transparent zone in phagocytized *Mycobacterium avium* and other mycobacteria: formation, persistence and role in bacterial survival. Ann Inst Pasteur Microbiol 1986; 137B:239–257.

19. Mizuguchi Y, Ogawa M, Udou T. Morphological changes induced by β-lactam antibiotics in *Mycobacterium avium-intracellulare* complex. Antimicrob Agents Chemother 1985; 27:541–547.

20. Jarlier J, Gutmann L, Nikaido H. Interplay of cell wall barrier and β-lactamase activity determines high resistance to β-lactams antibiotics in *Mycobacterium chelonae*. Antimicrob Agents Chemother 1991; 35:1937–1939.

21. Cambau E, Sougakoff W, Revel V, Jarlier V. Amplification and nucleotide sequence of a mycobacterial DNA fragment homologous to the quinolone resistance determining region (QRDR) in the *gyrA* gene of *Escherichia coli* and *Staphylococcus aureus*. 33rd Intersci Conf Antimicrob Agents Chemother 1993, New Orleans, Louisiana; Abstr. 1093.

22. Douglass J, Steyn LM. A ribosomal gene mutation in streptomycin-resistant *Mycobacterium tuberculosis* isolates. J Infect Dis 1993; 167:1505–1506.

23. Udou T, Mizuguchi Y, Yamada T. Biochemical mechanisms of antibiotic resistance in a clinical isolate of *Mycobacterium fortuitum*. Am Rev Respir Dis 1986; 133:653–657.

24. Hui J, Gordon N, Kajioka R. Permeability barrier to rifampin in mycobacteria. Antimicrob Agents Chemother 1977; 11:773–779.

25. McNeil MR, Brennan PJ. Structure, function and biogenesis of the cell envelope of mycobacteria in relation to bacterial physiology, pathogenesis and drug resistance; some thoughts and possibilities arising from recent structural information. Res Microbiol 1991; 142:451–463.

26. Draper P. The anatomy of mycobacteria. In: Ratledge T, Stanford J, eds. The Biology of Mycobacteria. London: Academic Press, 1982:9–52.

27. Petit JF, Lederer E. The structure of the mycobacterial cell wall. In: Kubica GP, Wayne LG, eds. The Mycobacteria. A Sourcebook. New York: Marcel Dekker, 1984:301–311.

28. Daffé M, Brennan PJ, McNeil M. Predominant structural features of the cell wall arabinogalactan of *Mycobacterium tuberculosis* as revealed through characterization of oligoglycosyl alditol fragments by gas chromatography/mass spectrometry and by ^1H and ^{13}C NMR analysis. J Biol Chem 1990; 265:6734–6743.

29. Minnikin DE. Lipids: complex lipids, their chemistry, biosynthesis and roles. In: Ratledge C, Stanford J, eds. The Biology of Mycobacteria. London: Academic Press, 1982:95–184.

30. Chatterjee D, Hunter SW, McNeil M, Brennan PJ. Liporabinomannan. Multiglycosylated form of the mycobacterial mannosylphosphatidylinositols. J Biol Chem 1992; 266:6228–6233.

31. Chatterjee D, Bozic CM, McNeil M, Brennan PJ. Structural features of the arabinan component of the lipoarabinomannan of *Mycobacterium tuberculosis*. J Biol Chem 1992; 266:9652–9660.

32. Hunter SW, Brennan PJ. Evidence for the presence of a phosphatidylinositol anchor on the lipoarabinomannan and lipomannan of *Mycobacterium tuberculosis*. J Biol Chem 1990; 265:9272–9279.

33. Venisse A, Berjeaud JM, Chaurand P, Gilleron M, Puzo G. Structural features of lipoarabinomannan from *Mycobacterium bovis* BCG. J Biol Chem 1993; 268:12401–12411.

34. Rastogi N. Recent observations concerning structure and function relationships in the mycobacterial cell envelope: elaboration of a model in terms of mycobacterial pathogenicity, virulence and drug resistance. Res Microbiol 1991; 142:355–486.

35. Rastogi N, Hellio R. Evidence that the capsule around mycobacteria grown in axenic media contains mycobacterial antigens: implications at the level of cell envelope architecture. FEMS Microbiol Lett 1990; 70:161–166.

36. David HL, Lévy-Frébault V, Thorel MF. Characterization of distinct layers of the *Mycobacterium avium* envelope in respect of their composition by fatty acids, proteins, oligosaccharides and antigens. Zentralbl Bakteriol Mikrobiol Hyg[A] 1988; 268:193–208.

37. Nikaido H, Kim S-H, Rosenberg EY. Physical organization of lipids in the cell wall of *Mycobacterium chelonae*. Mol Microbiol 1993; 8:1025–1030.

38. Trias J, Jarlier V, Benz R. Porins in the cell wall of mycobacteria. Science 1992; 258:1479–1481.

39. Trias J, Benz R. Characterization of the channel formed by the mycobacterial porin in lipid bilayer membranes. Demonstration of voltage gating and of negative point charges at the channel mouth. J Biol Chem 1993; 268:6234–6240.

40. Hall RM, Sritharan M, Messenger AJM, Ratledge C. Iron transport in *Mycobacterium smegmatis*: occurrence of iron-regulated envelope proteins as potential receptors for iron uptake. J Gen Microbiol 1987; 133:2107–2114.
41. Barrow WW, Wright EL, Goh KS, Rastogi N. Activities of fluoroquinolone, macrolide, and aminoglycoside drugs combined with inhibitors of glycosylation and fatty acid and peptide biosynthesis against *Mycobacterium avium*. Antimicrob Agents Chemother 1993; 37:652–661.
42. Takayama K, Kilburn JO. Inhibition of synthesis of arabinogalactan by ethambutol in *Mycobacterium smegmatis*. Antimicrob Agents Chemother 1989; 33:1493–1499.
43. Tsukamura M, Mizuno S, Miyama A. Different correlation of drug susceptibilities to colonial morphology in *Mycobacterium avium* complex strains. Microbiol Immunol 1989; 33:1001–1011.
44. Jarlier V, Nikaido H. Permeability barrier to hydrophilic solutes in *Mycobacterium chelonei*. J Bacteriol 1990; 172:1418–1423.
45. Trias J, Dufresne J, Levesque RC, Nikaido H. Decreased outer membrane permeability in imipenem-resistant mutants of *Pseudomonas aeruginosa*. Antimicrob Agents Chemother 1989; 33:1201–1206.
46. Nikaido H, Rosenberg EY, Foulds J. Porin channels in *Escherichia coli*: studies with β-lactams in intact cells. J Bacteriol 1983; 153:232–240.
47. Nicas TI, Hancock REW. *Pseudomonas aeruginosa* outer membrane permeability: isolation of a porin protein F-deficient mutant. J Bacteriol 1983; 153:281–285.
48. Nikaido H. Transport through the outer membrane of bacteria. Methods Enzymol 1986; 125:265–278.
49. Stock JB, Rauch B, Roseman S. Periplasmic space in *Salmonella typhimurium* and *Escherichia coli*. J Biol Chem 1977; 252:7850–7861.
50. Naser SA, McCarthy CM, Smith GB, Tupponce AK. Low temperature protocol for efficient transformation of *Mycobacterium smegmatis* spheroplasts. Curr Microbiol 1993; 27:153–156.
51. Udou T, Ogawa M, Mizuguchi Y. Spheroplast formation of *Mycobacterium smegmatis* and morphological aspects of their reversion to the bacillary form. J Bacteriol 1982; 151:1035–1039.
52. Udou T, Ogawa M, Mizuguchi Y. An improved method for the preparation of mycobacterial spheroplasts and the mechanism involved in the reversion to their bacillary form: electron microscopy and physiological study. Can J Microbiol 1983; 29:60–68.
53. Hancock, R.E.W. Aminoglycoside uptake and mode of action—with special reference to streptomycin and gentamicin. I. Antagonist and mutants. J Antimicrob Chemother 1981; 8:249–276.
54. Beggs WH, Williams NE. Streptomycin uptake by *Mycobacterium tuberculosis*. Appl Microbiol 1971; 21:751–753.
55. Ross DL, Riley CM. Physicochemical properties of the fluoroquinolone antimicrobials V. Effect of fluoroquinolone structure and pH on the complexation of various fluoroquinolones with magnesium and calcium ions. Int J Pharm 1993; 93:121–129.

56. Zhang Y, Heym B, Allen B, Young D, Cole S. The catalase-peroxidase gene and isoniazid resistance in *Mycobacterium tuberculosis*. Nature 1992; 358:591–593.

57. Banerjee A, Dubnau E, Quemard A, Jacobs WR. A novel *M. tuberculosis* gene conferring resistance to isoniazid and ethionamide. Mol Mech Drug Resistance 1993. 1993 Albany Conference.

58. Beggs WH, Jenne JW. Capacity of tubercle bacilli for isoniazid accumulation. *Am Rev Respir Dis* 1970; 102:92–96.

59. Rastogi N, Goh KS. Action of 1-isonicotinyl-2-palmitoyl hydrozine against the *Mycobacterium avium* complex and enhancement of its activity by *m*-fluorophenylalanine. Antimicrob Agents Chemother 1990; 34:2061–2064.

60. Telenti A, Imboden P, Marchesi F, Lowrie D, Cole S, Colston MJ, Matter L, Schopfer K, Bodmer T. Detection of rifampicin-resistance mutations in *Mycobacterium tuberculosis*. Lancet 1993; 341:647–650.

61. David HL, Clavel-Seres S, Clement F, Goh KS. Uptake of selected antibacterial agents in *Mycobacterium avium*. Zentralbl Bakteriol Mikrobiol Hyg[A] 1987; 265:385–392.

62. Yamori S, Tsukamura M. Paradoxical effect of Tween 80 between the susceptibility to rifampicin and streptomycin and the susceptibility to ethambutol and sulfadimethoxine in the *Mycobacterium avium–Mycobacterium intracellulare* complex. Microbiol Immunol 1991; 35:921–926.

63. Udou A, Mizuguchi Y, Yamada T. Biochemical mechanisms of antibiotic resistance in a clinical isolate of *Mycobacterium fortuitum*. Am Rev Respir Dis 1986; 133:653–657.

64. Mizuguchi Y, Udou T, Yamada T. Mechanism of antibiotic resistance in *Mycobacterium intracellulare*. Microbiol Immunol 1983; 27:425–431.

65. David HL. Resistance to D-cycloserine in the tubercle bacilli: mutation rate and transport of alanine in parental cells and drug resistant mutants. Appl Microbiol 1971; 21:888–892.

66. Nikaido H, Thanassi DG. Penetration of lipophilic agents with multiple protonation sites into bacterial cells: tetracyclines and fluoroquinolones as examples. Antimicrob Agents Chemother 1993; 37:1393–1399.

67. Silve G, Valero-Guillen P, Quemard A, Dupont MA, Daffe M, Laneellle G. Ethambutol inhibition of glucose metabolism in mycobacteria: a possible target of the drug. Antimicrob Agents Chemother 1993; 37:1536–1538.

68. Takayama K, Armstrong EL, Kunugi KA, Kilburn JO. Inhibition by ethambutol of mycolic acid transfer into the cell wall of *Mycobacterium smegmatis*. Antimicrob Agents Chemother 1979; 16:240–242.

69. Doster B, Murray FJ, Newman R, Woolpert SF. Ethambutol in the initial treatment of pulmonary tuberculosis. Am Rev Respir Dis 1973; 107:177–190.

70. Hoffner SE, Kratz M, Olsson-Liljequist B, Svenson SB. In-vitro synergistic activity between ethambutol and fluorinated quinolones against *Mycobacterium avium* complex. J Antimicrob Chemother 1989; 24:317–324.

71. Hoffner SE, Svenson SB, Beezer AE. Microcalorimetric studies of the initial interaction between antimycobacterial drugs and *Mycobacterium avium*. J Antimicrob Chemother 1990; 25:353–359.

72. Rastogi N, Goh KS, David H. Enhancement of drug susceptibility of *Mycobacterium avium* by inhibitors of cell envelope synthesis. Antimicrob Agents Chemother 1990; 34:759–764.
73. Ji B, Truffot-Pernot C, Grosset J. In vitro and in vivo activities of sparfloxacin (AT-4140) against *Mycobacterium tuberculosis*. Tubercle 1991; 72:181–186.
74. Cohen Y, Perrone C, Truffot-Pernot C, Grosset J, Vildé JL, Pocidalo JJ. Activities of WIN-57273, minocycline, clarithromycin, and 14-hydroxy-clarithromycin against *Mycobacterium avium* complex in human macrophages. Antimicrob Agents Chemother 1992; 36:2104–2107.
75. Lazard T, Perrone C, Truffot-Pernot C, Grosset J, Vildé JL, Pocidalo JJ. Clarithromycine, minocycline, and rifabutin treatments before and after infection of C57BL/6 mice with *Mycobacterium avium*. Antimicrob Agents Chemother 1993; 37:1690–1692.

10

Bacterial Transport as an Import Mechanism and Target for Antimicrobials

Robert E. W. Hancock
*University of British Columbia, Vancouver, British Columbia,
Canada*

I. INTRODUCTION

In the past 50 years, literally tens of thousands of antibacterial compounds
have been chemically synthesized or isolated from soil microorganisms,
plant, aquatic, or other natural sources, and systematically modified.
However, it is becoming clear that, as rapidly as compounds are developed, subsets of bacteria are developing resistance.

To my knowledge, no fundamentally new, useful antibiotic structures
have been developed in the past 25 years, with the possible exception of
the cationic peptides (1). In the search for clinically useful compounds,
two strategies hold significant promise. One is to devise methodologies
that can be employed to increase uptake by overcoming the intrinsic impermeability of bacterial cells toward potential antimicrobial chemicals.
Such a strategy, involving piggybacking on natural bacterial transport systems, is considered in Section II. A second strategy involves the identification of novel targets for antibiotics (e.g., transport; see Sec. III) that can be
used to devise targeted screens for the identification of novel compounds.

A. Barrier Function in Bacteria

Generally speaking, antimicrobials can be divided into those that are selective for gram-positive bacteria, those that have superior activity against

gram-negative bacteria, and the broad-spectrum antimicrobials. Although certain bacteria represent special cases, for example, mycobacteria (see Chap. 9), mycoplasma, and ureaplasma, and selective antibiotic-resistant organisms (e.g., *Xanthomonas maltophilia*), these antibacterial specificities can usually be explained as follows. Antibiotics that are relatively selective for gram-positive bacteria tend to be excluded by the unique outer membrane of the gram-negative bacteria. For example, the poor susceptibility of gram-negative bacteria to vancomycin, bacitracin, erythromycin, the ionophores, rifampin, clindamycin, fusidic acid, penicillin G, methicillin, and novobiocin, can be simply explained by the barrier effect of the outer membrane (2). In contrast, the few antimicrobials with better gram-negative activity are generally those, such as polymyxin, the octapeptins, and certain of the cationic peptides, that interact with the outer membrane as the first step in their action on cells (3). The physiological basis for these two observations is described later (see Sec. II.A.3). Those compounds with equivalent activities against both gram-negative and gram-positive bacteria generally pass through the outer membrane efficiently [although not freely, since a 4- to 16-fold disparity in minimum inhibitory concentrations (MICs) is common]. Even these antibacterial compounds, however, can be rendered clinically less effective against gram-negative bacteria, such as *Pseudomonas aeruginosa*, with intrinsically poorly permeable outer membranes (3).

B. Substrate Transport Systems

Although not all bacteria grow at equivalent rates, many important pathogens can double their masses (and numbers) every 30 min–1 h. Similar rapid rates of mass doubling can occur in either optimized culture media or in vivo (4,5). To support such rates of mass increase, bacteria require efficient uptake mechanisms for a variety of nutrients, including a source of carbon, reducing equivalents, nitrogen, oxygen, phosphorus, sulfur, potassium, sodium, magnesium, iron, chlorine, and trace elements, including Co, Zn, Mo, Cu, and Mn, as micronutrients. All of these represent essential building blocks and must be imported by specific transport systems. Many of these transport systems have been well studied in *Escherichia coli* and other bacteria (6) and are described in overview here. With certain prominent exceptions (e.g., iron uptake, see later discussion), we know little about the actual chemical form of these elements that are utilized in vivo. Nor do we understand which transport mechanisms are actually employed by bacteria growing inside eukaryotic hosts. A further complication is posed by regulatory mechanisms in bacteria that optimize growth efficiently. For example, the presence in a bacterium's environment of a building block for macromolecular synthesis, often leads to down-regulation of metabolic synthesis (by allosteric end-product inhibition or transcriptional down-regulation of synthesis of key enzymes), followed by uptake of the building block from the environment. Such a transport system would not make a good target for inhibition, since loss of uptake would generally lead to a counterbalancing adjustment of metabolic activity. Similarly, when multiple alternative uptake systems exist (e.g., for specific carbon sources, since bacteria can generally use a range of carbon sources), there is little prospect for isolation of a transport inhibitor. With these prefacing remarks, it is worth briefly describing the nature of bacterial uptake systems.

There are three major classes of uptake systems: passive diffusion, facilitated diffusion, and active (energized) transport (7,8). A fourth class would be porin-mediated passive diffusion, whereby small hydrophilic substances cross the outer membranes of gram-negative bacteria through nonspecific, water-filled channels of proteins, termed porins. This is passive diffusion in the sense that it obeys Fick's law, although there are some restrictions to free diffusion owing to frictional, steric, and charge interactions (see Chap. 6). With this addendum to traditional classes of transport systems, a summary of bacterial transport systems is presented in Table 1. For a more detailed description, the reader is referred to specific reviews (7,8). In general, similar types of transport systems exist in eukaryotic host cells. However, the active transport of substrates is more common in bacterial cells, which require such concentrative mechanisms to permit growth at the usual rapid rate of bacterial doubling, whereas the nutrient supply of the cells of the complex eukaryotes is often accomplished through either facilitated diffusion or pinocytosis (7,8).

C. Known Targets of Antimicrobial Drugs

The targets of antimicrobial compounds must be such that their inhibition either causes growth cessation (*bacteriostatic compounds*) or loss of cellular integrity or ability to form colonies (*bactericidal compounds*). There are relatively few classes of targets for bactericidal antimicrobials (9). These include destruction of peptidoglycan, leading to osmotic lysis; loss of cytoplasmic membrane integrity; or irreversible damage to DNA, (including double-stranded breaks, certain base modifications, cross-linking, or presumptive loss of DNA membrane attachment. However, many bactericidal antibiotics have modes of action that are difficult to assign to a single, specific inhibitory step and may be quite complex (10). In contrast, the action of bacteriostatic drugs is often more easily defined and can involve any essential metabolic event in bacterial cells.

Table 1 Bacterial Transport Systems

Uptake mechanism	Description	Natural substrates	Antibiotic substrate (ref.)
Passive diffusion	Free movement across lipid bilayers	H_2O, N_2, NH_3	Hydrophobic antibiotics (2); fluoroquinolones; tetracyclines (45)
Porin-mediated passive diffusion	Diffusion through the aqueous channels of outer membrane porin proteins	Small hydrophilic or charged substrates (amino acids, ions, sugars)	β-Lactams (3,24)
Facilitated diffusion	Passage along a concentration gradient across a lipid bilayer membrane using a specific substrate-binding protein (e.g., specific porins in the outer membrane)	Varies among bacteria (e.g., maltose, nucleotides, phosphate, glucose, fatty acids, specific iron–siderophore complexes)	Imipenem (48); cathechol β-lactams (15,19); albomycin (9); albicidin (52)
Active transport	Concentrative uptake dependent on energy expenditure, and a substrate-binding protein (e.g., cytoplasmic membrane "carriers")	Amino acids, metal cations, sugars, nucleotides	Aminoglycosides (3); D-cycloserine (9); phosphomycin (9); alaphosphin (9)

II. KNOWN SUBSTRATE TRANSPORT PATHWAYS AS ROUTES OF ANTIBIOTIC UPTAKE

There are two categories of substrate transport systems that can be employed to increase uptake of antimicrobial compounds (Table 2). One is the promiscuous uptake systems. These involve transport systems that will take up a wide variety of compounds (within parameters that are presumably set by the physical constraints imposed by channel architecture) provided they contain a specific prosthetic group. The second, and

Table 2 Known Substrate Transport Pathways as Routes of Antibiotic Uptake

Pathway	Location	Antibacterial transported
Ferrichrome	Outer membrane (FhuA)	Albomycin, rifamycin, CGP4832
Other iron uptake	Outer membrane	Ferrioxamine B, ferrimycin, ferrocin
Basic amino acids	Outer membrane	Imipenem
Nucleotide	Outer membrane (Tsx)	Albicidin
Self-promoted uptake	Outer membrane	Nourseothricin, melittin, cecropins, defensins, polymyxin, colistin, aminoglycosides, azithromycin, teicoplanin aglycones
Phosphate	Cytoplasmic membrane	Arsenate
Iron scavenging	Outer membrane (Cir, Fiu)	Catechol β-lactams (BRL 41897A, GR69153, E-0702)
Oligopeptide	Cytoplasmic membrane (Opp)	Compounds IV, V, VI; alaphosphin
Alanine	Cytoplasmic membrane	D-Cycloserine
α-Glycerophosphate	Cytoplasmic membrane	Phosphomycin
Peptide permease	Cytoplasmic membrane	Alaphosphin

perhaps less useful, category of transport systems is the narrow-specificity systems. These generally accept only closely related analogues.

A. Promiscuous Uptake System

1. Catechol–Iron Complex Uptake

Bacteria are obligately dependent on iron for growth. However, iron exists in nature largely in insoluble complexes and in host fluids and tissues complexed to transport proteins, such as transferrin and lactoferrin. Thus, the amount of freely available iron is minimal, and bacteria have evolved efficient means of capturing and importing ferric iron for use in redox enzymes and cytochromes. Generally speaking, three types of iron transport systems exist: siderophore–iron uptake, transferrin– or lactoferrin–iron uptake, and the scavenger systems.

Siderophore–iron uptake (11) involves the synthesis and secretion of compounds (siderophores) with high affinities ($K_a = 10^{21}$ M) for Fe^{3+}. Siderophores usually fit into one of two general classes of iron-binding core structures, hydroxamates or catechols. However, the prosthetic groups attached to the core structures can vary in such a way that they confer host specificity during uptake of the iron–siderophore complex.

This is accomplished in gram-negative bacteria by the synthesis of a specific, coregulated, outer membrane receptor protein (e.g., FepA for ferri-enterochelin uptake in *E. coli*) (11). Translocation across the outer membrane has been proposed to require an energized event involving the cytoplasmic membrane proton motive force and a cytoplasmic membrane protein TonB that spans the periplasm and contacts a region (the TonB box) of the outer membrane receptor. The bacterial components involved in siderophore synthesis and ferri–siderophore complex uptake and processing are up-regulated by iron deficiency, which is the normal growth condition of pathogenic bacteria in their host.

Siderophore–iron-uptake systems are usually quite specific. For example, the peptide catechol siderophores of fluorescent *Pseudomonas* species tend to be quite strain-specific (12). Nevertheless, at least one system, the iron–hydroxamate (ferrichrome)-uptake system, is flexible enough to permit uptake of analogues that have antibiotics attached. Thus, the semi-synthetic rifamycin derivative CGP4832 913 and the ferrichrome analogue albomycin have MICs in iron-depleted medium of 0.02–0.005 μg/ml. However, mutations that prevent ferrichrome uptake, including loss of the outer membrane receptor FhuA, or of the energy transducing protein TonB, lead to MICs for both compounds of 8–16 μg/ml.

A second class of uptake systems involves the direct binding of transferrin– or lactoferrin–iron complexes to outer membrane receptor proteins on the surface of such bacteria as *Neisseria*, *Haemophilus*, *Pasteurella*, and others (14). The subsequent mechanisms involved in ferric iron uptake are poorly understood, and there are no known antimicrobial compounds that utilize this system.

The third class of iron-uptake systems involve the scavenger systems. In *E. coli*, in which these systems have been best studied, the relevant outer membrane proteins involved are Cir (the colicin I receptor) and Fiu (15,16). For example, these proteins can mediate uptake of iron complexed to dihydroxybenzoyl-serine, a degradation product of enterochelin (11). These proteins seem to be able to function in uptake of a broad range of β-lactam compounds with appended catechol substituents (15–18). As with the siderophore–iron-uptake systems, the scavenger iron-uptake systems are dependent on TonB and are up-regulated in low iron medium. Similarly, the catechol-β-lactams that utilize the scavenger pathway work preferably in low iron growth environments (i.e., host conditions) and are TonB-dependent.

2. Oligopeptide Uptake

Salmonella typhimurium and *E. coli* contain a promiscuous transport system for uptake of oligopeptides (*opp*; 19,20). The oligopeptide permease system transports di- to pentapeptides, although this may partly reflect the exclusion limit of the outer membrane. The system involves four proteins, a periplasmic-binding protein OppA of molecular weight 52,000, and three membrane-associated proteins OppB, OppC, and OppD (the latter being an ATP-binding protein). The genes for these proteins constitute an operon in both *E. coli* and *S. typhimurium* and are expressed constitutively. The oligopeptide permease system is quite promiscuous and has been used to promote uptake of certain phosphorylated intermediates (21,22) and cytidine monophosphate (CMP)-α-keto-3-deoxyoctanate (KDO) synthase inhibitors (compounds IV, V, and VI) (23). In addition, dipeptide-linked CMP-KDO synthase inhibitors were active against many *Enterobacteriaceae* and *Pseudomonas* species, suggesting that the *opp* uptake system is broadly distributed, although MICs of only 5–100 μg/ml were recorded, suggesting a certain minimal efficiency. Unfortunately, it appears that mutants lacking the system can be selected with high frequency. Thus, the oligopeptide permease route does not seem to be broadly useful for antimicrobial drug delivery.

3. Self-Promoted Uptake

The outer membranes of gram-negative bacteria are stabilized, in part, by divalent cation cross-bridging between adjacent surface-localized, negatively charged lipopolysaccharide (LPS) molecules (3,24,25). This explains the ability of the outer membrane to resist detergents and bile salts and to exclude hydrophobic compounds (3,24); chemicals that disrupt the cross-bridging, such as the divalent cation chelator EDTA, result in loss of barrier function for these compounds. Hancock et al. (26) proposed that the interaction of (poly)cationic antibiotics, such as aminoglycosides, at cross-bridging sites on LPS is the first step in "self-promoted uptake." This uptake route involves the initial interaction of polycations with the divalent cation-binding sites on LPS at the bacterial surface (3,37). Polycationic antibiotics, such as polymyxin B and the aminoglycosides, have affinities for these LPS sites that are two to three orders of magnitude higher than the native divalent cations (usually Ca^{2+} or Mg^{2+}) and, thus, can competitively displace them. Since the competing polycations are bulkier than the native divalent cations, they alter the outer membrane packing, resulting in blebs or transient cracks (3). This permits enhanced uptake of certain probe molecules, including the chromogenic β-lactam nitrocefin, the hydrophobic fluorophore 1-*N*-phenyl-1-naphthylamine (NPN), and the peptidoglycan-degrading enzyme lysozyme, across the permeabilized outer membrane (3). Therefore, it was hypothesized that polycationic antimicrobials promote their own uptake across the outer membrane, and the process was termed "self-promoted uptake."

Three major lines of evidence suggest that self-promoted uptake is relevant to eventual cell killing by polycationic antibiotics. First, outer membrane mutants that have reduced interaction with such polycationic antibiotics are resistant to killing by these antibiotics (27), whereas those with enhanced interactions are hypersusceptible (28). Second, for the aminoglycosides, there is a linear relation between the affinity of different aminoglycoside antibiotics for the cell surface and the MIC (29). Third, excess divalent cations that inhibit the interactions of polycationic antibiotics with the cell surface increase the MIC (3,29). With this in mind, self-promoted uptake has been demonstrated for a wide variety of polycations, including polymyxins, aminoglycosides, the macrolide azithromycin, teichoplanin aglycones, nourseothricin (streptothricin), and several cationic peptides, in a range of gram-negative bacteria (1,3,30–32).

The ability of polycations to promote their own uptake across the outer membrane as well as to promote the uptake of other probe molecules suggests two potential methods of improving antibiotic uptake into gram-negative bacteria. The first method for utilizing self-promoted uptake is to enhance the cationic character of the antibiotic in question. Two clear examples exist in the literature. The dibasic macrolide azithromycin was created chemically from the monobasic macrolide erythromycin by expansion of the 14-membered ring to include one extra methylamine with a positive charge. Azithromycin had substantially improved activity against *E. coli* (33) and appeared to be taken up by self-promoted uptake (31). In preliminary studies, a tribasic analogue had even better activity against gram-negative bacteria. The second example involved the glycopeptide antibiotic teicoplanin that has three negative charges and one positive charge and no useful activity against *E. coli* or *P. aeruginosa*. Removal of the sugar moieties deleted the negative charges and led to some anti-*E. coli* activity, whereas modifications at carbon 56 to add polyamines resulted in good activity against *E. coli* and *P. aeruginosa*, and uptake by the self-promoted uptake pathway (32). For the polycationic peptides, of which there are many (1), amidation of the COOH-terminal carboxyl is essential for the antimicrobial activity of certain peptides (34), whereas positive charge chain extension yields peptides with improved antibacterial activities (35,36). This has not yet been proved to be linked to self-promoted uptake, although self-promoted uptake has been implicated in the uptake of certain polycationic peptides.

The second method for enhancing antibiotic uptake, based on a knowledge of self-promoted uptake, is to use the ability of polycations to promote uptake of certain other molecules (including the β-lactam nitrocefin) (37). Of special note is the deacylated derivative of polymyxin B, termed polymyxin B nonapeptide (PMBN). Vaara and colleagues (38) have demonstrated that this compound can substantially enhance the anti–gram-negative bacterial activity of a range of antibiotics, especially hydrophobic ones that are normally excluded (2). Interestingly, the parent compound shows limited ability to enhance antibiotic activity. However, there is a simple explanation for these data. The PMBN is unable to form channels in artificial membranes and, presumably, in the cytoplasmic membrane of bacteria, in marked contrast to polymyxin B (39); consequently, PMBN has little antibiotic activity. Thus, it may be able to enhance the activity of other antibiotics because it can achieve a concentration sufficient to permeabilize the outer membrane, whereas at concentrations at which polymyxin B permeabilizes the outer membrane to other compounds, it self-promotes its own uptake, leading to killing. This would suggest that if the goal of such a compound was to enhance the uptake of other antibiotics, it should be designed so it interacts strongly with the outer membrane, but does not have intrinsically high antibacterial activity. As an example of such design limitations, we have synthesized by recombinant procedures a peptide, CEMA, that is a modification of a cationic *cecropin–me*littin hybrid (CEME), in that it contains two extra positively charged amino acids at the COOH-terminus (36). This hybrid has a threefold higher affinity for LPS and superior permeabilizing ability, but decreases the MIC of co-added antibiotics only twofold whereas CEME is not synergistic with other antibiotics. Instead, the antibiotic with which the cationic peptide antimicrobials are maximally synergistic is polymyxin, presumably because they act synergistically at divalent cation-binding sites.

Other classes of compounds can disrupt outer membrane integrity and, together with the polycations just described, bear the group name "permeabilizers." In a survey study (37), it was demonstrated that organic monovalent cations and chelators, as well as ascorbate and acetylsalicylate, were capable of permeabilizing the outer membrane, although generally at much higher concentrations than those required for the better polycations.

4. Other Uptake Routes

It has been demonstrated that the gram-negative bacterial outer membrane is reasonably permeable to certain compounds for which there is no adequate description of an uptake route. Such compounds include certain steroids (40) and the fluoroquinolones, such as ciprofloxacin (41). For the latter antibiotics, uptake has been proposed to involve, in part, passage through porins in *E. coli*, although this may depend to some extent on the physiochemical character of the individual fluoroquinolone (42). For example, it has been proposed that fluoroquinolones utilize a novel nonporin pathway in *P. aeruginosa* (43), whereas the limited influence of porin deficiency on *E. coli* susceptibility to fluoroquinolones (44) is also consistent with a nonporin pathway of uptake. This then may explain the excellent antimicrobial activity of the hybrid quinolone-β-lactams (44), which appear to be too bulky to pass rapidly through the channels of porins. This uptake mechanism bears some study, since it represents a hypothetical promiscuous-uptake system.

A better understood process of promiscuous uptake is passive diffusion across the cytoplasmic membrane (see Table 1). Any hydrophobic compound with significant lipid solubility (i.e., a suitably high partition coefficient) will partition into the cytoplasmic membrane (2). However, recently it has been convincingly argued (45) that fluoroquinolones and tetracyclines undergo a pH-dependent equilibrium between forms with different net charges and forms with zwitterionic or uncharged character. Furthermore, it has been suggested that only the uncharged form is membrane-permeable by passive diffusion. Despite the relatively low abundance of this uncharged form, it must be sufficient to permit a lethal concentration to accumulate in the cytoplasm, partly because of a higher pH in the cytoplasm that tends to shift the equilibrium toward the charged forms, which become trapped inside the cell.

B. Narrow Specificity Uptake Systems

1. Amino Acid Transport

A very wide variety of amino acid analogues exist (46). In certain cases, these have been demonstrated to be competitive inhibitors for uptake of the amino acid they resemble (9,47). Their actual mode of action often depends on the translational synthesis of inactive proteins. Some of these amino acids are toxic, presumably because they are transported also by mammalian cells. The best-studied bacteria-selective amino acid analogue is cycloserine, which has some useful antituberculosis activity. Cycloserine is specifically transported by the high-affinity, energized D,L-alanine transport system of *Streptococcus faecalis* and the D-alanine transport system of *E. coli* (9). This antibiotic works by inhibiting D-alanine racemase and D-alanine-D-alanine synthase, two enzymes involved in peptidoglycan side chain biosynthesis. Other antibiotics that are amino acid analogues include hadacin (an L-aspartate analogue) and azaserine and diazo-oxonorleucine (DON) (glutamine analogue). However, to my knowledge, their transport has not been studied.

Recently it has been demonstrated that *P. aeruginosa* (48) synthesizes an outer membrane protein, OprD (also known as D2), that enhances uptake of the β-lactam imipenem and related zwitterionic carbapenems.

OprD forms channels across the outer membrane, with a binding site for basic amino acids and zwitterionic carbapenems. This probably reflects the fact that although these carbapenems, like other β-lactams, are dipeptide analogues, they uniquely resemble the preferred dipeptide substrate of *oprD*, since apparently, no other β-lactams can use this channel (48,49).

2. Other Metabolites

Phosphomycin, a peptidoglycan biosynthesis inhibitor, is an α-glycerophosphate analogue, reported to access the cytoplasmic membrane uptake system for this compound (9). Its ability to access the hexose-6-phosphate permease is, however, somewhat more difficult to understand. Arsenate, an antimicrobial substance that is also a general metabolic poison and phosphate analogue, can use the phosphate uptake pathways of the cytoplasmic membrane (50) and outer membrane (51). Although not studied, one can assume that nucleotide analogues with antibacterial activity, such as psicofuranine, decoyinine, the hydroxyphenyl-azidopyrimidines—iododeoxyuridine, arabinosylcytosine, and arabinosyladenosine (9)—use normal nucleotide uptake pathways across the cytoplasmic membrane. In addition, the antibiotic albicidin utilizes the Tsx protein, a nucleotide-specific channel, to cross the *E. coli* outer membrane (52).

III. TRANSPORT AS A TARGET

There are no instances known to me in which an antimicrobial agent acts exclusively by inhibiting bacterial transport. Thus, the following represents a general discussion of inhibitory compounds, both known and potential.

A. Inhibition of Bacterial Energization

Bacteria generate energy for various cellular functions in one or both of the following ways: through substrate level phosphorylation (fermentation), leading to ATP production; or by generation of a proton gradient across the cytoplasmic membrane, oriented internally negative and alkaline relative to the outside (53). The latter, called the proton motive force, involves protons pumped across the cytoplasmic membrane by the cytoplasmic membrane-bound electron transport chain, or the movement of protons through membrane-bound ATPase as a result of ATP hydrolysis. One important use of the energy generated by these processes is for active transport of compounds from the extracellular milieu. Thus, any inhibitor of cellular energization has the potential, by definition, to be an inhibitor of transport, although transport is by no means the only process inhibited.

Active transport systems can be broadly divided into those energized directly by ATP and requiring a specific periplasmic binding protein [so-called (osmotic) shock-sensitive systems]; those (shock-resistant systems) energized by the proton motive force (or by one or other of the components of it—namely, the electrical potential gradient or the pH gradient); and those energized by direct phosphorylation, using the process of group translocation (8). Those systems that require high-energy phosphates (shock-sensitive system or group translocation) are inhibited by the phosphate analogue arsenate, which inhibits ATP formation through substrate-level phosphorylation or by dicyclohexylcarbodiimide (DCCD), which inhibits ATP synthesis directed by the proton motive force, mediated by the Na^+, K^+-ATPase. The shock-resistant systems are inhibited by ionophores, which shuffle monovalent cations or protons across the cytoplasmic membrane to neutralize the proton motive force. Such ionophores (9,54) include the known antibiotics, valinomycin, nonactin, monensin, and nigericin; the channel-forming antibiotic gramicidin A acts similarly. In addition, under conditions in which cells are energized through electron transport (i.e., respiration), electron transport inhibitors (e.g., KCN) block transport. Nevertheless, all of the foregoing agents tend to be quite toxic, owing to their effects on mammalian energy generation. Therefore, with the exception of monensin, which has been used as a feed additive for chickens, they are now used only as biochemical tools for studying energetics.

B. Inhibiting Uptake of Essential Metabolites

For metabolite transport to be considered a target, the transport system must be obligately required for bacterial growth. Given the multitude of transport systems for carbon sources and the intrinsic ability of most bacteria to synthesize all amino acids and nucleotides, this is a substantial constraint. There are, however, selected bacteria that are amino acid auxotrophs. For example, the multiply antibiotic-resistant bacterium *Xanthomonas maltophilia* is a natural methionine auxotroph, whereas the obligate intracellular pathogen *Chlamydia trachomatis* is unable to synthesize cysteine, histidine, or ATP. Thus, these significant pathogens are potential targets for amino acid or ATP analogues that inhibit uptake of these required amino acids or ATP. Phosphate and sulfate are also required by bacteria, and known transport inhibitors include arsenate (50), for phosphate, and thiosulfate and vanadate (55), for sulfate. However, it is likely that such agents would also inhibit mammalian cell transport, making them potentially toxic.

Another essential metabolite is iron. Iron uptake was previously discussed in detail (see Sec. II.A.1). Despite the substantial heterogeneity of iron uptake systems, two potential classes of inhibitors could be envisaged. One class would include inhibitors of the function of TonB, the central player in energization of siderophore–iron uptake. A second class would comprise inhibitors of the binding of transferrin–iron or lactoferrin–iron complexes to their specific outer membrane receptors in bacteria (including several important pathogens) that transport iron by this route. No such inhibitors have yet been reported. A third possible site of intervention is in the global regulation of iron transport that is mediated through a central aporepressor, Fur.

C. Channel-Forming Compounds

Although not, strictly speaking, transport inhibitors, the channel-forming compounds destroy cytoplasmic membrane integrity and, thereby, prevent transport and encourage leakage of internal cell constituents. Such compounds include the related cationic antibiotics polymyxin B and colistin (39), the cationic antiseptic chlorhexidine (9), the cyclic decapeptides gramicidin S and the tyrocidins (9), and the antimicrobial cationic peptides magainins, cecropins, defensins, and others (1). Several of these are used medicinally or are being considered for commercial application; for example, the magainin (MSI-78) is currently in Phase III clinical trials.

D. Secretion Mechanisms

There are two general classes of secretion systems in bacteria, both of which involve the passage of molecules across bacterial membranes. One class involves export of molecules to cell compartments beyond the cytoplasmic membrane. The second involves excretion of molecules into the environment of the bacterium. The former involves export of proteins (56) by a conserved system involving a cytoplasmic membrane apparatus and an NH_2-terminal leader sequence on the exported protein, as well as export of lipopolysaccharides, peptidoglycan precursors, and other carbohydrate-containing molecules. These would appear to be potential targets for antimicrobials and, indeed, the antibiotics enduracidin A, vancomycin, monomycin, and tunicamycin, all cause accumulation of membrane-bound undecaprenol lipid intermediates required in the biosynthesis and export of peptidoglycan (and lipopolysaccharide O-antigen) precursors (9).

The second class involves excretion of proteins involved in the pathogenesis of certain bacteria, including extracellular proteases, lipases, hemolysins, and toxins. The generally high level of conservation of these excretion systems, especially the general secretory pathway and the hemolysin-like secretory pathway (56), seems to offer opportunities for antimicrobial intervention, possibly leading to decreased pathogenic potential, rather than bacterial death or stasis. Cerulenin, an inhibitor of fatty acid synthase, exhibits such activity (57).

E. ATP-Requiring Transport Systems

Bacterial shock-sensitive transport systems contain a peripheral membrane protein, with a conserved motif that is involved in ATP binding and energization of transport (47). This motif is shared by two highly important mammalian cells for drug intervention; namely, the multidrug resistance (MDR) protein and the cystic fibrosis transmembrane regulator (CFTR) proteins (58). Given that pharmaceutical companies are directing considerable effort toward finding inhibitors for the MDR protein, this may offer a potential source of compounds active against the homologous bacterial proteins involved in energization of shock-sensitive transport systems.

ACKNOWLEDGMENTS

Transport research in the author's laboratory is funded by the Medical Research Council of Canada, by the Canadian Cystic Fibrosis Foundation, and through the Canadian Bacterial Diseases Network.

REFERENCES

1. Hancock REW, Falla T, Brown MH. Cationic antimicrobial peptides. Adv Microb Physiol 1995; (in press).
2. Nikaido H. Outer membrane of *Salmonella typhimurium*. Transmembrane diffusion of some hydrophobic substances. Biochim Biophys Acta 1976; 433:118–132.
3. Hancock REW, Bell A. Antibiotic uptake into gram-negative bacteria. Eur J Clin Microbiol Infect Dis 1988; 7:713–720.
4. Day SEJ, Vasil KK, Russell RJ, Arbuthnott JP. A simple method for the study of bacterial growth and accompanying host response. J Infect 1980; 2:39–51.
5. Kelly NM, Battershill JL, Kuo S, Arbuthnott JP, Hancock REW. Colonial dissociation and susceptibility to phagocytosis of *Pseudomonas aeruginosa* grown in a chamber implant model in mice. Infect Immun 1987; 55:2841–2843.
6. Silver S, Walderhaug M. Gene regulation of plasmid and chromosome-determined inorganic ion transport in bacteria. Microbiol Rev 1992; 56:195–228.

7. Jain MK, Wagner RC. Introduction to Biological Membranes. New York: John Wiley & Sons, 1980.

8. Cronan JE, Gennis RB, Maloy SR. Cytoplasmic membrane. In: Ingraham JL, Low KB, Magasanik B, Schaechter M, Umbarger HE, eds. *Escherichia coli* and *Salmonella typhimurium*. Cellular and Molecular Biology. Vol 1. Washington DC: American Society for Microbiology, 1987:31–55.

9. Franklin TJ, Snow GA. Biochemistry of Antimicrobial Action, 3rd ed. London: Chapman & Hall, 1981.

10. Hancock REW. Aminoglycoside uptake and mode of action—with special reference to streptomycin and gentamicin. II. Effects of aminoglycosides on cells. J Antimicrob Chemother 1981; 8:429–445.

11. Braun V. Genetics of siderophore biosynthesis and transport. In: Kleinkauf H, Dohren H, eds. Biochemistry of Peptide Antibiotics. Berlin: Walter de Gruyter, 1990:103–129.

12. Bakker PAHM, van Peer R, Schippers B. Specificity of siderophores and siderophore receptors and biocontrol by *Pseudomonas* spp. In: Hornby D, ed. Biological Control of Soil-borne Plant Pathogens. Wallingford: CAB International, 1990:131–142.

13. Pugsley AP, Zimmerman W, Wehrli W. Highly efficient uptake of a rifamycin derivative via the FhuA–TonB-dependent uptake route in *Escherichia coli*. J Gen Microbiol 1987; 133:3505–3511.

14. Morton DJ, Williams P. Siderophore-independent acquisition of transferrin-bound iron by *Haemophilus influenzae* type b. Infect Immun 1990; 136:927–933.

15. Curtiss NAC, Eisenstadt RL, East SJ, Cornford RJ, Walker LA, White AJ. Iron-regulated outer membrane proteins of *Escherichia coli* K-12 and mechanism of action of catechol-substituted cephalosporins. Antimicrob Agents Chemother 1988; 32:1879–1886.

16. Nikaido H, Rosenberg EY. Cir and Fiu proteins in the outer membrane of *Escherichia coli* catalyse transport of monomeric catechols: study with β-lactam antibiotics containing catechol and analogous groups. Antimicrob Agents Chemother 1990; 172:1361–1367.

17. Watanabe N, Nagasu T, Katsu K, Kitoh K. E-0702, a new cephalosporin, is incorporated into *Escherichia coli* cells via the tonB-dependent iron transport system. Antimicrob Agents Chemother 1987; 31:497–504.

18. Silley P, Griffiths JW, Monsey D, Harris AM. Mode of action of GR69153, a novel catechol substituted cephalosporin and its interaction with the tonB-dependent iron transport system. Antimicrob Agents Chemother 1990; 34:1806–1808.

19. Higgins CF, Hardie MM. Periplasmic protein associated with the oligopeptide permeases of *Salmonella typhimurium* and *Escherichia coli*. J Bacteriol 1983; 155:1434–1438.

20. Higgins CF. Peptide transport systems of *Salmonella typhimurium* and *Escherichia coli*. In: Leive L, Schlessinger D, eds. Microbiology, 1984. Washington DC: American Society for Microbiology, 1984:17–20.

21. Ames BN, Ames GF, Young JD, Tsuchiyd D, Lecocq J. Illicit transport: the oligopeptide permease. Proc Natl Acad Sci USA 1973; 70:456–458.

22. Fickel TE, Gilvarg C. Transport of impermeant substances in *E. coli* by way of oligopeptide permeases. Nature 1973; 241:161–163.

23. Goldman R, Kohlbrenner W, Lartey P, Pernet A. Antibacterial agents specifically inhibiting lipopolysaccharide synthesis. Nature 1987; 329:162–164.

24. Nikaido H, Vaara M. Molecular basis of bacterial outer membrane permeability. Microbiol Rev 1985; 49:1–32.

25. Hancock REW, Egli C, Karunaratne N. Molecular organization and structural role of outer membrane macromolecules. In: Ghuysen JM, Hakenbeck R, eds. Bacterial Cell Envelope, pp 263–279. Amsterdam: Elsevier Science Publishers, 1994.

26. Hancock REW, Raffle VJ, Nicas TI. Involvement of the outer membrane of *Pseudomonas aeruginosa* in gentamicin and streptomycin uptake and killing in *Pseudomonas aeruginosa*. Antimicrob Agents Chemother 1981; 19:777–785.

27. Paterson AA, Fesik SW, McGroarty EJ. Decreased binding of antibiotics to lipopolysaccharides from polymyxin-resistant strains of *Escherichia coli* and *Salmonella typhimurium*. Antimicrob Agents Chemother 1987; 31:230–237.

28. Rivera M, Hancock REW, Sawyer JG, Haug A, McGroarty EJ. Enhanced binding of polycationic antibiotics to lipopolysaccharide from an aminoglycoside-supersusceptible *tolA* mutant strain of *Pseudomonas aeruginosa*. Antimicrob Agents Chemother 1988; 32:649–655.

29. Loh B, Grant C, Hancock REW. Use of the fluorescent probe 1-*N*-phenylnaphthylamine to study the interactions of aminoglycoside antibiotics with the outer membrane of *Pseudomonas aeruginosa*. Antimicrob Agents Chemother 1984; 26:546–551.

30. Seltmann G, Wolter E. Effect of nourseothricin (streptothricin) on the outer membrane of sensitive and resistant *Escherichia coli* strains. J Basic Microbiol 1987; 3:139–146.

31. Farmer S, Li Z, Hancock REW. Influence of outer membrane mutations on susceptibility of *Escherichia coli* to the dibasic microlide azithromycin. J Antimicrob Chemother 1992; 29:27–33.

32. Hancock REW, Farmer S. Mechanism of uptake of deglucoteicoplanin amide derivatives across the outer membranes of *Escherichia coli* and *Pseudomonas aeruginosa*. Antimicrob Agents Chemother 1993; 37:453–456.

33. Retsema J, Girard A, Schelkly W, et al. Spectrum and mode of action of azithromycin (CP-62,993) a new 15-membered–ring macrolide with improved potency against gram-negative organisms. Antimicrob Agents Chemother 1987; 31:1939–1947.

34. Callaway JE, Lai J, Haselbeck B, Baltaian M, Bonnesen SP, Weickmann J, Wilcox G, Cei S. Modification of the C terminus of cecropin is essential for broad-spectrum antimicrobial activity. Antimicrob Agents Chemother 1993; 37:1614–1619.

35. Bessalle R, Haas H, Goria A, Shalit I, Fridkin M. Augmentation of the antibacterial activity of magainin by positive charge chain extension. Antimicrob Agents Chemother 1992; 36:313–317.

36. Piers KL, Brown MH, Hancock REW. Improvement of the outer membrane-permeabilizing and lipopolysaccharide-binding activities of an antimicrobial cationic peptide by C-terminal modification. Antimicrob Agents Chemother 1994; (in press).

37. Hancock REW, Wong PGW. Compounds which increase the outer membrane permeability of *Pseudomonas aeruginosa*. Antimicrob Agents Chemother 1984; 26:546–551.

38. Vaara M, Vaara T. Polycations sensitize enteric bacteria to antibiotics. Antimicrob Agents Chemother 1983; 24:107–113.

39. Schroeder G, Brandenburg K, Seydel U. Polymyxin B induces transient permeability fluctuations in assymetric planar lipopolysaccharide/phospholipid bilayers. Biochemistry 1992; 31:621–630.

40. Plesiat P, Nikaido H. Outer membranes of gram-negative bacteria are permeable to steroid probes. Mol Microbiol 1992; 6:1323–1333.

41. Hancock REW, Bellido F. Antibiotic uptake: unusual results for unusual molecules. J Antimicrob Chemother 1992; 29:235–243.

42. Hirai K, Aoyama H, Irikura T, Iyobe S, Matsuhashi S. Differences in susceptibility to quinolones in outer membrane mutants of *Salmonella typhimurium* and *Escherichia coli*. Antimicrob Agents Chemother 1986; 29:535–538.

43. Young ML, Hancock REW. Fluoroquinolone supersusceptibility mediated by OprH overexpression in *Pseudomonas aeruginosa*: evidence for involvement of a non-porin pathway. Antimicrob Agents Chemother 1992; 36:2566–2568.

44. Georgopapadakou NH, Bertasso A. Mechanisms of action of cephalosporin 3′-quinolone esters, carbamates and tertiary amines in *Escherichia coli*. Antimicrob Agents Chemother 1993; 37:559–565.

45. Nikaido H, Thanassi DG. Penetration of lipophilic agents with multiple protonation sites into bacterial cells: tetracyclines and fluoroquinolones as examples. Antimicrob Agents Chemother 1993; 37:1393–1399.

46. Meister A. Biochemistry of the Amino Acids. Vol. 1, 2nd ed. New York: Academic Press, 1965.

47. Furlong CE. Osmotic shock-sensitive transport systems. Cytoplasmic membrane. In: Ingraham JL, Low KB, Magasanik B, Schaechter M, Umbarger HE, eds. *Escherichia coli* and *Salmonella typhimurium*. Cellular and Molecular Biology. Vol 1. Washington DC: American Society for Microbiology, 1987; 768–796.

48. Trias J, Nikaido H. Outer membrane protein D2 catalyzes facilitated diffusion of carbapenems and penems through the outer membrane of *Pseudomonas aeruginosa*. Antimicrob Agents Chemother 1990; 34:52–57.

49. Huang H, Hancock REW. Genetic definition of the substrate selectivity of outer membrane porin protein OprD of *Pseudomonas aeruginosa*. J Bacteriol 1993; 175:7793–7800.

50. Willsky GR, Malamy MH. Effect of arsenate on inorganic phosphate transport in *Escherichia coli*. J Bacteriol 1980; 144:366–374.
51. Hancock REW, Benz R. Demonstration and chemical modification of a specific phosphate binding site in the phosphate-starvation-inducible outer membrane porin protein OprP of *Pseudomonas aeruginosa*. Biochim Biophys Acta 1986; 860:699–707.
52. Birch RG, Pemberton JM, Basnayake WVS. Stable albicidin resistance in *Escherichia coli* involves an altered outer membrane nucleoside uptake system. J Gen Microbiol 1990; 136:51–58.
53. Ingraham JL, Low KB, Magasanik B, Schaechter M, Umbarger HE, eds. *Escherichia coli* and *Salmonella typhimurium*. Cellular and Molecular Biology. Washington DC: American Society for Microbiology, 1987.
54. Bakker EP. Ionophore antibiotics. In: Hahn FE, ed. Mechanism of Action of Antibacterial Agents. Berlin: Springer-Verlag, 1979:67–97.
55. Pardee AB, Prestidge LS, Whipple MB, Dreyfuss J. A binding site for sulfate and its relation to sulfate transport into *Salmonella typhimurium*. J Biol Chem 1966; 241:3962–3969.
56. Pugsley AP. The complete general secretory pathway in gram-negative bacteria. Microbiol Rev 1993; 57:50–108.
57. Paton, JC, May BK, Elliott WH. Cerulenin inhibits production of extracellular proteins but not membrane proteins in *Bacillus amyloliquefaciens*. J Gen Microbiol 1980; 118:179–187.
58. Riordan JR, Rommens JM, Kerem B, Alan N, Rozmahel R, Grzelczak Z, Zielenski J, Lok S, Plavsic N, Chou J, Drum ML, Iannuzzi MC, Collins FS, Tsui L. Identification of the cystic fibrosis gene. Cloning and characterization of complementary DNA. Science 1989; 245:1066–1073.

11

Internalization of Amphotericin B and Other Polyene Antifungals in Mammalian Cells: A Possible Origin of Their Toxicity

Jacques Bolard and Aline Vertut-Doï
Université Pierre et Marie Curie, Paris, France

I. INTRODUCTION

Amphotericin B (AmB) and nystatin (Fig. 1) are the most widely used drugs in the treatment of systemic fungal infections. Other polyenes, such as mepartricin or hamycin, are less frequently used, as their higher toxicity limits their usefulness, despite their higher activity. The polyene antibiotics were discovered 40 years ago and, therefore, could be considered old drugs, not deserving further attention. Actually, this is not true for the following reasons:

1. Systemic fungal diseases occur primarily in individuals with defective immune response and thus are becoming prevalent as the population of immunosuppressed, acquired immunodeficiency syndrome (AIDS), cancer, and transplant patients increases. For example, a recent study has shown that AmB use increased almost tenfold between 1978 and 1988 at Duke University Medical Center (1).
2. The clinically used formulation of AmB, Fungizone, has several serious side effects, especially severe nephrotoxicity. Therefore, it would be highly desirable to design new formulations with decreased host toxicity. Indeed, new derivatives of AmB are currently in clinical trials, as are new delivery systems, particularly liposomes. One liposomal formulation is already commercially available.

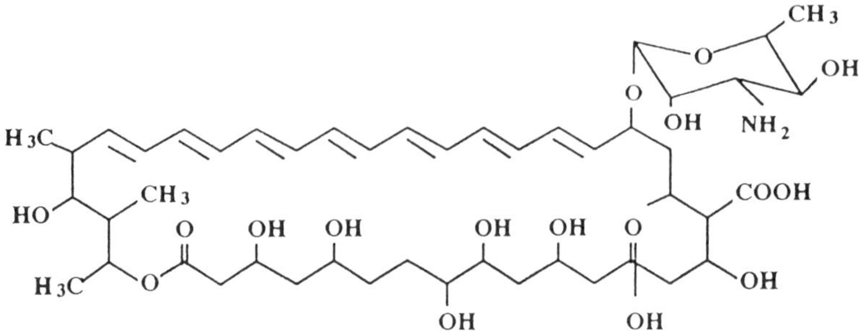

Amphotericin B

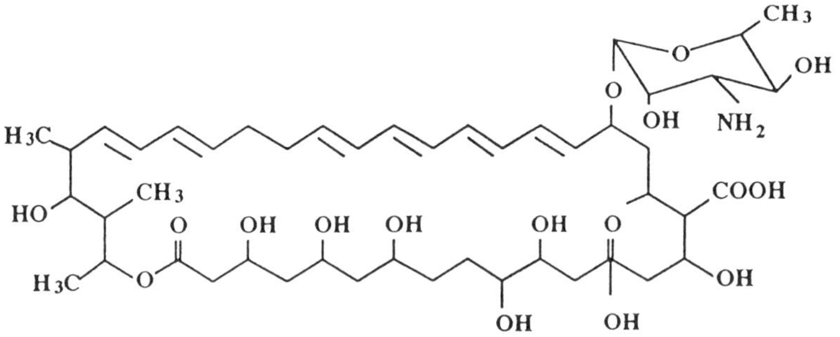

Nystatin A$_1$

Figure 1   Structures of amphotericin B and nystatin A$_1$.

The polyene macrolide antibiotics possess a large lactone ring that contains a nonpolar, transconjugated, double-bond system, and a polar polyhydroxylic region (see Fig. 1). The macrolide ring structure of AmB contains 37 carbon atoms. There are seven conjugated double bonds and seven free hydroxyls on the ring structure. A mycosamine is bound to the hydroxyl group at carbon 19. Nystatin is a tetraene that also contains a mycosamine. In addition, it has two double bonds not conjugated with the four that qualify it as a tetraene.

Because AmB is an amphoteric molecule having a hydrophobic part (the polyene chain) and a polar part (the OH groups and mycosamine), it is difficult to predict its overall hydrophobicity. Nevertheless, it appears that AmB is very poorly soluble in water, and aqueous solutions are usually made from a stock solution in dimethyl sulfoxide or as mixed micelles with deoxycholate (commercially available Fungizone). At concentrations below 0.1 μM, amphotericin B is present in water as soluble monomers, but beyond this concentration, soluble oligomers and aggregates of oligomers begin to appear (2). The three forms (monomers, oligomers, micelles) are not in true equilibrium, the equilibrium between the non–water-soluble aggregates and the other forms are slow to be established (3). The first specific action of AmB described was the induction of permeability through sterol-containing membranes (ergosterol in fungi, cholesterol in mammalian cells). Indeed, permeability to monovalent cations is strongly enhanced by the one-sided addition of the antibiotic. Therefore, it is not surprising that numerous studies have addressed the interaction of AmB and nystatin with membranes. To what extent this phenomenon is the cause of their activity will be discussed later; but it is certain that the model of transmembrane pores formed by AmB–sterol complexes, a model proposed in the 1970s, has been well established. We shall also see that its success tends to obscure other well-demonstrated mechanisms of action, such as lipid peroxidation, blockade of membrane enzyme and, a topic of this chapter, intracellular activity. We shall also see that the structure proposed for the transmembrane pores has increased in complexity.

II. BIOLOGICAL ACTIVITIES OF AMPHOTERICIN B

A. Antifungal Activity

In spite of the advent of azole derivatives, AmB remains the gold standard for the therapy of acute systemic fungal infections, including candidiasis, coccidioidomycosis, cryptococcal meningitis, histoplasmosis, and blastomycosis. Amphotericin B has also been used in the treatment of amebic meningoencephalitis, leishmaniasis, and vaginal trichomoniasis. The aggressive candidal and aspergillar infections associated with leukemia are treated very early, using protocols for empirical therapy with AmB (4). Although liposomal formulations of AmB as well as the triazole compounds (fluconazole, itraconazole), have proved effective in several types of infections, some mycoses, such as invasive aspergillosis in neutropenic patients and bone-marrow transplant recipients, remain a real therapeutic problem.

Amphotericin B may be given orally or, more usually, intravenously by infusing the antibiotic over several hours (5). Conventionally, AmB is administered as a short infusion over 3–4 h, with daily increases in dose until therapeutic levels are reached. Peak serum AmB concentrations of 2–3 μM are achieved by the end of infusion. The drug achieves high concentrations in most visceral organs, and peritoneal fluid levels are nearly as high as those in serum. However, AmB penetrates very poorly into cerebrospinal fluid, urine, and the interior of the eye. In humans, infusion of AmB is often associated with nausea, anemia, fever, and kidney damage.

Nystatin is used successfully in the topical treatment of candidal infection of the skin, nails, and mucosal surfaces. It is a common choice for the treatment of oral and vaginal forms of candidiasis. Oral ingestion of nystatin is a safe procedure in the therapy of esophageal candidiasis and the prophylactic treatment of candidiasis in neutropenia; given orally, it rapidly clears candidiasis of the alimentary tract.

B. Potential in Cancer Chemotherapy

Several in vitro studies have shown that AmB can increase the cytotoxicity of different antitumor agents. In particular, reversal of cisplatin resistance (6–8) has been recently observed in a non–small-cell lung cancer cell lines and in human ovarian cancer cell lines. This potentiation of the cytotoxicity to tumor cells has also been described in vivo (9), in particular against a transplantable AKR mouse leukemia, for which AmB enhanced 180-fold the antitumor effect of cyclophosphamide, 330-fold of doxorubicin (Adriamycin), 209-fold of nitrogen mustard, and over 1000-fold of lomustine (CCNU). Two mechanisms have been considered responsible for this effect: stimulation of the immune system of the host (with antitumor agents presenting little or no immunosuppressive effects) and direct potentiation of cytotoxicity by an increase of uptake of the anticancer agents through the membrane-permeabilizing effect of AmB. The proposed stimulation of the immune system stems from the observation that sublethal doses of AmB have a stimulatory effect on fungal as well as mammalian cells. Prompted by these in vitro experiments and findings with animal tumors, trials (10), or retrospective studies (11) were done to examine whether AmB also had therapeutic effects on cancer patients. These studies produced conflicting results. However, murine studies have shown that both AmB dose and schedule are important parameters in obtaining maximum potentiation of antineoplastic agents (12).

C. Immunomodulation

We have seen that, at sublethal doses, AmB has stimulatory effects on fungal cells as well as on mammalian cells. Its action is, therefore, complex and, in addition to toxicity, stimulation of the cells of the immune system can be expected (see Refs. 13,14). Under these conditions, the selectivity of AmB action between fungal and host cells could be indirect; it would result from the high specificity of the immune system against foreign organisms. Numerous in vivo studies have shown that the cellular and humoral arms of the immune response may be affected by AmB, or by AmB methyl ester. The drugs enhance the response in most of the common inbred mouse strains.

The possible enhancement of the phagocytic activity of macrophages by AmB was first demonstrated in vivo on peritoneal macrophages of AKR mice (15,16). The tumoricidal (17,18) and candidicidal (19) capability of activated macrophages could be demonstrated in vitro. Amphotericin was shown to enhance the production of superoxide anion and surface expression of I_a antigen of *human* monocyte-derived macrophages (20), to induce secretion of tumor necrosis factor alpha (TNF-α; 21,22) by *murine* macrophages in vitro, and to completely block germ tube formation of *Candida albicans* in macrophages (23). However, in human monocyte-derived macrophages, phagocytosis appeared reduced (20), and AmB greatly suppressed mouse resident peritoneal macrophage differentiation and in vitro effector functions at doses of approximately 1 μM (24).

Numerous in vitro studies have examined the influence of AmB on the activity of polymorphonuclear leukocytes, with conflicting results. The contribution of the experimental conditions to these discrepancies has been discussed (13).

Stimulation of murine B cells in culture by AmB has also been reported in several studies. In contrast, one study indicated inhibition of lipopolysaccharide (LPS)-induced activation of BALB/c B lymphocytes. Mitogen- and antigen-induced stimulation of human lymphocytes is suppressed by AmB in vitro, although AmB stimulated interleukin-1β (IL-1β) expression by peripheral blood mononuclear cells (25). Human peripheral blood lymphocytes showed a decreased natural killer activity in the presence of AmB.

Murine T cells were not stimulated by AmB. Proliferation of freshly obtained guinea pig and rat antigen-specific T lymphocytes was inhibited, but the effect was different with a cultured cell line (26).

Recent observations indicating a strong correlation between the magnitude of the in vitro effects and the in vivo adjuvant effects of AmB or AmE in different mouse strains, have provided new perspectives on the variability in the results. Most of the common inbred mouse strains show AmB-induced immunostimulation (AmB high-responders), but mice of the C 57 BL strains are AmB low-responders. On the other hand, lymphoid cells and macrophages (27) from AmB high-responder strains exhibit greater resistance to H_2O_2 toxicity in vitro, compared with cells from AmB low-responders. This result led to an evaluation of differences in the tissue catalase levels of AmB high- and low-responder strains. The C 57 BL mouse strains expressed low levels of tissue catalase activity, whereas several AmB high-responder strains had high levels of spleen cell, macrophage, and liver catalase. It was suggested, therefore, that cellular peroxidation is a major determinant of the genetic regulation of AmB-induced immunostimulation.

D. Toxicity

Unfortunately, amphotericin B causes a variety of adverse effects, including fever, chills, nausea, vomiting, hypokalemia, anemia, and phlebitis (reviewed in Ref. 5). The most important complication of therapy with AmB is nephrotoxicity, which is manifested by changes in renal hemodynamics and alterations in renal tubular cell function. The acute nephrotoxicity of AmB appears to be mediated by its effect on the luminal aspect of the tubular membrane, altering permeability to small solutes, sharply modifying glomerular filtration rate and renal plasma flow through increased solute delivery to the macula densa, and activating the tubuloglomerular feedback mechanism. Amphotericin B may also directly affect the glomerular mesangial cells and the afferent or efferent arterioles.

III. MECHANISM OF ACTION OF AMPHOTERICIN B

A. Mode of Action at the Cellular Level

The type of interaction between AmB and cells depends on the concentration of the drug. Membrane permeability alterations are considered to be the first toxic event and occur before cell death, which results from osmotic imbalances and additional mechanisms. Early events, which precede actual toxicity, are stimulatory effects and morphological alterations of the cells.

1. Stimulatory Effects

Brajtburg et al. (28) showed that exposure of *C. albicans* to AmB concentrations lower than those causing detectable potassium leakage, increased the plating efficiency of yeasts, although the precise mechanisms have remained unknown. Other studies showed that AmB stimulates several cellular functions: increases in DNA, RNA, and protein synthesis have been demonstrated in several cell types (29,30). Although it has been hypothesized (31) that changes in intracellular concentrations of monovalent cations could affect DNA synthesis through stimulation of ATPase, Brajtburg et al. showed that the stimulatory effect of AmB does not depend on its permeabilizing effect (32).

2. Membrane Permeability Alterations

Polyenes, such as AmB, with a large macrolide ring induce, at least at the onset of their action, specific membrane changes that permit potassium efflux from the cells. Intact cells release K^+ after a short exposure to low doses of AmB. Potassium leakage is easy to measure, and this method has allowed determination of the sensitivities of different cell types to the drug (33). At low concentrations of AmB, a repair mechanism ensures that the initial intracellular K^+ level is more or less restored. Different mechanisms have been postulated for this repair process: disruption of membrane pathways, degradation or internalization of the polyene, stimulation of the Na^+, K^+-ATPase, explaining the beneficial effect of an available energy source (34,35). When erythrocytes are exposed to AmB, the increase in cell permeability to monovalent cations may lead to swelling and hemolysis. It has been suggested that the increase in intracellular osmotic pressure is not the only mechanism responsible for cell death; conversely, permeabilizing effects of AmB may exist without cell death.

3. Oxidative Mechanisms

Evidence for the role of active oxygen species in the lytic activity of AmB was obtained in experiments which showed that AmB injury to cells could be reduced by hypoxia or extracellular catalase (36,37). Neither hypoxia nor extracellular scavengers affect the AmB-induced intracellular K^+ leakage. AKR mouse erythrocytes, which have high levels of catalase activity, are less sensitive to lysis by AmB than are C 57 BL/6 mouse erythrocytes, which have lower levels of this enzymatic activity. These in vitro results have been confirmed by in vivo experiments that showed that AKR mice were more resistant to the toxic effects of AmB than C 57 BL/6 mice (38). The specific nature of the oxidative insult to cells, as well as the actual mechanism of the irreversible damage, remain to be clarified. Lipid peroxidation may render the membrane more fragile, thereby making the cell more sensitive to osmotic shock.

4. Modulation of Cellular Enzymatic Activities and Other Effects

Amphotericin B-induced inhibitory effects were observed on alkaline phosphatase from the membrane fraction of *C. albicans*, on chitin synthesis, and on several membrane enzymes of *C. albicans* (reviewed in Ref. 14). By contrast, AmB may stimulate some enzymes. The Na^+, K^+-ATPase of human erythrocytes deserves special mention because this enzyme is membrane-associated, and its activity is influenced by the intracellular sodium concentration that AmB is likely to alter. It has been shown that AmB exerts a direct inhibitory effect on this enzyme (39). Amphotericin exhibits a direct vasoconstrictor effect that is probably initiated by depolarization-induced opening of Ca^{2+} channels (40).

6. Endocytosis

This is the topic of this chapter and will be developed in the following sections.

B. Mode of Action at the Membrane Level

1. Binding to Membranes

Despite what is generally written in the literature, different studies with model membranes (41) or isolated cell membranes (34,42) have shown that the affinity of AmB for membranes is often limited. Only the interaction with ergosterol-containing membranes is strong and well defined, with an ergosterol–AmB stoichiometry of 1:1. With cholesterol-containing membranes, a saturation of binding is observed at a ratio of approximately 1 AmB to 30 cholesterol molecules. Binding to pure phospholipids is still weaker, unless phospholipids are in the gel state. These observations have led to the proposal that, in membranes, a sterol–AmB complex exists only with ergosterol. With cholesterol, there is no proof of the existence of such an entity in membranes at concentrations at which biological activity is observed.

2. Binding to Serum Components

When used clinically, AmB circulates in the blood bound to lipoproteins and other serum proteins. This aspect has been generally neglected when considering the mode of action of AmB although, as we shall see from the following, it may totally change it by favoring the endocytosis of AmB through the low-density lipoprotein (LDL) receptor. At 25°C, AmB binds equally well to LDL and to very low-density lipoprotein (VLDL), with equivalent lipoprotein–cholesterol contents, but to a lesser extent to high-density lipoprotein (HDL) (43). It also binds to lipoprotein-deficient serum and human serum albumin. In contrast, another study (44) showed that AmB binds equally well to LDL and to HDL at 25°C. Even at 37°C, after 1 h of incubation, more than 75% of the AmB bound to lipoproteins was recovered in the HDL fraction.

3. Induction of Permeability and Formation of Pores

This topic has been the subject of many studies, but a clear conclusion is difficult to reach because different experimental conditions have been used: two-sided addition of the antibiotic versus one-sided; ergosterol- or cholesterol-containing membranes; model membranes, with different radii of curvature and phospholipids (in gel or liquid crystalline state, with lipid acyl chains of various lengths, saturated or not); and different temperatures. Nevertheless, under conditions corresponding to those used for antifungal activity (one-sided addition of AmB, phospholipids in liquid crystalline state, drug concentration about 1 μM, 37°C) the following two models can now be proposed (45–47):

1. With ergosterol-containing membranes (fungal cells), the model proposed in the 1970s is valid; that is, a pore spanning the membrane is formed by several AmB–ergosterol complexes.
2. With cholesterol-containing membranes (mammalian cells), a pore spanning the membrane is formed by oligomers (dimers?) of AmB, without direct interaction with the cholesterol molecules.

The nature of the permeability changes induced by AmB, therefore, is different, depending on the presence of ergosterol or cholesterol. In particular, calcium ions can pass through the former pores (48), but not through the latter ones. So far, this is the only difference likely to account for the selectivity of AmB action against fungal cells.

IV. METHODS FOR MEASURING THE INTERACTION OF AMPHOTERICIN B WITH MEMBRANES AND ITS INTERNALIZATION

A. Interaction with Membranes

Two types of methods, direct and indirect, may be used to measure AmB interaction with membranes. They deal either with the spectroscopic characteristics of the molecule, or with the effect of the antibiotic. Methods used in model systems have been thoroughly described (33); therefore, we will concentrate on techniques used in cell studies.

1. Indirect Methods

We have seen that there are three distinct cellular effects of polyene antibiotics, in particular AmB: stimulation, permeabilization, and killing. The first effect will not be discussed here, since it has not yet been shown to be related to AmB action at the plasma membrane level. Permeability measurements, mainly K^+ retention or continuous leakage, can be monitored, depending on the antibiotic concentration, temperature, and number of cells, using either atomic absorption or a selective K^+ electrode

(49,50). Unfortunately, the results already published and presented in the form of dose–response curves are difficult to compare owing to the different protocols used. The different methods used to assess the cell death induced by polyene antibiotics have been reviewed (51).

Cation fluxes induced by AmB result in changes in membrane potential (52). This parameter can be assessed with a fluorescent probe, such as bisoxonol or carbocyanine dyes that are permeant-charged molecules. These and related compounds undergo potential-dependent distribution between extracellular medium and cell, with a quantum yield (i.e., fluorescence intensity) change when the probe moves from hydrophilic to hydrophobic environment or self-associates.

Finally, the interaction of AmB with plasma membrane may be followed by fluorescence energy transfer from the fluorescent 1-[4-(trimethylammonio)phenyl]-6-phenylhexa-1,3,5-triene (TMA-DPH) to the polyene. The dye is rapidly incorporated into cell membranes, when added to living cells, according to a partition equilibrium. The overlap of the absorption spectrum of AmB with the emission of TMA-DPH allows one to assess the amount of polyene bound to the cell from the experimental energy transfer efficiency measurement (42,53).

2. Direct Methods

Direct methods are based on the spectroscopic properties of the antibiotic (i.e., UV-visible absorption and circular dichroism) (CD). For instance, free AmB and related compounds exhibit strong CD spectra that are highly sensitive to the antibiotic aggregation state. At low concentrations (below 0.1 μM), small positive bands are observed between 410 and 345 nm. When the concentration of AmB is increased, an intense doublet centered at about 345 nm appears. The CD spectra of the bound forms are modified; in particular, they are strongly reduced in comparison with the doublet of the free form. Therefore, for a total AmB concentration above 1 μM, it is possible to measure, from the intensity of the doublet, the amount of drug remaining free in the presence of cells, neglecting the CD of the bound species. In these experiments, 1.5 (42) to 16% (34) of the total antibiotic interacted with plasma membranes.

Absorption spectra are less useful for binding measurements in the presence of cells because the spectrum of AmB does not present high-intensity bands specific for a species and, in addition, light scattering represents an important problem. However, the total content of antibiotic bound to adherent cells may be easily measured by absorption spectrophotometry, after removal of the medium by aspiration and treatment of the cells with detergent to solubilize the drug. Concentration is determined from the optical density, using the molar extinction coefficient of AmB in the detergent.

Radioactive AmB derivatives have been synthesized to allow direct-binding measurements (50), but unfortunately no comparison can be made with AmB. Similarly, a fluorescent derivative of AmB has been synthesized, but the characteristic biological properties of the polyene have been altered by the process (54).

B. Measurement of the Internalization

The determination of the localization of drugs inside cellular compartments after their internalization is of high interest, and many techniques have recently been developed, mainly using separation on sucrose or Percoll gradients (55,56). Thus, to assess drug internalization inside cells, one has to separate intracellular organelles, mainly plasma membrane, endosomes, and lysosomes, that are the main targets of the polyene antibiotic, since the drug cannot penetrate the cells by mechanism other than endocytosis (57). Postnuclear supernatants may be prepared after cell homogenization, mixed with a suspension of Percoll (final concentration 20%), and layered on a 1-ml cushion of 60% sucrose (57). The tubes are centrifuged at 50,000 g for 45 min at 4°C, and fractions are collected from the gradients, starting from the bottom of the tube. The formation of a gradient may be verified by using density marker beads under identical conditions. Specific labels, such as fluorescent concanavalin A for plasma membrane, or sulforhodamine B for endosomes and lysosomes, enable one to determine the location of organelles within the gradient. Amphotericin B is measured in each fraction spectrophotometrically in the presence of detergent.

The development of fluorescence microscopy and enhanced video microscopy have allowed visualization of movement inside cells or localization of organelles, such as endosomes, lysosomes, phagolysosomes, and others. More recently, a nondestructive approach, laser microspectrofluorimetry, has allowed detection of fluorescent molecules and their metabolites inside living cells at a subcellular level (59). Unfortunately, these powerful techniques are so far limited to fluorescent molecules or fluorescent-labeled ones. Problems arise when the compound of interest is nonfluorescent and cannot be labeled without losing its properties. These molecules may be detected spectrophotometrically, but with lower sensitivity, owing to their absorption properties. With this approach, we have been able to measure, under the microscope, liposomal AmB internalized inside phagosomes of J774 macrophages (60). Unfortunately, we could not detect internalized nonliposomal AmB because of its low local concentration.

V. INTERNALIZATION OF AMPHOTERICIN B

A. Fungal Cells

As yet, it has not been possible to prove or assess the presence of AmB inside fungal cells. The main reason seems to be the low dose of antibiotic required to kill the fungus, which makes its measurement difficult. However, an endocytic process occurs in fungal as in mammalian cells, and the possibility that internalization of polyene antibiotics in fungus happens cannot be dismissed.

B. Mammalian Cells

1. Macrophages and Liposomal Amphotericin B

Two mechanisms can be used by the cells to internalize external compounds: endocytosis, receptor-mediated or not, and phagocytosis for larger particles ($> 1 \mu$m). Because of the relatively low selectivity of AmB for fungal cells, research has focused on improving its therapeutic index with suitable vectors. A recent study from our laboratory (61) compared the behavior of nine different formulations, proposed in the literature, in an effort to better understand the mechanism of their internalization and fate inside the macrophage cell line J774. From the nine different preparations (termed below according to literature), some were negatively charged, multilamellar liposomes containing 5, 10, or 33% AmB ($> 1 \mu$m; L-AmpB, L-AmpB10, and ABLC), or negative, small unilamellar or positive oligolamellar vesicles containing 5 or 10% antibiotic ($< 0.2 \mu$m; AmBisomes and ampholiposomes). Other preparations were negatively charged disks of cholesteryl sulfate–AmB at a molar ratio $1:1$ (0.12μm; ABCD), mixed micelles of lecithin and detergent containing 3–4% of AmB (EDAM and EGAM), or γ-cyclodextrin inclusion complexes of AmB ($<0.1 \mu$m). Two types of pharmacokinetic behavior could be distinguished in animal studies, depending on size and overall charge of the formulations: (1) Encapsulated antibiotic in the form of L-AmpB, L-AmpB10, ABLC, and ABCD had substantially decreased serum half-life, with an avid intake by the reticuloendothelial system. Indeed, these preparations accumulate well inside macrophages, up to 500-fold the extracellular concentration. (2) AmBisomes and ampholiposomes allowed a longer half-life of AmB in the blood stream, but were poorly concentrated in cells, less than pure

AmB, as were the mixed micelles EDAM, EGAM, and cyclodextrin inclusion complexes. In the presence of an inhibitor of the phagocytic process, the uptake of the larger liposomes was strongly reduced, suggesting that this process is responsible for the large accumulation of the drug in the macrophage. It should be emphasized that the toxicity of all these preparations is much less than that of pure AmB. In light of our results, the weaker internalization of AmBisomes, ampholiposome, EDAM, and EGAM, is sufficient to explain their weaker toxicity.

2. Other Cells

Fibroblasts: *Internalization of LDL* The LDL receptor pathway is the principal mechanism of sterol biosynthesis in cultured cells. The LDL, bound to receptors at the cell surface, is internalized, and the released cholesterol suppresses sterol synthesis. Amphotericin B binds to serum proteins and, more specifically, to cholesterol of lipoproteins. This binding results in a reduction of AmB toxicity (measured as K^+ leakage) for red blood cells, but not for *C. albicans* (43). A study with human skin fibroblasts (62), showed that there were no differences in the ability of the AmB–LDL complex to bind to the LDL receptors, nor to be internalized and degraded, when compared with native LDL. These results establish a route for AmB internalization without disruption of the pathway.

CHO Cells: *Endocytosis of AmB* Endocytosis of AmB by Chinese hamster ovary cells (CHO-K1) has been investigated using Percoll gradient separation of the plasma membrane, endosomes, and lysosomes after different incubation times with the drug (57). After 10 min, AmB was present only in the plasma membrane fraction (Table 1). After 30 and 60 min, at lower drug concentrations, AmB was localized in three fractions, with about half in plasma membrane, whereas at higher concentrations, accumulation was observed in endosomal fractions, but no longer

Table 1 Localization of AmB After Interaction with CHO-K1 Cells

AmB conc (μM)	Incubation time (min)	Plasma membrane	Endosomes	Lysosomes
		Total AmB (%)		
5–100	10	100	0	0
5	30	56	24	20
5	60	62	18	20
25	60	42	49	9
50	30	55	36	9
50	60	30	61	9

in the lysosomes. At 5°C, even after 60 min, the drug was associated with only the plasma membrane fraction: LDL receptor-mediated endocytosis was involved in this process. Observation under fluorescence microscope showed, in the presence of AmB, a great accumulation of sulforhodamine in dots scattered in the cell cytoplasm.

The first conclusion to be drawn from these experiments is that AmB is indeed endocytosed by the cells in a distinct manner, dependent on the drug concentration. The second point is that high concentrations induce an accumulation of the drug in the endosomal fraction and a decrease in the lysosomal one. This point indicates a direct effect of the polyene on the endocytotic process itself, since the transit to lysosomes is greatly reduced. These data are confirmed by the measurement of sulforhodamine accumulation in cells, observed by both microscopy and fluorescence spectrometry. Finally, we can show an accumulation of the drug in the lysosomal fraction only at low concentration of AmB or for cells grown in LDL-free medium.

The most striking point is that the increase of sulforhodamine uptake corresponded to a 90% release of cellular K^+. Indeed, it had been shown in 3T3 L1 fibroblasts (63) that receptor-mediated endocytosis was inhibited by depletion of intracellular K^+, 40% below normal by hypotonic shock. However, in rat Kupffer cells (64), the depletion of intracellular K^+ caused a marked reduction in the rate of the endocytosis of receptor-bound hyaluronan, whereas no effect was found on sucrose internalization.

This study shows that polyene antibiotics penetrate the cellular compartment and that AmB accumulates in the endosomes when cells are incubated in the presence of high concentrations of antibiotic. The results are supported by the increase of AmB concentration detected in the endosomal fraction, the increase of total uptake of a water-soluble marker, and its partition in treated and untreated cells. This event is related to the endocytotic processes: pinocytosis and receptor-mediated endocytosis. This could explain drastic metabolic changes in the cells owing to the specific properties of this molecule, in particular, permeability. At first the internalization of AmB could be related to a homeostatic mechanism for removing the drug from circulation, but as a result, the drug itself would have a drastic effect on these processes, perhaps by blocking the fusion between early endosomes.

Monocytes Accumulation of AmB in human monocytes has been proposed to be responsible for the potentiation of killing of phagocytosed *C. albicans* (58). Although it was not possible to find a difference between the levels of AmB associated with the cells at 37° and at 4°C, internalization was assumed to occur, because killing enhancement was always lower at 4°C.

VI. CONCLUSIONS AND FUTURE DIRECTIONS

Several recent studies (57,58,61,62) indicate that the internalization of AmB into mammalian cells does occur and should be considered as a possible source for the toxicity of the drug. The role of lipoproteins, to which AmB binds, seems to be essential in this mechanism. These proposals are new, insofar as AmB action has always been considered to be localized at the membrane level. Starting from this last hypothesis, numerous studies have been carried out with model membranes or erythrocytes, conditions under which it is not possible to test the role of LDL receptors. When studies were done on mammalian cells, they were often performed in lipoprotein-free media. In the small number of studies for which lipoproteins were taken into account, it was noted only that their presence partially inhibited membrane events, such as induced K^+ leakage, which is true. One can understand why the mechanism of internalization was missed.

The mechanism of endocytosis of the drug and its consequences should be refined. In particular, the following points need to be clarified:

1. The respective weight of the membrane events and endocytosis. Should induction of transmembrane permeability by AmB be considered as not relevant to in vivo toxicity, or does it contribute to it? AmB-induced lipid peroxidation is essential to membrane disruption. Does it still develop in the presence of lipoproteins?
2. The respective role of lipoproteins and their receptors. In particular, does the decrease of the number of LDL receptors at the cell surface decrease or increase AmB toxicity?
3. The extent of applicability of this mechanism to different mammalian cell types.
4. The mechanism of AmB internalization in fungal cells—does it also occur?
5. The relative importance of endocytosis and phagocytosis in the internalization of liposomal formulations.

Answers to these questions may lead to an improvement in the efficacy of AmB treatment by furnishing clues for the development of new lipid formulations of the drug and the modulation of their optimal conditions of administration.

REFERENCES

1. Gross MHP, Perfect JR. Retrospective review of amphotericin B use in a tertiary-care medical center. Am J Hosp Pharm 1987; 44:1353–1357.
2. Mazerski J, Borowski E. Influence of net charge on the aggregation and solubility behaviour of amphotericin B and its derivatives in aqueous media. Eur Biophys J 1990; 18:1–6.
3. Lamy-Freund MT, Peitzsch R, Reed WF. Characterization and time dependence of amphotericin B: deoxycholate aggregation by quasi elastic light scattering. J Pharm Sci 1991; 80:262–266.
4. Graybill JR. Overview of management of fungal infections. 2. Clin Infect Dis 1993; 17(suppl 2):S513–S514.
5. Hammond SM. Biological activity of polyene antibiotics. Prog Med Chem 1977; 14:106–179.
6. Masuda H, Tanaka T, Kido A, Kusaba I. Potentiation of cisplatin against sensitive and resistant human ovarian cancer cell line by amphotericin B. Cancer J 1991; 4:119–124.
7. Morikage T, Ohmori T, Nishio K, Fujiwara Y, Takeda Y, Saijo N. Modulation of cisplatin sensitivity and accumulation by amphotericin-B in cisplatin-resistant human lung cancer cell lines. Cancer Res 1993; 53:3302–3307.
8. Kikkawa F, Kojima M, Oguchi H, et al. Potentiating effect of amphotericin-B on five platinum anticancer drugs in human cis-diamminedichloroplatinum(II) sensitive and resistant ovarian carcinoma cells. Anticancer Res 1993; 13:891–896.
9. Medoff G, Valeriote F, Dieckman J. Potentiation of anticancer agents by amphotericin B. JNCI 1981; 6:131–135.
10. Presant CA, Bartolucci AA, Lowenbraun S. Effects of amphotericin B on combination chemotherapy of metatstatic sarcomas. Cancer 1984; 53:214–218.
11. Borer B, Sauter C. Acute myelogenous leukemia: improvement of induction, results and median survival by amphotericin B. A retrospective study of 98 patients. Cancer J 1992; 5:224–225.
12. Valeriote F, Dieckman J, Chabot, G. Schedule-dependent potentiation of lomustine cytotoxicity by amphotericin B in mice. JNCI 1986; 76:521–524.
13. Bolard J. Modulation of the immune defenses against fungi by amphotericin B and its derivatives. In: Yamaguchi H, Kobayashi GS, Takakashi H, eds. Recent Progress in Antifungal Chemotherapy. New York: Marcel Dekker, 1991:293–304.
14. Bolard J. Mechanism of action of an anti-candida drug: amphotericin B and its derivatives. In: Prasad R, ed. *Candida albicans*: Cellular and Molecular Biology. Berlin: Springer-Verlag, 1991:210–238.
15. Lin HS, Medoff G, Kobayashi GS. Effects of amphotericin B on macrophages and their precursors cells. Antimicrob Agents Chemother 1977; 11:154–158.
16. Wolf JE, Massof SE. In vitro activation of macrophage oxidative burst activity by cytokines and amphotericin B. Infect Immun 1990; 58:12296–12300.

17. Chapman H, Jand A, Hibbs JB Jr. Modulation of macrophage tumoricidal capability by polyene antibiotics: support for membrane lipid as a regulatory determinant of macrophage function. Proc Natl Acad Sci USA 1978; 75:4349–4353.

18. Perfect JR, Granger, Durack DT. Effects of antifungal agents and gamma interferon on macrophage cytotoxicity for fungi and tumor cells. J Infect Dis 1987; 156–160.

19. Vecchiarelli AVG, Perito S, Marconi P, Bistoni F. Involvement of host macrophages in the immunoadjuvant activity of amphotericin B in a mouse fungal infection model. J Antibiot 1986; 39:846–855.

20. Wilson E, Speert TL, David P. Enhancement of macrophage superoxide anion production by amphotericin B. Antimicrob Agents Chemother 1991; 35:796–800.

21. Chia JKS, Pollack M. Amphotericin B induces tumor necrosis factor production by murine macrophages. J Infect Dis 1989; 159:113–116.

22. Gelfand JA, Kimball K, Burke JF, Dinarello CA. Amphotericin B induces tumor necrosis factor and interleukin-1. Clin Res 1988; 36:456–462.

23. van't Wout J, Meynaar I, Linde I, Poell R, Mattie H, van Furth R. Effect of amphotericin B, fluconazole and itraconazole on intracellular *Candida albicans* and germ tube development in macrophages. Antimicrob Agents Chemother 1990; 25:803–814.

24. Mehta K, Claringbold P, Lopez-Berestein G. Amphotericin B inhibits the serum-induced expression of tissue transglutaminase in murine peritoneal macrophage. J Immunol 1986; 136:4206–4212.

25. Cleary JD, Chapman SW, Nolan RL. Pharmacologic modulation of interleukin-1 expression by amphotericin B-stimulated human mononuclear cells. Antimicrob Agents Chemother 1992; 36:977–981.

26. Boggs JM, Chang NH, Goundalkar A. Liposomal amphotericin B inhibits in vitro T-lymphocyte response to antigen. Antimicrob Agents Chemother 1991; 35:879–885.

27. Wolf JE, Little KD, Abegg AL, Little JR. Amphotericin B selectively stimulates macrophages from high responder mouse strains. Immunopharmacol Immunotoxicol 1991; 13:221–235.

28. Brajtburg J, Elberg S, Medoff G, Kobayashi GS. Increase in colony forming units of *Candida albicans* after treatment with polyene antibiotics. Antimicrob Agents Chemother 1981; 19:199–205.

29. Foresti M, Amati, P. Influence of amphotericin B on leucine uptake in 3T3 cells. Biochim Biophys Acta 1983; 732:251–255.

30. Kitagawa T, Andoh T. Stimulation by amphotericin B of uridine transport, RNA synthesis and DNA synthesis in density-inhibited fibroblasts. Exp Cell Res 1978; 115:37–46.

31. Rozengurt E, Mendoza S. Monovalent ion fluxes and the control of cell proliferation in cultured fibroblasts. Ann NY Acad Sci 1980; 339:175–190.

32. Brajtburg J, Elberg S, Medoff J, Kobayashi GS, Schlessinger D, Medoff G. Stimulatory, permeabilizing and toxic effects of amphotericin B on L cells. Antimicrob Agents Chemother 1984; 26:892–898.

33. Bolard J. How do the polyene macrolide antibiotics affect the cellular membrane permeability? Biochim Biophys Acta 1986; 864:257–304.

34. Binet A, Bolard J. Recovery of hepatocytes from attack by the pore former amphotericin B. Biochem J 1988; 253:435–440.

35. Malewicz B, Jenkin HW, Borowski E. Repair of membrane alterations induced in baby hamster kidney cells by polyene macrolide antibiotics. Antimicrob Agents Chemother 1981; 19:238–247.

36. Brajtburg J, Elberg S, Schwartz DR, Vertut-Croquin A, Schlessinger D, Kobayashi G, Medoff G. Involvement of oxidative damage in erythrocyte lysis induced by amphotericin B. Antimicrob Agents Chemother 1985; 27:172–176.

37. Sokol-Anderson ML, Brajtburg J, Medoff G. Amphotercin B-induced oxidative damage and killing of *Candida albicans*. J Infect Dis 1986; 154:76–82.

38. Brajtburg J, Elberg S, Kobayashi GS, Medoff G. Toxicity and induction of resistance to *Listeria monocytogenes* by amphotericin B in inbred strains of mice. Infect Immun 1986; 54:303–306.

39. Vertut-Doï A, Hannaert P, Bolard J. The polyene antibiotic amphotericin B inhibits the Na^+/K^+ pump of human erythrocytes. Biochem Biophys Res Commun 1988; 157:692–696.

40. Saways BP, Wehlprecht H, Campbell WR, Lorenz JN, Webb RC, Briggs RC, Schnermann J. Direct vasoconstriction as a possible cause for amphotericin B-induced nephrotoxicity in rats. J Clin Invest 1991; 87:2097–2107.

41. Milhaud J, Hartmann M-A, Bolard J. Interaction of the polyene antibiotic amphotericin B with model membranes: differences between small and large unilamellar vesicles. Biochimie 1989; 71:49–56.

42. Henry-Toulmé N, Séman M, Bolard J. Interaction of amphotericin B and its *N*-fructosyl derivative with murine thymocytes: a comparative study using fluorescent membrane probe. Biochim Biophys Acta 1989; 982:245–252.

43. Brajtburg J, Elberg S, Bolard J, Kobayashi GS, Levy RA, Ostlund RE, Schlessinger D, Medoff G. Interaction of plasma proteins and lipoproteins with amphotericin B. J Infect Dis 1984; 149:986–997.

44. Wasan KM, Brazeau GA, Keyhani A, Hayman A, Lopez-Berestein G. Roles of liposome composition and temperature in distribution of amphotericin B in serum lipoproteins. Antimicrob Agents Chemother 1993; 37:246–250.

45. Bolard J, Legrand P, Heitz F, Cybulska B. One-sided action of amphotericin B on cholesterol-containing membranes is determined by its self-association in the medium. Biochemistry 1991; 30:5707–5715.

46. Legrand P, Romero E, Cohen BE, Bolard J. Effects of aggregation and solvent on the activity of amphotericin B on human erythrocytes. Antimicrob Agents Chemother 1992; 36:2518–2522.

47. Lambing HE, Wolf BD, Hartsel SC. Temperature effects on the aggregation state and activity of amphotericin B. Biochim Biophys Acta 1993; 1152:185–188.

48. Ramos H, Attias de Murciano A, Cohen BE, Bolard J. The polyene antibiotic amphotericin B acts as a Ca^{2+} ionophore in sterol-containing liposomes. Biochim Biophys Acta 1989; 982:303–306.

49. Vertut-Croquin A, Brajtburg J, Medoff G. Two mechanisms of synergism when amphotericin B is used in combination with actinomycin D or 1-(2-chloroethyl)-3-cyclohexyl-1-nitrosourea against the human promyelocytic leukemia cell line HL-60. Cancer Res 1986; 46:6054–6058.

50. Wietzerbin J, Szponarski W, Borowski E, Gary-Bobo CM. Kinetic study of interaction between [^{14}C]amphotericin B derivatives and human erythrocytes: relationship between binding and induced K$^+$ leak. Biochim Biophys Acta 1990; 1026:93–98.

51. Joly V, Bolard J, Yéni P. In vitro models for studying toxicity of antifungal agents. Antimicrob Agents Chemother 1992; 36:1799–1804.

52. Henry-Toulmé N, Sarthou P, Bolard J. Early membrane potential and cytoplasmic calcium changes during mitogenic stimulation of WEHI 231 cell line by polyene antibiotics, lipopolysaccharide and anti-immunoglobulin. Biochim Biophys Acta 1990; 1051:285–292.

53. Joly V, Saint-Pierre-Chazalet M, Saint-Julien L, Bolard J, Carbon C, Yeni P. Inhibiting cholesterol synthesis reduces the binding and toxicity of AmB against rabbit renal tubular cells in primary culture. J Infect Dis 1992; 165:337–343.

54. O'Neill LJ, Miller JG, Petersen NO. Evidence of nystatin micelles in L-cells membranes from fluorescence photobleaching measurements of diffusion. Biochemistry 1986; 25:177–181.

55. Dunn WA, Connolly TP, Hubbard AL. Receptor-mediated endocytosis of epidermal growth factor by rat hepatocytes: receptor pathway. J Cell Biol 1986; 102:24–36.

56. Lippincott-Schwartz J, Fambrough DM. Lysosomal membrane dynamics: structure and inter-organellar movement of a major lysosomal membrane glycoprotein. J Cell Biol 1986; 102:1593–1605.

57. Vertut-Doï A, Bolard J, Ohnishi SI. The endocytic process in CHO cells, a toxic pathway of the polyene antibiotic amphotericin B. Antimicrob Agents Chemother 1994; 38:2373–2379.

58. Martin E, Stuben A, Gorz A, Weller U, Bhakdi S. Novel aspect of amphotericin B action: accumulation in human monocytes potentiates killing of phagocytised *Candida albicans*. Antimicrob Agents Chemother 1994; 38:13–22.

59. Sureau F, Chinsky L, Amirand C, Ballini JP, Duquesne M, Laigle A, Turpin PY, Vigny P. An ultraviolet micro-Raman spectrometer: resonance Raman spectroscopy within single living cells. Appl Spectrosc 1990; 44:1047–1051.

60. Vertut-Doï A, Legrand P, Sureau F, Seksek O, Laigle A, Chinsky L, Amirand C, Ballini JP, Turpin PY, Duquesne M, Vigny P, Bolard J. Microspectrophotometry absorption measurements at subcellular level: application to amphotericin B and benanomycin A. (submitted).

61. Legrand P, Vertut-Doï A, Bolard J. Comparative internalization and recycling of different amphotericin B formulations by macrophage-like cell line J774. (submitted).

62. Levy RA, Ostlung RE, Brajtburg J. The effects of amphotericin B on lipid metabolism in cultured human skin fibroblasts. In Vitro Cell Dev Biol 1985; 21:21–31.

                                                            Bolard and Vertut-Doï

63. Larkin JM, Brown MS, Goldstein JL, Anderson RGW. Depletion of intracellular potassium arrests coated pit formation and receptor-mediated endocytosis in fibroblasts. Cell 1983; 33:273–285.
64. Alston-Smith J, Pertoft H, Laurent TC. Endocytosis of hyaluronan in rat Kupffer cells. Biochem J 1992; 286:519–526.

12

Azole Antifungals

Patrick Boiron
Institut Pasteur, Paris, France

I. INTRODUCTION

A. Perspective and Definitions

The azole antifungals, with their broad-spectrum activity and relative lack of toxicity, are distinct from other agents, such as amphotericin B and flucytosine (5-fluorocytosine), and are the most rapidly expanding group of antifungals. These drugs have contributed significantly to the treatment of both superficial and systemic fungal infections (1).

The basic structure of the antifungal azoles is a five-membered azole ring attached by a carbon–nitrogen bond to other side chains (Fig. 1). The early imidazole antifungals, such as clotrimazole, miconazole, and econazole, showed good topical activity, but were of only limited value for systemic administration (Table 1). Ketoconazole was the first imidazole to achieve broad use for deep mycoses. It was synthesized and developed by Janssen Pharmaceutica in 1977 (2,3) and is still the most widely used systemic antifungal azole.

A major advance in the development of systemic antifungal therapy was the insertion of an extra nitrogen into the imidazole ring, creating triazoles, a class of drugs with a longer half-life, owing to decreased metabolism. In general, the triazole derivatives appear to have a broader spec-

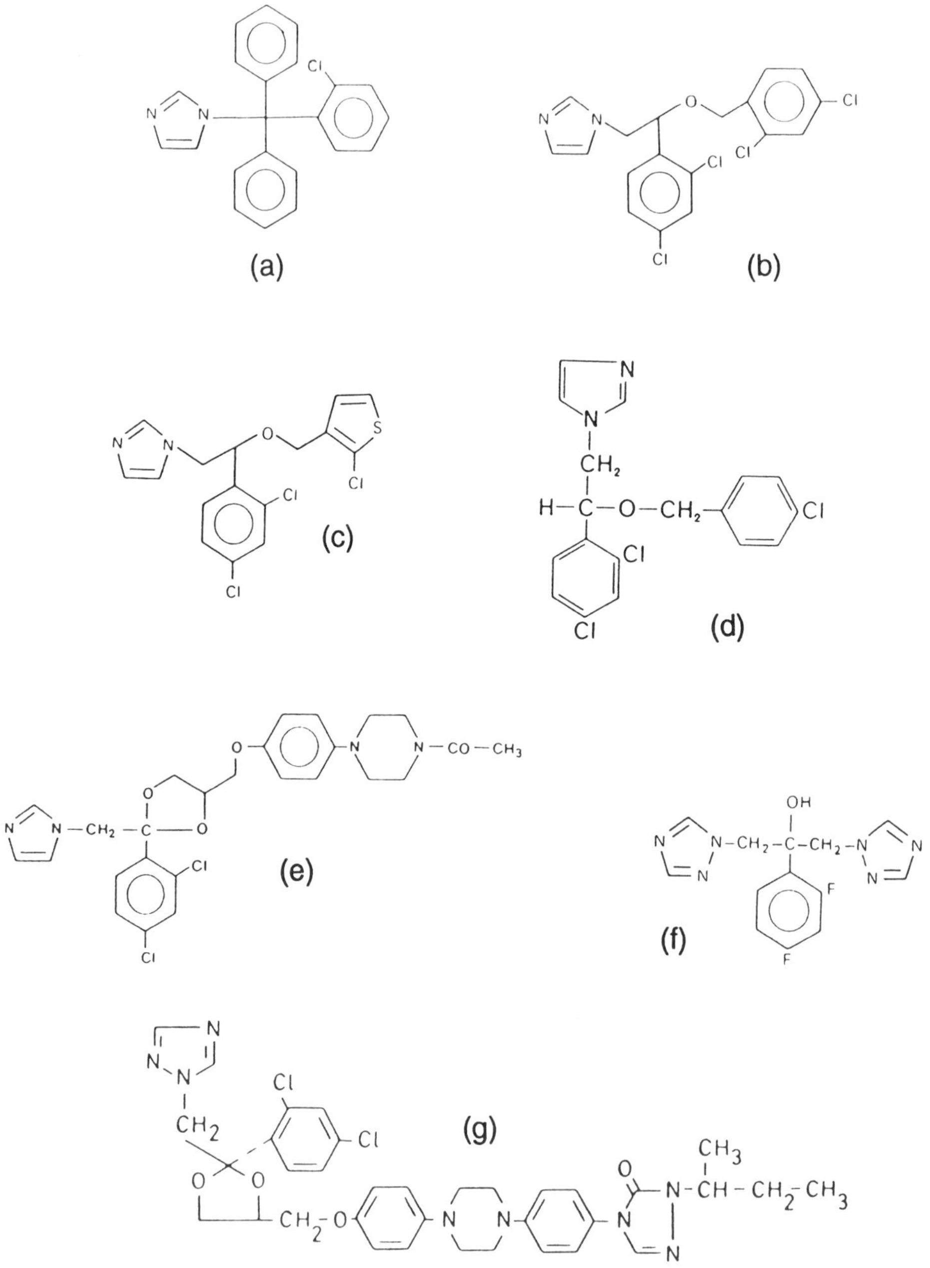

Figure 1 Chemical structure of some principal azoles. (a) clotrimazole; (b) miconazole; (c) tioconazole; (d) econazole; (e) ketoconazole; (f) fluconazole; (g) itraconazole.

Table 1 Principal Azoles Used in the Treatment of Fungal Infections

Generic name	Route of administration	Indications
Imidazoles		
Clotrimazole	Topical	Superficial fungal infections, including dermatophytoses, tinea versicolor, and cutaneous and vaginal candidiasis
Miconazole	Intravenous	Systemic fungal infections, including coccidioidomycosis, candidiasis, cryptococcosis, paracoccidioidomycosis, pseudallescheriosis, and chronic mucocutaneous candidiasis
	Topical	Superficial fungal infections, including dermatophytoses, tinea versicolor, and cutaneous and vaginal candidiasis
Econazole	Topical	Superficial fungal infections, including dermatophytoses, tinea versicolor, and cutaneous and vaginal candidiasis
Ketoconazole	Oral	Superficial fungal infections, including blastomycosis, certain forms of coccidioidomycosis and histoplasmosis, chronic mucocutaneous candidiasis, chromoblastomycosis, paracoccidioidomycosis, and pseudallescheriosis; *not* recommended for fungal meningitis
	Topical	Superficial fungal infections, including dermatophytoses and tinea versicolor
Tioconazole	Topical	Superficial fungal infections, including dermatophytoses, tinea versicolor, and cutaneous and vaginal candidiasis
Triazoles		
Fluconazole	Oral, IV	Superficial and mucosal candidiasis and cryptococcal meningitis
Itraconazole	Oral	Superficial fungal infections, including dermatophytoses, tinea versicolor,

(*continued*)

Table 1 (*Continued*)

Generic name	Route of administration	Indications
		and oral and vaginal forms of candidiasis Promising in systemic fungal infections, including aspergillosis, blastomycosis, chromoblastomycosis, histoplasmosis, paracoccidioidomycosis, and sporotrichosis

trum of antifungal activity in vivo and reduced toxicity, when compared with the imidazole group.

Fluconazole is an antifungal agent, developed by Pfizer UK, with a bistriazole structure that is remarkably different from other azole antifungal agents (4); for example, it is less lipophilic and has excellent penetration into cerebrospinal fluid and various tissues (5,6). Its long elimination half-life and other pharmacokinetic properties explain the success of this agent in the treatment of both superficial and systemic fungal infections (7,8).

Itraconazole is also a triazole antifungal agent, developed by Janssen Pharmaceutica (9). Similar to ketoconazole and fluconazole, it has excellent oral bioavailability. Its potential advantages over ketoconazole include better pharmacokinetics, a broader spectrum of antifungal activity, particularly in aspergillosis and sporotrichosis, and less toxicity.

B. Mechanism of Action and Toxicity of Azoles

1. *Mechanism of Action*

Biochemical Effects on Fungi   Early studies of miconazole and clotrimazole showed that, at *fungicidal* concentrations, these compounds directly damage the fungal cell membrane (10). At *fungistatic* concentrations, the compounds inhibit biosynthesis of ergosterol, the major sterol found in the membranes of yeasts and other fungi (11). Currently used systemic antifungal azoles—ketoconazole, itraconazole, and fluconazole—show only the second mechanism of action and thus, are exclusively fungistatic.

Ergosterol is essential for normal growth in fungi. The removal of the C-14α methyl group of lanosterol, as formic acid, is a key step in the pathway to ergosterol (fungi) or cholesterol (mammals) and is catalyzed by a cytochrome P-450-dependent lanosterol 14-demethylase system ($P450_{14DM}$) (12) that acts as a monooxygenase. Cytochrome P-450, a class of heme proteins that participate in a wide variety of important metabolic processes, is widely distributed in nature, from bacteria to higher plants and animals, and has been found in the microsomal fraction of yeasts.

Despite their varied structures, all antifungal azoles appear to have a similar major mechanism of action (i.e., inhibition of ergosterol synthesis) (12,13). This inhibition originates from the interaction of azole derivatives with microsomal cytochrome $P450_{14DM}$ (Fig. 2). Cytochrome $P450_{14DM}$

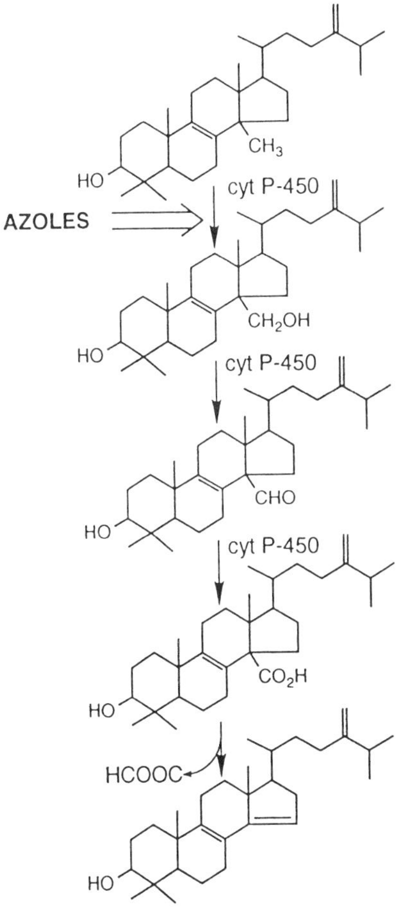

Figure 2 Mechanism of action of azole antifungals.

can be purified from microsomes after solubilization with sodium cholate in the presence of 20% glycerol, followed by precipitation with ammonium sulfate (14). The concentrated cytochrome is then chromatographed on aminohexyl-Sepharose 4B, hydroxyapatite, and CM-Sephadex C-50 columns to obtain a purified preparation. Oxidized cytochrome P-450 shows a Soret band at 417 nm and no absorption band at 650 nm. The Soret band of the reduced cytochrome P-450–carbon monoxide complex is at 448 nm.

Azole antifungals form one-to-one complexes with oxidized cytochrome $P450_{14DM}$ and induce a type II spectral change in the cytochrome (15,16); namely, a peak at about 430 nm (425–435 nm) and a trough at about 398 nm (390–405 nm). From the spectrum observed—in particular, peak 8 of the Soret band—it can be deduced that the unhindered nitrogen (i.e., N^3 in the imidazole and N^4 in the triazole ring) binds to the heme iron atom at the sixth coordination position. In the active state, this position is normally taken by the activated oxygen needed to hydroxylate the methyl group. Thus, by occupying this position, the azole derivatives inhibit the hydroxylation of the C-14α-methyl group of lanosterol, the first step in the demethylation process. The high affinity of the antifungal azoles for cytochrome $P450_{14DM}$ ($K_d < 0.01$ μM) suggests that they interact not only with the heme iron, but also at some additional site in the apoprotein (17).

The reduced form of cytochrome $P450_{14DM}$ combines avidly with carbon monoxide and forms the reduced carbon monoxide complex. The interference of azole antifungals was assessed by measuring the absorbance increment between 448 and 490 nm using an extinction coefficient of 91 $cm^{-1} \cdot mM^{-1}$ to calculate the cytochrome $P450_{14DM}$ content (17). Vanden Bossche (12) reported that azole derivatives interact with the reduced cytochrome $P450_{14DM}$, leading to interference with the appearance of the Soret band at 448 nm in the reduced carbon monoxide difference spectrum. These observations indicate that azole compounds interfere with binding of carbon monoxide to the reduced cytochrome $P450_{14DM}$ and suggest that these agents inhibit oxygen activation by cytochrome $P450_{14DM}$.

Inhibition of C-14 demethylation results in only two classes of sterols (C-4,4′,14 trimethyl and C-4,14 dimethyl) being synthesized. Assessment of the ability of antifungals to cause accumulation of C-14-methyl sterols is based on analysis of nonsaponifiable lipids (sterol and sterol precursors) (18). Azole antifungals are added at various concentrations to growing fungal cells, and sterol synthesis is followed using sodium [^{14}C]acetate or [^{14}C]mevalonate as radioactive precursors. Radioactive components are located by autoradiography or by the use of a Berthold thin-layer plate scanner, and radioactivity is assayed by scintillation counting.

Accumulation of 14α-methylated sterol intermediates and depletion of ergosterol have several effects, including inhibition of membrane-bound enzymes (19), and modulation of membrane fluidity, permeability, and transport functions (20,21). The protein components of the microsomal cytochrome $P450_{14DM}$ systems are deeply embedded in the membrane, and one of the roles of the membrane matrix in cytochrome $P450_{14DM}$ catalysis is to provide a hydrophobic environment that is suitable for the bulk of hydrophobic substrates for cytochrome $P450_{14DM}$ (22).

There is convincing evidence that some imidazole antifungals have two distinct antifungal actions. At low concentrations, and in common with all azole derivatives, they inhibit sterol synthesis, resulting in fungistasis, whereas at higher concentrations, and depending on growth phase, they damage fungal cell membranes directly, and are fungicidal, as was demonstrated with miconazole and clotrimazole, but not with ketoconazole (23). Some secondary effects of azoles may be drug-specific, such as inhibition of cytochrome c peroxidase and catalase, leading to accumulation of hydrogen peroxide (24), blocking electron transport in the respiratory chain (25,26), and inhibition of hyphae formation.

The greater affinity of some azole derivatives for cytochrome $P450_{14DM}$ of yeast, relative to mammalian microsomes, may be partly due to a tighter association of these antifungals with the fungal membrane. However, other factors could also be involved in this selectivity, such as interaction of the nonligating portion of antifungal azoles with lipophilic subsites(s) on the cytochrome $P450_{14DM}$ apoprotein. The architecture of the binding site could be different, or the phospholipids in the membrane could provide a different environment for the enzyme to bind the azole drug (13).

Synergy with the Host Immune System Polymorphonuclear leukocytes and monocytes are important components of the host defense system against fungal infections. The synergism between phagocytic cell functions and antifungal drugs is often crucial to the successful treatment of these infections, particularly in immunosuppressed patients. There is evidence that there may be a synergistic action between ketoconazole and polymorphonuclear cells, with subsequent enhanced killing of fungi by host defense cells (27,28). This may explain the effectiveness of ketoconazole in eradicating some deep candidal infections, since plasma concentrations of the antifungal agent that are inhibitory to both growth and germ tube formation in *Candida albicans* are readily achievable after a single daily dose (20).

It has been demonstrated that the dimorphic yeast *C. albicans* may resist intracellular killing by phagocytes through the formation of germ tubes inside the phagocytes (29). Thus, antifungal agents that inhibit intracellular germ tube formation could facilitate the host defense against *C. albicans*. Fluconazole and itraconazole inhibited significantly, although incompletely, germ tube formation of *C. albicans* cells both in macrophages and extracellularly. Accordingly, it has been suggested that an in vitro test that uses the mycelial form of *C. albicans* might provide a better indication of the therapeutic value of the azole antifungal agents than a test in which the inoculum is the blastospore (yeast) form (30).

2. Toxicity of Azoles

Ketoconazole   A variety of adverse effects of ketoconazole have been reported, such as toxicity and interactions with other drugs. Dose-related nausea and vomiting have limited use of this drug at dosages above 400 mg daily. This common side effect occurs in up to 50% of patients receiving oral doses of more than 800 mg, but can be reduced by giving the drug with food or at bedtime.

High dosages of ketoconazole ($\geq$ 800 mg daily) depress certain endocrine functions, particularly testosterone and adrenocorticoids, the biosyntheses of which also involve cytochrome P-450-dependent enzymes (31). Clinical manifestations of interference with testosterone synthesis include gynecomastia, impotence, and loss of hair. High-dose ketoconazole should be avoided in patients with tuberculosis, histoplasmosis, paracoccidioidomycosis, or AIDS, as it can aggravate these infections, which are often associated with hypoadrenalism.

The most concerning dose-limiting adverse reaction is serious, even fatal, hepatoxicity (32), that occurs at an incidence of 1:10,000–1:15,000 (33,34). Most cases have been reported in patients treated for onychomycosis or chronic recalcitrant dermatophytosis. It requires the vigilance of physicians, even though this adverse reaction has proved rare and is usually reversible within several months following discontinuation of ketoconazole treatment (35). In animal toxicity studies, rats treated with ketoconazole showed hepatomegaly, accompanied by liver vacuolation and cell necrosis (36). Deposition of lipofuscin, an end product of lipid peroxidation, was reported in the adrenal glands, lymph nodes, thymus, and ovaries, as well as in liver, where it may initiate the development of toxigenic liver cell injury.

Serum levels of ketoconazole are substantially reduced in patients receiving rifampin, isoniazid, cimetidine, ranitidine, or drugs that reduce gastric acid secretion (antacids, anticholinergics, H_2-antagonists). Ketoconazole can also raise serum levels of other drugs, such as cyclosporine and warfarin.

Fluconazole   Fluconazole appears to be a well-tolerated, almost nontoxic, azole derivative (37). Minor side effects, such as nausea and vomiting, occur in a few patients. Therapeutic dose level of fluconazole administered long-term did not affect adrenal or testicular steroid metabolism.

Fluconazole had activity comparable with that of ketoconazole in the inhibition of fungal C-14 demethylase (i.e., inhibition of ergosterol biosynthesis), but was significantly less potent in the inhibition of the mammalian enzymes (38). In animal models, it was less potent than ketoconazole in liver enzyme induction, inhibition of steroid biosynthesis, and induction of fetal malformations and teratological effects. When fluconazole was administered orally to mice, rats, and dogs, only the liver showed microscopically detectable changes, with minimal increases in fat (37). Small increases in weight, cytochrome $P450_{14DM}$, and proliferation of the smooth endoplasmic reticulum were also observed at the higher dose levels. At the highest doses, there was a slight increase in plasma transaminase levels in the high-dose groups in the mice, rats, and dogs, that was reversible in the former after drug withdrawal. This suggests the presence of a minimal cytotoxic injury. In other studies, fluconazole was not mutagenic or teratogenic, even at dose levels that were toxic to the mother.

Several drug interactions have been reported for fluconazole. Phenytoin serum concentration can increase to toxic levels, presumably owing to inhibition of phenytoin metabolism (39). Cyclosporine concentration in blood has also been reported to be elevated in patients receiving fluconazole (40). Fluconazole can potentiate the anticoagulant effect of warfarin and prolong the serum half-life of chlorpropamide, glibenclamide, glipizide, and tolbutamide.

Itraconazole Itraconazole has the same spectrum of adverse effects, with less nausea and virtually no adrenal or testicular steroid suppression. Other minor side effects, such as headache and abdominal pain, occur in a few patients. Hepatitis and adverse drug interactions also appear to be infrequent (approximately 1:12,000 patients). Transient asymptomatic elevations of liver function tests have been seen in a few patients. It is advisable not to give the drug to patients with liver disease, or to patients who have experienced hepatotoxic reactions with other drugs. The necessity for oral administration remains a substantial limitation in cases of deep candidiasis in patients with severe mucositis, abdominal surgery, sedation, or nausea; or of cryptococcal meningitis, in patients with nausea, confusion, or obtundation.

From toxicity studies, the potential drug-specific target in both rats and dogs was the mononuclear phagocytosing cell system and the adrenal glands (41). These effects might be therapeutically important, since many systemic fungal infections are accompanied by mononuclear cell infiltrations or by granuloma formation. No alterations of hepatic structure and function in dogs was observed up to high-dose levels, indicating that itraconazole was less hepatotoxic than ketoconazole. Teratogenicity studies showed that itraconazole at high-dose levels was embryotoxic and teratogenic in rats, but not in rabbit, similar to ketoconazole. Therefore, itraconazole is absolutely contraindicated in pregnant women. Mutagenicity studies showed that itraconazole has no genotoxic potential in nonmammalian and mammalian test systems.

Itraconazole concentrations are decreased following concomitant administration of phenytoin, rifampicin, antacids, and H_2-antagonists. Administration of itraconazole leads to elevations in concentration of cyclosporine, digoxin, and terfenadine, the latter resulting rarely in life-threatening cardiac dysrhythmias. It has been reported that itraconazole enhances the anticoagulant effect of warfarin.

C. Antifungal Activity Spectrum and Potential in Cancer Chemotherapy

1. Antifungal Activity Spectrum

Ketoconazole   Ketoconazole is a broad-spectrum antifungal agent active against a variety of pathogenic fungi, including *Blastomyces dermatitidis*, *Coccidioides immitis*, *Histoplasma capsulatum*, *Paracoccidioides brasiliensis*, and *Candida* species (42,43).

Ketoconazole has proved useful in certain forms of histoplasmosis (particularly in disseminated and chronic pulmonary forms), blastomycosis, paracoccidioidomycosis, petriellidiosis, some forms of coccidioidomycosis, and chronic mucocutaneous candidiasis. It should not be used for the *oral* treatment of dermatophytosis, such as griseofulvin-resistant ringworm of the glabrous skin, or relapsing cases of vulvovaginal candidiasis, because of its possible effects on the liver and on steroid metabolism. However, it could be a useful *topical* drug for dermatophytoses, cutaneous candidiasis, pityriasis versicolor, and seborrheic dermatitis. Ketoconazole is rarely useful in aspergillosis, mucormycosis, sporotrichosis, and deep candidiasis.

Shadomy et al. demonstrated that there was no apparent clinical emergence of ketoconazole-resistant fungi, although in vitro data did not necessarily correlate with the clinical outcome of treatment (44). As with many other ergosterol synthesis inhibitors, in vitro activity of ketoconazole is affected by several factors, including pH, culture medium, presence of serum, temperature and time of incubation, and growth phase of the fungus (45,46).

Fluconazole   Fluconazole has a broad activity spectrum, including *Blastomyces dermatitidis*, *Coccidioides immitis*, *Cryptococcus neoformans*, *Histoplasma capsulatum*, and *Paracoccidioides brasiliensis*. It is active against *Candida albicans*, *C. tropicalis*, and *C. parapsilosis*, but many strains of *C. krusei* and *C. glabrata* (previously classified as *Torulopsis glabrata*) appear to be resistant. Fluconazole appears to be ineffective against *Aspergillus* and Mucorales species. It is active against dermatophytes. Resistant strains of *C. albicans* have been recovered from AIDS patients receiving long-term treatment with fluconazole for oropharyngeal or esophageal candidiasis (47).

Fluconazole is indicated for the treatment of acute cryptococcal meningitis and can be used as maintenance treatment to prevent relapse of cryptococcosis in AIDS patients. It can also be used to treat oropharyngeal and cutaneous forms of candidiasis.

Itraconazole Itraconazole has been used successfully to treat a variety of deep-seated mycoses in animals and humans, including those achieved by ketoconazole, and additionally in some patients, invasive aspergillosis and cutaneous sporotrichosis. It appears to be a useful drug in blastomycosis, chromoblastomycosis, histoplasmosis, paracoccidioidomycosis, and perhaps coccidioidomycosis. In animal models, itraconazole has been effective in the treatment of cryptococcal meningitis, despite undetectable drug levels in the cerebrospinal fluid (48). These studies were confirmed in human cases of cryptococcal meningitis (49). Possible explanations for the efficacy of itraconazole in the treatment of central nervous system infections include immune stimulation of host cells, or intracellular accumulation of drug not detectable in drug assays of biological fluids (50).

2. *Potential in Cancer Chemotherapy*

Interestingly, the endocrine effects of ketoconazole have suggested a new use for the drug: the treatment of prostatic cancer (51,52). Administration of exogenous estrogens in the treatment of advanced prostatic cancer has proved successful in lowering circulating levels of testosterone and inducing a clinical remission. However, the use of estrogens is associated with undesirable side effects, such as a marked increase in morbidity and mortality, owing to an increased incidence of thromboembolic events.

Among nonestrogenic drugs, such as progestational agents, agonist analogues of the luteinizing hormone-releasing hormone, and antiandrogens, found to confer the anticancer benefits of estrogens, without the associated side effects, none has proved superior to estrogens. Ketoconazole has been demonstrated to reduce adrenal and testicular androgen production in animals and men (53). This agent markedly reduces adrenal as well as testicular androgen production, which might confer a survival advantage to patients. High-dosage ketoconazole therapy (400 mg every 8 h) may induce and maintain a remission in patients with advanced prostatic cancer. By 24 h of treatment, serum testosterone had decreased to the castrate level, the adrenal androgens—androstenedione and dihydroepiandrosterone—were also reduced significantly, and 17-hydroxyprogesterone, luteinizing hormone, and follicle-stimulating hormone were increased. By 1 week of treatment, clinical response was observed and side effects (weakness and lethargy) were few.

II. METHODS FOR MEASURING CELL UPTAKE OF AZOLES

The ability of azole antifungal agents to penetrate and accumulate within fungal cells and phagocytic and nonphagocytic cells, although critical to their mechanism of action and resistance, has not been extensively studied. For fungal pathogens, studies have focused so far on the intracellular accumulation of ketoconazole in *C. albicans*. For mammalian cells, several studies were performed with itraconazole and fluconazole. Various types of cells were investigated, such as polymorphonuclear leukocytes, macrophages (monocytes), and epithelial cells.

Determination of antifungal uptake can be obtained by measuring cellular drug concentration in comparison with extracellular concentration (54). The easiest way of determination is based on use of radiolabeled antifungal agent. Cells are incubated in medium containing several concentrations of radiolabeled drug. After different incubation periods, cells are separated from the extracellular solution by filtration or centrifugation. In the filtration method, samples of the incubation mixture are removed at time intervals, filtered on filters compatible with radioactivity measurement, washed with a solution of unlabeled drug at high concentration to completely remove the unbound labeled compound, and then with sterile distilled water, and filters are counted for radioactivity (55). The cells can also be separated from the extracellular solution by a velocity gradient centrifugation technique, described by Klempner and Styrt (56). Centrifugation is performed through a water-impermeable silicone–oil barrier in a microcentrifuge tube. An aliquot of the extracellular medium and the entire cell pellet, obtained by cutting off the portion of the microcentrifuge tube containing the pellet, are counted in a liquid scintillation counter.

The intracellular water space must be previously measured by using tritiated water, since calculation of cellular drug concentration is based on intracellular volume. This can be estimated by adding radiolabeled water to the cell suspensions, allowing the suspensions to reach equilibrium, and then directly counting the unincorporated radioactivity in the supernatant. All intracellular volume is assumed to be available for uptake: this is not entirely accurate because, in most biological systems, the intracellular fluids account for approximately 80% of the cell volume. From the values obtained by these procedures, cell-associated concentrations of antimicrobial agents can be calculated and expressed as the ratio of intracellular to extracellular concentration (C/E).

A. Determination of Ketoconazole Uptake by *Candida albicans*

Cells must be incubated with [³H]ketoconazole at a concentration equal to the minimal inhibitory concentration (MIC) previously determined for the strain tested (55). The cell–ketoconazole mixture is incubated at 37°C, or at the optimal growth temperature for the fungus being tested.

Elucidation of the mechanism of ketoconazole uptake requires the determination of several characteristics; for example, the necessity of cell viability (to determine if the drug penetration is a passive or active phenomenon), the effect of temperature and pH, and the effectiveness of various metabolic inhibitors, such as sodium azide, sodium fluoride, or 2,4-dinitrophenol. The use of various metabolic inhibitors, such as sodium fluoride, an inhibitor of glycolysis; sodium azide, an inhibitor of oxidized cytochrome oxidase; and 2,4-dinitrophenol, an uncoupler of oxidative phosphorylation, can further elucidate the active transport system involved in [³H]ketoconazole uptake.

Displacement of intracellular [³H]ketoconazole can also be attempted using high concentrations of unlabeled ketoconazole or other antifungal agents (clotrimazole, miconazole, econazole, itraconazole, amphotericin B, or flucytosine).

Kinetic analysis of ketoconazole accumulation in cells also needs to be performed by exposing the cells to a wide range of drug concentration for a short time (e.g., 2 min). The velocity of transport is determined for each concentration, after subtraction of the energy-independent uptake and binding as measured on killed cells, and by construction of a double-reciprocal (Lineweaver–Burk) plot of uptake velocity versus concentration.

Displacement of other intracellular azoles can similarly be attempted on cells that have been incubated in buffer containing radiolabeled azole, by the addition of unlabeled drug to the incubation mixture.

B. Determination of Fluconazole and Itraconazole Uptake by Mammalian Cells

Polymorphonuclear leukocytes may be recovered from heparinized venous blood of healthy donors. Alveolar macrophages can be obtained by lung lavage from rabbits that had received *Mycobacterium bovis* BCG intravenously (57). Tissue culture epithelial cells can be obtained from human synovial fluid (58).

Polymorphonuclear leukocytes, macrophages, and epithelial cells are incubated in Hanks' balanced salt solution containing different concentrations of radioactive antifungal drug. Cells are layered over a phthalate bed in microcentrifuge tubes and incubated in 5% CO_2 at 37°C, generally for 10 min (57). The cells are pelleted through phthalate and lysed in a 0.5% deoxycholate solution. Radioactivity is then measured in the supernatants and lysed cells.

To elucidate the mechanism of fluconazole uptake, the effect of cell viability must be studied by using cells killed by exposure to 10% formalin. The influence of temperature, pH, metabolic inhibitors (sodium fluoride, an inhibitor of glycolysis; sodium cyanide, an inhibitor of mitochondrial oxidative metabolism; carbonylcyanide-*m*-chlorophenylhydrazone, a blocker of the proton gradient; 2,4-dinitrophenol, an uncoupler of oxidative phosphorylation) and potential competitive inhibitors should also be evaluated.

For a quantitative measurement of biological activity of intracellular itraconazole, alveolar macrophages are incubated with high concentrations of drug for 2 h, washed extensively, and then lysed. Itraconazole concentration in the lysate is assayed by placing the lysate into agar wells with *Candida* spp. added to the medium as an index organism.

III. UPTAKE AND EFFLUX

A. Characterization of Ketoconazole Uptake in *Candida albicans*

Although the metabolism and antifungal effect of ketoconazole have been extensively studied, little is known about the cellular penetration of this drug. Studies designed to evaluate [³H]ketoconazole uptake revealed that it is an active, energy-requiring process; it is characterized by a requirement for cellular viability, physiological temperature (37°C) and, at least in part, glycolytically derived energy (55).

The uptake of [³H]ketoconazole is rapid: more than 30% enters the cells within the first minute, and 60% of the total uptake occurs during the first 10 min. [³H]Ketoconazole is concentrated by cells: the maximal intracellular concentration reached is nearly 80 times the extracellular concentration within the 30-min incubation period.

The dependence of drug uptake on cell viability is suggestive of an active transport of [³H]ketoconazole. Moreover, the effect of changing incubation temperature on [³H]ketoconazole uptake (at low extracellular concentrations, drug accumulation is slower at 27° than at 37°C; Fig. 3A), adds support to the notion that an active metabolic process concentrates drug in cells. Among various metabolic inhibitors used to elucidate the active transport system involved in [³H]ketoconazole uptake, sodium flu-

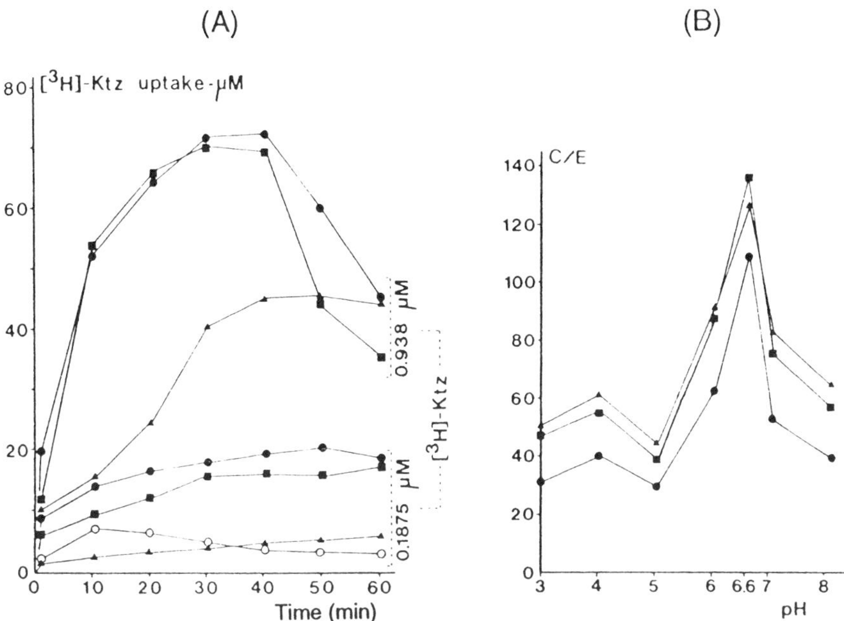

Figure 3 Dependence of [³H]ketoconazole (Ktz) uptake on (A) temperature and cell viability; (B) pH. [³H]Ketoconazole concentration: 0.1875 mM.

oride significantly reduced uptake at low extracellular drug concentration, whereas sodium azide and 2,4-dinitrophenol had no effect. The uptake of [³H]ketoconazole is pH-dependent; intracellular concentration is maximal at pH 6.6 (see Fig. 3B) (59).

A double-reciprocal (Lineweaver–Burk) plot of uptake velocity versus concentration showed [³H]ketoconazole uptake to be saturable and characterized by a high binding affinity (K_m = 50 nM) and a high maximum velocity (V_{max} = 1.4 mol/min per 10^{-7} cells) for concentrations equal to or lower than the MIC. The saturability of drug uptake suggests a carrier-mediated transport. At higher concentrations, [³H]ketoconazole enters cells by a simple diffusion process, as evidenced by the lack of effect on drug uptake with sodium fluoride.

[³H]Ketoconazole appears tightly—possibly covalently—bound to cellular component(s). Unlabeled ketoconazole added at concentration 100- to 500-fold greater than that of [³H]ketoconazole did not result in significant efflux of the labeled drug. Efflux experiments with other antifungal drugs (clotrimazole, miconazole, econazole, itraconazole, amphotericin B, flucytosine) revealed that the [³H]ketoconazole remains bound to C.

albicans cells. Moreover, all these drugs, particularly amphotericin B, increased [^{3}H]ketoconazole uptake when used at subinhibitory concentrations. This last effect is not surprising with amphotericin B, which has been shown to facilitate the entry of the second agent into the fungal cell when used in combination (60,61).

B. Characterization of Fluconazole and Itraconazole Uptake in Mammalian Cells

1. *Fluconazole*

Fluconazole rapidly penetrates into polymorphonuclear leukocytes and macrophages, the maximal cellular concentration being reached within 7 min. The maximal intracellular concentrations were twice as high as the extracellular ones (58,62). The intracellular penetration of fluconazole was significantly higher when formalin-killed cells were used. Temperature, pH, or different metabolic inhibitors did not affect fluconazole uptake. The kinetics of efflux revealed that the reversibility of fluconazole binding is rapid, with 83% of the cell-associated drug being lost by 5 min. Phagocytosis (ingestion of opsonized *C. albicans* or zymosan) or other cell membrane stimuli (phorbol myristate acetate) do not affect the penetration of fluconazole.

After 4 h, at concentrations between 5 and 20 μg/ml), fluconazole did not significantly affect the intracellular survival of *C. albicans* in polymorphonuclear leukocytes and macrophages. However, the germination of blastospores was significantly reduced in polymorphonuclear leukocytes, and in macrophages a marked reduction in the elongation of the germ tubes was observed. After a 24-h incubation, fluconazole prevented the formation of mycelia and significantly reduced the growth of the phagocytosed fungi in macrophages. By comparison, amphotericin B showed significant intracellular activity at concentrations of 2 and 10 mg/L, completely blocking germ tube formation of *C. albicans*. All these data indicate that the uptake of fluconazole by leukocytes probably occurs by a passive mechanism, in line with its high lipid solubility. The fluconazole that becomes cell associated is still recoverable in a fully active form.

The distribution of fluconazole in the various compartments of human phagocytic cells has been investigated by electron microscopic autoradiography (63). Quantitative analysis of electron micrographs after incubation with 4 μg/ml of [^{3}H]fluconazole at 37°C for 10 min revealed a nonrandom distribution of silver grains. Compared with the surrounding resin, grain density in neutrophil polymorphonuclear leukocytes and monocytes was respectively 5- and 20-fold higher. This result demonstrates that fluconazole penetrates the cell membrane and reaches the intracellular space of the phagocytic cells. Moreover, silver grains were evenly distributed over cytoplasm and nucleus. Thus, the antimycotic activity of the compound necessary for the control of ingested fungi appears to be available where it is required.

2. *Itraconazole*

The uptake of itraconazole by alveolar macrophages is both rapid and passive (57; i.e., it is not an active, energy-requiring process). Varying the pH of the medium (from 4 to 9) or temperature (from 4° to 37°C) has no substantial effect on the uptake.

In the presence of 5% serum in the medium, the ratio of intracellular to extracellular drug concentration is approximately 18, compared with a ratio of over 70 in cells placed in serum-free medium. This significant effect of serum on itraconazole uptake can be explained by the presence of proteins that bind over 90% of the drug. When cells are placed in 100% serum, drug accumulation continues, despite competitive binding by extracellular serum proteins, but the uptake ratio drops further to 3 (57).

Itraconazole does not require live cells for uptake, since formalin-treated cells accumulate drug. Metabolic inhibitors, such as carboxylcyanide-*m*-chlorophenylhydrazone (CCCP), and potassium fluoride, do not change uptake of itraconazole by viable macrophages. Very little itraconazole is spontaneously released from the cells after uptake. When intact, viable macrophages are examined for efflux of entrapped itraconazole over a 60-min period, less than 1% of drug is released into the medium. By comparison, clindamycin is continuously released from the cells into the extracellular medium over this period. These data suggest a primary physicochemical interaction of itraconazole, such as simple partitioning of this hydrophobic compound into the lipid bilayer, rather than a specific receptor-mediated event, or an active metabolic process, such as occurs with clindamycin.

Itraconazole appears to facilitate its own binding to cells. When cells are preincubated with unlabeled itraconazole, there is a two- to fourfold increase in intracellular uptake of [^{3}H]itraconazole in the presence of cold drug. The facilitated accumulation may account for its uptake ratio being higher than those of other lipid-soluble antimicrobial agents.

Finally, pathogenic fungi may face a much higher concentration of itraconazole when they are taken up by host cells than is present in extracellular fluids, such as serum and cerebrospinal fluid. This result may help explain its effectiveness in infections, despite its low levels in biological fluids.

IV. TRANSPORT-ASSOCIATED AZOLE RESISTANCE

Since the introduction of the azole antifungal agents in the early 1970s, only a few *C. albicans* strains resistant to these drugs have been described (64–70). Most isolates were from patients with chronic mucocutaneous candidiasis who relapsed after prolonged treatment with ketoconazole. Further studies suggest that resistance was due to change in the properties of the cell membrane (71). Two azole-resistant isolates contained more nonesterified sterol, resulting in a phospholipid/sterol ratio of about half that of azole-susceptible isolates (72). The mechanism of resistance of another isolate (73), was investigated. The drug target, cytochrome $P450_{14DM}$, was less susceptible to the triazole antifungal agent ICI 153,066, but this property did not correlate quantitatively with growth inhibition (74). Isolates from the same patient contained much higher amounts of fecosterol relative to the amounts in susceptible isolates (75). Another isolate was less susceptible (66) and had an altered cytochrome $P450_{14DM}$, with reduced affinity for miconazole, ketoconazole, itraconazole, and fluconazole (76). Although the antifungal activity of ketoconazole can be influenced by its ability to enter fungal cells (11), it is not known to what extent the emergence of azole-resistant fungal isolates is associated with decreased transport (71).

Since the introduction of fluconazole in clinical practice in the mid-1980s, the number of resistant yeast strains appears to be increasing. A *C. albicans* strain, isolated from a patient with AIDS, was resistant to fluconazole (68), but remained susceptible to ketoconazole and itraconazole. Decreased susceptibility to fluconazole has been described in four AIDS patients with oropharyngeal or esophageal candidiasis (77). Clinical resistance to fluconazole has been observed in some patients treated orally with 50 mg of fluconazole per day to 400 mg/day intravenously (78). Five other *C. albicans* isolates resistant to fluconazole were obtained from patients after 4–36 months of treatment (79).

Resistant strains are rare in clinical practice and difficult to obtain in the laboratory (67,76). The *diploid* nature of *C. albicans* and the absence of a known sexual cycle are suspected to be the major reasons. In contrast, a strain of the *haploid* yeast *C. glabrata* that had become resistant to fluconazole after 9 days of treatment with 400 mg once daily was isolated (70), and resistance to azole antifungal agents can be induced more readily in this species (80,81).

In an attempt to elucidate the mechanism of resistance, differences in uptake, efflux, or intracellular distribution of drug between azole-resistant and azole-susceptible strains were measured. In one study, *C. glabrata* cells were unable to take up [^{3}H]fluconazole (82). Moreover, fluconazole potency against demethylase in lysates from resistant cells was very similar to that in lysates from susceptible cells. These results suggested that resistance was due to a permeability barrier to fluconazole, rather than to changes in the target P450$_{14DM}$ enzyme. The phospholipid/nonesterified sterol ratio may considerably influence the physical and biochemical properties of membranes and could change membrane fluidity. This was suggested after comparing ICI 153,066 uptake in yeast and mycelial forms of different strains of *C. albicans* (83).

In contrast, in another study, fluconazole entered into both types of cells of *C. glabrata* (69). Although the cellular fluconazole content was 1.5- to 3-fold lower in resistant than in susceptible cells, the difference in the fluconazole content between the two types of strains was lower than the susceptibility difference. Moreover, when the azole-resistant strain was repeatedly subcultured on drug-free medium, both cytochrome P450$_{14DM}$ content and ergosterol synthesis decreased, concomitantly with increased susceptibility to itraconazole and, more slightly, to fluconazole. Thus, a mechanism in addition to decreased drug uptake may be involved in fungal resistance to azoles. The fact that ergosterol synthesis in subcellular fractions of the azole-resistant strain was 2.4-fold less sensitive to itraconazole than in the azole-susceptible strain suggests that differences in the target P450$_{14DM}$ enzyme may be responsible for resistance. The resistant strain synthesized more lanosterol from squalene or mevalonate than did the susceptible strain. Increased ergosterol synthesis, together with decreased sensitivity to demethylase inhibitors, may result from a higher constitutive demethylase level, or from induced overexpression of the enzyme. Consequently, higher concentrations of inhibitors of ergosterol biosynthesis, especially P450$_{14DM}$, would be required to inhibit ergosterol synthesis and fungal growth.

V. CONCLUSIONS AND FUTURE DIRECTIONS

The synthetic azole derivatives are characterized by an *N*-substituted imidazole or triazole group as the reactive functional moiety, linked to a hydrophobic moiety that may contribute to the interaction of the drug with the plasma membrane. The primary target of these compounds is the cytochrome P450$_{14DM}$, involved in the 14α-demethylation of lanosterol. The result is inhibition of ergosterol biosynthesis in susceptible fungi and accumulation of methylated sterol intermediates that, in turn, adversely affect the permeability and transport functions of the cytoplasmic membrane and lead to inhibition of growth and, eventually, cell death.

Less well understood are the secondary antifungal effects of azoles that range from inhibition of ATPase, cytochrome c oxidase, and peroxidase, to physicochemical damage of the membrane barrier function. Some of these effects are not common to all azole derivatives. Nevertheless, they may be relevant to their overall mechanism of action and resistance and, thus, need to be sorted out. In addition, systematic studies are needed to address the contribution of membrane permeability to the mechanism of action and resistance of azole derivatives in different fungal pathogens. Such studies may lead to useful structure–permeability relationships and, eventually, to the development of more potent azole antifungals.

REFERENCES

1. Fromtling RA. Overview of medically important antifungal azole derivatives. Clin Microbiol Rev 1988; 1:187–217.
2. Heeres J, Backx LJJ, Mostmans JH, et al. Antimycotic imidazoles. 4. Synthesis and antifungal activity of ketoconazole, a new potent orally active broad-spectrum antifungal agent. J Med Chem 1979; 22:1003–1005.
3. Thienpont D, Van Cutsem J, Van Gerven F, et al. Ketoconazole, a broad-spectrum orally active antimycotic. Experientia 1979; 35:606–607.
4. Henderson JT. Fluconazole—a significant advance in the management of human fungal disease. In: Fromtling RA, ed. Recent Trends in the Discovery, Development and Evaluation of Antifungal Agents. Barcelona: JR Prous Science Publishers, 1987:77–79.
5. Humphrey MJ, Jevons S, Tarbit MH. Pharmacokinetics of UK-49,858, a metabolically stable triazole antifungal drug in animals and humans. Antimicrob Agents Chemother 1985; 28:648–653.
6. Rogers TE, Galgiani JN. Activity of fluconazole (UK 49,858) and ketoconazole against *Candida albicans* in vitro and in vivo. Antimicrob Agents Chemother 1986; 30:418–422.
7. Sugar AM, Saunders C. Oral fluconazole as suppressive therapy of disseminated cryptococcosis in patients with acquired immunodeficiency syndrome. Am J Med 1988; 85:481–489.
8. Wit S, de Goosens H, Weert D, et al. Comparison of fluconazole and ketoconazole for oropharyngeal candidiasis in AIDS. Lancet 1989; 1:746–747.
9. Heeres J, Backx LJJ, Van Cutsem J. Antimycotic azoles. 7. Synthesis and antifungal properties of a series of novel triazol-3-ones. J Med Chem 1984; 27:894–900.
10. Taylor FR, Rodriques RJ, Parks LW. Relationship between antifungal activity and inhibition of sterol biosynthesis in miconazole, clotrimazole, and 15-azasterol. Antimicrob Agents Chemother 1983; 23:515–521.
11. Pye GW, Marriott MS. Inhibition of sterol C14-demethylation by imidazole-containing antifungals. Sabouraudia 1982; 20:325–331.
12. Vanden Bossche H. Biochemical targets for antifungal azole derivatives:

hypothesis on the mode of action. In: McGinnis MR, ed. Current Topics in Medical Mycology. Vol 1. New-York: Springer-Verlag, 1985:313–351.

13. Vanden Bossche H. Itraconazole: a selective inhibitor of the cytochrome P-450-dependent ergosterol biosynthesis. In: Fromtling RA, ed. Recent Trends in the Discovery, Development and Evaluation of Antifungal Agents. Barcelona, JR Prous Science Publishers, 1987:207–221.

14. Yoshida Y, Aoyama Y. Yeast cytochrome P450 catalyzing lanosterol 14α-demethylation. I. Purification and spectral properties. J Biol Chem 1984; 259:1655–1660.

15. Vanden Bossche H, Willemsens G, Marichal P, et al. The molecular basis for the antifungal activities of *N*-substituted azole derivatives. Focus on R51 211. In: Trinci APJ, Riley JF, eds. Mode of Action of Antifungal Agent. Symposium of the British Mycological Society, Cambridge: Cambridge University Press, 1984:321–341.

16. Yoshida Y, Aoyama Y. Interaction of azole fungicides with yeast cytochrome P450 which catalyzes lanosterol 14-demethylation. In: Iwata K, Vanden Bossche H, eds. In Vitro and In Vivo Evaluation of Antifungal Agents. Amsterdam: Elsevier Science Publishers, 1986:123–134.

17. Yoshida Y. Cytochrome P450 of fungi: primary target for azole antifungal agents. In McGinnis MR, ed. Current Topics in Medical Mycology. Vol. 2. New York, Springer-Verlag, 1988:388–418.

18. Marriott MS. Inhibition of sterol biosynthesis in *Candida albicans* by imidazole-containing antifungals. J Gen Microbiol 1980; 117:253–255.

19. Surarit R, Shepherd MG. The effects of azole and polyene antifungals on the plasma membrane enzymes of *Candida albicans*. J Med Vet Mycol 1987; 25:403–413.

20. Borgers M, Vanden Bossche H, De Brabander M. The mechanism of action of the new antimycotic ketoconazole. Am J Med 1983; 74(suppl 1B):2–8.

21. Vanden Bossche H, Willemsens G, Cools W, et al. Biochemical effects of miconazole on fungi. II. Inhibition of ergosterol biosynthesis in *Candida albicans*. Chem Biol Interact 1978; 21:59–78.

22. Ingelman-Sundberg M. Cytochrome P-450 Organization and Membrane Mechanism and Biochemistry. New York, Plenum Press, 1986:119–160.

23. Sud IJ, Feingold DS. Mechanisms of action of the antimycotic imidazoles. J Invest Dermatol 1981; 76:438–441.

24. De Nollin S, Van Belle H, Goossens F, et al. Cytochemical and biochemical studies of yeast after in vitro exposure to miconazole. Antimicrob Agents Chemother 1977; 11:500–513.

25. Shigematsu ML, Uno J, Arai T. Effect of ketoconazole on isolated mitochondria from *Candida albicans*. Antimicrob Agents Chemother 1982; 21:919–924.

26. Uno J, Shigematsu ML, Arai T. Primary site of action of ketoconazole on *Candida albicans*. Antimicrob Agents Chemother 1982; 21:912–918.

27. De Brabander M, Aerts F, Van Cutsem J, et al. The activity of ketoconazole in mixed cultures of leukocytes and *Candida albicans*. Sabouraudia 1980; 18:197–210.

28. Roilides E, Walsh TJ, Rubin M, et al. Effects of antifungal agents on the function of human neutrophils in vitro. Antimicrob Agents Chemother 1990; 34:196–201.

29. Peterson EM, Calderone RA. Growth inhibition of *Candida albicans* by rabbit alveolar macrophages. Infect Immun 1977; 15:910–915.

30. Van't Wout JW, Meynaar I, Linde I, et al. Effect of amphotericin B, fluconazole and itraconazole on intracellular *Candida albicans* and germ tube development in macrophages. J Antimicrob Chemother 1990; 25:803–811.

31. Loose DS, Kan PB, Hirst MA, et al. Ketoconazole blocks adrenal steroidogenesis by inhibiting cytochrome p450-dependent enzymes. J Clin Invest 1983; 71:1495–1499.

32. Duarte PA, Chow CC, Simmons F, et al. Fatal hepatitis associated with ketoconazole therapy. Arch Intern Med 1984; 144:1069–1070.

33. Janssen PAJ, Symoens JE. Hepatic reactions during ketoconazole treatment. Am J Med 1983; 74(suppl 1B):80–85.

34. Lewis JH, Zimmerman HJ, Benson GD, et al. Hepatic injury associated with ketoconazole therapy: analysis of 33 cases. Gastroenterology 1984; 86:503–513.

35. Lake-Bakaar G, Scheuer PJ, Sherlock S. Hepatic reactions associated with ketoconazole in the United Kingdom. Br Med J 1987; 294:419–422.

36. Nishikawa S, Hara T, Miyazaki E, et al. Studies on the safety of KW-1414: studies of the effects on reproduction. Clin Rep 1984; 18:313–328.

37. Tachibana M, Noguchi Y, Monro AM. Toxicology of fluconazole in experimental animals. In: Fromtling RA, ed. Recent Trends in the Discovery, Development and Evaluation of Antifungal Agents. Barcelona, JR Prous Science Publishers, 1987:93–102.

38. Shaw JTB, Tarbit MH, Troke PF. Cytochrome P-450 mediated sterol synthesis and metabolism: differences in sensitivity to fluconazole and other azoles. In: Fromtling RA, ed. Recent Trends in the Discovery, Development and Evaluation of Antifungal Agents. Barcelona, JR Prous Science Publishers, 1987:125–139.

39. Blum RA, Wilton JH, Hilligoss DM, et al. Effect of fluconazole on the disposition of phenytoin. Clin Pharmacol Ther 1991; 49:420–425.

40. Torregrosa V, De la Torre M, Campistol JM, et al. Interaction of fluconazole with cyclosporin A. Nephron 1992; 60:125–126.

41. Van Cauteren H, Coussement W, Vandenberghe J, et al. The toxicological properties of itraconazole. In: Fromtling RA, ed. Recent Trends in the Discovery, Development and Evaluation of Antifungal Agents. Barcelona, JR Prous Science Publishers, 1987:263–271.

42. Drouhet E, Dupont B. Laboratory and clinical assessment of ketoconazole in deep-seated mycoses. Am J Med 1983; 74(suppl 1B):30–47.

43. Van Cutsem J. The antifungal activity of ketoconazole. Am J Med 1983; 74(suppl 1B):9–15.

44. Shadomy S, White SC, Yu HP, Dismukes WE, NIAID Mycoses study group. Treatment of systemic mycoses with ketoconazole: in vitro susceptibilities

of clinical isolates of systemic and pathogenic fungi to ketoconazole. J Infect Dis 1985; 152:1249–1256.

45. Odds FC. Laboratory evaluation of antifungal agents. A comparative study of five imidazole derivatives of clinical importance. J Antimicrob Chemother 1980; 6:749–761.

46. Hoeprich PD, Merry JM. Influence of culture medium on susceptibility testing with BAY no 7133 and ketoconazole. J Clin Microbiol 1986; 24:269–71.

47. Bart-Delabesse E, Boiron P, Carlotti A, et al. *Candida albicans* genotyping in studies with patients with AIDS developing resistance to fluconazole. J Clin Microbiol 1993; 31:2933–2937.

48. Perfect JR, Savani DV, Durack DT. Comparison of itraconazole and fluconazole in treatment of cryptococcal meningitis and candida pyelonephritis in rabbits. Antimicrob Agents Chemother 1986; 29:579–583.

49. Denning DW, Tucker RM, Hanson LH, et al. Itraconazole therapy for cryptococcal meningitis and cryptococcosis. Arch Intern Med 1989; 149:2301–2308.

50. Perfect JR, Granger DL, Durack DT. Effects of antifungal agents and gamma interferon on macrophage cytotoxicity for fungi and tumor cells. J Infect Dis 1987; 156:316–323.

51. Amery WK, De Coster R, Caers I. Ketoconazole: from an antimycotic to a drug for prostate cancer. Drug Dev Res 1986; 8:299–307.

52. Trachtenberg J. Ketoconazole therapy in advanced prostatic cancer. J Urol 1984; 132:61–63.

53. Pont A, Williams PL, Azhar S, et al. Ketoconazole blocks testosterone synthesis. Arch Intern Med 1982; 142:2137.

54. Boiron P, Drouhet E, Dupont B, et al. Etude de la pénétration du kétoconazole dans les cellules de *Candida albicans*. Bull Soc Fr Mycol Med 1986; 15:255–260.

55. Boiron P, Drouhet E, Dupont B, et al. Entry of ketoconazole into *Candida albicans*. Antimicrob Agents Chemother 1987; 31:244–248.

56. Klempner MS, Styrt B. Clindamycin uptake by human neutrophils. J Infect Dis 1981; 144:472–475.

57. Perfect JR, Savani DV, Durack DT. Uptake of itraconazole by alveolar macrophages. Antimicrob Agents Chemother 1993; 37:903–904.

58. Pascual A, Garcia I, Conejo C, et al. Uptake and intracellular activity of fluconazole in human polymorphonuclear leukocytes. Antimicrob Agents Chemother 1993; 37:187–190.

59. Boiron P, Drouhet E, Dupont B, et al. Effect of pH on the mode of action of ketoconazole in *Candida albicans*. In: Iwata K, Vanden Bossche H, eds. In Vitro and In Vivo Evaluation of Antifungal Agents. Amsterdam: Elsevier Science Publishers, 1986:135–142.

60. Medoff G, Comfort M, Kobayashi GS. Synergistic action of amphotericin B and 5-fluorocytosine against yeast-like organisms. Proc Soc Exp Biol Med 1971; 138:571–574.

61. Beggs WH, Sarosi GA, Walker MI. Synergistic action of amphotericin B and rifampicin against *Candida* species. J Infect Dis 1976; 133:206–9.

62. Wildfeuer A, Laufen H, Haferkamp O. Interaction of fluconazole and human phagocytic cells. Uptake of the antifungal agent and its effects on the survival of ingested fungi in phagocytes. Arzneimittel forsching 1990; 40:1044–1047.

63. Wildfeuer A, Reisert I, Laufen H. Subcellular distribution and antifungal effects of fluconazole in human phagocytic cells. Demonstration of the antifungal agent in neutrophil polymorphonuclear leucocytes and monocytes by autoradiography and electron micrography. Arzneimittel forsching 1992; 42:1049–1052.

64. Holt RJ, Azmi A. A miconazole resistant *Candida*. Lancet 1978; 1:50–51.

65. Horsburgh CRJ, Kirkpatrick CH. Long-term therapy of chronic mucocutaneous candidiasis with ketoconazole: experience with twenty-one patients. Am J Med 1983; 74(suppl 1B):23–29.

66. Smith KJ, Warnock DW, Kennedy CTC, et al. Azole resistance in *Candida albicans*. J Med Vet Mycol 1986; 24:133–144.

67. Kerridge D, Fasoli M, Wayman FJ. Drug resistance in *Candida albicans* and *Candida glabrata*. Ann NY Acad Sci 1988; 544:245–259.

68. Kitchen VS, Savage M, Harris JRW. *Candida albicans* resistance in AIDS. J Infect 1991; 22:204–205.

69. Vanden Bossche H, Marichal P, Odds FC, et al. Characterization of an azole-resistant *Candida glabrata* isolate. Antimicrob Agents Chemother 1992; 36:2602–2610.

70. Warnock DW, Burke J, Cope NJ, et al. Fluconazole resistant in *Candida glabrata*. Lancet 1988; 2:1310.

71. Ryley JF, Wilson RG, Barrett-Bee K. Azole resistance in *Candida albicans*. Sabouraudia 1984; 22:53–63.

72. Hitchcock CA, Barrett-Bee KJ, Russell NJ. The lipid composition of azole-sensitive and azole-resistant strains of *Candida albicans*. J Gen Microbiol 1986; 132:2421–2431.

73. Johnson EM, Richardson MD, Warnock DW. In vitro resistance to imidazole antifungals in *Candida albicans*. J Antimicrob Chemother 1984; 13:547–558.

74. Hitchcock CA, Barrett-Bee KJ, Russell NJ. Inhibition of 14-α-sterol demethylase activity in *Candida albicans* Darlington does not correlate with resistance to azole. J Med Vet Mycol 1987; 25:329–333.

75. Howell SA, Mallet AI, Noble WC. A comparison of the sterol content of multiple isolates of the *Candida albicans* Darlington strain with other clinically azole-sensitive and -resistant strains. J Appl Bacteriol 1990; 69:692–696.

76. Vanden Bossche H, Marichal P, Gorrens J, et al. Mutation in cytochrome P-450-dependent 14α-demethylase results in decreased affinity for azole antifungals. Biochem Soc Trans 1990; 18:56–59.

77. Willocks L, Leen CLS, Brettle RP, et al. Fluconazole resistance in AIDS patients. J Antimicrob Chemother 1991; 28:937–939.

78. Dupont B. Antifungal therapy in AIDS patients. In: Bennett JE, Hay RJ,

Peterson PK, eds. New Strategies in Fungal Disease. Edinburgh: Churchill Livingstone, 1992:290–300.

79. Dupouy-Camet J, Paugam A, Di Donato C, et al. Résistance au fluconazole en milieu hospitalier. Concordance entre la résistance de *Candida albicans* in vitro et l'échec thérapeutique. Presse Med 1991; 20:1341.

80. Nicholas RO, Burton JA, Kerridge D, et al. Isolation of mutants of *Candida glabrata* resistant to miconazole. Crit Rev Microbiol 1987; 15:103–110.

81. Nobre G, Mendes E, Charrua MJ, et al. Ketoconazole resistance in *Torulopsis glabrata*. Mycopathologia 1989; 107:51–55.

82. Hitchcock CA, Pye GW, Troke PF, et al. Fluconazole resistance in *Candida glabrata*. Antimicrob Agents Chemother 1993; 37:1962–1965.

83. Hitchcock CA, Barrett-Bee KJ, Russell NJ. The lipid composition and permeability to the triazole antifungal antibiotic ICI 153066 of serum-grown mycelial cultures of *Candida albicans*. J Gen Microbiol 1989; 135:1949–1955.

13

Chloroquine Transport in the Malarial Parasite Plasmodium falciparum

**Stephen Andrew Ward, Patrick G. Bray,
and Graeme Y. Ritchie**
University of Liverpool, Liverpool, England

I. INTRODUCTION

Malaria has been and remains one of the most important diseases of humans in terms of both mortality and morbidity. Despite the recognition of malaria for over 2000 years, progress toward the treatment, control, and eradication of the disease has been modest. The extensive eradication program of the 1950s and 1960s, based on the insecticide control of the vector, can claim some limited success (1). However, the most recent statistics from the World Health Organization (WHO) state that over 40% of the world's population are at risk of malaria infection. About 25% of those at risk live in tropical Africa, where endemic malaria remains stable, with intense transmission and few control programs (2). Global incidence is thought to be in the order of 110 million, with 250 million people infected, 90% of whom are found in Africa. In all cases, treatment relies solely on the use of an effective antimalarial drug.

There are four species of *Plasmodium* that can cause malaria in humans: *P. falciparum*, *P. vivax*, *P. ovale*, and *P. malariae*. All follow a basic course of development through both vertebrate and invertebrate hosts, although there are variations in the individual life cycles of different malarial species. For this discussion, we will limit ourselves to the species of malarial parasite that is responsible for the bulk of clinical infections and that has proved most deadly and difficult to control, *P. falciparum*. The parasites are transmitted to humans in the form of sporozoites that are inoculated into the blood by the bite of an infected female anopheline mosquito. The sporozoites invade the parenchymal cells of the liver, where they undergo multiplication or schizogony, to become exoerythrocytic or tissue schizonts containing merozoites. Toward the end of the incubation period of the infection, large numbers of merozoites from ruptured tissue schizonts are released into the blood circulation.

Liberated tissue merozoites invade erythrocytes or reticulocytes and undergo erythrocytic schizogony, a phase of growth and multiplication. Nuclear division occurs in the schizont stage: the fully developed schizont ruptures and releases merozoites that invade fresh erythrocytes, initiating a new cycle of schizogony. It is this erythrocytic stage of the life cycle that is responsible for the clinical manifestations of the disease.

Following invasion of the host erythrocyte, some merozoites develop into male and female gametocytes. These gametocytes give rise to male and female gametes, which initiate the sporogonic or sexual cycle if they are taken up by a susceptible female anopheline mosquito. The sporogonic cycle results in the release of sporozoites that travel to the salivary glands of the insect and can thus be transmitted to humans, completing the life cycle.

A. The Role of Chloroquine in the Treatment of Malaria

Of all the drugs developed for the treatment of malaria, none has found as much use as the 4-aminoquinoline chloroquine (7-chloro-4-(-4-diethylamino-1-butylamino)quinoline (Fig. 1). First synthesized in 1934, it has been the most extensively used drug for the treatment of *P. falciparum* infections from the 1940s to the present day. Since the 1960s, however, the development and rapid spread of resistance to this drug has severely limited its effectiveness.

With the exception of drug-resistant *P. falciparum*, chloroquine is highly effective against the asexual erythrocytic stages of all species of *Plasmodium* that cause human malaria. The drug is inactive against sporozoites and primary and secondary exoerythrocytic stages of all strains. Chloroquine has gametocytocidal activity against *P. vivax*, *P. ovale*, and *P. malariae*, but is active against only immature gametocytes of *P. falciparum* (1,3).

The drug is well tolerated, with minimal host toxicity at the antimalarial dose level, although nausea and vomiting may occur if the drug is taken on an empty stomach. Headache and difficulty in visual accommodation

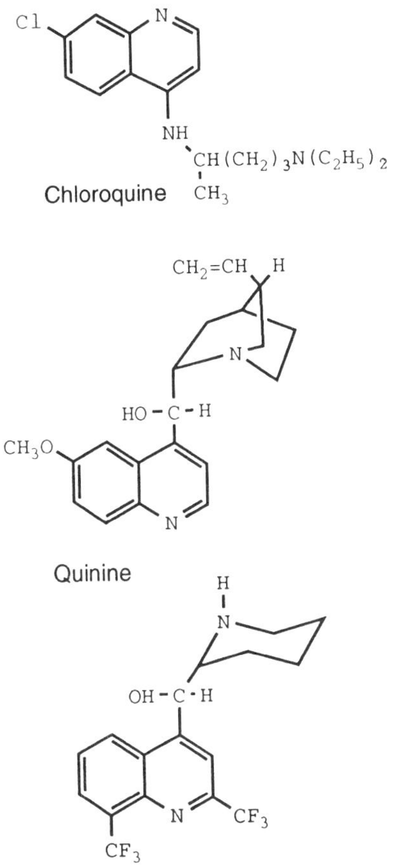

Chloroquine

$CH(CH_2)_3N(C_2H_5)_2$

CH_3

Quinine

Mefloquine

Figure 1 Structures of classic antimalarials: chloroquine, quinine, and mefloquine.

have been reported in some patients. Pruritus of the palms, soles, and scalp that is not relieved by antihistamines has been reported in up to 20% of Africans using chloroquine. Long-term exposure to chloroquine may produce other side effects, particularly when higher doses are used. These side effects are reversible on drug withdrawal and include visual disturbances, weight loss, skin problems, headache, bleaching of hair, and electrocardiographic changes (1,4).

Chloroquine is a fast-acting antimalarial, usually reducing fever after 24 h. The drug is usually given orally in a 3-day course for the curative treatment of chloroquine-susceptible *P. falciparum* and *P. malariae* and for termination of an acute attack of *P. vivax* or *P. ovale* malaria. There is no evidence that increasing the dose of chloroquine increases the clinical cure rate in areas of developing chloroquine-resistant *P. falciparum* malaria. Chloroquine can also be used for clinical prophylaxis or suppressive treatment of all human plasmodial species, where the drug is given before tissue or blood infection occurs. In this case, the clinical symptoms are prevented or eliminated by the early destruction of the erythrocytic parasites. If the response to chloroquine of a *P. falciparum* infection is slow or incomplete, chloroquine resistance is indicated.

B. Epidemiology of Chloroquine Resistance

Strains of *P. falciparum* resistant to antimalarial treatment are considered to arise from drug-induced selection, although natural variations in drug susceptibility of strains from different parts of the world has been recognized for many years (5).

Drug-induced selection results from spontaneous mutations, which reduce the susceptibility of a proportion of the parasites to the drug, followed by selection of the resistant parasites in the bloodstream by subcurative drug concentrations. This may occur a number of different times in different parasite populations, resulting in differing levels of resistance. Resistance is propagated by active transmission of malaria. As drug resistance is genetically determined, gametocytes arising from resistant parasites will produce resistant offspring.

Drug resistance was defined by the WHO as "the ability of a parasite strain to multiply or survive in the presence of concentrations of a drug that normally destroys parasites of the same species or prevents their multiplication" (6). Resistance may be relative (yielding to increased doses of the drug tolerated by the host), or complete (withstanding the maximum doses tolerated by the host).

Since the first recognized cases in 1959–1960, strains of *P. falciparum* resistant to chloroquine have been reported in most areas of the world where malaria is endemic. However, the level and frequency of chloroquine resistance are not constant from region to region, but depend on the intensity of drug pressure in addition to the extent of malaria transmission. A high level and frequency of chloroquine resistance has been observed in Thailand, Kampuchea, and Vietnam (7–9).

Chloroquine resistance was slower to emerge in Africa, with the first documented cases being reported in the mid-1970s. It has been suggested that chloroquine resistance in this continent went undetected for many years owing to the semi-immune status of the population and the differing dose–response of African isolates to chloroquine (5,10). As yet, there have been few conclusive reports of chloroquine resistance in species causing human malaria other than *P. falciparum.*

The rapid spread of chloroquine resistance and the development of resistance to all other classes of currently used blood schizontocides, together with the lack of interest of the drug companies in developing new antimalarials, underscores the need for reevaluation of currently available drugs. A thorough understanding of both the mode of action of chloroquine and the means by which the parasite becomes resistant to the drug should pinpoint the sites at which pharmacological intervention may reverse resistance. In addition, this information may be useful in the rational design and use of future antimalarials, thereby improving malarial chemotherapy.

C. Mechanism of Chloroquine Action

Many theories have been put forward to explain the mode of action of chloroquine (for reviews see Refs. 11,12). A common feature of all of the hypotheses proposed are the observations that chloroquine accumulates selectively into parasitized erythrocytes, and that the parasite-feeding process is inhibited. The recent work by Slater and colleagues (13) appears to provide an explanation of chloroquine action that is consistent with most of the experimental data available. They demonstrated that heme, a toxic hemoglobin breakdown product produced during parasite feeding, is converted to nontoxic hemozoin (a crystalline substance also known as malaria pigment) by an enzyme-dependent polymerization in the acid food vacuole of the parasite. Chloroquine and related aminoquinolines inhibit this polymerization in vitro at concentrations that correlate with antimalarial activity. These observations have since been confirmed in both *P. falciparum* (14) and the rodent malarial parasite *P. bergei* (15). Interestingly, it has been reported that heme polymerization is similarly susceptible to chloroquine in both chloroquine-susceptible and chloroquine-resistant parasites.

D. Chloroquine Resistance

The mechanisms proposed to explain chloroquine resistance have been traditionally associated with theories on its mode of action. Studies on the polymerization of heme suggest that this association is unfounded, and that drug resistance is independent of the mechanism of action. Furthermore, numerous investigations have shown that chloroquine-resistant parasites accumulate less drug than their susceptible counterparts (16–21). This suggests that drug resistance is associated with altered drug transport. However, one study has failed to show any relation between chloroquine accumulation and resistance (22). Therefore, it would appear that transport and accumulation of chloroquine into the parasite are not only the essential features for activity, in terms of achieving concentrations necessary to inhibit the polymerization process, but are also intimately associated with the resistance phenotype.

II. DRUG TRANSPORT INTO THE MALARIAL PARASITE

A. General

Chloroquine accumulates selectively into parasitized erythrocytes several hundredfold when compared with uninfected erythrocytes, which accumulate drug less than tenfold (23). This accumulation is primarily associated with the acid food vacuole, or lysosome, of the parasite, as demonstrated by electron microscope autoradiography (24). Indeed, the first morphological changes noted after treatment of parasites with chloroquine involve disruption of the lysosomal system within the parasite (25). Initially, lysosomes show characteristic swelling and vesiculation, followed by the accumulation of endocytic vacuoles containing undigested hemoglobin (26–29).

Chloroquine accumulation is energy-dependent, saturable, and competitively inhibited by other 4-aminoquinolines (19,30; Fig. 2). These findings have been interpreted as evidence for the existence of an intracellular high-affinity receptor for binding 4-aminoquinolines in malaria-infected erythrocytes. The dissociation constant (K_d) for the interaction of chloroquine with this proposed receptor is estimated to be approximately 10^{-8} M (31). It was proposed that this high-affinity receptor was ferriprotoporphyrin IX (thought to be a major constituent of malarial pigment). This ''drug–receptor'' interaction was originally put forward as the basis for chloroquine's antimalarial action. Since that time, many lines of evidence have been presented refuting the role of this complex in the drug's mode of action and pointing out that it cannot explain the total level of drug accumulation observed experimentally (32). However, it is conceivable that an interaction between chloroquine and some component of hemazoin may contribute to the global steady-state concentrations of drug achieved. Some investigators refute this possibility completely, because ammonium chloride can almost completely displace the drug from the infected cell, without affecting the complexation of drug to heme (33). Recent studies from this laboratory (Ward SA, unpublished results) have indicated that, after treatment of chloroquine-loaded parasites with proton ionophores,

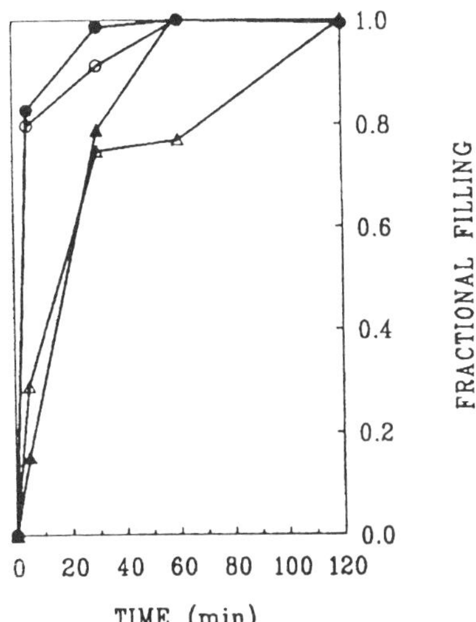

Figure 2 Kinetics of chloroquine uptake by susceptible (filled symbols) and resistant (empty symbols) parasites. The external concentration of chloroquine was 10^{-7} (triangles) and 10^{-8} M (circles). (From Ref. 54.)

there is an almost instantaneous loss of drug from the parasite. However, after the reestablishment of distribution equilibrium, significant concentrations of drug remain within the parasite, independent of the environmental pH. We have concluded that this must indicate an intraparasitic binding site for the drug, which, therefore, must contribute to the concentrations achieved at steady state.

It was suggested by Homewood (34) that chloroquine accumulates within the parasite as a consequence of its weak base properties. Chloroquine is a weak base with two protonation sites with pK_a of 10.2 and 8.3. Consequently, it can exist as either the unprotonated membrane-permeant form, or as the mono- or diprotonated membrane-impermeant forms. In the presence of a pH gradient between the extracellular milieu and acidic compartments, such as lysosomes, unprotonated drug would be expected to distribute equally across all compartments. The resulting protonation of the weak base at lower pH within the lysosome has the effect of trapping the membrane-impermeant protonated base and maintaining the concentration gradient for the inward movement of unprotonated drug. This results in selective drug accumulation within acid compartments. Furthermore, it was suggested that the accumulation of drug within the lysosome caused an increase in vacuolar pH. This would result in the inactivation of proteases essential for parasite viability, as described for mammalian systems by deDuve et al. (35).

Several groups have measured pH of the parasite's food vacuole using different techniques, giving a pH value between 5 and 5.4 for this compartment (22,36,37). The mechanism by which this acidic pH is maintained is unknown, although the inhibition of chloroquine uptake into infected erythrocytes by metabolic poisons is suggestive of the functional presence of an ATP-driven proton pump (17,38). In mammalian cells, Mg^{2+}-dependent, ATP-driven, proton pumps, located on lysosome membranes, are responsible for the acidification of lysosomes, by translocating protons into the lysosomal interior at the expense of metabolic energy (39–42). An Mg^{2+}-dependent ATPase has recently been purified from vacuolar membranes of *P. falciparum*. Although this protein has been only partially characterized, the results show it to be inhibited by the classic proton pump inhibitors N-ethylmaleimide (NEM) and 7-chloro-4-nitrobenzo-2-oxa-1,3-diazole (NBD-Cl) (43). Furthermore, Karcz et al. (44) have recently sequenced a gene from *P. falciparum* that shows significant sequence homology with the A subunit of the vacuolar ATPase of a wide range of organisms.

Chloroquine accumulation in both *P. berghei* and *P. falciparum* is absolutely dependent on the existence of a pH gradient between the accumulating compartment and the extracellular milieu (19,33). Despite arguments to the contrary (45), it should be emphasized that many workers have demonstrated that the extent (although possibly not the rate) of chloroquine accumulation into *P. falciparum* can be fully accounted for by the weak base effect (22,46,47). Since chloroquine is a diprotic weak base, it accumulates into acidic compartments as a function of the square of the pH gradient (46) and, if we assume a vacuolar pH of 5.2, chloroquine should accumulate 60,000-fold in the fold vacuole of the parasite. If we further assume that the food vacuole occupies approximately 3% of the volume of the infected red cell (36), then it is possible that the full extent of chloroquine accumulation by the infected cell can be explained by proton trapping, although there is some evidence for an intracellular binding component to chloroquine accumulation (18).

Even though proton trapping can provide the explanation for the extent of chloroquine accumulation by the infected cell, there is some evidence that a chloroquine carrier may be required to explain the kinetics of chloroquine transport. Early studies with parasite-infected red cells appeared to demonstrate a saturable component of chloroquine transport (19). In addition, Yayon and Ginsburg demonstrated saturable chloroquine transport across uninfected red cell membranes (48). These observations were interpreted as supporting the existence of a carrier system in the red cell membrane capable of moving drug, irrespective of its protonation state. It was assumed that a chloroquine-specific transport mechanism was essential to explain the very rapid movement of drug across membranes at physiological pH, where the drug is predominantly (>99%) in a protonated, membrane-impermeant form. This hypothesis is not supported by the fact that the chloroquine inward permeability coefficient is approximately 100-fold higher than permeability coefficients of other substrates known to exhibit facilitated diffusion across erythrocyte membranes (49). Indeed, a subsequent investigation demonstrated that chloroquine uptake by human erythrocytes could be fully explained by passive diffusion of the nonionized species (23). These authors explained that some of the discrepancies between their observation and those of Yayon and Ginsburg could be due to the differing methodologies employed.

B. Drug Efflux

1. *Biochemical Evidence for a Rapid Efflux Phenotype*

Several investigators have suggested marked similarities between chloroquine resistance in *P. falciparum* and multidrug resistance (MDR) in mammalian cancer cells (see Chaps. 17 and 18), indicating a common resistance mechanism in these two cell types. The most striking similarity is the ability of chemically unrelated compounds (termed chemosensitizers) to promote a return to susceptibility of drug-resistant strains. The ability of verapamil to reverse chloroquine resistance of several *P. falciparum* isolates prompted the comparison of chloroquine resistance in this parasite with multidrug resistance (MDR) in mammalian cancer cell lines (50). Anticancer drugs, such as daunorubicin and vinblastine, can increase chloroquine accumulation in *P. falciparum* (21); conversely, antimalarial compounds, such as chloroquine and quinine, can sensitize MDR tumor cells by increasing the concentration of the antitumor drug (51,52). These findings provide compelling evidence for common resistance reversal mechanisms in the two cell types and, despite limited experimental evidence, inhibition of a chloroquine-exporting protein by verapamil, with a concurrent increase in steady-state accumulation of chloroquine, was proposed as the mechanism by which reversal of chloroquine resistance is achieved in *P. falciparum* (21). The rate of efflux of preaccumulated chloroquine from resistant parasites was some 40 times faster than the rate of efflux from drug-susceptible parasites ($t_{1/2}$ of 2 vs. 75 min; 21). Additionally, verapamil at 10 μM reduced the rate of efflux selectively in resistant parasites. This explanation of resistance and susceptibility enhancement, based on active drug efflux as seen in MDR cancer, is appealing in its simplicity; however, it fails to explain all of the observations reported to date.

Studies carried out in our laboratory using a variety of *P. falciparum* isolates have demonstrated efflux rates for preaccumulated chloroquine of approximately 2 min, irrespective of drug susceptibility (53). Indeed, the mathematical model of Ginsburg and Stein for chloroquine accumulation (54) states that the rate of drug efflux is a function of vacuolar concentration, irrespective of the forces for uptake or efflux. Hence, according to the model, simple efflux rate measurements do not provide sufficient information to allow the resistance mechanism to be studied. Somewhat paradoxically, it would seem that actual measurement of efflux rate may not necessarily be able to identify an enhanced efflux capability. Ginsburg and Stein (54) supported the use of fractional fill analysis to differentiate forces of uptake from forces of efflux. They concluded that the differences in drug accumulation observed for resistant and susceptible parasites could be explained purely in terms of differences in uptake force (Fig. 2). Similar treatment of our own data suggests that there is a small, but measurable, efflux component to chloroquine transport in resistant parasites. This force can be inhibited by verapamil, but is present only at pharmacologically irrelevant chloroquine concentrations. As chloroquine concentrations are increased across the range used in standard in vitro susceptibility assays, the ability of a fixed verapamil concentration to enhance chloroquine accumulation is diminished (55). Moreover, at chloroquine concentrations in the therapeutic range, verapamil has no effect on chloroquine accumulation, yet it can still enhance susceptibility. The observation of reduced chloroquine overaccumulation as chloroquine concentrations are increased in the presence of a fixed concentration of verapamil is not unusual if it is assumed that both compounds are competing for a common site on a transporter. This line of argument would suggest (if we accept that resistant parasites selectively efflux chloroquine) that verapamil accumulation must be lower in chloroquine-resistant isolates than in chloroquine-sensitive isolates. The observations we have made on our susceptible and resistant isolates fail to reveal any significant differences in the extent of verapamil accumulation (53). Despite these disparities, it is clear that chloroquine-resistant parasites have a limited efflux capacity that is sensitive to the action of verapamil and other chemosensitizers. This has been demonstrated by the small, but significant, increases in steady-state chloroquine concentration achieved in energy-deprived resistant parasites compared with energy-deprived susceptible parasites in which accumulation of chloroquine is significantly reduced (53,56). Additionally, it is striking that all antimalarials for which susceptibility can be enhanced by verapamil (e.g., quinine, mepacrine) show some degree of cross-resistance to chloroquine in vitro, and all are themselves chemosensitizers of anticancer drugs, the resistance mechanisms of which have been shown to be MDR-dependent.

2.   Molecular Evidence for a Rapid Efflux Phenotype

The parallels between chloroquine resistance in *P. falciparum* and the MDR phenotype in tumor cell lines aroused intense interest in the molecular basis of drug resistance in malarial parasites. The mammalian MDR phenotype is usually accompanied by amplification of *mdr* genes, leading to increased expression of P-glycoprotein, although there are examples of cells that exhibit increased P-glycoprotein without *mdr* gene amplification (57). The search for *mdr* homologues in *P. falciparum* uncovered two genes, termed *pfmdr1* and *pfmdr2*, which have sequence and predicted protein structure similar to the *mdr* gene family.

The *pfmdr2* gene encodes a 110-kDa protein that has 61% similarity to the heavy-metal tolerance, *hmt1* gene of yeast (58). The *pfmdr2* protein product is predicted to comprise ten membrane-spanning domains and one ATP-binding site. There is little evidence to suggest a link with chloroquine resistance, although one study reported increased transcription of *pfmdr2* in chloroquine-resistant isolates (59).

In contrast, a considerable amount of promising, but at times baffling, data has implicated *pfmdr1* in the mechanism of drug resistance. The *pfmdr1* gene encodes a 162-kDa protein, P-glycoprotein homologue 1 (Pgh1), which consists of two homologous halves separated by a hinge region (60). Each half of the protein is proposed to contain six transmembrane domains and a nucleotide-binding fold. The predicted amino acid sequence has a 54% similarity to human *mdr1* (60).

Quantitative Southern blotting of chromosomal DNA from *P. falciparum* isolates with varying degrees of chloroquine susceptibility, revealed amplification of *pfmdr1* in some chloroquine-resistant isolates, resulting in increased transcription, but in none of the chloroquine-susceptible lines (60). In a separate study, *pfmdr1* amplification was observed in a strain subjected to pressure with the related quinoline antimalarial mefloquine (61).

Detailed investigation of *pfmdr1* amplification in one of the chloroquine-resistant lines, B8, revealed that the gene is amplified five times on amplicons of 105 kb, configured head to tail. Sequencing of the breakpoints followed by polymerase chain reaction analysis of 16 other strains that have amplified *pfmdr1*, demonstrated the uniqueness of the B8 breakpoint. This indicated that *pfmdr1* amplification has arisen as a number of independent events, suggesting that the gene is under some selective pressure (62).

Examination of the *pfmdr1* protein product by immunofluorescence and immunoelectron microscopy revealed that Pgh1, which is expressed throughout the erythrocytic cycle, is located in trophozoites, predominantly on the vacuolar membrane (63). Since the digestive vacuole is the principal site of chloroquine accumulation, the protein is found in a location consistent with its putative role as a chloroquine transporter. Contrary to the hopeful initial observations, however, quantitation of Pgh1 by immunoblot analysis disclosed no correlation between overexpression and drug resistance, with equivalent amounts of Pgh1 in several chloroquine-resistant and -susceptible lines. The chloroquine-resistant clone FAC8, differed in expressing approximately threefold more Pgh1 than other isolates (as a consequence of a threefold gene amplification), but was no more resistant to chloroquine than some strains expressing less Pgh1 (63). More recent work, measuring transcription of *pfmdr1*, has broadly confirmed this picture; although mRNA levels varied between strains, there was a poor correlation with chloroquine susceptibility (59). The T9-94R strain (growth IC_{50} for chloroquine 265 nM), for example, had a level of transcription four times higher than the K1 strain (growth IC_{50} for chloroquine 338 nM).

With no apparent association of chloroquine resistance and Pgh1 expression, the possibility that chloroquine-resistant strains possess specific mutations in *pfmdr1* that are associated with the resistance phenotype was investigated. In an extensive study, Foote and his co-workers compared the *pfmdr1* sequences of chloroquine-resistant and chloroquine-susceptible isolates and identified two "alleles" related to chloroquine resistance (64). One involved a single amino acid change (Tyr-86), and the other three amino acid substitutions (Cys-1034, Asp-1042, Tyr-1246). On the basis of these, the chloroquine resistance status of 34 of 36 isolates was correctly predicted in a blinded study. Additionally, a 3' polymorphism pattern was associated with the resistance phenotype.

The significance of these findings, however, is questionable; recent analysis of chloroquine-resistant strains isolated from Thailand revealed none with the *pfmdr1* mutations identified in the former study (65). In addition, the 3' polymorphisms distinguished in this more recent work were considerably more variable than those described by Foote et al. (64). Taken together, these observations suggest that the isolates used by Foote may have been more closely related than originally appreciated.

A genetic cross between the chloroquine-susceptible HB3 and chloroquine-resistant Dd2 clones (66) generated independent offspring that exhibited the drug response characteristics of either the resistant or the susceptible parent. This suggests that a single genetic locus may be responsible for the drug susceptibility phenotype. A restriction-fragment polymorphism enabled the parental origin of *pfmdr1* in the offspring to be identified. This analysis of the inheritance pattern revealed that the parental *pfmdr1* did not segregate with the drug response of the progeny. Likewise, *pfmdr2* inheritance showed no linkage with chloroquine resistance. The interpretation given to these results was that chloroquine resistance is independent of the *mdr* genes. Contrary to this, it was argued that the HB3 parent strain possesses one of the mutations (Asp-1042) proposed to be associated with resistance, and that this may confer competence for resistance when coexpressed with other gene products in what is likely to be a multigenic phenomenon.

The progeny of the genetic cross were further examined using restriction fragment length polymorphism markers, which were able to distinguish inheritance from the chloroquine-resistant and chloroquine-susceptible parents (67). An exhaustive search of the 14 chromosomes disclosed the perfect linkage of the chloroquine resistance phenotype to a single genetic locus of about 400 kb on chromosome 7. As yet, no likely "chloroquine resistance" genes have been reported from the search of this locus.

Although the link between chloroquine resistance and *pfmdr1* is unclear, several studies have implicated *pfmdr1* amplification in resistance to mefloquine. A mefloquine-resistant strain (W2-Mef) was selected from a chloroquine-resistant parent by exposure to sequential increases in mefloquine concentration (68), and was found to have amplified *pfmdr1* (61). The decrease in susceptibility to mefloquine was accompanied with increased chloroquine susceptibility. Consistent with this, a more recent study of three strains selected for mefloquine resistance showed that *pfmdr1* was amplified in all three cases (cited in Ref. 69). In two of the parent lines, *pfmdr1* was already amplified, but selection resulted in further gene amplification. Again, increased mefloquine resistance was concomitant with an increase in chloroquine susceptibility.

Furthermore, Barnes et al. showed that selection of the chloroquine-resistant strain FAC8 to a tenfold higher level of chloroquine resistance resulted in deamplification of *pfmdr1* from three copies of the gene to one (70). This was accompanied by increased susceptibility to mefloquine, strengthening the link of *pfmdr1* gene amplification with resistance to mefloquine and, by implication, halofantrine and quinine, which show a degree of cross-resistance. Indeed, an association between both mefloquine and halofantrine resistance and *pfmdr1* overexpression was the conclusion of a study of drug-resistant isolates from Thailand (65).

The deamplification of *pfmdr1* in strains adapted to conditions of high chloroquine concentration, and the increase in chloroquine susceptibility in lines that have amplified *pfmdr1* in response to mefloquine pressure, implies that *pfmdr1* amplification may be incompatible with high-level chloroquine resistance, and that Pgh1 may indeed confer a degree of chloroquine susceptibility.

This putative "chloroquine-sensitizing" role of Pgh1 has been examined in heterologous expression systems. Chinese hamster ovary cells (CHO) transfected with *pfmdr1* expressed intracellular Pgh1 that was associated with increased susceptibility of the CHO cells to chloroquine and hydroxychloroquine (71). The Pgh1 expression was reported to be accompanied by an increased energy-dependent influx of drug which, for hydroxychloroquine, was enantiospecific, suggesting a transport process. Expression of *pfmdr1* in the protozoan parasite *Leishmania* resulted in Pgh1 being localized on intracellular membranes, and was concomitant with a significant increase in chloroquine susceptibility (and, perhaps paradoxically, a slight increase in mefloquine susceptibility; 72). Taken together, these studies raise interest in the possible role of Pgh1 as a chloroquine concentrator.

III. DIFFERENCES IN THE RATE OF CHLOROQUINE UPTAKE AS A RESISTANCE MECHANISM

A. Is a Carrier Required?

In our opinion, the rate of chloroquine accumulation by uninfected red cells can be fully explained by passive diffusion of the un-ionized species. However, the question remains of whether the rate of drug accumulation by parasitized red cells can also be explained in terms of simple diffusion of unprotonated drug, or if additional specialized transport processes are required. On the basis of the belief that vacuolar drug accumulation by proton trapping would be unlikely in the absence of a continuous pH gradient, Warhurst suggested the existence of an active carrier, or "permease," capable of moving ionized drug across parasites' membranes (73). The need to invoke such a permease is in itself unnecessary if we accept that the ability of drug to concentrate as a function of proton trapping does not require a continuous pH gradient. However, support for a chloroquine transporter, at least in some strains, has been provided by Ferrari and Cutler (74). Their kinetic analysis of chloroquine uptake data obtained by Geary et al. (22) indicated that the rate of uptake of chloroquine by erythrocytes infected with a chloroquine-susceptible strain is substantially higher than can be predicted by passive diffusion. In contrast, drug uptake by the resistant strain could be explained adequately by passive diffusion. This kinetic model was based on first-order exchange of chloroquine between the four main compartments of an infected erythrocyte (Fig. 3). In the absence of experimental data, the model was normalized, assuming similar passive permeability of both parasite and erythrocyte membranes to chloroquine. This assumption seems reasonable, as similar chloroquine permeability coefficients have been reported for membranes of other cell types (75). Increases in the inward permeability coefficient for the drug across any of the barrier membranes, while leaving the outward permeability coefficient unchanged, could generate an excellent fit to the data observed by Geary et al. (22) for chloroquine-susceptible strains. This analysis was interpreted as evidence for a drug importer specifically in the susceptible strain. Our own data indicate that chloroquine resistance in *P. falciparum* can be attributed (at least in part) to a reduction of energy-dependent drug accumulation, possibly the loss of a unidirectional chloroquine carrier, although our interpretation of these results favors impaired vacuolar acidification by resistant parasites (53,55,76). Studies described in the foregoing with transfected CHO cells also exhibited increased energy-dependent chloroquine accumulation, suggesting that Pgh1 acts as a chloroquine carrier in these cells. The recent demonstration that selection for high-level chloroquine resistance results in reduced expression of Pgh1 in *P. falciparum* (70) raises the intriguing prospect of Pgh1 acting as a functional energy-dependent chloroquine carrier selectively in some chloroquine-susceptible isolates. If this were true, chloroquine resistance could arise either through reduced expression of Pgh1, or through mutations of the *pfmdr1* gene that decrease the ability

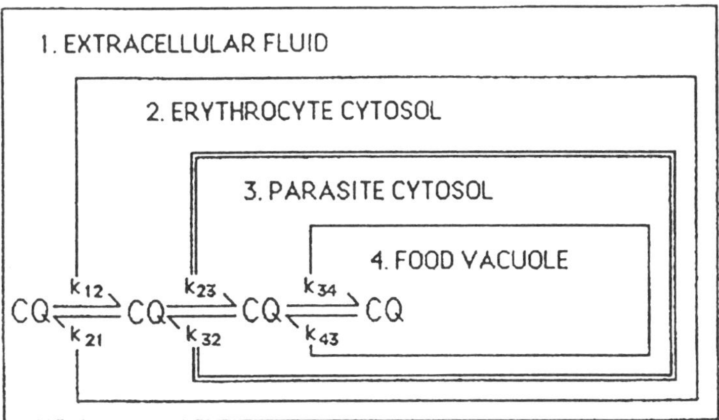

Figure 3 Four-compartment model of a malaria-infected erythrocyte showing kinetics of chloroquine (CQ) uptake. (From Ref. 74.)

of Pgh1 to concentrate chloroquine. Although this theory can explain some of the apparently contradictory chloroquine transport data from susceptible and resistant parasites, it is unlikely to provide a satisfactory explanation of the ability of verapamil and other compounds to sensitize chloroquine-resistant *P. falciparum*. Chloroquine resistance reversers have the ability to increase chloroquine accumulation by the resistant parasite, even though these increases appear to be insufficient to explain the degree of sensitization (55). If this transport effect is important for chloroquine sensitization, then it is inconceivable that the site of action is Pgh1 or is a related molecule that functions as an inward chloroquine carrier.

B. The Role of Vacuolar pH Homeostasis

Chloroquine is predicted to accumulate within acidic compartments by virtue of its weak base properties. The extent of chloroquine accumulation and, consequently, parasite susceptibility, is altered by changes in the magnitude of the pH gradient between the extracellular space and the parasite's food vacuole. This effect has been demonstrated with both altered external pH (33,46) and alkalinization of the food vacuole with ammonium chloride or inhibitors of acidification (33,76).

It has been demonstrated that chloroquine accumulation is largely energy dependent and that the magnitude of the energy-dependent component is reduced in resistant parasites (19,53,77). By analogy with other eukaryotic systems, the maintenance of an acidic vacuolar pH requires a vacuole-specific proton pump that is also energy-dependent (78). This has led to the hypothesis that chloroquine resistance can result from an elevation of basal vacuolar pH in the resistant parasite (46). An elevation of as little as 0.3 of a pH unit would be sufficient to explain most reported differences in both chloroquine susceptibility and accumulation. Although direct vacuolar pH measurement has been attempted (36,37,47), none of these studies compared absolute vacuole pH between chloroquine-susceptible and chloroquine-resistant parasites. Additionally, some of the reported data have been criticized on methodological grounds.

Geary et al. reported the inhibitory effect of chloroquine to be directly proportional to medium pH (46). According to weak base theory, if the only force responsible for accumulation of a diprotonated drug, such as chloroquine, is the pH gradient, the relation between the log–dose response and external pH should be linear with a slope of -2, irrespective of chloroquine susceptibility. This relation has been reported to hold for at least one strain of *P. falciparum* (46). Similar experiments carried out in our own laboratory have shown that this relation holds only for chloroquine-susceptible isolates. Chloroquine-resistant isolates also exhibited

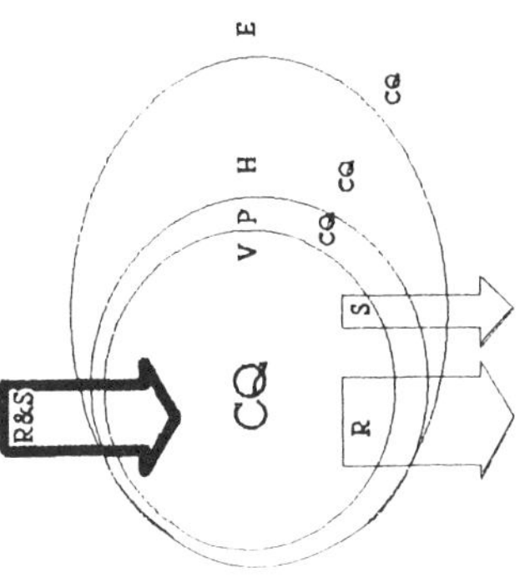

Figure 4 Mechanisms of chloroquine (CQ) resistance in a malaria-infected erythrocyte. Chloroquine uptake is represented by bold arrows, efflux by fine arrows. E, extracellular space; H, host erythrocyte; P, malaria parasite; V, vacuole; S, susceptible parasite; R, resistant parasite. (From Ref. 76.)

a linear relation between susceptibility and medium pH, but with a significantly reduced slope. Our interpretation of these findings is that in the resistant parasite, there is a reduced buffering capacity for chloroquine. Similar observations have been obtained with the 4-aminoquinoline amodiaquine, using both chloroquine-susceptible and chloroquine-resistant isolates, although the differences were less marked. Some of this reduced-buffering capacity could reflect selective efflux of drug from resistant parasites. An argument against this explanation is the finding that amodiaquine accumulation and susceptibility are not influenced by either verapamil or other reported chloroquine chemosensitizers (P.G. Bray et al., in preparation). Alternatively, these findings may support an argument for lysosomotropic actions of chloroquine selectively in the resistant parasite. This argument may explain the recent observations of Orjih and Fitch (14). In their paper, chloroquine was reported to inhibit the growth of resistant parasites without reducing the production of hemozoin, suggesting a mechanism of action unrelated to heme polymerase in the resistant strain.

Although changes in basal vacuolar pH or buffering capacity can potentially explain the differential susceptibility of parasites to chloroquine, it is difficult to reconcile the sensitization of resistant parasites by agents such as verapamil. According to pH theory, these chemosensitizers would have to decrease vacuolar pH, either directly or indirectly, by reducing proton leak, specifically in the resistant parasite. Chemosensitizers can only partially restore chloroquine susceptibility in *P. falciparum*, although a direct comparison between resistant and susceptible parasite clones derived from a common parent line has not been carried out. In contrast, the MDR phenotype is often completely reversed in cancer cells (57). This, together with the data discussed earlier, may suggest the involvement of both drug efflux and reduced pH-dependent uptake in the resistance phenotype displayed in *P. falciparum* (Fig. 4).

IV. CONCLUSIONS AND FUTURE DIRECTIONS

The evidence presented here clearly indicates altered drug transport in the chloroquine-resistance phenomenon. There is some evidence for an MDR-type drug efflux process in *P. falciparum*, particularly in the area of chemosensitization, although major genetic and biochemical differences exist between chloroquine resistance in *P. falciparum* and MDR in cancer cells. Similarly, there is good evidence to support a role for altered vacuolar pH homeostasis as a basis for chloroquine resistance. We should not forget the possibility that the two processes may be linked. For example, recent evidence has linked P-glycoprotein transporters with Cl⁻ channel activity, a factor that could be important in the maintenance of vacuolar pH. Clearly, significant effort is required to unravel these complexities. As in the field of cancer chemotherapy, it is essential that we fully understand the biochemical and molecular basis of drug resistance in *P. falciparum* if we hope to provide effective chemotherapeutic strategies to treat this important disease.

ACKNOWLEDGMENTS

SAW is a Wellcome Trust Study Leave fellow, PGB and GYR are both supported by the Wellcome Trust.

REFERENCES

1. Bruce-Chwatt LJ, Black RH, Canfield CJ, Clyde DF, Peters W, Wernsdorfer WH. Chemotherapy of Malaria, 2nd ed. Geneva: World Health Organization, 1986.
2. World Health Organization. World malaria situation in 1989. Weekly Epidemiology Rec 1991; 65:189–196.
3. Anand N. Chemotherapy of malaria. In: Sharma VP, ed. Proceedings of the Indo-UK Workshop on Malaria. New Delhi: Malaria Research Centre (ICMR), 1984.
4. Canfield CJ. Antimalarial aminoalcohol alternatives to mefloquine. Acta Trop 1980; 37:232–237.
5. Peters W. Drug resistance in malaria—a perspective. Trans R Soc Trop Med Hyg 1969; 63:25–45.
6. World Health Organization. Terminology of malaria and of malaria eradication. Report of drafting committee. Geneva: World Health Organization, 1963.
7. World Health Organization. Advances in Malaria Chemotherapy. Tech Rep Ser 711. Geneva: World Health Organization, 1984.
8. Wernsdorfer WH. Drug resistant malaria. Endeavour 1984; 8:166–171.
9. Thaithong S, Beale GK, Chutmongkonkul M. Susceptibility of *Plasmodium falciparum* to five drugs: an in vitro study of isolates mainly from Thailand. Trans R Soc Trop Med Hyg 1983; 77:228–231.
10. Peters W. Chemotherapy of malaria. In: Kreier JP, ed. Malaria. Vol. 1. New York: Academic Press, 1980.
11. Ward SA. Mechanisms of chloroquine resistance in malarial chemotherapy. Trends Pharmacol Sci 1988; 9:241–246.
12. Ginsburg H, Krugliak M. Quinoline-containing antimalarials: mode of action, drug resistance and its reversal. Biochem Pharmacol 1992; 43:63–70.
13. Slater AFG. Chloroquine: mechanism of drug action and resistance in *Plasmodium falciparum*. Pharmacol Ther 1993; 57:203–236.

14. Orjih AU, Fitch CD. Hemozoin production by *Plasmodium falciparum*: variation with strain and exposure to chloroquine. Biochim Biophys Acta 1993; 1157:270–274.

15. Chou AC, Fitch CD. Heme polymerase: modulation by chloroquine treatment of a rodent malaria. Life Sci 1992; 51:2037–2078.

16. Macomber PB, O'Brien RL, Hahn FE. Chloroquine: physiological basis of drug resistance in *Plasmodium berghei*. Science 1966; 152:1374–1375.

17. Polet H, Barr CF. Uptake of chloroquine-3-^{3}H by *Plasmodium knowlesi* in vitro. Pharmacol Exp Ther 1969; 168:187–192.

18. Fitch CD. *Plasmodium falciparum* in owl monkeys. Drug resistance and chloroquine binding capacity. Science 1970; 169:289–290.

19. Fitch CD, Yunis NG, Chevli R, Gonzales Y. High affinity accumulation of chloroquine by mouse erythrocytes infected with *P. berghei*. J Clin Invest 1974; 54:24–33.

20. Verdier F, Le Bras J, Clavier F, Hatin I, Blayo M. Chloroquine uptake by *Plasmodium falciparum*-infected human erythrocytes during in vitro culture and its relationship to chloroquine resistance. Antimicrob Agents Chemother 1985; 27:561–564.

21. Krogstad DJ, Gluzman IY, Kyle DE, Oduola AMJ, Martin SK, Milhous WK, Schlesinger PH. Efflux of chloroquine from *Plasmodium falciparum*: mechanism of chloroquine resistance. Science 1987; 235:1283–1285.

22. Geary TG, Jensen JB, Ginsburg H. Uptake of ^{3}H chloroquine by drug-sensitive and resistant strains of the human malarial parasite *Plasmodium falciparum*. Biochem Pharmacol 1986; 35:3805–3812.

23. Ferrari V, Cutler DJ. Uptake of chloroquine by human erythrocytes. Biochem Pharmacol 1990; 39:753–762.

24. Aikawa M. High resolution autoradiography of malarial parasites treated with ^{3}H chloroquine. Am J Pathol 1972; 67:277–280.

25. Macomber PB, Sprinz H, Tousimis AJ. Morphological effects of chloroquine on *Plasmodium berghei* in mice. Nature 1967; 214:937–939.

26. Yayon A, Ginsburg H. Chloroquine inhibits the degradation of endocytic vesicles in human malaria parasites. Cell Biol Int Rep 1983; 7:895.

27. Yayon A, Timberg R, Friedman S, Ginsburg H. Effects of chloroquine on the feeding mechanism of the intraerythrocytic human malaria parasite *Plasmodium falciparum*. J Protozool 1984; 31:367–372.

28. Zhang Y, Just WW. A comparative study on the effect of chloroquine and ammonium chloride on the feeding process of *Plasmodium falciparum* in vitro. Parasitol Res 1987; 73:475–478.

29. Zhang Y, Hempelmann E. Lysis of malaria parasites and erythrocytes by FPIX-chloroquine and the inhibition of this effect by proteins. Biochem Pharmacol 1987; 36:1267–1273.

30. Fitch CD, Chevli R, Gonzales Y. Chloroquine resistant *Plasmodium falciparum*: effect of substrate on chloroquine and amodiaquine accumulation. Antimicrob Agents Chemother 1974; 6:757–762.

31. Chou AC, Chevli R, Fitch CD. Ferriprotoporphyrin IX fulfills the criteria for identification as the chloroquine receptor of malaria parasites. Biochemistry 1980; 19:1543–1549.

32. Ginsburg H, Geary TG. Current concepts and new ideas on the mechanism of action of quinoline-containing antimalarials. Biochem Pharmacol 1987; 40:1567–1576.

33. Yayon A, Cabantchik ZI, Ginsburg H. Susceptibility of human malaria parasites to chloroquine is pH dependent. Proc Natl Acad Sci USA 1985; 82:2784–2788.

34. Homewood CA, Warhurst DC, Peters W, Baggaley VC. Lysosomes, pH and the antimalarial action of chloroquine. Nature 1972; 235:50–52.

35. de Duve C, deBarsy T, Poole B, Trouet A, Tulkens P, van Hoof F. Lysosomotropic agents. Biochem Pharmacol 1974; 23:2495–2531.

36. Yayon A, Cabathik ZI, Ginsburg H. Identification of the acidic compartment of *P falciparum* infected human erythrocytes as the target for the antimalarial drug chloroquine. EMBO J 1984; 3:2695–2700.

37. Krogstad DJ, Schlesinger PH, Gluzman IY. Antimalarials increase vesicle pH in *Plasmodium falciparum*. J Cell Biol 1985; 101:2302–2309.

38. Krogstad DJ, Schlesinger PH. A perspective on antimalarial action: effects of weak bases on *Plasmodium falciparum*. Biochem Pharmacol 1986; 35:547–552.

39. Mego JL. The ATP dependent pump in lysosome membranes (still a valid hypothesis). FEBS Lett 1979; 107:113–116.

40. Schneider DL. ATP dependent acidification of intact and disrupted lysosomes. J Biol Chem 1981; 256:3858–3864.

41. Ohkuma S, Moriyama Y, Takana T. Identification and characterisation of a proton pump on lysosomes by fluorescein isothionate–dextran fluorescence. Proc Natl Acad Sci USA 1982; 79:2758–2762.

42. Kakinuma Y, Ohsumi Y, Anraku Y. Properties of H^+-translocating adenosine triphosphate in vacuolar membrane of *Saccharomyces cerevisiae*. J Biol Chem 1981; 256:10859–10863.

43. Choi I, Mego JL. Intravacuolar proteolysis in *Plasmodium falciparum* digestive vacuoles is similar to intralysosomal proteolysis in mammalian cells. Biochim Biophys Acta 1987; 926:170–176.

44. Karcz SR, Herrmann VR, Cowman AF. Cloning and characterization of a vacuolar ATPase A subunit homologue from *Plasmodium falciparum*. Mol Biochem Parasitol 1993; 58:333–345.

45. Krogstad DJ, Schlesinger PH. The basis of antimalarial action: nonweak base effects of chloroquine on acid vesicle pH. Am J Trop Med Hyg 1987; 36:213–220.

46. Geary TG, Divo AD, Jensen JB, Zangwill M, Ginsburg H. Kinetic modelling of the response of *Plasmodium falciparum* to chloroquine and its experimental testing in vitro. Implications for mechanism of action and resistance to the drug. Biochem Pharmacol 1990; 40:685–691.

47. Ginsburg H, Nissani E, Krugliak M. Alkalinisation of the food vacuole of malaria parasites by quinoline drugs and alkylamines is not correlated with their antimalarial activity. Biochem Pharmacol 1989; 38:2645–2654.

48. Yayon A, Ginsburg H. The transport of chloroquine across human erythrocyte membranes is mediated by a simple symmetric carrier. Biochim Biophys Acta 1982; 686:197–203.

49. Stein WD. Transport and Diffusion Across Cell Membranes. Orlando, FL: Academic Press, 1986.

50. Martin SK, Oduola AMJ, Milhous WK. Reversal of chloroquine resistance in *Plasmodium falciparum* by verapamil. Science 1987; 235:899–901.

51. Rogan AM, Hamilton TC, Young RC, Klecker RW Jr, Ozols RF. Reversal of Adriamycin resistance by verapamil in human ovarian cancer. Science 1984; 244:994–996.

52. Fojo AT, Akiyama S, Gottesman MM, Pastan I. Reduced drug accumulation in multiply drug-resistant human carcinoma cell lines. Cancer Res 1985; 45:3002–3007.

53. Bray PG, Howells RE, Ritchie GY, Ward SA. Rapid chloroquine efflux phenotype in both chloroquine-sensitive and chloroquine-resistant *Plasmodium falciparum*. Biochem Pharmacol 1992; 44:1317–1324.

54. Ginsburg H, Stein WD. Kinetic modelling of chloroquine uptake by malaria infected erythrocytes. Biochem Pharmacol 1990; 41:1463–1470.

55. Bray PG, Boulter MK, Ritchie GY, Howells RE, Ward SA. Resistance reversal in *Plasmodium falciparum* independent of global drug transport. Mol Biochem Parasitol 1994; 63:87–94.

56. Krogstad DJ, Gluzman IY, Herwaldt BL, Schlesinger PH, Wellems TE. Energy-dependence of chloroquine accumulation and chloroquine efflux in *Plasmodium falciparum*. Biochem Pharmacol 1992; 43:57–62.

57. Endicott JA, Ling V. The biochemistry of P-glycoprotein mediated multidrug resistance. Annu Rev Biochem 1989; 58:137–171.

58. Zalis MG, Wilson CM, Zhang Y, Wirth DF. Characterisation of the *pfmdr2* gene for *Plasmodium falciparum*. Mol Biochem Parasitol 1993; 62:83–93.

59. Ekong RM, Robson KJH, Baker DA, Warhurst DC. Transcripts of the multidrug resistant genes in chloroquine sensitive and chloroquine resistant *P. falciparum*. Parasitology 1993; 106:107–115.

60. Foote SJ, Thompson JK, Cowman AF, Kemp DJ. Amplification of the multidrug resistance gene in some chloroquine resistant isolates of *P. falciparum*. Cell 1989; 57:921–930.

61. Wilson CM, Serrano AE, Wasley A, Bogenshutz MP, Shankar AH, Wirth DF. Amplification of a gene related to mammalian *mdr* genes in drug resistant *P. falciparum*. Science 1989; 244:1184–1186.

62. Triglia T, Foote SJ, Kemp DJ, Cowman AFC. Amplification of the multidrug resistant gene, *pfmdr1* in *Plasmodium falciparum* has arisen as multiple independent events. Mol Cell Biol 1993; 11:5244–5250.

63. Cowman AF, Karcz S, Galatis D, Culvenor JG. A P-glycoprotein homologue

of *Plasmodium falciparum* is localised on the digestive vacuole. J Cell Biol 1991; 113:1033–1045.

64. Foote SJ, Kyle DE, Martin RK, Oduola AMJ, Forsyth K, Kemp DJ, Cowman AF. Several alleles of the multidrug resistance gene are closely linked to chloroquine resistance in *Plasmodium falciparum*. Nature 1990; 345:255–258.

65. Wilson CM, Violkman SK, Thaithong S, Martin RK, Kyle DE, Milhous WK, Wirth DF. Amplification of *pfmdr1* associated with mefloquine and halofantrine resistance in *Plasmodium falciparum* in Thailand. Mol Biochem Parasitol 1993; 57:151–160.

66. Wellems TE, Panton LJ, Gluzman IY, de Rosario VE, Gwadz RW, Walker-Jonah A, Krogstad DJ. Chloroquine resistance not linked to to *mdr*-like gene in a *Plasmodium falciparum* cross. Nature 1990; 345:253–255.

67. Wellems TE, Walker-Jonah A, Panton LJ. Genetic mapping of the chloroquine resistance locus on *Plasmodium falciparum* chromosome 7. Proc Natl Acad Sci USA 1991; 88:3382–3386.

68. Oduola AMJ, Weatherly NF, Bowdre JH, Desjardins RE. *Plasmodium falciparum*: cloning by single erythrocyte micromanipulation and heterogeneity in vitro. Exp Parasitol 1988; 66:86–95.

69. Cowman AF, Karcz S. Drug resistance and the P-glycoprotein homologues of *Plasmodium falciparum*. Semin Cell Biol 1993; 4:29–35.

70. Barnes DA, Foote SJ, Galatis D, Kemp DJ, Cowman AF. Selection for high-level chloroquine resistance results in deamplification of the *pfmdr1* gene and increased sensitivity to mefloquine in *Plasmodium falciparum*. EMBO J 1992; 11:3067–3075.

71. van Es HHG, Karcz S, Cowman A, Gros P, Schurr E. CHO cells expressing the *pfmdr1* gene show altered chloroquine uptake characteristics. In: Resistance Against Anticancer Drugs: Molecular Mechanisms and Clinical Opportunities. Toronto: General Motors Cancer Research Foundation, 1993:F14.

72. Karcz S, Cappai R, Handman E, Cowman AF. Altered sensitivity to antimalarial drugs in *Leishmania* expressing a *Plasmodium falciparum* P-glycoprotein homologue. In: Resistance Against Anticancer Drugs: Molecular Mechanisms and Clinical Opportunities. Toronto: General Motors Cancer Research Foundation, 1993:F8.

73. Warhurst DC. Antimalarial schizontocides: why a permease is necessary. Parasitol Today 1986; 2:331–334.

74. Ferrari V, Cutler DJ. Simulation of kinetic data on the influx and efflux of chloroquine by erythrocytes infected with *Plasmodium falciparum*. Biochem Pharmacol 1991; 42:S167–S179.

75. MacIntyre AC. Studies on Chloroquine Distribution in Tissues. Ph.D. dissertation, University of Sydney, 1989.

76. Bray PG, Howells RE, Ward SA. Vacuolar acidification and chloroquine sensitivity in *Plasmodium falciparum*. Biochem Pharmacol 1992; 43:3100–3109.

77. Diribe CO, Warhurst DC. A study of the uptake of chloroquine in malaria-infected erythrocytes: high and low affinity uptake and the influence of glucose and its analogues. Biochem Pharmacol 1986; 34:3019–3027.

78. Forgac M. Structure and function of vacuolar class of ATP-driven proton pumps. Physiol Rev 1989; 69:765–796.

14

Transport of Antifolates and Antimonials in Drug-Resistant Leishmania

Marc Ouellette, Barbara Papadopoulou, Annas Haimeur, Katherine Grondin, Eric Leblanc, Danielle Légaré, and Gaétan Roy
Centre Hospitalier de l'Université Laval, Laval, Quebec, Canada

I. *LEISHMANIA*

The protozoan parasite *Leishmania* belongs to the order Kinetoplastidae and the family Trypanosomatidae. The parasite was first described independently in 1903 by Leishman and Donovan (reviewed in Ref. 1). The Leishman–Donovan bodies were then recognized as the etiologic agents of leishmaniasis, a term used to describe various diseases. Leishmania has a relatively simple life cycle that includes two basic life stages. The flagellated promastigote leishmania is found in the insect vector, the phlebotomine sandfly. Promastigotes in the proboscis of a female sandfly are introduced into a vertebrate host during a blood meal. The promastigotes are engulfed by the host macrophages, differentiate into the intracellular aflagellated amastigote form, and multiply within phagolysosomes. The cycle is completed when sandflies feed on infected individuals, and the amastigotes transform into promastigotes in the gut of the fly.

A. Epidemiology

Leishmania species are distributed worldwide and are endemic around the Mediterranean littoral, North and East Africa, the Near and Middle

East, India, China, South and Central America, and Russia. Between 10 and 15 million people have clinical symptoms, and 400,000 new cases are diagnosed each year (2). As an important percentage of the population living in endemic areas is seropositive for leishmania infection, but is either asymptomatic or exhibits subclinical manifestations of the diseases (3), the number of infected persons probably far exceeds the number usually cited. Increases in traveling and intervention in regional conflicts has raised the number of leishmanial cases in nonendemic areas. Indeed, several cases of leishmaniasis were reported in veterans from "Operation Desert Storm" (4), and, as incubation periods can be very long, more cases may be reported in the future. Leishmania has also emerged as a serious opportunistic pathogen in human immunodeficiency virus (HIV)-infected humans (5).

At least 12 *Leishmania* species infect humans, and these can be grouped into four main complexes: *L. donovani*, *L. tropica*, *L. mexicana*, and the *L. braziliensis* complex. The clinical manifestations of infections vary with the species, encompassing cutaneous leishmaniasis (oriental sore), characterized by skin lesions that can self-heal, generally within 1 year; mucocutaneous leishmaniasis (espundia), caused by *L. braziliensis* and presenting destructive lesions of nasopharyngeal tissues that rarely heal by themselves; and visceral leishmaniasis (kala azar), the most severe form of leishmaniasis, which is usually fatal if left untreated and is caused mainly by species of the *L. donovani* complex.

B. Chemotherapy

The treatment of choice for all forms of leishmaniasis is based on pentavalent antimonial [Sb(V)]-containing drugs, such as sodium stibogluconate (Pentostam) and meglumine (N-methylglucamine; Glucantime; Fig. 1). Most clinical studies have focused on optimizing treatment regimens of pentavalent antimony. The World Health Organization currently recommends 20 mg of antimony per kilogram per day for 4 weeks. However, resistance to antimonials is increasing (6), and development of new drugs is essential. Although Sb(V)-containing drugs are relatively safe, they require intramuscular administration and are expensive. Second-line drugs, such as pentamidine and amphotericin B (see Fig. 1), are available, but do not have a therapeutic index as favorable as that of Sb(V) and often induce toxic effects. Cheaper, easily administered drugs are urgently needed for the treatment of all forms of leishmaniasis. Several gene-regulation mechanisms and biochemical differences exist between leishmania and the host organism, suggesting that it should be feasible to find specific drugs against these parasites.

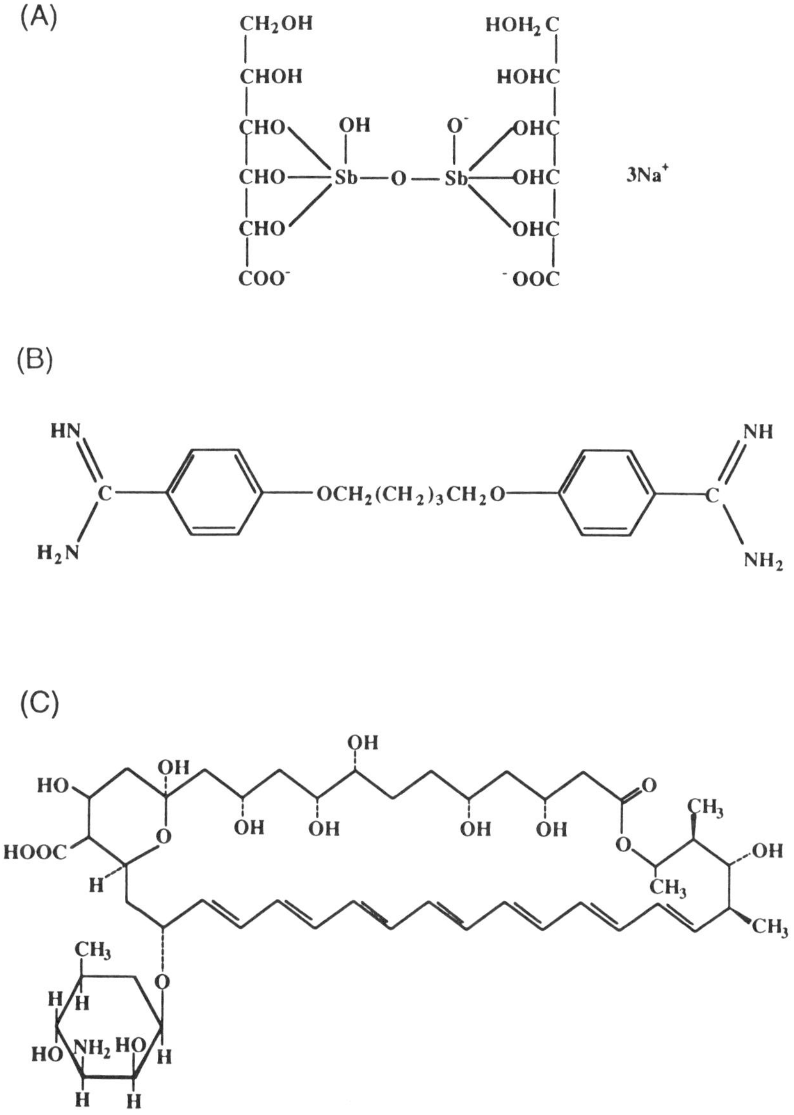

Figure 1 Structure of drugs used for the treatment of leishmaniasis. (A) Stibogluconate [Pentostam; with N-methylglucamine (Glucantime)] is the drug of choice in the treatment of all forms of leishmaniasis. Shown here is the textbook structure where two molecules of gluconate are complexed to two molecules of antimony by oxygens. However, analysis of stibogluconate structure has revealed that it is a mixture of carbohydrates derived from gluconic acids complexed to antimony (44): (B) pentamidine; (C) amphotericin B.

In this chapter, we examine folate and antifolate metabolism and transport into leishmania and describe novel pathways that might serve as targets for chemotherapy. An overview of the transport properties of antimonials and other oxyanions and of the putative mechanism of resistance to these compounds is also presented.

II. ANTIFOLATES

A. Folate Metabolism

Folates serve as cofactors in a variety of one-carbon transfer reactions in most cells. Extensive work has been done with the key enzyme dihydrofolate reductase (DHFR), which reduces dihydrofolate to tetrahydrofolate, the latter being an essential one-carbon donor for the synthesis of DNA precursors. The primary structures of DHFR from a variety of organisms share very little homology, suggesting that specific inhibitors (antifolates) against this enzyme could be found. Indeed, antifolates are widely used antimicrobial and antineoplasic agents; their use includes infections caused by *Plasmodium* and *Toxoplasma* species. Antifolates have not yet proved useful, however, in the treatment of leishmaniasis. Because the folate pathway in leishmanias is poorly understood, the basis for this ineffectiveness is unknown. Nevertheless, the classic bacterial antifolate trimethoprim and the antiprotozoan pyrimethamine (Fig. 2) are poor inhibitors of the leishmanial DHFR (7), explaining in part the inefficacy of these antifolates against leishmania. The primary structure of the DHFR of leishmania is known (8,9). As in other protozoa, it is fused to the thymidylate synthetase (TS) protein, resulting in one bifunctional protein (10,11). In rich medium, notably one containing pterin derivatives, the exclusive role of DHFR is to provide thymidylate precursors to cells. This was first demonstrated by the reversion of methotrexate (MTX; see Fig. 2) cytotoxicity on addition of thymidylate precursors (12–14). More recently, a null mutant of the *dhfr-ts* gene of an *L. major* laboratory strain was obtained by gene targeting, and its only phenotype was thymidine auxotrophy (15). The antifolate MTX, a potent inhibitor of the leishmanial DHFR (11), is toxic to leishmanias, but more so to mammalian cells, precluding its clinical use for leishmaniasis. Coupling MTX to a carrier molecule for more effective delivery to macrophages resulted in greatly enhanced antileishmanial activity both in vitro and in vivo (16). Other antifolates showed more selective toxicity against *Leishmania* strains (Santi D, personal communication), suggesting that antifolates might be useful drugs for leishmaniasis. Moreover, the biochemistry and regulation of both transport and folate synthesis from pterin derivatives are novel (see fol-

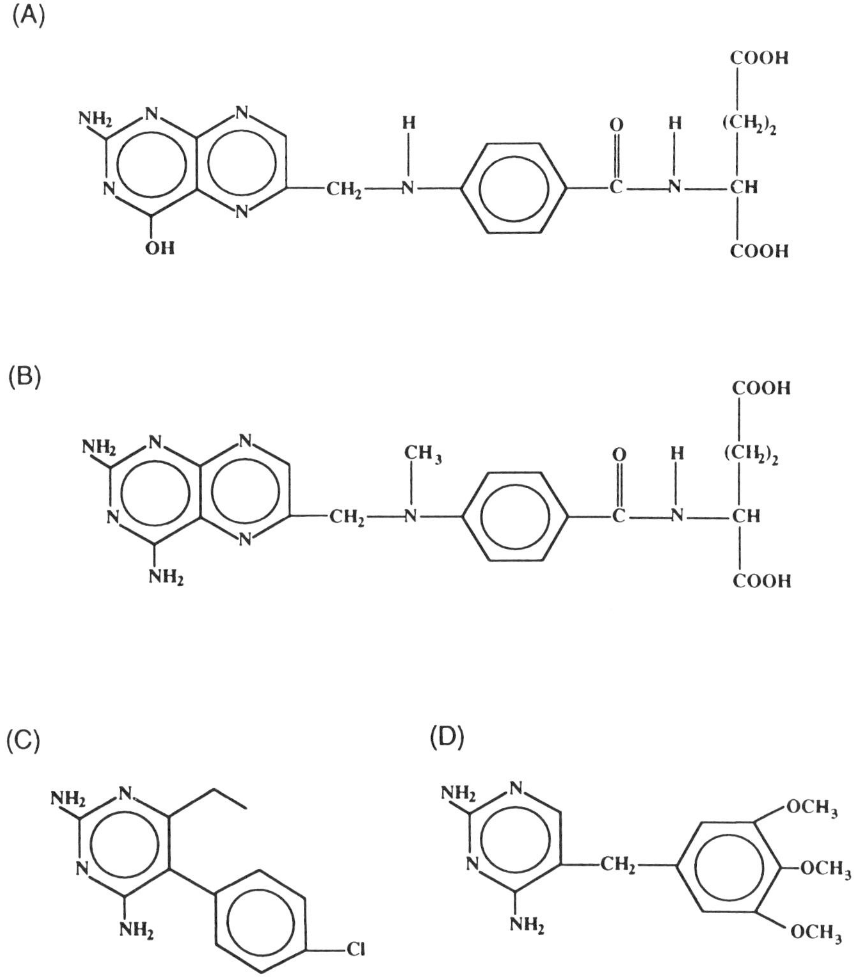

Figure 2 Structure of folate and antifolates. (A) Folate is composed of three building blocks: a pterin derivative, *para*-amino benzoic acid, and glutamic acid. In leishmania the predominant metabolite of folate is the pentaglutamate conjugate (84). (B) The folate analogue methotrexate. (C) The antiprotozoan pyrimethamine. (D) The bacterial dihydrofolate reductase inhibitor trimethoprim.

lowing section), opening the possibility that drugs specific for one of these processes could be developed against leishmania.

B. Biochemistry of Transport

Growth in defined medium has revealed that leishmania is auxotrophic for folates (12,13,17). However, ample evidence now exists that leishmania is capable of synthesizing folates from pterins (18,19) and, although the precise mechanism is not understood, genes involved in this process are beginning to be isolated (20).

Leishmanias contain a high-affinity folate uptake system, with K_m ranging from 0.23 to 0.7 μM, depending on the species (13,21). Folate uptake occurs against a concentration gradient, and is dependent on cellular energy and the growth phase of the organism (21). Uptake is competitively inhibited by 5-methyltetrahydrofolate, 5-formyltetrahydrofolate, p-aminobenzoic acid (PABA)-glutamate, dihydrofolate, tetrahydrofolate, and the antifolate MTX (21,22). Several lines of evidence indicate that the high-affinity folate uptake system also represents the main source for MTX uptake. Indeed, the transport of both folate and MTX is competitively inhibited by the same compounds (21), and cell lines selected for MTX resistance and showing a decrease in the accumulation of MTX also exhibited a parallel decrease in folate uptake (13,23).

The common folate–MTX transporter from leishmania has been studied in greater detail by using affinity labeling with activated radioactive MTX or folate (22). A 46-kDa protein, enriched in the membrane fraction, was labeled specifically with the activated ligand. Competitive inhibitors of folate or MTX transport prevented the labeling of the activated ligand. Finally, no reactive band was detectable in MTX-resistant mutants that are defective in folate–MTX transport (22). This 46-kDa protein has been isolated and partially sequenced (B. Ullman, personal communication), and cloning and transfection of the corresponding gene should reveal whether it indeed corresponds to the MTX–folate transporter.

Secondary folate–MTX transporters cannot be excluded, as cell lines with no detectable uptake of folate or MTX under experimental conditions used were, nevertheless, able to grow in defined medium supplemented with folates (13). Selection of *Leishmania* mutants for MTX resistance suggests that several types of mutations can lead to decreased uptake of the drug (24). It is not known whether these mutations affect the same or different loci.

C. Resistance Mechanisms

The study of resistance mechanisms of *Leishmania* mutants selected for MTX resistance has contributed to our understanding of folate metabolism and transport in leishmanias. Two main mechanisms were observed: gene amplification and transport mutations. Because of the relatively small genome size of leishmania (50,000 kb), gene amplification could be easily observed by careful examination of ethidium bromide-stained gel of restriction digests of DNA isolated from wild-type and mutant strains (11). At least two different loci, termed the *R* and *H* locus, were found amplified in MTX-resistant mutants.

1. Gene Amplification

The R Locus   The *R* locus encodes the gene for the bifunctional target DHFR-TS, and transfection of the *dhfr-ts* gene has indicated that it is capable by itself of conferring MTX resistance (25). Amplification of the *R* locus has been observed primarily in *L. major* selected for MTX resistance (23), but not in *L. donovani* or in *L. tarentolae* wild-type cells selected in a step-by-step fashion (13,24,26). It is not known why *dhfr-ts* is not amplified in *L. tarentolae*, but the reason might be related to the lack of optimal repeated sequences in the vicinity of the *dhfr-ts* gene, as gene amplification in leishmania always occurs by homologous recombination (reviewed in Ref. 27). Amplification of this locus was also described after selection with the TS inhibitor CB3717 (28).

The H Locus   Amplification of the *H* locus has been observed in several *Leishmania* species selected for resistance to MTX (24,26,29–32) (Fig. 3). The copy number of the H circles correlated well with the level of MTX resistance (26,30), and *Leishmania* mutants selected for resistance to drugs unrelated to MTX and exhibiting *H* locus amplification were cross-resistant to MTX (27,32–34). Amplification of the *H* locus did not correlate with elevated levels of DHFR-TS (26), with changes in the steady-state accumulation of MTX (23,35), or with gross modification of MTX (14,36). From gene transfection experiments, the *H* locus-associated MTX resistance gene was isolated and characterized. The gene *ltdh* (also called *hmtxr*) belongs to the family of short-chain dehydrogenases (14,25), a family of enzymes involved in a variety of oxidoreduction reactions (reviewed in Ref. 37).

The mechanism by which LTDH confers resistance is beginning to be understood. We have proposed that LTDH, when overproduced, is capable of providing reduced folates to the cells even when DHFR is blocked (14,27,35). Gene transfection and gene knockout experiments by homologous recombination provided clear evidence that LTDH is involved in the conversion of pterin derivatives into reduced folates (20). Although the exact mechanism remains to be elucidated, the evidence suggests that leishmania might be capable of de novo folate synthesis. The novelty and uniqueness of LTDH opens the possibility of developing specific inhibitors of parasites.

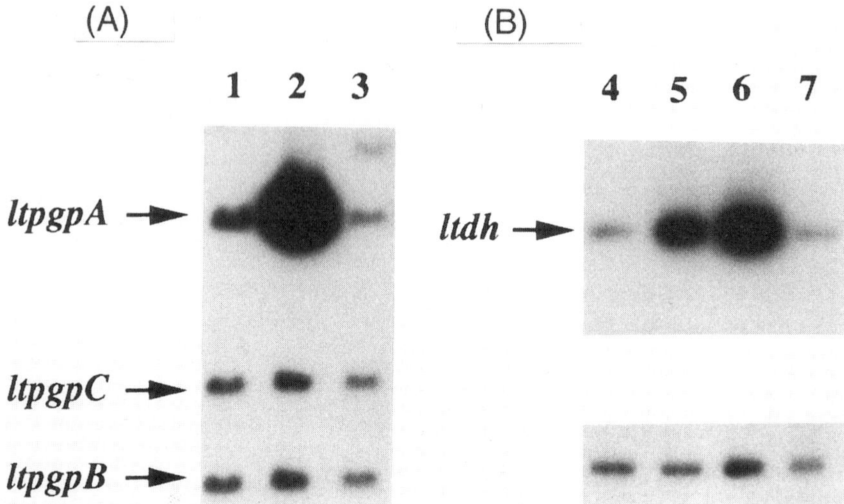

Figure 3 *H* locus amplification in arsenite-resistant and methotrexate (MTX)-resistant mutants. DNA isolated from *Leishmania* cells was run on agarose gel, blotted, and hybridized to (A) a nucleotide-binding site probe recognizing the P-glycoprotein gene family in leishmania (62) or (B) to a probe recognizing the MTX resistance gene *ltdh* (14). (A) 1, TarIIWT (wild-type); 2, an arsenite-resistant mutant with *ltpgpA* amplification; 3, an arsenite-resistant mutant without gene amplification. (B) 4, TarIIWT; 5 and 6, MTX-resistant mutants with *ltdh* amplification; 7, a MTX-resistant mutant without gene amplification. The probe was stripped off and the blot was rehybridized to a *ltpgpE*-specific probe to monitor the amount of DNA in each lane.

2.   Transport Mutations

Amplification of *ltdh* is a frequent event in wild-type cell lines selected in a stepwise manner for MTX resistance (24). Five *L. tarentolae* homozygous *ltdh* null clones were selected in a stepwise selection procedure for MTX resistance. As expected, amplification of the *H* locus was not observed. In one mutant the *R* locus encoding the *dhfr-ts* gene was amplified (E. Leblanc, B. Papadopoulou, G. Roy, and M. Ouellette, unpublished data), suggesting that when a preferred mechanism of resistance is disrupted, a secondary mechanism can be used. In the four remaining MTX-resistant clones, a decrease in the steady-state accumulation of MTX was observed (E. Leblanc, B. Papadopoulou, G. Roy, and M. Ouellette, unpublished data). Although gene amplification is a frequent event in leishmania cells selected for MTX resistance, it is only observed in 50–60% of cells (23,24). The remaining cells failed to show DNA amplification, but every independent cell line studied exhibited a decrease in the steady-state accumulation of MTX (23,24). Therefore, transport mutations seem to be very frequent in MTX-selected cell lines.

Reduced Uptake of MTX Every *Leishmania* cell line selected for MTX resistance, whether it had DNA amplification or not, exhibited reduced accumulation of the drug (13,23,24,38). This decreased accumulation was attributed to mutations in the common high-affinity folate MTX carrier (13,23). In every *L. major* MTX-resistant cell line studied, a two- to fourfold decrease of the V_{max} of the MTX influx was observed, but it did not always correlate with the level of MTX resistance (23). In contrast, a clone of a mutagenized *L. donovani* population that was selected for high-level MTX resistance showed a pronounced decrease in MTX accumulation (13). Transport studies in several *L. tarentolae* cells selected in a step-by-step fashion to MTX resistance indicated that two different transport mutant phenotypes exist (24). The first category, as in *L. major*, showed a 4.5-fold decrease in the accumulation of MTX, whereas the reduction in accumulation was more pronounced in the second category. Biochemical and genetic analyses have revealed one main common folate MTX transporter, but other minor transporters could not be excluded (13; see foregoing). It is not known whether the mutations leading to the observed differences in MTX accumulation concern the same locus, or whether different mutations influence a high-affinity or low-affinity folate–MTX transporter. Both types of mutations are stable and are retained in mutants grown in the absence of MTX for prolonged periods (13,24). The cloning of the folate–MTX transporter could help elucidate the molecular mechanism of reduced accumulation of MTX in leishmania.

Link with Pterin Metabolism *Leishmania donovani* MTX-resistant mutants, with less than 1% of the uptake of folate and MTX of wild-type cells, were capable of growing in defined medium supplemented with folates, suggesting that other transporters are also present in leishmania. Unlike wild-type cells, however, these mutants were incapable of thriving in defined medium supplemented with pterins (13,18). A revertant of one mutant selected for its capacity to grow in a defined medium supplemented with pterin was obtained from a mutagenized population. This revertant regained folate and MTX transport capability (18), suggesting that a single locus is involved in both the transport of folates and the conversion of pterins into folates. The identity of this gene is unknown. It does not appear to be *ltdh*, because although it is required for growth in defined medium supplemented with pterins, folate–MTX transport is unaffected in *ltdh* overproducer (35) or *ltdh* null mutant (E. Leblanc, B. Papadopoulou, and M. Ouellette, unpublished data).

In summary, the folate metabolism of leishmanias is considerably different from the mammalian host they infect. Although both are capable of using folate from their environment, leishmanias can in addition synthesize folates de novo from pterins, although the details of this mechanism remain to be elucidated. This suggests that drugs could be developed that would specifically inhibit the parasite's folate pathway. Studies on antifolate resistance have revealed that, as in mammalian cells (39,40), several mechanisms occur in leishmania, including amplification of the target gene *dhfr-ts* or the short-chain dehydrogenase gene *ltdh* and, in all resistant cells, a defect in the uptake of the drug. At least two types of transport mutations exist: one leading to a moderate decrease in the steady-state accumulation of MTX, the other in a more pronounced (>50-fold) decrease. Future work will answer the question of whether or not these mutations affect the same locus.

III. ANTIMONIALS AND OTHER OXYANIONS

The arsenical salvarsan, developed by Paul Erlich at the beginning of this century, was the first antimicrobial agent designed specifically for chemotherapy. More selective drugs are now available to treat most infections, but oxyanions, in the form of aromatic arsenicals or drugs containing the related metal antimony, are still widely used in the treatment of some protozoan infections. Pentavalent antimonials in the form of sodium stibogluconate (Pentostam) and N-methylglucamine (meglumine; Glucantime) are still the drugs of choice in the fight against leishmaniasis. The rapid clearance of Sb(V) avoids acute toxicity, but requires high doses for prolonged periods (1,41). High initial antimony concentrations, rather than sustained levels, seem important for parasite clearance (42). The Sb(V) drugs might be metabolized in vivo into trivalent antimonials, which may be the active form (43).

The mode of action of Sb(V) drugs in leishmanias is poorly understood, but, as with most heavy metals, it is likely to be multifactorial; this is substantiated by the binding of Sb(V) to several leishmanial proteins (44). One of the mechanisms seems to involve the inhibition of enzymes involved in glycolysis and in fatty acid β-oxidation (45), although studies with *L. mexicana* failed to show an inhibition of glycolytic enzymes by antimonials (46).

A. Biochemistry of Transport

1. Pentavalent Antimonials

In attempts to understand the mechanism of action of Sb(V), accumulation studies of Sb(V)-containing drugs were performed (42,43,47,48), and resistant mutants were generated in vitro in a stepwise fashion (49–51).

Accumulation studies in leishmania were first done with radiolabeled preparations of Pentostam (43,47). More recently, electrothermal—or hydride generation—atomic absorption spectroscopy has been used to study Sb(V) accumulation in leishmania (48) or tissue distribution of stilboglucanate in animal models (42). Pentavalent antimony was thought to be more active against intracellular amastigotes than against promastigotes (52,53); the greater accumulation of Sb(V) drugs in amastigotes, compared with promastigotes, determined by uptake experiments with [^{125}Sb]stibogluconate, was consistent with this premise (43,47). The foregoing finding was obtained by comparing free-living promastigotes in culture media and intracellular amastigotes in macrophage cell lines (52,53). However, when the susceptibility of promastigotes and amastigotes to Sb(V) was measured in identical medium, it was identical (45). More recently, the influx rate of Sb(V) across a unit area of membrane appeared similar in promastigotes and amastigotes (48).

Drug uptake by cells can occur by simple or facilitated diffusion or, as with MTX, by active transport. Uptake of Sb(V) is proportional to drug concentration (47) and with time up to 8 h (48), supporting the idea that stibogluconate is transported, at least in the species tested, mainly by a passive diffusion mechanism.

2. Other Oxyanions

The trivalent antimonial [Sb(III)] antimony potassium tartrate was used before Sb(V)-containing drugs, and it has been suggested that Sb(V) derivatives are metabolized in vivo into active Sb(III) compounds (43). Antimonite is chemically similar to arsenite (54), and mutants selected for resistance to one of the oxyanion are cross-resistant to other oxyanions at various levels (51). This finding has led to the study of transport properties of Sb(III) (48) and of arsenite in leishmania (51).

The influx of Sb(III) drug into promastigotes was very rapid and reached a plateau after 2 h, whereas the efflux was much slower (48), raising the possibility that this drug does not enter the cell solely by passive diffusion, but also by an active transport system, although tight binding of Sb(III) derivatives to parasite molecules cannot be excluded. Influx of trivalent antimony drug in amastigote, however, was linear for at least 8 h (48). Wild-type *L. tarentolae* cells accumulated $^{73}AsO_2^-$ in a time-dependent manner, reaching a plateau in 10 min, with the steady-state level of accumulation remaining constant for at least 20 min (51).

B. Mechanisms of Resistance

The emergence of drug resistance in protozoan parasites is a major obstacle to their control. Unresponsiveness to Sb(V) drugs in mucocutaneous and visceral leishmaniasis has long been recognized and is now becoming a common problem, occurring in 5–70% of the patients in some endemic areas (55,56). Although unresponsiveness to Sb(V) drugs has not always been attributed to drug resistance of the parasite, Sb(V) resistant parasites have been isolated from patients who did not respond to therapy (55,56). The mechanisms of drug resistance are not well understood, but the development of drug-resistant parasite cell lines in vitro has contributed to our understanding of the possible mechanisms of oxyanion resistance in *Leishmania* strains. As with the antifolates, two main mechanisms of resistance were found in in vitro selected oxyanion-resistant mutants: one mechanism involves gene amplification, and the other implicates transport mutations. Sodium arsenite, an oxyanion related to antimony, is a potent inducer of gene amplification in leishmania (27,57,58). Trivalent and pentavalent antimonials are less potent inducers of gene amplification, but an amplicon was recently observed in a stibogluconate-resistant cell line (A. Haimeur, M. Ouellette, unpublished data).

1. Gene Amplification

P-Glycoprotein Gene Amplification   A number of bands reacting with the monoclonal antibody C-219, specific for a conserved hexapeptide in the mammalian P-glycoprotein (59), were detected in higher amounts in Sb(V)-resistant leishmania cells than in controls (60). Most of these C-219-reacting bands were too small to encode a P-glycoprotein, and more work is needed to correlate this observation with resistance. P-glycoproteins are large plasma membrane proteins that extrude hydrophobic drugs from mammalian cells (61). The *H* locus of *Leishmania* species (see Ref. 6 for review) is amplified in more than half of the mutants selected for arsenite resistance (58). The first gene described on the amplified *H* locus was the P-glycoprotein-related gene *ltpgpA* (62). The *ltpgpA* gene product is a member of the superfamily of transport systems that includes the P-glycoprotein and the cystic fibrosis transmembrane regulator (CFTR); its closest homologue is the recently described MRP protein found in multidrug-resistant small-cell lung cancer (63). The *ltpgpA* gene is part of a large gene family in leishmania, with at least six other genes separated on chromosomes of 800 and 1400 kb (64). LtpgpA is not associated with drugs that are part of the typical multidrug-resistant phenotype caused by mammalian P-glycoproteins (62). However, another leishmanial P-glycoprotein gene, _ldmdr_, seems to be involved in a typical mammalian multidrug-resistant phenotype (65).

Several observations suggested that LtpgpA might be involved in oxyanion resistance (summarized in Ref. 27). These speculations were recently tested by gene transfection, and the _pgpA_ genes of _L. tarentolae_ and _L. major_ were found to be involved in low-level resistance to oxyanions (66,67). The resistance phenotype is specific to arsenite and antimony compounds and in this respect resembles the Ars ATPase of _Escherichia coli_ (54). The _ltpgpA_ gene is amplified in mutants that are highly resistant to arsenite (see Fig. 3), but transfection indicated that it was capable of conferring only low-level resistance. Transfection of _ltpgpA_ alleles, derived from arsenite-resistant mutants of whole _ltpgpA_-containing amplicons or of _pgpA_ genes in partial revertants, indicated that LtpgpA is involved only in low-level resistance to oxyanions, and that no other cooperating factors, either physically linked or unlinked to _ltpgpA_, are contributing to higher levels of resistance (67). Although the _L. major_ _pgpA_ gene was not capable of conferring resistance to stibogluconate, the _L. tarentolae_ gene did (66,67). This difference could be explained by point mutations changing substrate specificity, as encountered in mammalian P-glycoprotein (68,69), by subtle differences in the level of expression, owing to different vectors and recipient strains, or by subtle differences in protein modification (70). As a member of a superfamily of transporters, LtpgpA would be expected to confer resistance by increasing drug extrusion. Preliminary data by Callahan and Beverley (66) indicated that _lmpgpA_ transfectants accumulated twofold less trivalent antimony than control cells, but this decrease was not directly correlated with the level of resistance (66). In contrast, no difference in the steady-state accumulation of radioactive arsenite was noted between _ltpgpA_ transfectants and controls (67). The source of the difference in results is as yet unclear. Two distinct methodologies were used, radioisotopes versus atomic absorption, to measure arsenite and Sb(III), and these could partly account for the differences noted (see, e.g., Ref. 48).

Other Gene Amplifications   Another locus not encoding _ltpgpA_, but derived from the same 800-kb chromosome, was also frequently amplified in arsenite-resistant _Leishmania_ strains (58). The amplicon present in these mutants is linear, 50-kb long, and lost in partial revertants grown in the absence of selective pressure (58). Transfection of the whole linear amplicon in wild-type cells did not lead to an increase in arsenite resistance, whereas transfection in a partial revertant restored the resistance level of the parents (K. Grondin and M. Ouellette, unpublished data). This result suggests that the resistance gene present on the linear amplicon acts cooperatively with another mutation, absent in the wild-type cells but present in the partial revertant, to confer resistance. Another uncharacterized amplicon unrelated to *ltpgpA* or to the linear amplicon was also noted in an arsenite-resistant mutant (A. Haimeur and M. Ouellette, unpublished data). A novel amplicon was observed in a mutant selected for high-level resistance to Sb(V). This circular amplicon is derived from an 1800-kb chromosome. The role of this amplicon in resistance is being investigated by transfection experiments. Preliminary results indicated that when a 7-kb fragment derived from this amplicon is transfected in wild-type cells, it confers a two- to fourfold increase in arsenite, Sb(III), and Sb(V) resistance (A. Haimeur and M. Ouellette, unpublished data). In total, therefore, four different loci are amplified after oxyanion stepwise selection. Transfection experiments suggest that most of these amplicons are involved in low-level resistance. The study of the contribution of the amplicons in resistance should reveal possible modes of action and resistance to oxyanions, a class of molecules useful in treating this protozoan infection.

2. Transport Mutations

Gene amplification occurs only late during stepwise selection for oxyanion resistance (58,67), and some mutants highly resistant to arsenite did not show any DNA amplification, suggesting that additional mechanisms may be involved in resistance. Gene amplification has not yet been observed in cell lines selected for resistance to Sb(III) and is rare in cell lines selected for stibogluconate resistance (49–51).

Efflux of Oxyanions   Initial uptake studies with ^{125}Sb failed to show a difference in steady-state accumulation between Sb(V)-resistant and Sb(V)-sensitive mutants (45). However, uptake experiments of resistant promastigotes from which the resistant amastigotes were derived showed a two- to fourfold decrease in steady-state accumulation of Sb(V) compared with the parent strain (60). Although the difference between amastigote and promastigote remains unexplained, decreased accumulation of the drug might be involved in resistance. As Sb(V) seems to enter cells by passive diffusion (47), it is likely that increased extrusion, rather than reduced uptake, is responsible for decreased accumulation, although direct evidence for increased extrusion is lacking.

Steady-state accumulation of radioactive arsenite has been studied in arsenite- and antimonite-resistant *Leishmania* strains. Oxyanion-resistant cell lines exhibiting various levels of arsenite cross-resistance all showed a marked decrease in the steady-state accumulation of radioactive arsenite. This phenotype was independent of *ltpgpA* amplification and also of the presence of the linear amplicon (51). Arsenite-resistant cells lacking drug accumulation and parent cell lines were depleted of endogenous energy reserves with metabolic inhibitors and then loaded with radioactive arsenite. Rapid and nearly complete efflux of arsenite was observed only from arsenite-resistant cells, following the addition of glucose (51). The nature of the oxyanion efflux system in leishmania remains to be identified. It could resemble the arsenite resistance ATPase found in *E. coli*, as eukaryotic homologues to the pump proteins, have been identified (54). Another possibility is that point mutations could change the substrate specificity of an existing pump. Cloning of the gene(s) responsible for this phenotype should clarify the matter.

Reversal of Oxyanion Resistance   Resistance conferred by the mammalian P-glycoprotein or by the putative efflux system responsible for chloroquine resistance in *Plasmodium* is reversed by calcium channel

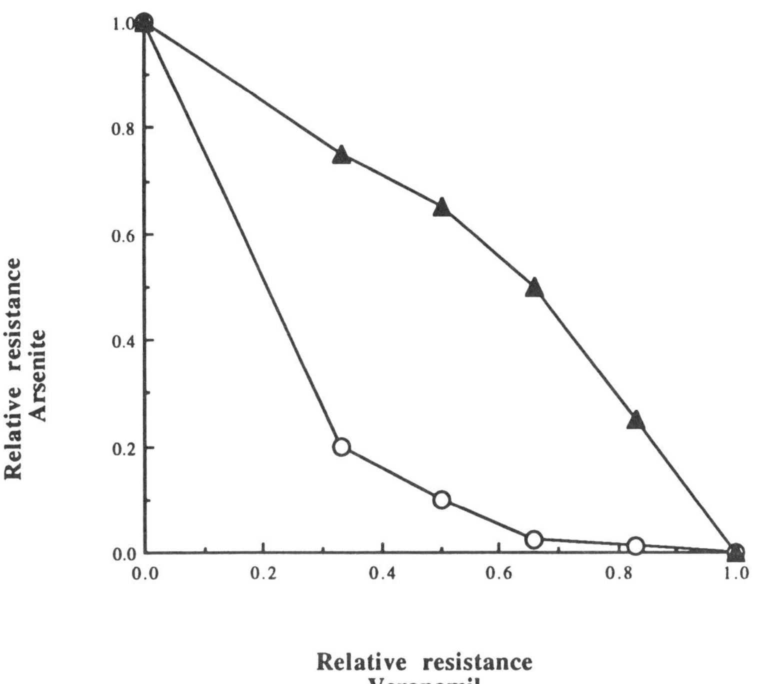

Figure 4   Isobologram analysis (73) of verapamil and arsenite in a wild-type cell (▲) and in an arsenite-resistant mutant (○) without gene amplification.

blockers, such as verapamil, and by other chemosensitizers (61,70,71). Resistance conferred by LtpgpA is not reversed by verapamil (62,66; A. Haimeur and M. Ouellette, unpublished data). Verapamil reverts Sb(V) resistance in vitro and in vivo in leishmania (72), but it is not known by which mechanism. The combination of verapamil and arsenite was studied in one arsenite-resistant mutant and in wild-type cells by isobologram analysis (Fig. 4). The linear curve in wild-type cells indicated that verapamil and arsenite were acting in an additive fashion, but the concave shape of the curve in the mutant indicated that they were acting synergistically (73). This reversal of resistance was found in a strain without DNA amplification that showed increased extrusion of arsenite. Therefore, arsenite is extruded outside the cell in an energy-dependent manner, and resistance is reversed with verapamil.

The parallel between oxyanion resistance in leishmania and chloroquine resistance in plasmodium is intriguing. In both organisms, P-glycoprotein amplification is frequent (58,74,75), but apparently plays only a minor role in resistance (66,67,76). Nevertheless, in both cases, an efflux system seems involved (51,77), which is reverted by agents that revert P-glycoprotein-mediated multidrug resistance in cancer cells. Therefore, it is possible that genes responsible for oxyanion resistance or chloroquine resistance are part of the superfamily of transporters to which the P-glycoprotein belongs. This would not be so surprising for oxyanion resistance, as plasmid-mediated resistance to arsenite and antimonite in *E. coli* is due to an ATPase that is analogous to a P-glycoprotein in structure and confers resistance by ATP-dependent efflux (54).

IV. CONCLUSIONS AND FUTURE DIRECTIONS

Several studies have dealt with *Leishmania* cells selected for drug resistance in vitro (see Table 1). *Leishmania* mutants selected in a stepwise manner always showed a decrease in the steady-state accumulation of the drug used for selection (see Table 1). This decrease in accumulation can be attributed either to a reduced uptake or to an active efflux, and an example of each has been described here. Mutations leading to transport defects always seem to occur early during the selection process (24), whereas gene amplification occurs at a higher drug concentration (24,67) when transport mutations might not be sufficient to confer resistance. Genes responsible for resistance are now being isolated, which will permit elucidating their role in resistant clinical strains.

Antimonials have been used to treat human leishmaniasis since the beginning of the century. Clinical studies have brought better treatment

Table 1 Mechanisms of Drug Resistance in *Leishmania*[a]

Drug class	Mechanism of resistance	Ref.
Oxyanions	Decreased accumulation	
	Reduced accumulation	60, 66
	Increased efflux	51
	Gene amplification	
	P-glycoprotein *ltpgpA*	32, 57, 58, 66, 67
	Linear 50-kb amplicon	58, unpub.[b]
	Other loci	unpub.[b]
Antifolates	Decreased accumulation	
	Low-level (4.5-fold) reduced uptake	23, 24
	High-level (>50-fold) reduced uptake	13, 24
	Gene amplification	
	Target overproduction; *R* locus (*dhfr-ts*)	23, 28, 29, unpub.[b]
	Target bypass *H* locus (*ltdh*)	14, 24–26, 29–32
Nucleoside analogues	Decreased accumulation	
	Guanosine transporter	85, 88
	Adenosine transporter	85, 88
	Gene amplification	
	Reduced uptake system	90

[a] Drugs listed are those mentioned in the text. Several other drugs have also been used to select for drug-resistant mutants, and one mechanism of resistance frequently encountered is gene amplification (see Ref. 6 for recent review).
[b] Ouellette M, Haimeur A, Grondin K, Leblanc E, unpublished results.

regimens of Sb(V) but, in some regions where resistance levels are high, the antimonials have been pushed to their limits of safety and tolerability (41): new drugs are clearly needed. Nevertheless, studies on transport properties and resistance mechanisms to antimonials are warranted, as these drugs will still be widely used in the future, and the drug resistance problem will have to be dealt with shortly.

A. Improved Drug Delivery

Pentavalent antimony is directed against the intracellular amastigote stage of the parasite that is found inside macrophages. Liposomes have been proposed as an effective way to target drugs at macrophages. Liposomes containing antimonial compounds have been more effective in the treatment of leishmaniasis (78,79). One of the second-line drugs, amphotericin

B (see Fig. 1C), is rarely used because of its toxicity. In animal models, amphotericin B incorporated into liposomes was highly effective against leishmaniasis, with low toxicity (80). Liposomal amphotericin B was also used successfully in the treatment of human visceral leishmaniasis (81).

In addition to liposomes, other drug delivery systems that target drugs to macrophages have also shown their usefulness in the treatment of leishmaniasis. Niosomes (nonionic liposomes) in addition to liposomes were also effective against parasites in a mouse model of visceral leishmaniasis. They were especially superior to the free drug in reaching spleen and bone marrow parasites and were less toxic (82). When the antifolate MTX is coupled to bovine serum albumin, it is taken up efficiently through the scavenger receptors present on macrophages. The drug conjugate was nearly 100 times as effective as free MTX in eliminating intracellular parasites in tissue culture and was also highly effective against experimental leishmaniasis in animal models (16).

B. Drug Combinations

Antimonials have been used in combination with other drugs (41). The nucleoside analogue allopurinol or the aminoglycoside paromomycin, two drugs currently used in the treatment of leishmanial infection, were shown, at least in vitro, to act synergistically with Sb(V) drugs, although the biochemical basis of this synergy is unknown (41). The cytokine interferon gamma has also been used in combination with Pentostam to treat difficult cases of leishmaniasis (83). Interferon gamma is thought to enhance the intracellular killing of leishmania, and the combination cytokine and antimony was highly effective and well tolerated in patients (83). If resistance to antimonials in resistant parasites isolated from the field is due to an efflux system, as found in in vitro-selected resistant cells, it might be possible to use antimonials in combination with chemosensitizers that would inhibit efflux.

C. Novel Drugs

Although antimonials are still effective, the problem of resistance is increasing and leishmanial cases, particularly in AIDS patients, are more difficult to treat. Clearly cheaper and more easily administered drugs are needed to treat leishmaniasis. The studies on folate metabolism and transport presented here have indicated novel properties that could be exploited for the treatment of leishmaniasis. In addition to the folate pathway, several biochemical pathways are different between the parasite and the host they infect. Of particular interest is the use of purine analogues or inhibitors of sterol metabolism (reviewed in Refs. 1,41).

1. Purine Analogues

Leishmania, similar to every protozoal parasite yet characterized, is auxotrophic for purines and must scavenge host purines to meet its requirements. Therefore, leishmania cells must transport host purine nucleosides across their plasma membrane. At least two nucleoside transporters that are distinguished by their substrate specificity have been identified in leishmania (85). The apparent K_m values for the transport of nucleosides specific for each transporter were at least two orders of magnitude lower than values obtained for the transport of purine nucleosides by mammalian cells (85). Several nucleoside or nucleobase analogues are metabolized through the salvage system and are cytotoxic toward leishmania (86). The purine analogue allopurinol has been used in clinical trials against leishmania and was effective against American cutaneous leishmaniasis (87), although several reports have questioned the efficacy of allopurinol in the treatment of leishmaniasis (reviewed in Ref. 41).

Several *Leishmania* mutants resistant to purine analogues have been described (88–90). Two separate mutations confer defects in transport capacity; the first in the transport of inosine, guanosine, and their analogues, and the second in the transport of adenosine and its analogues (85,88). Recently, an extrachromosomal amplified circle was found in leishmania cells selected for resistance to inosine dialdehyde or tubercidin, two nucleoside analogues. Gene transfection experiments have shown that a gene present on this amplified circle had the ability to confer resistance on wild-type cells to nucleoside analogues and, interestingly, the transfectants also exhibited a decreased ability to accumulate purine nucleosides (90).

2. Sterol Biosynthesis Inhibitors

The lipids in leishmania that are the basis for new chemotherapeutic agents are the sterols. In mammalian cells cholesterol is the major demethylated sterol. In leishmania, just as in several fungi, such as *Candida albicans*, ergostane sterols are the major demethylated sterols. Several fungal inhibitors are directed against the sterol pathways, and this explained why inhibitors such as amphotericin B (see Chap. 11) and ketoconazole (see Chap. 12) are active against *Leishmania* species (80,81,91). However, some *Leishmania* species when inside macrophages are capable of utilizing host sterols, including cholesterol (1), suggesting that some inhibitors might not be as effective as expected. For instance, ketoconazole was effective against human infections caused by *L. mexicana*, but not by *L. braziliensis* (91). Nevertheless, with all the antifungals available that affect sterol metabolism, it should be possible to find one compound that would be very active against *Leishmania* strains; therefore, animal studies to discover cheap and easily administered drugs to treat leishmaniasis are warranted (41).

ACKNOWLEDGMENTS

The collaboration of S. Dey and B. P. Rosen on arsenite transport properties is acknowledged. The reading of the manuscript by D. Castilaw is also acknowledged. Work in the laboratory is supported by NSERC, MRC, FCAR, and by the UNDP/World Bank/WHO Special Programme for Research and Training in Tropical Diseases. MO and BP are chercheur boursier junior of the Fonds de Recherche en Santé du Québec.

REFERENCES

1. Berman JD. Chemotherapy for leishmaniasis: biochemical mechanisms, clinical efficacy, and future strategies. J Infect Dis 1988; 10:560–586.
2. Ashford RW, Desjeux P, deRaadt P. Estimation of population at risk of infection and number of cases of leishmaniasis. Parasitol Today 1992; 8:104–105.
3. Badaro R, Jones TC, Carvalho EM, Sampaio D, Reed SG, Barral A, Teixeira R, Johnson WD Jr. New perspectives on a subclinical form of visceral leishmaniasis. J Infect Dis 1986; 154:1003–1011.
4. Magill AJ, Grögl M, Gasser RA, Wellington S, Oster C. Visceral infection caused by *Leishmania tropica* in veterans of Operation Desert Storm. 1993; N Engl J Med 328:1383–1387.
5. Altes J, Salas A, Riera M, Udina M, Galmés A, Balanzat J, Ballesteros A, Buades J, Salva F, Villalonga C. Visceral leishmaniasis: another HIV-associated opportunistic infection? Report of eight cases and review of the literature. AIDS 1991; 5:201–207.
6. Ouellette M, Papadopoulou B. Mechanisms of drug resistance in *Leishmania*. Parasitol Today 1993; 9:150–153.
7. Hightower RC, Santi DV. Drug action and drug resistance: antifolate resistance in parasitic protozoa. In: Leech JH, Sande MA, Root RK, eds. Parasite Infections. New York: Churchill Livingstone, 1988:81–94.
8. Beverley SM, Ellenberger TE, Cordingley JS. Primary structure of the gene encoding the bifunctional dihydrofolate reductase–thymidylate synthetase of *Leishmania major*. Proc Natl Acad Sci USA 1986; 83:2584–2588.
9. Grumont R, Washtien WL, Caput D, Santi DV. Bifunctional thymidylate synthase–dihydrofolate reductase from *Leishmania*: sequence homology with the corresponding monofunctional proteins. Proc Natl Acad Sci USA 1986; 83:5387–5391.
10. Ferone R, Roland S. Dihydrofolate reductase: thymidylate synthetase a bifunctional polypeptide from *Crithidia fasciculata*. Proc Natl Acad Sci USA 1980; 77:5802–5806.

11. Coderre JA, Beverley SM, Schimke RT, Santi DV. Overproduction of a bifunctional thymidylate synthetase–dihydrofolate reductase and DNA amplification in methotrexate-resistant *Leishmania tropica*. Proc Natl Acad Sci USA 1983; 80:2132–2136.

12. Petrillo-Peixoto ML, Beverley SM. In vitro activity of sulfonamides and sulfones against *Leishmania major* promastigotes. Antimicrob Agents Chemother 1987; 31:1575–1578.

13. Kaur K, Coons T, Emmet K, Ullman B. Methotrexate-resistant *Leishmania donovani* genetically deficient in the folate–methotrexate transporter. J Biol Chem 1988; 263:7020–7028.

14. Papadopoulou B, Roy G, Ouellette M. A novel antifolate resistance gene on the amplified H circle of *Leishmania*. EMBO J 1992; 11:3601–3608.

15. Cruz A, Coburn CM, Beverley SM. Double targeted gene replacement for creating null mutants. Proc Natl Acad Sci USA 1991; 88:7170–7174.

16. Mukhopadhyay A, Chaudhuri G, Arora SK, Sehgal S, Basu SK. Receptor-mediated drug delivery to macrophages in chemotherapy of leishmaniasis. Science 1989; 244:705–707.

17. Scott DA, Coombs GH, Sanderson BE. Folate utilisation by *Leishmania* species and the identification of intracellular derivatives and folate-metabolising enzymes. Mol Biochem Parasitol 1987; 23:139–149.

18. Beck JT, Ullman B. Nutritional requirements of wild-type and folate transport-deficient *Leishmania donovani* for pterins and folates. Mol Biochem Parasitol 1990; 43:221–230.

19. Beck JT, Ullman B. Biopterin conversion to reduced folates by *Leishmania donovani* promastigotes. Mol Biochem Parasitol 1991; 49:21–28.

20. Papadopoulou B, Roy G, Mourad W, Leblanc E, Ouellette M. Changes in folate and pterin metabolism after disruption of the *Leishmania H* locus short-chain dehydrogenase gene. J Biol Chem 1994; 269:7310–7315.

21. Ellenberger TE, Beverley, SM. Biochemistry and regulation of folate and methotrexate transport in *Leishmania major*. J Biol Chem 1987; 262:10053–10058.

22. Beck JT, Ullman B. Affinity labeling of the folate–methotrexate transporter from *Leishmania donovani*. Biochemistry 1989; 28:6931–6937.

23. Ellenberger TE, Beverley SM. Reductions in methotrexate and folate influx in methotrexate-resistant lines of *Leishmania major* are independent of R and H region amplification. J Biol Chem 1987; 262:13501–13506.

24. Papadopoulou B, Roy G, Ouellette M. Frequent amplification of a short chain dehydrogenase gene as part of circular and linear amplicons in methotrexate resistant *Leishmania*. Nucleic Acids Res 1993; 21:4305–4312.

25. Callahan HL, Beverley SM. A member of the aldoketo reductase family confers methotrexate resistance in *Leishmania*. J Biol Chem 1992; 267:24165–24168.

26. White TC, Fase-Fowler F, van Luenen H, Calafat J, Borst P. The H circles of *Leishmania tarentolae* are a unique amplifiable system of oligomeric DNAs associated with drug resistance. J Biol Chem 1988; 263:16977–16983.

27. Ouellette M., Borst P. Drug resistance and P-glycoprotein gene amplification in the protozoan parasite *Leishmania*. Res Microbiol 1991; 142:737–746.

28. Garvey EP, Coderre JA, Santi DV. Selection and properties of *Leishmania* resistant to 10-propargyl-518-dideazofolate, an inhibitor of thymidylate synthase. Mol Biochem Parasitol 1985; 17:79–91.

29. Beverley SM, Coderre JA, Santi DV, Schimke RT. Unstable DNA amplification in methotrexate-resistant *Leishmania* consist of extrachromosomal circles which relocalize during stabilization. Cell 1984; 38:431–439.

30. Hightower RC, Ruiz-Perez LM, Lie Wong M, Santi, DV. Extrachromosomal element in the lower eukaryote *Leishmania*. J Biol Chem 1988; 263:16970–16976.

31. Petrillo-Peixoto ML, Beverley SM. Amplified DNAs in laboratory stocks of *Leishmania tarentolae*: extrachromosomal circles structurally and functionally similar to the inverted *H* region amplification of methotrexate-resistant *Leishmania major*. Mol Cell Biol 1988; 8:5188–5199.

32. Ouellette M, Hettema E, Wust D, Fase-Fowler F, Borst P. Direct and inverted repeats associated with P-glycoprotein gene amplification in drug resistant *Leishmania*. EMBO J 1991; 10:1009–1016.

33. Ellenberger TE, Beverley SM. Multiple drug resistance and conservative amplification of the *H* region in *Leishmania major*. J Biol Chem 1989; 264:15094–15103.

34. Katakura K, Chang K-P. *H* DNA amplification in *Leishmania* resistant to both arsenite and methotrexate. Mol Biochem Parasitol 1989; 34:189–192.

35. Papadopoulou B, Ouellette M. Amplification of a short-chain dehydrogenase confers high level of resistance to antifolates in *Leishmania*. In: Ayling JE, Nair MG, Baugh CM, eds. Chemistry and Biology of Pteridines and Folates. New York: Plenum Publishing, 1993:559–562.

36. Ellenberger TE, Wright JE, Rosowsky A, Beverley SM. Wild type and drug-resistant *Leishmania major* hydrolyze methotrexate to *N*-10-methyl-4-deoxy-4-aminopteroate without accumulation of methotrexate polyglutamates. J Biol Chem 1989; 264:15960–15966.

37. Persson B, Krook M, Jornvall H. Characteristics of short-chain alcohol dehydrogenases and related enzymes. Eur J Biochem 1991; 200:537–543.

38. Dewes H, Ostergaard HL, Simpson L. Impaired drug uptake in methotrexate resistant *Crithidia fasciculata* without changes in dihydrofolate reductase activity or gene amplification. Mol Biochem Parasitol 1986; 19:149–161.

39. Assaraf ZJ, Feder JN, Sharmal RC, Wright JE, Rosowsky A, Shane B, Schimke RT. Characterization of the coexisting multiple mechanisms of methotrexate resistance in mouse 3T6 R50 fibroblasts. J Biol Chem 267:5776–5784.

40. Li WW, Lin JJ, Tong WP, Trippett TM, Brennan MF, Bertino JR. Mechanisms of natural resistance to antifolates in human soft tissue sarcomas. Cancer Res 1992; 52:1434–1438.

41. Olliaro PL, Bryceson ADM. Practical progress and new drugs for changing patterns of leishmaniasis. Parasitol Today 1993; 9:323–328.

42. Collins M, Carter KC, Baillie AJ. Visceral leishmaniasis in the BALB/c mouse: antimony tissue disposition and parasite suppression after the administration of free stibogluconate. Ann Trop Med Parasitol 1992; 86:34–40.

43. Croft SL, Neame KD, Homewood CA. Accumulation of [^{125}Sb] sodium stibogluconate by *Leishmania mexicana amazonensis* and *Leishmania donovani* in vitro. Comp Biochem Physiol 1981; 68C:95–98.

44. Berman JD, Grogl M. *Leishmania mexicana*: chemistry and biochemistry of sodium stibogluconate (Pentostam). Exp Parasitol 1988; 67:96–103.

45. Berman JD, Edwards N, King M, Grögl M. Biochemistry of Pentostam resistant *Leishmania*. Am J Trop Med Hyg 1989; 40:159–164.

46. Mottram JC, Coombs GH. *Leishmania mexicana*: enzyme activities of amastigotes and promastigotes and their inhibition by antimonials and arsenicals. Exp Parasitol 1985; 59:151–160.

47. Berman JD, Gallalee JV, Hansen BD. *Leishmania mexicana*: uptake of sodium stibogluconate (Pentostam) and pentamidine by parasite and macrophages. Exp Parasitol 1987; 64:127–131.

48. Roberts WL, Rainey PM. Antimony quantification in *Leishmania* by electrothermal atomic absorption spectroscopy. Anal Biochem 1993; 211:1–6.

49. Grögl M, Odula AMJ, Cordero LDC, Kyle DE. *Leishmania* spp.: development of Pentostam-resistant clones in vitro by discontinuous drug exposure. Exp Parasitol 1989; 69:78–90.

50. Ullman B, Carrero-Valenzuela E, Coons T. *Leishmania donovani*: isolation and characterization of sodium stibogluconate (Pentostam)-resistant cell lines. Exp Parasitol 1989; 69:157–163.

51. Dey S, Papadopoulou B, Haimeur A, Roy G, Grondin K, Dou D, Rosen BP, Ouellette M. High level arsenite resistance in *Leishmania* is mediated by an active extrusion system. Mol Biochem Parasitol 1994; 67:49–57.

52. Berman JD, Wyler DJ. An in vitro model for investigation of chemotherapeutic agents in leishmaniasis. J Infect Dis 1980; 142:83–86.

53. Coombs GH, Hart DT, Capaldo J. *Leishmania mexicana*: drug sensitivities of promastigotes and transforming amastigotes. J Antimicrob Chemother 1983; 11:151–162.

54. Rosen BP, Dey S, Dou D, Ji G, Kaur P, Ksenzenko MY, Silver S, Wu J. Evolution of an ion-translocating ATPase. Ann NY Acad Sci 1992; 671:257–272.

55. Jackson JE, Tally JD, Ellis WY, Mebrahtu YB, Lawyer PG, Were JB, Reed SG, Panisko DM, Limmer BL. Quantitative in vitro drug potency and drug susceptibility evaluation of *Leishmania* spp. from patients unresponsive to pentavalent antimony therapy. Am J Trop Med Hyg 1990; 43:464–480.

56. Grögl M, Thomason TN, Franke ED. Drug resistance in leishmaniasis: its implication in systemic chemotherapy of cutaneous and mucocutaneous disease. Am J Trop Med Hyg 1992; 47:117–126.

57. Detke S, Katakura K, Chang K-P. DNA amplification in arsenite-resistant *Leishmania*. Exp Cell Res 1989; 180:161–170.

58. Grondin K, Papadopoulou B, Ouellette M. Homologous recombination be-

tween direct repeat sequences yields P-glycoprotein containing circular amplicons in arsenite resistant *Leishmania*. Nucleic Acids Res 1993; 21:1895–1901.

59. Georges E, Bradley G, Gariepy J, Ling V. Detection of P-glycoprotein isoforms by gene-specific monoclonal antibodies. Proc Natl Acad Sci USA 1990; 87:152–156.

60. Grögl M, Martin RK, Odula AMJ, Milhous WK, Kyle DE. Characteristics of multidrug resistance in *Plasmodium* and *Leishmania*: detection of P-glycoprotein-like components. Am J Trop Med Hyg 1991; 45:98–111.

61. Gottesman MM, Pastan I. Biochemistry of multidrug resistance mediated by the multidrug transporter. Annu Rev Biochem 1993; 62:385–427.

62. Ouellette M, Fase-Fowler F, Borst P. The amplified *H* circle of methotrexate-resistant *Leishmania tarentolae* contains a novel P-glycoprotein gene. EMBO J 1990; 9:1027–1033.

63. Cole SPC, Bhardwaj G, Gerlach JH, Mackie JE, Grant CE, Almquist KC, Stewart AJ, Kurz EU, Duncan AMV, Deely RG. Overexpression of a transporter gene in a multidrug-resistant human cancer cell line. Science 1992; 258:1650–1654.

64. Légaré D, Hettema E, Ouellette M. The P-glycoprotein related gene family in *Leishmania*. Mol Biochem Parasitol 1994; 68:81–91.

65. Henderson DM, Sifri CD, Rodgers M, Wirth DF, Hendrickson N, Ullman B. Multidrug resistance in *Leishmania donovani* is conferred by amplification of a gene homologous to the mammalian *mdr1* gene. Mol Cell Biol 1992; 12:2855–2865.

66. Callahan HL, Beverley SM. Heavy metal resistance: a new role for P-glycoproteins in *Leishmania*. J Biol Chem 1991; 266:18427–18430.

67. Papadopoulou B, Roy G, Dey S, Rosen BP, Ouellette M. Contribution of the *Leishmania* P-glycoprotein related gene *ltpgpA* to oxyanion resistance. J Biol Chem 1994; 269:11980–11986.

68. Choi K, Chen C-J, Kriegler M, Roninson IB. An altered pattern of cross-resistance in multidrug-resistant human cells results from spontaneous mutations in the *mdr1* (P-glycoprotein) gene. Cell 1988; 53:519–529.

69. Gros P, Dhir R, Croop J, Talbot F. A single amino acid substitution strongly modulates the activity and subtrate specificity of the mouse mdr1 and mdr3 drug efflux pumps. Proc Natl Acad Sci USA 1991; 88:7289–7293.

70. Endicott JA, Ling V. The biochemistry of P-glycoprotein-mediated multidrug resistance. Annu Rev Biochem 1989; 58:137–171.

71. Martin SK, Oduola AMJ, Milhous WK. Reversal of chloroquine resistance in *Plasmodium falciparum* by verapamil. Science 1987; 235:899–901.

72. Neal RA, Van Bueren J, McCoy NG, Iwobi M. Reversal of drug resistance in *Trypanosoma cruzi* and *Leishmania donovani* by verapamil. Trans R Soc Trop Med Hyg 1989; 83:197–198.

73. Krogstadt DJ, Moellering RC. Antimicrobial combinations. In: Lorian V, ed. Antibiotics in Laboratory Medicine. Baltimore: Williams & Wilkins, 1986:537–578.

74. Foote SJ, Thompson JK, Cowman AF, Kemp DJ. Amplification of the multi-

drug resistance gene in some chloroquine-resistant isolates of *Plasmodium falciparum*. Cell 1989; 57:921–930.

75. Wilson CW, Serrano AE, Wasley A, Bogenschutz MP, Shankar AH, Wirth DF. Amplification of a gene related to mammalian *mdr* genes in drug resistant *Plasmodium falciparum*. Science 1989; 244:1184–1186.

76. Wellems TE, Panton LJ, Gluzman IY, de Rosario VE, Gwadz RW, Walker-Jonah A, Krogstad DJ. Chloroquine resistance not linked to *mdr*-like genes in a *Plasmodium falciparum cross*. Nature 1990; 345:253–255.

77. Krogstadt DJ, Gluzman IY, Kyle DE, Odoula AM, Martin SK, Milhous WK, Schlesinger PH. Efflux of chloroquine from *Plasmodium falciparum*: mechanism of chloroquine resistance. Science 1987; 238:1283–1285.

78. Alving CR, Steck EA, Chapman WL, Waits VB, Hendricks LS, Swartz GM, Hanson WL. Therapy of leishmaniasis: superior efficacies of liposome-encapsulated drugs. Proc Natl Acad Sci USA 1978; 75:2959–2963.

79. New RRC, Chance ML, Thomas SC, Peters W. Antileishmanial activity of antimonials entrapped in liposomes. Nature 1978; 272:55–56.

80. Croft SL, Davidson RN, Thornton EA. Liposomal amphotericin B in the treatment of visceral leishmaniasis. J Antimicrob Chemother 1991; 28(suppl B):111–118.

81. Davidson RN, Croft SL, Scott A, Maini M, Moody AH, Bryceson AD. Liposomal amphotericin B in drug-resistant viseral leishmaniasis. Lancet 1991; 337:1061–1062.

82. Carter KC, Dolan TF, Alexander J, Baillie AJ, McColgan C. Visceral leishmaniasis: drug carrier characteristics and the ability to clear parasites from the liver, spleen, and bone marrow in *Leishmania donovani* infected BALB/c mice. J Pharm Pharmacol 1989; 41:87–91.

83. Badaro R, Falcoff E, Badaro FS, Carvalho EM, Pedral-Sampaio D, Barral A, Carvalho JS, Barral-Netto M, Brandely M, Silva L, Bina JC, Teixeira R, Falcoff R, Rocha H, Ho, JL, Johnson, WD. Treatment of visceral leishmaniasis with pentavalent antimony and interferon gamma. N Engl J Med 1990; 322:16–21.

84. Santi DV, Nolan P, Shane B. Folylpolyglutamates in *Leishmania major*. Biochem Biophys Res Commun 1987; 146:1089–1092.

85. Aronow B, Kaur K, McCartan K, Ullman B. Two high affinity nucleoside transporters in *Leishmania donovani*. Mol Biochem Parasitol 1987; 22:29–37.

86. Marr JJ, Berens RL, Nelson DJ, Krenitsky TA, Spector T, LaFon SW, Elion, GB. Antileishmanial action of 4-thiopyrazolo(3,4-*d*)pyrimidine and its ribonucleoside. Biochem Pharmacol 1982; 31:143–148.

87. Martinez S, Marr JJ. Allopurinol in the treatment of American cutaneous leishmaniasis. N Engl J Med 1992; 326:741–744.

88. Iovannisci DM, Kaur K, Young L, Ullman B. Genetic analysis of nucleoside transport in *Leishmania donovani* Mol Cell Biol 1984; 4:1013–1019.

89. Rainey P, Santi DV. Formycin B resistance in *Leishmania*. Biochem Pharmacol 1984; 33:1374–1377.

90. Kerby BR, Detke S. Reduced purine accumulation is encoded on an ampli-

fied DNA in *Leishmania mexicana amazonensis* resistant to toxic nucleosides. Mol Biochem Parasitol 1993; 60:171–186.

91. Navin TR, Arana BA, Arana FE, Berman JD, Chajon JF. Placebo-controlled clinical trial of sodium stibogluconate (Pentostam) versus ketoconazole for treating cutaneous leishmaniasis in Guatemala. J Infect Dis 1992; 165:528–534.

15

Nucleoside Transport

Carol E. Cass
University of Alberta, Edmonton, Alberta, Canada

I. INTRODUCTION

A. Historical Perspective and Chapter Overview

Mammalian cells require the presence of nucleoside transport (NT) proteins in their plasma membranes for cellular uptake or release of adenosine, uridine, and other physiological nucleosides. Mediated transport of nucleosides in mammalian cells was first characterized in studies conducted with human erythrocytes in the early 1970s and, for a decade, the erythrocytic transporter, which is equilibrative and exhibits broad permeant selectivity, was considered the prototype. In the 1980s, with the application of rapid-assay technologies that provided unequivocal initial rates of uptake, NT processes that differed significantly in their functional characteristics from the erythrocytic transporter were identified. Today, seven functionally distinct NT processes have been described, and it is likely that others will yet be discovered. The functional heterogeneity of NT processes in the various cells and tissues that have now been studied suggests the existence of a complex family of transporter proteins, with diverse physiological functions.

Although most nucleoside drugs are highly hydrophilic and thus do not readily permeate the lipid bilayer of biological membranes in the absence of functional NT processes, a few (e.g., azidothymidine) are sufficiently hydrophobic that substantial permeation into target cells also occurs by passive diffusion. The role of NT processes in the cellular pharmacology of nucleoside drugs varies considerably, depending on the extent to which the nucleoside, as a consequence of its inherent diffusibility and its transportability, permeates plasma membranes. In the decade that has passed since the publication of a comprehensive review of the transport of nucleoside drugs (1), there have been major advances in the understanding of NT processes, most notably, the recognition of multiple transporter types, with quite different characteristics. Although there is much yet to be learned about the transportability of nucleoside drugs, it is clear that expression of functionally active NT proteins in target cells is a prerequisite for pharmacological activity of many nucleoside drugs. This chapter focuses on the characteristics of the multiple NT processes, with particular emphasis on the transportability of adenosine, because of its unique role among nucleosides in signaling processes, and of nucleoside drugs with established clinical roles in treatment of human diseases. The reader is also referred to previous review articles that summarize early studies of NT processes of erythrocytes (2), methodologies for NT assays (3,4), and results of extensive kinetic (5–8) and mutational (9) analyses of equilibrative NT processes. There are several recent overview articles that deal with the emerging heterogeneity of nucleoside transporter types in cultured cells and peripheral tissues (10–12) and in the central nervous system (13).

The issue of greatest current interest, and the key to understanding the physiological roles of NT processes, is identification of the proteins responsible for the functionally distinct transport processes that have been documented in kinetic studies of nucleoside fluxes. The proteins that mediate NT processes are minor membrane components (see Ref. 14 for review), and purification to homogeneity has been achieved only for the equilibrative transporters of erythrocytes (15). Efforts to identify other NT proteins by molecular cloning have only just begun to produce results. Proteins with NT activity have been identified by molecular cloning and expression of cDNAs from rabbit (16), rat (17,18), and mouse (19,20). The sequences of the proteins predicted by these cDNAs are a clear indication of the heterogeneity of NT processes, since they are not at all related to each other. Two of the cloned proteins are Na^+–nucleoside cotransporters of the plasma membrane, whereas the third is expressed in organellar membranes and appears to accept nucleotides as well as nucleosides as permeants. The beginnings of an understanding of the molecular structure of NT proteins is also reviewed in this chapter.

B. Relationships Between Nucleoside Transport and Metabolism

Cellular uptake of nucleosides is a multifactorial process. Depending on the nucleoside, it involves (1) permeation across the plasma membrane, by passive diffusion and one or more mediated mechanisms; and (2) metabolism, by either anabolic (e.g., nucleoside kinases) or catabolic enzymes (e.g., nucleoside deaminases, nucleoside phosphorylases). For most nucleosides, transport and metabolism are independent events, and intracellular metabolism is usually rate-limiting in the uptake process. In general, the enzymes of nucleoside metabolism exhibit much narrower substrate selectivities than NT processes. A review of relationships between transport and phosphorylation of nucleosides in cultured cell lines was published some years ago (21).

The role of nucleosides in nucleotide metabolism, although well understood in terms of pathways (e.g., see Refs. 21–26), continues to be the subject of intense investigation, particularly relative to physiological function and regulatory mechanisms. Salvage of nucleosides by conversion to nucleotides through the action of various kinases is energetically favored for support of anabolic processes over de novo synthesis. For cell types that lack de novo pathways, such as hematopoietic cells in the bone marrow, acquisition of purines and pyrimidines through salvage of nucleosides and bases is essential for production of nucleotides in the quantities required for intermediary metabolism and specialized cellular functions (27). The major route for salvage of pyrimidine nucleosides is by action of the highly selective nucleoside kinases, whereas purine nucleosides are salvaged primarily by the successive action of purine nucleoside phosphorylase and either adenine or hypoxanthine–guanine phosphoribosyltransferase. The metabolic fate of physiological nucleosides within cells is complex and can be understood only by utilization of in situ approaches that permit analyses of metabolic processes within intact cells. Although detailed consideration of nucleoside metabolism is beyond the scope of this review, recent advances pertinent to the role of NT processes in nucleoside physiology and pharmacology are summarized briefly.

Nucleoside kinases are almost always required for the intracellular activation of purine and pyrimidine nucleosides with antiviral or anticancer activity. There are exceptions; for example, 2′,3′-dideoxyinosine is phosphorylated by 5′-nucleotidase (28). Among the nucleoside kinases, perhaps the most important for activation of nucleoside drugs are thymidine kinase and deoxycytidine kinase. Mammalian and viral thymidine kinases have been studied extensively, and the substantial differences in substrate specificities between human and various viral-encoded enzymes have been exploited in the design of selective antiviral drugs, such as the acyclo-nucleosides (see Refs. 29,30 for reviews). In cancer cells, thymidine kinase may also be a selective drug target, since its expression is increased at the G_1/S phase boundary of the cell cycle (31,32); consequently, there is a strong correlation between enzyme activity and tumor growth fraction (33). Excess thymidine is growth-inhibitory to mammalian cells by virtue of the regulatory effects of dTTP on DNA synthesis (34). Deoxycytidine kinase, which catalyzes the phosphorylation of a variety of clinically active anticancer nucleosides, including cytarabine (arabinosyl cytosine) and fludarabine (arabinofuranosyl-2-fluoroadenine; 35–37), has broad substrate specificity and phosophorylates both purine and pyrimidine deoxyribonucleosides. The cDNA, as well as genomic sequences, for human deoxycytidine kinase have recently been cloned (38,39), making possible studies of drug resistance that involve changes in enzyme structure (40) and regulation of expression (41). Changes in the activities of the various nucleoside kinases have profound effects on cellular uptake of nucleosides, and decreases in kinase activities have been associated with resistance to particular nucleoside drugs (42–44). It is possible that there may be coordinate regulation of nucleoside kinase and transport activities in some cell types.

Adenosine deaminase and purine nucleoside phosphorylase are widely distributed in tissues and, together with adenosine kinase, 5'-nucleotidase, and S-adenosyl-L-homocysteine hydrolase, play a major role in the metabolism of adenosine and its structural analogues (26). Because genetic deficiencies in either adenosine deaminase or purine nucleoside phosphorylase give rise to severe combined immunodeficiency diseases in newborns, the pathophysiological effects of the natural substrates of these enzymes have been studied extensively (see Refs. 45–49 for reviews). The crystal structures of human adenosine deaminase (50) and purine nucleoside phosphorylase (51) are known, and both are considered to be key targets in the development of anticancer drugs (52–54).

Thymidine phosphorylase, a key catabolic enzyme of uracil and thymine-containing nucleosides (55), has recently been shown to be identical with a protein termed platelet-derived endothelial cell growth factor (PD-ECGF), that has mitogenic and chemotactic activity specific for endothelial cells and is thought to play a role in angiogenesis (56–58). The activity of platelet-derived thymidine phosphorylase is regulated by platelet agonists (59) and, because stimulation of thymidine phosphorylase activity of platelets enhances the uptake of thymidine by endothelial cells (57), it has been suggested that this enzyme modulates thymidine uptake and metabolism in endothelial cells (59). Although the biochemical basis of the effects of thymidine on endothelial cells remains to be determined, the newly recognized actions of thymidine phosphorylase suggest that it may function, together with NT processes, to regulate the levels of thymidine in plasma or interstitial fluids, or in both.

The possibility has been raised that there may be metabolic "channeling" of nucleosides in some cell types, possibly resulting from functional associations between NT proteins and nucleoside-metabolizing enzymes. Adenosine deaminase is sometimes associated with cell membranes (60–62), with its active site oriented toward the extracellular space (61,62). Association of adenosine deaminase with cell surfaces has recently been shown to be a consequence of its interaction with a serine protease (dipeptidyl peptidase IV), also known as the CD26 antigen, the function of which is important in T-cell activation (63,64). Several authors have proposed a role for cell surface adenosine deaminase in the transport of adenosine (65–67). A functional association between adenosine transporters and membrane-bound enzymes that generate nucleosides in hepatocytes has also been suggested, based on the canicular location of 5′-nucleotidase and Ca^{2+}, Mg^{2+} ecto-ATPase and the presence of inwardly directed concentrative NT activity (68,69). In the latter, an association between nucleotidases and NT processes, which would serve to conserve extracellular purines, may be related to the physiological role of liver as a source of preformed purines for export to cell types that are deficient in de novo purine synthesis. A complex kinetic model, relating anabolic and catabolic reactions of adenosine metabolism to adenosine transport, has been proposed (70). Even though such functional associations imply a physical interaction between NT proteins and enzymes of nucleoside metabolism, the demonstration of physical interactions awaits the molecular characterization of NT proteins and the subsequent development of appropriate experimental reagents (e.g., NT-specific antibodies) that could be used to detect physical association of transporter proteins with particular enzymes.

C. The Special Role of Adenosine in Mammalian Cells

Adenosine and adenine nucleotides are local signaling molecules that are released into the interstitium in response to appropriate stimuli and, because such stimuli are often stressful, have been termed "retaliatory metabolites" (71). Nucleoside transport processes play an important role in these signaling processes by mediating transmembrane fluxes of adenosine. The ability of adenosine and adenine nucleotides to regulate cellular function has long been recognized (72–75), and their physiological and pharmacological activities have been the subject of numerous monographs and review articles (e.g., Refs. 26,76–79). Such varied physiological processes as lipolysis, neurotransmitter release, platelet aggregation, coronary vasodilation, cardiac contractility, and renal vasoconstriction are regulated by adenosine or adenine nucleotides through interaction with a heterogeneous group of cell surface receptors, which can be identified in functional assays by the effects of diagnostic agonists and antagonists (80–84). The purinergic receptors, also termed "purinoceptors," have been classified as P_1 or P_2 receptors, depending on their preference, respectively, for adenosine or adenine nucleotides (81). In this classification, P_1 purinoceptors (adenosine > AMP > ADP > ATP) are selectively blocked by methylxanthines and act primarily, although not exclusively, through activation or inhibition of adenylate cyclase, whereas P_2 purinoceptors (ATP > ADP > AMP > adenosine) are unaffected by methylxanthines and apparently act through a variety of second-messenger systems, including G-protein-coupled cascades and ligand-gated ion fluxes (80,81,84–88). Some P_2 purinoceptors are also activated by uridine nucleotides.

During the past decade, functional studies with various agonists and antagonists had revealed a bewildering array of P_1 and P_2 receptor subtypes (80,89) and, although the nomenclature remains confusing, the molecular structure and potential signal transduction mechanisms of purinoceptors are being revealed by characterization and expression of cDNAs encoding P_1 (90–103) and P_2(104–108) receptor proteins and the development of agonists and antagonists with selectivity for particular receptors (83–85). Multiple representatives of each of the four major P_1 receptor subtypes (now termed A_1, A_{2a}, A_{2b}, and A_3) have been cloned from various species, including humans; the predicted proteins of the four subtypes exhibit the seven-transmembrane motif of G-protein-coupled receptors, and within a particular species (e.g., humans) there is considerable homology among receptor subtypes (109). The pharmacological identification of P_2 receptor subtypes remains controversial. Recent functional studies with a variety of ATP analogues indicate that there are several (possibly five) different receptor subtypes, distinguished by their signaling mechanisms. Two P_2 receptor subtypes (P_{2Y} and P_{2U}) have recently been cloned (104–108) and, although both are members of the G-coupled receptor superfamily to which the P_1 receptors also belong, their sequences are quite distinct from those of the P_1 receptor family.

The widespread distribution and complexity of purinoceptors may partly explain the apparent heterogeneity of NT processes, since controlled release and reuptake of adenosine and adenine nucleotides by cells, or secretory vesicles, with intact membranes requires the presence of functional transport systems. Much less is known about the mechanisms of release than of uptake. Extracellular adenosine arises by direct release from cells or vesicles (110) or, after release of adenine nucleotides, by the action of ecto-5'-nucleotidases (111). The release of adenosine from embryonic heart cells (110) and from spinal cord (112) and brain (113) synaptosomes in response to appropriate stimuli is, at least in part, transporter-mediated. In some tissues (e.g., heart), interstitial adenosine is produced primarily by rapid extracellular degradation by ecto-5'-nucleotidase of ATP that was released in response to ischemia (111,114). Even though release of adenine nucleotides from ischemic cells may be partly the result of nonspecific permeability changes, there is evidence that ATP release from affected cells may also be transporter-mediated. P-glycoprotein, which has been extensively studied relative to its role in multidrug resistance (see Ref. 115 and Chap. 17 for reviews), has recently been shown to mediate channel-like efflux of cellular ATP (116), giving rise to the suggestion that P-glycoprotein, or other members of the ABC family of transporter proteins (reviewed in Chap. 4), may be responsible for the release of adenine nucleotides for interaction with purinoceptors (117). The duration of interaction of adenosine and adenine nucleotides with purinoceptors is determined primarily by the rate of ligand removal from the vicinity of cell surface receptors by cellular reuptake of adenosine or its metabolites (Fig. 1). This uptake is mediated largely, if not exclusively, by NT processes (see Refs. 5,6,13 for reviews) and there is considerable interest in determining which NT process is most important. Indeed, NT

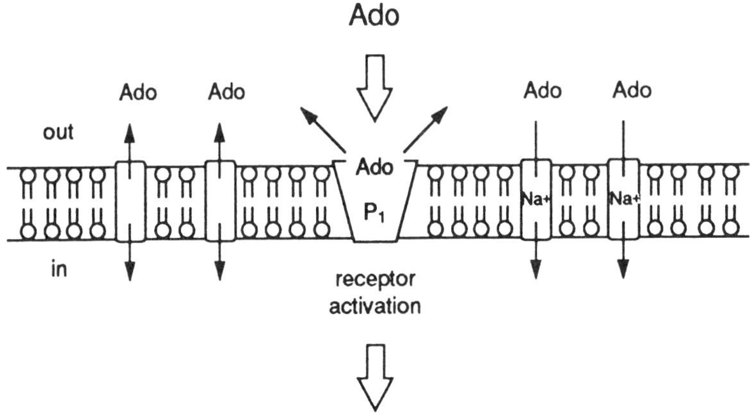

Figure 1 Interaction of adenosine with P₁ receptors is influenced by release and reuptake of adenosine by NT processes.

inhibitors have been proposed as therapeutic tools for treatment of ischemia by virtue of their ability to prolong the beneficial effects of adenosine activation of its receptors (e.g., see Refs. 113,114,118–122).

D. Nucleosides as Chemotherapeutic Agents

Nucleoside drugs have important clinical applications in therapy of hematological cancers and viral diseases (see Refs. 35–37,52,123–139 for recent reviews). The most important of these (Table 1) are used for treating leukemias, lymphomas, and cancers of the gastrointestinal tract, or a variety of viral diseases, including human immunodeficiency virus (HIV) and herpesvirus infections. A large number of nucleoside analogues with anti-

Table 1 Clinically Important Nucleoside Drugs

Drug[a]	Major use	Ref.[b]
Cladribine (chlorodeoxyadenosine, Cl-dAdo)	Leukemias, lymphomas	37,129,130
Cytarabine (arabinosylcytosine, araC)	Leukemias	35
2-Fludarabine (fluoroarabinosyladenine, F-araA)	Leukemias, lymphomas	37,131,132
Pentostatin (2'-deoxycoformycin, dCF)	Leukemias, lymphomas	130
Floxidine (fluorodeoxyuridine, F-dUrd)	Colorectal cancer	133,134
Didanosine (dideoxyinosine, ddIno)	HIV	135–138
Zalcitabine (dideoxycytidine, ddCyd)	HIV	136–138
Zidovudine (azidothymidine, AZT)	HIV	136–139
Acyclovir (Zovirax, ACV)	Herpes virus	123,125–128
Ganciclovir (Cytovene, GCV)	Herpes virus	123,125–128
Vidarabine (arabinosyladenine, araA)	Herpes virus	123,125–128
Idoxuridine (iododeoxyuridine, I-dUrd)	Herpes virus	123,125–128
Trifluridine (Viroptic; trifluoromethylthymidine, F$_3$-dThd)	Herpes virus	123,125–128
Ribavirin (Virazole, RBV)	RNA and DNA viruses	123,125–128

[a] Chemical names: ACV, 9-(2-hydroxyethoxymethyl)guanine; araA, 9-β-D-arabinofuranosyladenine; araC, 1-β-D-arabinofuranosylcytosine; AZT, 3'-azido-2',3'-dideoxythymidine; Cl-dAdo, 2-chloro-2'-deoxyadenosine; dCF, 3-(2-deoxy-β-D-*erythro*-pentofuranosyl)-3,6,7,7-tetrahydroimidazo[4,5-*d*]-[1,3]diazepin-8-ol; ddCyd, 2',3'-dideoxycytidine; ddIno, 2',3'-dideoxyinosine; F-araA, 9-β-D-arabinofuranosyl-2-fluoroadenine; F$_3$-dThd, 5-trifluoromethyl-2'-deoxyuridine; F-dUrd, 5-fluoro-2'-deoxyuridine; I-dUrd, 5-iodo-2'-deoxyuridine; GVC, 9-(1,3-dihydroxy-2-propoxymethyl)guanine; RBV, 1-β-ribofuranosyl-1,2,4-triazole-3-carboxamide.
[b] Recent review articles on the pharmacology and therapeutic uses of the drugs listed.

cancer or antiviral activity in experimental systems are currently in various stages of clinical development (123).

Most nucleoside drugs act intracellularly, after anabolic phosphorylation, by interfering, either directly or indirectly, with DNA synthesis. For those nucleosides that are hydrophilic, mediated transport systems (NT processes) are required for passage across the plasma membrane. In experimental systems, there is evidence that the activity of NT processes can be an important determinant of pharmacological action of cytotoxic nucleoside drugs. For example, cultured cells made incapable of transporting nucleosides by genetic mutations (140–144) or treatment with NT inhibitors (145–147) exhibit low levels of uptake of adenosine and other physiological nucleosides and are resistant to a variety of nucleoside analogues with anticancer activity. The permeant selectivities and mechanisms regulating distribution and expression of NT processes are important factors to be considered in the design of nucleoside analogues as therapeutic agents in human diseases.

II. NUCLEOSIDE TRANSPORT PROCESSES

A. Transporter Subclasses: How Many Transporters?

The current classification of NT processes is entirely based on functional and pharmacological characteristics and may not reflect underlying structural relations of the transporter proteins responsible for mediating nucleoside fluxes. The NT processes can be divided into two distinct classes, depending on whether they involve equilibrative or concentrative transport of nucleosides across plasma membranes. The equilibrative NT processes, which exhibit the typical features associated with facilitated diffusion (148), are driven by the concentration gradient of the nucleoside(s) being transported and presumably function in both uptake and release of nucleosides from cells, although most studies have focused on the characteristics of inwardly directed transport. The concentrative NT processes are secondary-active systems that are driven by transmembrane Na^+ gradients and, in isolated cells and vesicles, are inwardly directed Na^+–nucleoside cotransporters or symporters. Equilibrative NT processes are widely distributed among mammalian cells and tissues and may be ubiquitous, whereas concentrative NT processes are limited to specialized cell types, including intestine, kidney, spleen, lymphocytes, macrophages, and choroid plexus. Both equilibrative and concentrative NT processes have been observed in neoplastic cell types (12).

The total number of NT processes present in mammalian cells and tissues is uncertain. Seven subclasses (Table 2) are evident from the functional and pharmacological characteristics of permeant fluxes observed in studies with intact cells or plasma membrane vesicles from tissues (149–157). The characteristics that have been used to identify NT processes are (1) dependence on Na^+ gradients or an ability to translocate a nonmetabolized nucleoside against its concentration gradient; (2) sensitivity to inhibition by nitrobenzylthioinosine (NBMPR), one of several potent inhibitors of NT processes (Fig. 2); and (3) preference for purine or pyrimidine nucleosides as permeants. The classification of NT processes has evolved through comparisons of NT characteristics in cells or in vesicles from only a few mammalian species (humans, pigs, rabbits, rats, and mice). Although it is unlikely that all seven processes occur

Table 2 Functional Properties of Nucleoside Transporter Subclasses

| Trivial[c] | Equilibrative[a] | | Concentrative[b] | | | | |
| | | | *cif* | *cit* | | *cib* | *cs* |
Numerical[d]	*es*	*ei*	N1	N2	N4	N3	N5
Na^+-dependent	−	−	+	+	+	+	+
Na^+–nucleoside stoichiometry			1:1	1:1	1:1	2:1	ND[e]
Inhibited by							
NBMPR	+	−	−	−	−	−	+
Dipyridamole	+	+	−	−	−	−	+
Dilazep	+	+	−	−	−	−	+
Permeants							
Adenosine	+	+	+	+	+	+	+
Uridine	+	+	+	+	+	+	ND
Guanosine	+	+	+	−	+	+	ND
Inosine	+	+	+	−	−	+	ND
Formycin B	+	+	+	−	−	+	+
Tubercidin	+	+	−	−	ND	+	ND
Thymidine	+	+	−	+	+	+	ND

[a] The characteristics of equilibrative NT processes are reviewed in Refs. 1,2,6–8.
[b] Summarized from recent overview articles (11,12) and key functional studies of the *cif*/N1 (149–152), *cit*/N2 (149,152), *cib*/N3 (153,154), *cib*/N4 (155,156), and *cs*/N5 (157) processes.
[c] Adapted from Refs. 12,149.
[d] Adapted from Refs. 152–156; the designation "N5" has not been previously assigned to the newly discovered cs transporter (157).
[e] ND, not determined.

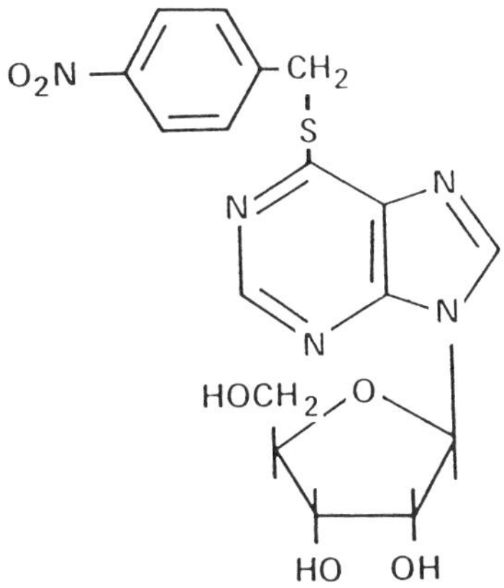

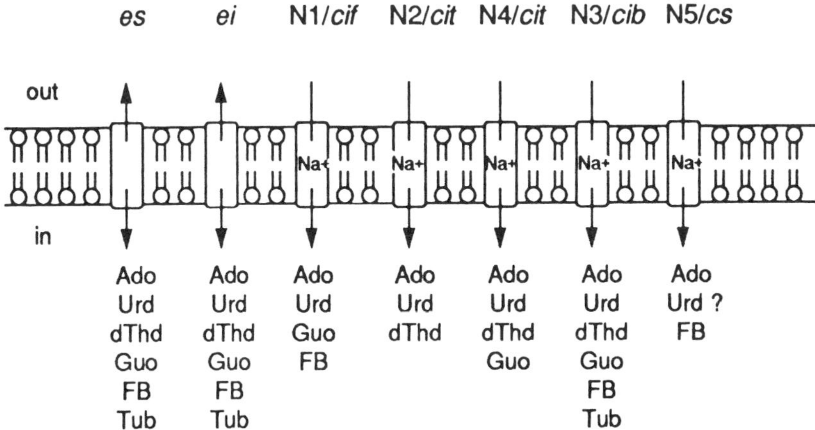

Figure 2 Structure of nitrobenzylthioinosine (NBMPR).

within a single species, thus far four functionally distinct NT processes have been observed in mice and five in rats and humans. L1210 leukemia cells simultaneously exhibit three different NT processes (158,159).

The classification schemes are based on functional characteristics (Fig. 3). A revised nomenclature, based on structural relations, may be more appropriate when the molecular structures of the transporter proteins are known. One classification scheme involves the use of trivial names that

Figure 3 Functional NT processes of mammalian cells.

are related to the functional characteristics of the various NT processes (12,149). In the initial version of this classification (149), letters were used to designate (1) the transport mechanism (e = equilibrative, c = concentrative); (2) the sensitivity to inhibition by NBMPR (s = sensitive, i = insensitive); and (3) the diagnostic nucleoside used to establish permeant selectivity (f = formycin B or purine selective; t = thymidine or pyrimidine selective) of concentrative transporters. When it was discovered that there are also concentrative NT processes that accept a variety of purine and pyrimidine nucleosides as permeants, the classification was expanded to include a third designation (b = broad) for the permeant selectivity of concentrative transporters (12). The classification of Belt (12) recognizes five subclasses of NT processes: equilibrative NBMPR-sensitive (es) transport; equilibrative NBMPR-insensitive (ei) transport; concentrative NBMPR-insensitive purine-selective (cif) transport; concentrative NBMPR-insensitive pyrimidine-selective (cit) transport; concentrative NBMPR-insensitive broadly selective (cib) transport. An inconsistency is the absence of an indicator for permeant selectivity in the trivial names used for equilibrative NT processes, which transport a heterogeneous array of purine and pyrimidine nucleosides and thus exhibit "broad" permeant selectivity. The recent observation (157) of NBMPR-sensitive concentrative transport of fludarabine in freshly isolated human leukemic cells suggests that there may also be concentrative NBMPR-sensitive (cs) transport. A second classification scheme, applicable only to the concentrative NT processes, involves numerical designations that signify the order of discovery (11,150–154).

The functional characteristics of the seven NT subclasses are outlined in Table 2. The two equilibrative processes of mammalian cells exhibit the classic features (148) of facilitated diffusion, including exchange diffusion and countertransport (160–165). The equilibrative NT processes are remarkably broad in their permeant selectivities and transport all of the exogenous nucleosides as well as a diverse group of structural analogues with various substituents in the base or sugar moieties (1,146,161–163). NBMPR, a tight-binding and highly specific inhibitor (166–169), has proved an invaluable chemical reagent for distinguishing between the two subclasses of equilibrative NT processes. Because of large differences (> 4-log) in sensitivity to inhibition by NBMPR among equilibrative NT processes (165,169–176), they are commonly subdivided into the two functionally distinct subclasses termed es and ei (170–172). The es NT processes are inhibited by low concentrations ($\leq$ 1 nM) of NBMPR as a direct result of a noncovalent interaction of NBMPR with high-affinity (K_d ~ 0.1 nM) binding sites (166) located on the extracellular face of the plasma membrane (177,178). In contrast, the ei NT processes are unaffected by

NBMPR at all, or are inhibited only by high (> 10 μM) concentrations (169–176) and, like *es* NT processes, accept a structurally diverse group of nucleosides as permeants (170,173). Both *es* and *ei* NT processes are inhibited by low concentrations (0.1–100 nM) of dipyridamole and dilazep (147,179–183), although there are differences among cell types and species (173,184–187). The *es* and *ei* NT processes exhibit different kinetic properties and different substrate specificities when present in the same cell type (174,188).

A comprehensive survey of the concentrative NT processes is presented in Table 3. It is evident that the five subclasses compose a heterogeneous group of processes, with a complex pattern of overlapping permeant selectivities. The concentrative NT processes have been defined primarily through differences observed in permeant selectivities, usually through an assessment of the ability of nonlabeled test permeants to block inward transport of radioactive tracer permeant (189–210). Of the many functional studies summarized in Table 3, only a few have used combinations of competing and tracer permeants that allow unambiguous assignment to a particular NT subclass. The most extensively studied processes, particularly in rodent cells and tissues, are N1/*cif* and N2/*cit*. These two processes share the ability to transport adenosine and uridine, but otherwise exhibit selectivity for purine nucleosides (N1/*cif*) or pyrimidine nucleosides (N2/*cit*). N1/*cif* activity has been found in mouse splenocytes (189,190) and macrophages (191,192) and in rat macrophages (192,199) and hepatocytes (68), as well as in several cultured cell types, including L1210 murine leukemia (151,158,183,193), Walker rat 256 carcinosarcoma (200), and IEC6 rat intestinal (211,212) cells. These various cell types have provided convenient model systems for analysis of the functional characteristics of N1/*cif* NT processes. By contrast, N2/*cit* activity has been observed only in freshly isolated mouse enterocytes (149) and in brush-border vesicles from epithelial cells of bovine (152), rat (198), and rabbit (207) kidney. The transporter protein responsible for mediating N2/*cit* activity in rat jejunum has recently been identified by molecular cloning and expression (17,18), and its characteristics are summarized later in Section II.B.2. Neither N1/*cif* nor N2/*cit* activity has been reported in human cells, raising the possibility of species differences in the functional characteristics of concentrative NT processes. Three distinct Na^+–nucleoside cotransport processes have been observed in human material, after considerable effort in surveying candidate cells and tissues. N3/*cib* activity has been observed in cultured colorectal (12) cells and, after induction of differentiation, in cultured human promyelocytic leukemia cells (209,210). A novel NT process, with a permeant selectivity similar to that of the N2/*cit* processes of rodents, except for the additional ability to transport guanosine, has

Table 3 Na$^+$-Dependent Nucleoside Transport Processes of Various Mammalian Cells and Tissues

Permeant/K_m (μM)	Sensitive[a] to	Resistant[a] to	Stoichiometry[b] of transport	Apparent subclass	Ref.
Mouse (intestinal enterocytes)					
FB[c]/45	Ado, dAdo, Guo Ino, Urd	Cyd, dThd NBMPR		N1	149
dThd	Ado, dAdo, Cyd	FB, Guo, Ino		N2	149
Mouse (splenocytes)					
FB/30	Ado, Ino, Urd	Cyd, dCyd, dThd DIP, NBMPR	1:1	N1	189
Urd/36	Ado, dAdo, FB Guo, Ino	Cyd, dCyd, dThd DIP, NBMPR	1:1	N1	189
Urd/38	Ado, dAdo, Guo Ino, dIno, Urd	Cyd, dCyd, dThd DIP, NBMPR		N1	190
Mouse (activated peritoneal macrophages)					
Ado	dAdo, Ino, dThd Urd	DIL, NBMPR		N1 + N2 or N3	191
FB	Guo, Ino, Urd	dCyd, dThd		N1	192
Mouse (cultured leukemia L1210 cells)					
Ado/9.4	dAdo, Ino	dCyd, dThd, Urd DIP, NBMPR	1:1	N1	151,193
FB	Ado, dAdo, Guo Ino, Urd	Cyd, dThd DIL, DIP, NBMPR		N1	158,183
Mouse (cultured lymphoma S49 cells)					
FB	Ado, Urd	dCyd, DIP, NBMPR dThd		N1	194
Rat (kidney brush-border membrane vesicles)					
Ado/2.9	dAdo, Guo, Ino Urd, DIP	NBMPR	1:1	N1 or N3	195
Ado/1.1	Urd	Cyd, dThd		N1	196,197
Cyd/3.8	Ado, dThd, Urd	NBMPR		N2 or N3	196,197
dThd/4.8	Ado	NBMPR		N2 or N3	196,197
Urd/9.7	Ado, dAdo, dUrd dThd, DIL	Guo, dGuo, dIno dIno, DIP, NBMPR	1:1	N2	198
Rat (hepatocytes or hepatocyte cancicular membrane vesicles)					
Ado/14	Ado, FB, Guo Ino, Urd	Cyd, dThd DIP, NBMPR	1:1	N1	68
Rat (macrophages)					
FB/6	Ado, dAdo, Guo Ino, Urd	Cyd, dCyd, dThd DIL, NBMPR	1:1	N1	192,199
Rat (cultured Walker 256 carcinosarcoma)					
FB	Ino	dThd, DIP, NBMPR		N1	200
Cow (renal brush-border membrane vesicles)					
Guo/11	Ado, dAdo, FB dGuo, Ino, dIno Urd, dUrd	Cyd, dCyd, dThd	1:1	N1	152
dThd/7	Ado, dAdo, Cyd dCyd, dThd, Urd dUrd	FB, Guo, dGuo Ino, dIno	1:1	N2	152

(continued)

Table 3 (*Continued*)

Permeant/K_m (μM)	Sensitive[a] to	Resistant[a] to	Stoichiometry[b] of transport	Apparent subclass	Ref.
Urd/11	Ado, Cyd, dCyd Guo, dGuo, Ino dThd, dUrd	DIL, DIP, NBMPR	1:1	N1 + N2	152
Rabbit (choroid plexus, intact or ATP-depleted slices)					
dCyd/15	Ado, dAdo, Cyd dThd, Urd, dUrd	NBMPR		N2 or N3	201
FB	dThd			N3	154
dThd/13	Cyd, FB, Guo Ino, Urd		2:1	N3	154
dThd/13.6	Ado, dAdo, Urd dUrd	DIP, NBMPR		N2 or N3	202
Urd/18	Ado, Cyd, FB dThd		2:1	N3	154
dUrd/7.2	Ado, dThd			N2 or N3	202,203
Rabbit (small intestinal brush-border membrane vesicles)					
Ado/17.3	Ino, Urd	NBMPR		N1 or N3	204
FB/27.6	Ado, Guo, Ino Urd	Cyd, dThd, NBMPR		N1	205
Urd/6.4	Ado, Cyd, Ino dIno, dThd, dUrd	DIL, DIP, NBMPR	1:1	N1 + N2 or N3	206
Rabbit (renal brush-border membrane vesicles)					
Urd/12	Ado, dCyd, Guo dGuo, Ino, dThd dUrd	DIL, DIP, NBMPR	1:1	N1 + N2 or N3	207
Guinea pig (intestinal enterocytes)					
Urd/46	Ado, Gyd, Guo			N1 + N2 or N3	208
Human (renal brush-border membrane vesicles)					
Urd/4.8	Cyd, dThd, dUrd	FB		N4	155
Urd			1:1	N4	156
dThd	Ado, Guo, Urd	FB, Ino		N4	155
dThd/2	Cl-Ado, F-dUrd I-dUrd			N4	156
Human (cultured promyelocytic leukemia HL-60 cells)					
Ado/1.1		NBMPR			209
Cyd/1.8					
Ino/2.1					
dThd/3.5					
Urd/1.1					
FB	Ado, dAdo, Cyd Guo, Ino, Urd dThd	DIP		N3	210
Human (cultured colorectal carcinoma CaCo cells)					
FB	Ado, dAdo, Cyd Guo, Ino, Urd dThd	DIP, NBMPR		N3	12

(*continued*)

Table 3 (*Continued*)

Permeant/K_m (μM)	Sensitive[a] to	Resistant[a] to	Stoichiometry[b] of transport	Apparent subclass	Ref.
Human (freshly isolated leukemic cells)					
FB[c]	DIP, NBMPR			N5	157
F-araA	DIP, NBMPR				
Cl-dAdo	DIP, NBMPR				

[a] NT processes were considered sensitive if >50% reductions were observed at compound concentrations of 50–100 μM, except dilazep (DIL), dipyridamole (DIP) and NBMPR, which were tested at $\leq$ 20 μM. Where possible, an assignment of transporter subclass has been made.

[b] Relative to Na^+.

[c] FB, formycin B (a nonmetabolized C-glycosidic analogue of inosine).

been observed in brush-border vesicles from human kidney (155,156); this process is designated in Table 2 as N4/*cit*. It is possible that the rodent N2/*cit* and human N4/*cit* processes are mediated by structurally related transporter proteins. Thus far, N5/*cs* activity has been observed only in freshly isolated human leukemic cells (157), and its permeant selectivity has not yet been established. With the obvious exception of the N5/*cs* process, which is highly sensitive to inhibition by low (<10 nM) concentrations of NBMPR and dipyridamole (157), there are no selective inhibitors for the concentrative NT processes. The N1/*cif*, N2/*cit*, N3/*cib*, and N4/*cit* processes are unaffected by high concentrations (> 10 μM) of either NBMPR or dipyridamole.

The coupling stoichiometries for Na^+ and nucleoside have been determined for several of the concentrative NT processes. A coupling stoichiometry of 1:1, indicating that the inward transport of each nucleoside molecule is driven by the cotransport of a sodium ion down its transmembrane gradient, has been reported for various N1/*cif* (68,151,152,189,192), N2/*cit* (152,198), and the recently described N4/*cit* processes (156). By contrast, a stoichiometry of 2:1 was observed for Na^+–nucleoside cotransport by the N3/*cib* process in ATP-depleted tissues slices of rabbit choroid plexus (154). Stoichiometries have not been reported for other N3/*cib* processes. Since most nucleosides are electroneutral molecules, operation of the various Na^+–nucleoside symporters in cells would be expected to be electrogenic, and experimental results suggesting nucleoside-dependent accumulation of positive charge have been obtained in studies with brush-border membrane vesicles of human (156) and rabbit (207) kidney.

B. Molecular Structure of Nucleoside Transport Proteins

1. Equilibrative Transporters

The molecular structure of the proteins that mediate equilibrative NT processes are poorly understood, and there is much current research directed toward identification and characterization of *es* and *ei* transporter proteins. Whereas the major structural features of *es* transporter proteins have been determined, nothing whatsoever is known about the protein(s) associated with *ei* NT processes. Although *es* and *ei* NT processes frequently occur in the same cell type (158,159,174) and exhibit many functional similarities (170,171), the existence of genetic variants that have lost one of the two equilibrative NT processes (9,144,150) has led to the speculation that they are mediated by distinct, but structurally related, proteins. However, it is also possible that *es* and *ei* processes are mediated by alternative forms of the same transporter protein, the relative levels of which are controlled by modifier protein(s). Resolution of these issues awaits determination of the primary structure and functional expression of the proteins responsible for *es*- and *ei*-mediated transport.

The *es* transporters of mammalian cells exhibit high affinities (K_d values, 0.1–1.0 nM) for NBMPR and its congeners (3,166–169). The tight binding of NBMPR, coupled with its remarkable specificity for *es* transporters (166–168) and its intrinsic photoreactivity (14,213), has permitted identification and quantification of transporter polypeptides in erythrocytes (15,214–221) and a variety of other cell types and tissues (159,165,222–226). Methods used for site-specific photolabeling of *es* transporter polypeptides with [^{3}H]-NBMPR are reviewed in Ref. 14. The number of high-affinity NBMPR-binding sites, determined by Scatchard analysis of binding of radiolabeled NBMPR to isolated membrane preparations or cell surfaces, is assumed to be a measure of the relative abundance of *es* transporter (8,166–169,227). Assuming a 1:1 relation between transporter abundance and NBMPR-binding sites, the number of *es* transporters varies considerably among various cell types, with relatively low numbers (10^2–10^4/cell) reported for erythrocytes (227) and lymphocytes (228) and extraordinarily high numbers ($> 10^7$/cell) for some cultured cell types (226). Even though NBMPR-binding site abundance is often equated with functional *es* transporters, mass law analysis of high-affinity binding of NBMPR to cells with internal membranes may overestimate the abundance of *es* transporters in the plasma membrane, if there is endocytotic internalization or sequestration of transporters inside cells (see discussion in Ref. 226).

Although *es* transporter polypeptides were identified in band 4.5 preparations of human erythrocyte membranes over a decade ago (214–216), their purification was delayed for several years because of low abundance in membrane preparations (about 11,000 copies per erythrocyte) and similarity in structure to glucose transporter polypeptides. The facilitative glucose transporters (GLUTs 1–6) of mammalian cells are members of a superfamily of related transporter proteins with amino acid sequences that contain 12 potential transmembrane-spanning domains (see Refs. 229,320 for recent reviews). In human erythrocytes, *es* and GLUT1 polypeptides are heterogeneously glycosylated proteins that comigrate in the "band 4.5" region (45–65 kDa) of sodium dodecyl sulfate (SDS) electrophoretograms of detergent-solubilized erythrocyte membranes, both before and after enzymatic deglycosylation (217,231). The two transporters copurify during DEAE-cellulose chromatography and, because GLUT1 polypeptides are 25-fold more abundant than *es* polypeptides in human erythrocytes, they have proved difficult to physically separate (15,231–233). Nonetheless, purification, followed by functional reconstitution, of *es* transporter polypeptides has been achieved by passage of band 4.5 preparations from human erythrocytes through columns of immobilized antibodies specific for GLUT1 polypeptides (15). Polypeptides so purified (1) migrate as a single broad band (about 55 kDa) on SDS-polyacrylamide electrophoretograms; (2) bind NBMPR with a stoichiometry of 1:1 and a K_d of 1.1 nM; (3) catalyze the uptake of uridine after reconstitution into large unilamellar phospholipid vesicles; and (4) are not recognized by antibodies specific for the glucose transporter. Although erythrocytes from fetal pigs exhibit both glucose and nucleoside transport activities (234,235), erythrocytes from adult pigs lack glucose transport activity (235), and their plasma membranes lack glucose transporter polypeptides (220). Band 4.5 preparations from adult pig erythrocytes have been used for purification and functional reconstitution of *es* transporter polypeptides (219,221) and for the isolation of *es*-specific monoclonal antibodies that do not cross-react with glucose transporter polypeptides (218,220). The general conclusion from these studies is that *es* transport is mediated by a single polypeptide species that is not immunologically related to the facilitative glucose transporter.

Electrophoretic analysis of NMBPR-photolabeled polypeptides isolated from membrane preparations from various cell types indicates considerable species- or tissue-related variations in size of *es* transporters (159,165,216–226,236–238), raising doubt about the extent of structural homology among transporter proteins. However, there is immunological evidence that *es* transporters from different mammalian species share sequence homology, since polyclonal antibodies specific for protein epitopes of the human *es* transporter also recognize *es* transporter polypeptides of pig and rabbit erythrocytes and rat liver (239). In some instances, the apparent heterogeneity in electrophoretic mobility of *es* transporters on SDS–polyacrylamide gels has been shown to be due to differences in glycosylation states (159,165,224,240). Results of peptide mapping experiments (240) have established structural conservation among several mammalian *es* transporters, showing that the sites of NBMPR covalent labeling, carbohydrate attachment, and trypsin cleavage are similar for *es* transporter polypeptides of erythrocytes, liver and lung from human, pig, rat, and guinea pig. The apparent structural similarity between the rat and human *es* transporters is of particular interest because it had been assumed that these transporters, which exhibit substantial functional differences (241), would also exhibit substantial differences in their amino acid sequences. The site of *N*-linked glycosylation of the *es* transporter of human erythrocytes has been localized to one end of the protein and the site of NBMPR photolabeling to within 16 kDa of the glycosylation site (240). An additional indication of structural homology between the human and pig erythrocytic *es* transporters is the recent finding of homology in the NH_2-terminal sequences of the human and pig proteins (242).

Despite the similarities in protein structure just described, clear structural differences have been demonstrated for the *es* transporters of pig and human erythrocytes (218–221,239,240). The glycosylated and deglycosylated *es* transporter polypeptides of pig erythrocytes exhibit relative molecular mass (M_r) values of 66,000 and 57,000, respectively, whereas those of human erythrocytes exhibit values of 55,000 and 45,000, respectively (216–218), suggesting that the pig transporter protein is larger than the human protein. Furthermore, monoclonal antibodies raised against the pig erythrocyte *es* transporter are pig-specific and do not cross-react with *es* transporter polypeptides of human or mouse erythrocytes, or of several cultured cell lines of human and rodent origins (218). The difference in size between the deglycosylated *es* transporter of human and pig erythrocytes appears to be due to a 10-kDa domain of the pig protein that is not present in the human protein (240). It seems likely that this 10-kDa domain contains the epitopes recognized by the pig-specific monoclonal antibodies isolated previously (218).

Results of an analysis of reactivity of polyclonal antibodies against the human erythrocyte *es* transporter with human placental tissue has raised the possibility that multiple *es* transporter isoforms exist within a single species and tissue (243). Brush-border and basal membranes of human placental syncytiotrophoblasts contain equal quantities of NBMPR-binding sites (244), yet erythrocyte *es*-specific antibodies recognize polypeptides in immunoblots prepared from brush-border membranes, but not from basal membranes (243). A similar conclusion has been reached from immunocytochemical studies in which the erythrocyte *es*-specific antibodies bind to brush-border surfaces, but not basolateral surfaces, of syncytiotrophoblasts (243).

The NBMPR-binding site of the *es* transporter is located at the extracellular face of the plasma membrane (177,178), at or near the permeant-binding site (168). The NBMPR-binding site appears to be superficially located and exposed to the aqueous microenvironment, since it is accessible to large, impermeant derivatives of nitrobenzyladenosine (10), which, like NBMPR, are potent inhibitors of *es*-mediated NT processes. These compounds are derivatives of S-(2-aminoethyl)-N^6-4-nitrobenzyl)-5′-thio-5′-deoxyadenosine (SAENTA), which was synthesized for use in preparation of affinity media for isolation of *es* transporter polypeptides (221). SAENTA can be derivatized through a spacer arm, at the 5′-position of the ribosyl moiety, to a variety of bulky substituents, without loss of ability to inhibit either *es*-mediated NT or NBMPR-binding activity (221). Several members of a family of 5′-substituted derivatives of SAENTA that are linked through spacer arms of different lengths to fluorescein inhibit *es*NT or NBMPR-binding activity, or both, in intact cells at low (< 100 nM) concentrations (10,245–247), indicating that the presence of a bulky hydrophilic substituent on the ribosyl moiety does not impede interaction with the *es* transporter. The fluorescein derivatives of SAENTA are useful flow cytometry probes for the identification within clinical samples of leukemic cells of subpopulations that express *es* transporters on their surfaces (10,245–247).

The primary sequence of *es* transporter proteins will most likely be determined by analysis and expression of cDNAs encoding *es* transporter polypeptides. Several cDNA fragments (2.0–2.3 kb), encoding polypeptides recognized by polyclonal antibodies specific for the human erythrocyte *es* transporter, have been isolated from a cDNA library prepared in a bacteriophage expression system (λgt11) from cultured human (BeWo) choriocarcinoma cells (248). BeWo cells have remarkable NT characteristics, with greatly elevated *es* NT activity and NBMPR-binding activity relative to other cell types (226). A comparison of BeWo and HeLa cells revealed a 30-fold difference in V_{max} values for thymidine and a 70-fold difference in the total number of NBMPR-binding sites, although BeWo cells possess two sets of NBMPR-binding sites (K_{d1}, 0.6 nM; K_{d2}, 14.5 nM) in roughly equal numbers. The high-affinity sites evidently represent typical *es* transporters (M_r value, 55,000), whereas the identity and location of the low-affinity sites is uncertain. BeWo cells also have an abundant supply of *es* transporter mRNA, since microinjection of BeWo mRNA into *Xenopus laevis* oocytes results in the acquisition by oocytes of low levels of BeWo-like *es* NT activity, with NBMPR sensitivity and permeant selectivity similar to that of the native transporter (249). Expression of BeWo *es* NT activity by injection of mRNA into *Xenopus* oocytes is being used to confirm the *es*-related identity of cDNA fragments cloned from a BeWo cDNA expression library by testing the ability of antisense RNA transcripts produced from these fragments to block expression of *es* NT activity in oocytes induced by microinjection of mRNA isolated from BeWo cells (248).

2. *Concentrative Transporters*

Proteins that mediate Na^+-dependent NT processes have not yet been physically purified, and specific immunological or chemical probes for concentrative NT proteins have not yet been developed. However, this situation will soon change with the recent successful cloning and expression of cDNAs encoding two different proteins with Na^+-dependent NT activities (16–18,250). Although the predicted proteins of the two cloned transporters (termed SNST1 and cNT1) are similar in size (73 and 71 kDa, respectively) and exhibit features typical of transporters of organic solutes, their amino acid sequences are completely unrelated. SNST1 (from rabbit kidney) belongs to a family of Na^+–organic solute cotransporters, the members of which are found in bacteria and mammals (16,230,150), whereas cNT1 (from rat intestine), which is not related to any known mammalian transporters, has some homology with a bacterial H^+–nucleoside cotransporter and thus belongs to a previously unrecognized family of transporter proteins (17,18).

SNST1 is encoded by a cDNA isolated from a rabbit kidney library by low-stringency hybridization with a probe derived from the Na^+–glucose cotransporter (termed SGLT1) of rabbit intestine (16). SNST1 is 61% identical and 80% similar in sequence to rabbit SGLT1 and, consequently, is considered to be a member of the SGLT family of transporters (16; see Ref. 251 for a review). When recombinant SNST1 is expressed in *Xenopus* oocytes, it exhibits low-to-moderate levels of Na^+–nucleoside cotransport activity with a permeant selectivity characteristic of *cib*/N3 NT processes (250). SNST1 mRNA is expressed in rabbit kidney and heart, but not in liver or intestine, and may function in reabsorption of nucleosides from the glomerular filtrate by proximal tubules (16). The physiological role of SNST1 in heart is unknown, since Na^+-dependent NT activity has not been observed in cardiac tissue. The SNST1 cDNA sequence predicts a protein of 672 amino acids (M_r, 73,161) with 3 potential *N*-linked glycosylation sites, 12 hydrophobic, potentially transmembrane domains and 2 amino acid residues that may be involved in Na^+ binding. Other members of the SGLT family of transporters are the Na^+–glucose cotransporters of human intestine (252) and pig kidney (LLC-PK) cells (253), the Na$^+$–*myo*-inositol of canine kidney (MDCK) cells (254), and the Na$^+$–proline (255) and Na$^+$–pantothenate (256) transporters of bacteria.

cNT1 is encoded by a cDNA that was isolated from a rat intestine cDNA library by expression selection in *Xenopus* oocytes (17,18). Functional expression in *Xenopus* oocytes has been used with striking success to isolate cDNAs encoding integral membrane proteins for which neither immunological or oligonucleotide probes were available (see Refs. 257–260, for example). This approach, which is warranted only if functional expression of the protein of interest can be achieved by microinjection of mRNA from a tissue known to express the protein, requires convenient procedures for assay of activity, since large numbers of oocytes must be injected and screened. Intestinal epithelial cells exhibit high levels of Na$^+$-dependent NT activity (149,204–206) and expression of N1/*cif*, N2/*cit*, and N3/*cib* activities can be achieved by microinjection of *Xenopus* oocytes with mRNA isolated from intestinal cells of rats and rabbits (153,261,262). cNT1 was isolated by screening RNA transcripts produced in vitro for their ability to stimulate Na$^+$-dependent uptake of uridine in injected oocytes (17). When expressed in *Xenopus* oocytes, the recombinant cNT1 transporter exhibits high levels (>20,000-fold stimulation) of NT activity with typical N2/*cit* characteristics, including the ability to transport the anti-HIV drugs azidothymidine and dideoxycytidine. The cDNA sequence of cNT1 predicts a protein of 648 amino acids (M$_r$, 71,000), with 14 potential transmembrane domains, high cysteine content (3.1%), three potential *N*-linked and four potential *O*-linked glycosylation sites, and four protein kinase C-dependent phosphorylation sites. cNT1 mRNA is detected in rat intestine and kidney, but not in heart, brain, spleen, lung, liver, or skeletal muscle. The absence of sequence homologies between the amino acid sequences of cNT1 and SNST1 or other transporter proteins of mammalian origin is intriguing and indicates an unexpected heterogeneity among Na$^+$-dependent NT proteins. cNT1 exhibits 27% identity in amino acid sequence with a bacterial transporter, the H$^+$–nucleoside symporter (NUPC) of *Escherichia coli* (263,264).

With the cloning and functional expression of SNST1 and cNT1 cDNAs, the prospect for significant advances in understanding of Na$^+$-dependent NT proteins is excellent. The N1/*cif* and N3/*cib* transporters of rat intestine (153) and the N2/*cit* transporter of rabbit intestine (262,263) are readily expressed in *Xenopus* oocytes by microinjection of mRNA, providing an approach to isolation of other Na$^+$–nucleoside cotransporters. It should also be possible to identify NT proteins structurally related to either SNST1 or cNT1 by a combination of hybridization selection and functional expression. For example, a cDNA probe that encodes amino acid residues 385–588 of cNT1 recognizes cNT1 mRNA (3.4 kb) and two additional mRNA species (1.9 and 2.5 kb) when hybridized with mRNA from rat intestine (17), raising the possibility, since rat intestine expresses N1/*cif* and N3/*cit* activities (153), that the 1.9- and 2.5-kb mRNAs may also encode NT proteins.

III. TRANSPORT OF NUCLEOSIDE DRUGS

Studies of the transportability of nucleoside drugs have involved measuring the uptake rates of radiolabeled analogues or, more commonly, the relative abilities of various analogues to block inwardly directed transport of a radiolabeled physiological nucleoside, such as adenosine or uridine (1,3,5,8). The presence of multiple NT processes in cells complicates the interpretation of results from such studies, unless the experimental design allows a clear separation of the various NT activities: by use of cells that express a single NT process naturally, as in erythrocytes (4,8); or by genetic or pharmacological elimination of all but one NT process, as in the NT-defective mutants of the L1210 leukemia (12,144,150,158). The results of "competition" assays are sometimes misleading, since an analogue can inhibit the transport process without itself also being transported. For example, the cytotoxic nucleoside tubercidin (7-deazaadenosine) inhibits, but is not actually a permeant, of the N1/*cif* transporter of L1210 leukemia cells (158). The "transportability" of nucleoside drugs that are in current clinical use is summarized in Table 4. It was compiled from an analysis of studies that involved direct determination of transport of radiolabeled drug, in most instances under conditions for which the identity of the operative transport process was known. Transportability by *es*-mediated NT processes has been established for most of the drugs of Table 4, either directly, by measurement of fluxes, or indirectly, by showing sensitivity of drug action to NBMPR. Transportability by the other NT processes remains largely undertermined, and there is clearly a need for more information.

Relationships have been established between the levels of *es*-mediated NT activity, NBMPR-binding activity, and antileukemic activity of cytarabine (araC) (see Refs. 228,275–279 for details); similar studies are currently in progress for *es*-, *ei*-, N1/*cif*-, and N5/*cs*-mediated transport of cladribine (Cl-dAdo; 157,273,274). Kinetic studies of antiviral nucleoside transport in erythrocytes and other cell types have led to recognition of the importance of both passive diffusion and nucleobase transport processes in cellular entry of zidovidine (AZT; 290,291), dideoxynucleosides (269,272), and acyclic nucleosides (266–268). For example, although there is little, if any, *es*-mediated transport of AZT in human erythrocytes and

Table 4 Transportability of Nucleoside Drugs[a]

Drug[b]	Accepted as permeant by[c]	Ref.
Cladribine (Cl-dAdo)	*es, ei*, N1/*cif*, N5/*cs*	157,273,274
Cytarabine (araC)	*es, ei*	228,275–279
2-Fludarabine (F-araA)	*es*, N1/*cif*, N5/*cs*	157,280–282[d]
Pentostatin (dCF)	*es*	283
Floxidine (F-dUrd)	*es, ei*	284[d],285
Didanosine (ddIno)	*es*, NB	272
Zalcitabine (ddCyd)	*es*, N2/*cit*	17,18,272,286–288
Zidovudine (AZT)	N2/*cit*	17,18
Acyclovir (ACV)	NB	266
Ganciclovir (GCV)	*es*, NB	268
Vidarabine (araA)	*es, ei*, N1/*cif*	183,289
Idoxuridine (I-dUrd)	*es*	285
Trifluridine (F₃-dThd)	ND[e]	
Ribavirin (RBV)	ND[e]	

[a] Included are only those NT processes for which there has been direct determination of transportability of drug, by assay of transporter-mediated passage of radiolabeled drug across plasma membranes.
[b] Chemical names are given in Table 1.
[c] NT processes are those defined in Table 2. Some nucleoside drugs are also permeants of nucleobase (NB) transport processes (265–272).
[d] Although this study demonstrated mediated transport of the analogue listed, it did not establish the NT process involved.
[e] ND, not determined.

lymphocytes, AZT entry by passive diffusion is sufficient to produce pharmacologically active intracellular pools of drug (290,291). However, the recent discovery of N2/*cit*-mediated transport of AZT (17,18) not only means that greater levels of AZT permeation will occur in N2/*cit*-expressing cells, but that factors that regulate expression of the N2/*cit* transporter may be important determinants of AZT entry. Although N2/*cit* activity has not yet been reported in human cells, it is likely that there are human NT proteins with similar permeant selectivities.

Until recently it was thought that the antiviral dideoxynucleosides didanosine and zalcitabine (ddIno and ddCyd) enter cells primarily by passive diffusion (e.g., see Refs. 290–295). However, results from two recent, independent studies involving human erythrocytes (269,272) and cultured leukemic cells (269) have implicated nucleobase transport processes in permeation of some dideoxynucleosides. Cellular entry of 2′,3′-dideoxyguanosine, an experimental antihepatitis drug, is mediated by a nucleobase transporter with selectivity for purines (272,269), whereas that of ddIno is mediated by both the nucleobase and *es* transporters (272). By contrast, cellular entry of 2,6-diaminopurine-2′,3′-dideoxyriboside, a prodrug form of 2′,3′-dideoxyguanosine, occurs by passive diffusion (269). Of interest is the finding from studies in human erythrocytes that cellular entry of carbovir, a carbocyclic analogue of 2′,3′-dideoxyguanosine, is mediated by both the nucleobase and *es* transporters (270). A similar spectrum of transportability has been found for the acyclic nucleosides, in that entry of acyclovir (ACV) is mediated almost entirely by the nucleobase transporter (266), entry of ganciclovir (GCV) is mediated primarily by the nucleobase transporter and to a much lesser extent by the *es* transporter (268), and entry of a new experimental acyclic nucleoside (desciclovir; DCV) occurs primarily by passive diffusion (267). The transport of nucleobases, such as hypoxanthine, guanine, or adenine, is mechanistically distinct from transport of the corresponding nucleosides (see Refs. 2,7,9 for reviews) and is presumed to involve different transporter proteins. Human erythrocytes and cultured leukemic cells evidently coexpress nucleobase and nucleoside transporters simultaneously (265,269,296).

The selectivities of the various NT processes provide a guide to important structural features that predict whether or not a nucleoside drug is likely to be a permeant. For example, extensive studies of *es* transporters have shown that nucleosides with either purine or pyrimidine bases and a variety of different five-carbon sugars, including ribose, 2′-deoxyribose, and arabinose, compete with adenosine (or uridine) for entry and are thus probably permeants (see Refs. 1,7,8 for reviews). The *es* transporter is highly stereoselective, with a strong preference for the D- over the L-enantiomer (297), and transportability is greatly decreased or eliminated by (1) the presence of ionized residues (298,299); (2) loss or substitution of the 3′-hydroxyl residue (290); or (3) addition of bulky, hydrophobic substituents at the N^6 position of the purine moiety (3). The importance of the 3′-hydroxyl group in determining transportability suggests that it may be involved in hydrogen binding of nucleosides to the transporter.

A molecular model of the permeant binding site of the *es* transporter has recently been developed (300) by application of an algorithm for analysis of the three-dimensional structures and physicochemical properties of various nucleoside permeants, as established from published quantitative structure–activity relationships (QSAR). Predictions from this three-dimensional (3D)-QSAR analysis of "pharmacophore" characteristics are that the permeant-binding site of the *es* transporter is sensitive to the size and hydrophobicity of the heterocyclic base moiety, prefers nucleosides in the *anti* conformation, and has residues that hydrogen bond with the 5′-OH of the sugar moiety. Although such attempts at molecular modeling are early, they promise to reveal structural criteria for the design of novel nucleoside drugs and competitive inhibitors of *es*-mediated NT processes. It should eventually be possible to use 3D-QSAR analysis to construct molecular models of permeant-binding sites of the other NT proteins.

IV. FUTURE DIRECTIONS

A. Regulation of Transport Activity

There are large differences in NT activities from one cell type to another (226,227), and in the same cell type with changes in growth state (209,212,301–305) or with neoplastic transformation (306). For example, induction of either granulocytic (303,304) or myeloid (209,301) differentiation of cultured HL-60 human leukemia cells is accompanied by decreased *es* NT activity and increased Na^+-dependent (N3/*cib*) NT activity (301–304). The up-regulation of N3/*cib* activity during granulocytic differentiation of HL-60 cells (1) is inhibited by pertussis toxin (303), suggesting involvement of a G-protein-coupled receptor in transporter regulation; and (2) is further enhanced by exposure of differentiated cells to a chemotactic peptide (*N*-formyl-Met-Leu-Phe), the receptor of which is coupled to phospholipase C (304), suggesting involvement of protein kinase C and mobilization of intracellular Ca^{2+} in transporter regulation. Another example of regulation can be found in the changes in *es* and *ei* NT activities when quiescent murine bone marrow macrophages are activated by exposure to colony-stimulating factor 1 (CSF-1) to enter the proliferative state (305); quiescent macrophages exhibit primarily *ei*-mediated transport, whereas proliferating macrophages exhibit primarily *es*-mediated transport. It is anticipated that future studies will identify other examples of physiological regulation of NT processes by hormones and growth factors. Cellular entry is a critical determinant of pharmacological activity of many nucleoside drugs, and it may be possible to harness regulatory phenomena to enhance therapeutic efficacy of nucleoside drugs, either by increasing drug uptake in diseased cells, or by decreasing drug uptake in dose-limiting normal cells.

B. Organelle Transport of Nucleosides

Since their discovery, the focus of research on NT processes in mammalian cells has been almost exclusively on transporters of the plasma membrane, and relatively little effort has been expended on transporters of intracellular membranes. The compartmentation of enzymes of nucleoside metabolism in organelles (307–315) implies mediated permeation of physiological nucleosides, which are highly hydrophilic molecules, across organelle membranes. Consistent with this view, a recently cloned protein that copurifies with Golgi membranes exhibits NT activity when expressed in *Xenopus* oocytes (19,20), a broadly selective NT process exists in lysosomes of cultured fibroblasts (316,317), and isolated liver mitochondria exhibit the capacity for uptake of thymidine and deoxyguanosine (318,319). Mitochondrial toxicity is emerging as an important dose-limiting side effect of chronic exposure to antiviral nucleosides, suggesting an important role for organelle NT processes in the "intracellular pharmacology" of nucleoside drugs.

The presumptive Golgi NT protein was identified by isolation of an L1210 leukemia-derived cDNA by phenotypic complementation of NT activity in yeast that lack the capacity for celluar uptake of thymidine (20,320). The original cDNA isolate, which lacks part of the 5' coding region, encodes a truncated protein that can be functionally expressed in plasma membranes of yeast and *Xenopus* oocytes and exhibits the ability to transport nucleosides. A comparison of the functional characteristics and cellular locations of either full-length or COOH- and NH$_2$-terminally truncated recombinant proteins and of endogeneously expressed native protein suggests that the truncated proteins are expressed in plasma membranes, whereas the native protein is a normal constituent of intracellular membranes, tentatively identified in the Golgi apparatus. The full-length cDNA encodes a 25-kDa protein with four potential membrane-spanning regions, and its coding sequence has no homology with that of other known transporter proteins. Golgi membrane vesicles exhibit the ability to catalyze coupled exchange of a variety of nucleotide-sugars with nucleotides (see Ref. 321 for review) and of ATP with AMP (322), and it is possible that the cloned protein is responsible for one of these activities.

The best characterized example of carrier-mediated transport of nucleosides in organellar membranes is that of adenosine uptake by lysosomes isolated from cultured human fibroblasts (316). The NT process(es) of lysosomes evidently function primarily in transfer of nucleosides produced by degradation of nucleic acids from lysosomes to cytosol (317). The lysosomal transporter of human fibroblasts exhibits broad permeant selectivity (purine and pyrimidine nucleosides, nucleobases), is moderately sensitive to inhibition by NBMPR and dipyridamole, and is unaffected by changes in pH. Its relation to nucleoside transporters of plasma membranes is unknown.

The importance of organellar uptake of nucleosides, or their activated metabolites, in the cellular pharmacology of nucleoside drugs is underscored by the mitochondrial toxicities seen during prolonged exposure of patients to some antiviral nucleosides. Serious muscle disorders, which resemble genetic mitochondrial myopathies, have been found in patients treated with AZT (323–326) and painful peripheral neuropathies in patients treated with ddCyd (327). Mitochondrial dysfunction in liver and kidney is thought to be the cause of several drug-induced deaths in clinical trials of 2′-F-arabinofuranosyl-5-iodouracil (FIAU) in patients with hepatitis B (328). Prolonged exposures of cultured cell lines to low concentrations of several antiviral nucleosides, including AZT and ddCyd, result in a reduction of mtDNA, evidently because of inhibition of mitochondrial DNA replication (329–332) and an increase in the proportion of damaged mitochondrial DNA in cells with preexisting mitochondrial mutations (333). The mechanism of mitochondrial uptake of nucleoside drugs is unclear. Isolated mitochondria that are incubated with AZT produce phosphorylated AZT (334), whereas most of the TTP that serves as precursor for mitochondrial DNA synthesis (335) and the ddCTP that inhibits mitochondrial replication (330) in proliferating cultured cells is produced in the cytosol. Thus, it has been suggested (328,330) that there are transport process(es) in mitochondria, other than the well-characterized and highly selective ATP–ADP translocator (336,337), that mediate uptake of the 5′-triphosphosphates of nucleosides and nucleoside analogues. It is possible that these, as yet uncharacterized, transport systems also mediate transport of nucleosides, as in the presumptive Golgi transport protein (19,20). A candidate mitochondrial transporter has recently been identified by isolation of a human kidney-derived cDNA that is capable of complementing NT-defective yeast (338); the cDNA sequence is identical with that of ND4, a mitochondrially encoded protein (see Ref. 339 for review) of unknown function, the predicted secondary structure of which is strikingly similar to that of the superfamily of transporters predicted to have 12 membrane-spanning domains.

C. Role of Nucleoside Transport Processes in Signal Transduction

The most significant achievement during the past decade of research on NT processes has been recognition of the considerable heterogeneity in functional characteristics of the transporters. The astonishing diversity of NT processes has implications for the complex physiology of nucleosides, particularly relative to the roles of adenosine and adenine nucleotides as extracellular signaling molecules, since the activity of NT processes determines the local concentration of signal in the vicinity of its receptors. With greater knowledge of functional interactions between purinoceptors and NT proteins, it may eventually be possible to manipulate cellular responses to adenosine and adenine nucleotides by selective inhibition of NT processes. The key to understanding the molecular basis of the functional heterogeneity of NT processes is the isolation and characterization of cDNAs encoding NT proteins. The recent successes in molecular cloning of purinoceptors and NT proteins, coupled with development of functional systems for analysis of NT activity, promise substantial progress in understanding of the role of membrane transport of nucleosides in signal transduction pathways.

REFERENCES

1. Paterson ARP, Cass CE. Transport of nucleoside drugs in animal cells. In: Goldman ID, ed. Membrane Transport of Antineoplastic Agents. Oxford: Pergamon Press, 1986:309–329.
2. Plagemann PGW, Wohlhueter RM. Permeation of nucleosides, nucleic acid bases, and nucleotides in animal cells. Curr Top Membr Transp 1980; 14:225–330.
3. Paterson ARP, Harley ER, Cass CE. Measurement and inhibition of membrane transport of adenosine. In: Paton DM, ed. Methods Used in Adenosine Research. New York: Plenum Publishing, 1985; 6:165–180.
4. Cabantchik ZI. Nucleoside transport across red cell membranes. Methods Enzymol 1989; 173:250–263.
5. Cass CE, Belt JA, Paterson ARP. Adenosine transport in cultured cells. Prog Clin Biol Res 1987; 230:13–40.
6. Jarvis SM. Adenosine transporters. In: Cooper DMF, Londos C, eds. Adenosine Receptors. New York: Alan R Liss, 1988:113–123.
7. Plagemann PGW, Wohlhueter RM, Woffendin C. Nucleoside and nucleobase transport in animal cells. Biochim Biophys Acta 1988; 947:405–443.
8. Gati WP, Paterson ARP. Nucleoside transport. In: Agre P, Parker JC, eds. Red Blood Cell Membranes. New York: Marcel Dekker, 1989:635–661.
9. Ullman B. Mutational analysis of nucleoside and nucleobase transport. In: Kessel D, ed. Resistance to antineoplastic drugs. Boca Raton, FL: CRC Press, 1989:293–315.
10. Paterson ARP, Clanachan AS, Craik JD, et al. Plasma membrane transport of nucleosides, nucleobases and nucleotides: an overview. In: Imai S, Nakazawa M, eds. Role of Adenosine and Adenine Nucleotides in Biological Systems. London: Elsevier Science Publishers, 1991:133–148.
11. Jarvis S. Multiple nucleoside transporters in animal cells. Physiol Soc Mag 1993; 7:35–38.
12. Belt JA, Marina NM, Phelps DA, et al. Nucleoside transport in normal and neoplastic cells. Adv Enzyme Regul 1993; 33:235–252.
13. Geiger JD, Fyda DM. Adenosine transport in nervous system tissues. In: Stone T, ed. Adenosine in the Nervous System. London: Academic Press, 1991:1–23.
14. Jarvis SM, Young JD. Photoaffinity labelling of nucleoside transport peptides. Pharmacol Ther 1987; 32:339–359.

15. Kwong FY, Davies A, Tse C-M, et al. Purification of the human erythrocyte nucleoside transporter by immunoaffinity chromatography. Biochem J 1988; 255:243–249.

16. Pajor AM, Wright EM. Cloning and functional expression of a mammalian Na^+/nucleoside cotransporter. A member of the SGLT family. J Biol Chem 1992; 267:3557–3560.

17. Huang QQ, Yao SYM, Ritzel MWL, et al. Cloning and functional expression of a complementary DNA encoding a mammalian nucleoside transport protein. J Biol Chem 1994; 269:17757–17760.

18. Young JD, Huang QQ, Yao SYM, et al. Cloning and functional expression of a cDNA encoding a mammalian sodium-dependent nucleoside transporter selective for adenosine pyrimidine nucleosides and anti-viral pyrimidine nucleoside analogs. Drug Dev Res 1994; 31:335.

19. Hogue DL. Functional and Molecular Studies of Eucaryotic Nucleoside Transporters. Ph.D. dissertation. University of Alberta, Edmonton, Alberta, Canada, 1994.

20. Hogue D, Ellison M, Young J, et al. Molecular characterization of an organelle-specific transporter protein. Biochem Cell Biol 1993: 71.

21. Wolhueter RM, Plagemann PGW. The roles of transport and phosphorylation in nutrient uptake in cultured animal cells. Int Rev Cytol 1980; 64:171–240.

22. Henderson JF, Paterson ARP. Nucleotide Metabolism. New York: Academic Press, 1973.

23. Jones ME. Pyrimidine nucleotide biosynthesis in animals: genes, enzymes, and regulation of UMP biosynthesis. Annu Rev Biochem 1980; 49:253–279.

24. Voet D, Voet JG. Nucleotide metabolism. In: Voet D, Voet JG, eds. Biochemistry. New York: John Wiley & Sons, 1990:740–768.

25. Fox M, Boyle JM, Kinsella AR. Nucleoside salvage and resistance to antimetabolite anticancer agents. Br J Cancer 1991; 64:428–436.

26. Stone TW, Simmonds HA. Purines: basic and clinical aspects. New York: Kluwer Academic Publishers, 1991.

27. Boss GR, Seegmiller JE. Genetic defects in human purine and pyrimidine metabolism. Annu Rev Genet 1982; 16:297–382.

28. Johnson MA, Fridland A. Phosphorylation of $2',3'$-dideoxyinosine by cytosolic $5'$-nucleotidase of human lymphoid cells. Mol Pharmacol 1989; 36:291–295.

29. De Clerq E. Antiviral agents: characteristic activity spectrum depending on the molecular target with which they interact. Adv Virus Res 1993; 42:1–15.

30. Gentry GA. Viral thymidine kinases and their relatives. Pharmacol Ther 1992; 54:319–355.

31. Gudas JM, Fridovich-Keil JL, Pardee AB. Posttranscriptional control of thymidine kinase messenger RNA accumulation in cells released from G_0–G_1 phase blocks. Cell Growth Differ 1993; 4:421–430.

32. McGinn CJ, Kinsella TJ. The experimental and clinical rationale for the use

of S-phase-specific radiosensitizers to overcome tumor cell repopulation. Semin Oncol 1992; 19:21–28.

33. Hallek M, Wanders L, Strohmeyer S, et al. Thymidine kinase: a tumor marker with prognostic value for non-Hodgkin's lymphoma and a broad range of potential clinical applications. Ann Hematol 1992; 65:1–5.

34. O'Dwyer PJ, King SA, Hoth DF, et al. Role of thymidine in biochemical modulation: a review. Cancer Res 1987; 47:3911.

35. Rustum YM, Raymakers RAP. 1-β-Arabinofuranosylcytosine in therapy of leukemia: preclinical and clinical overview. Pharmacol Ther 1992; 56:307–321.

36. Plunkett W, Huang P, Gandhi V. Metabolism and action of fludarabine phosphate. Semin Oncol 1990; 17:3–17.

37. Plunkett W, Saunders PP. Metabolism and action of purine nucleoside analogs. Pharmacol Ther 1991; 49:239–268.

38. Chottiner EG, Shewach DS, Datta NS, et al. Cloning and expression of human deoxycytidine kinase cDNA. Proc Natl Acad Sci USA 1991; 88:1531–5.

39. Song JJ, Walker S, Chen E, et al. Genomic structure and chromosomal localization of the human deoxycytidine kinase gene. Proc Natl Acad Sci USA 1993; 90:431–434.

40. Owens JK, Shewach DS, Ullman B, et al. Resistance to 1-β-D-arabinofuranosylcytosine in human T-lymphoblasts mediated by mutations within the deoxycytidine kinase gene. Cancer Res 1992; 52:2389–2393.

41. Mitchell BS, Song JJ, Johnson EE II, et al. Regulation of human deoxycytidine kinase expression. Adv Enzyme Regul 1993; 33:61–68.

42. Ullman B. Adenosine, deoxyadenosine, and deoxyguanosine. In: Gupta RS, ed. Drug Resistance in Mammalian Cells. Boca Raton, FL: CRC Press, 1989:69–88.

43. Gupta RS. Purine nucleoside analogs. In: Gupta RS, ed. Drug Resistance in Mammalian Cells. Boca Raton, FL: CRC Press, 1989; 89–110.

44. Buttin G, Debatisse M, de Saint Vincent, BR. Cytosine arabinoside, deoxycoformycin, and coformycin. In: Gupta RS, ed. Drug Resistance in Mammalian Cells. Boca Raton, FL: CRC Press, 1989:171–184.

45. Hirschhorn R. Overview of biochemical abnormalities and molecular genetics of adenosine deaminase deficiency. Pediatr Res 1993; 33:S35–S41.

46. Markert ML. Purine nucleoside phosphorylase deficiency. Immunodefic Rev 1991; 3:45–81.

47. Carson DA, Carrera CJ. Immunodeficiency secondary to adenosine deaminase deficiency and purine nucleoside phosphorylation deficiency. Semin Hematol 1990; 27:260–269.

48. Cournoyer D, Caskey CT. Gene therapy of the immune system. Annu Rev Immunol 1993; 11:297–329.

49. Ledley FD. Are contemporary methods for somatic gene therapy suitable for clinical applications? Clin Invest Med 1993; 16:78–88.

50. Wilson DK, Rudolph FB, Quiocho FA. Atomic structure of adenosine de-

aminase complexed with a transition state analog: understanding catalysis and immunodeficiency mutations. Science 1991; 252:1278–1284.

51. Montgomery JA. Purine nucleoside phosphorylase: a target for drug design. Med Res Rev 1993; 13:209–228.

52. Saven A, Piro LD. The newer purine analogs. Significant therapeutic advance in the management of lymphoid malignancies. Cancer 1993; 72:3470–3483.

53. Montgomery JA, Niwas S, Rose JD, et al. Structure-based design of inhibitors of purine nucleoside phosphorylase. 1. 9-(Arylmethyl)derivatives of 9-deazaguanine. J Med Chem 1993; 36:55–69.

54. Ealick SE, Babu YS, Bugg CE, et al. Application of x-ray crystallographic methods in the design of purine nucleoside phosphorylase inhibitors. Ann NY Acad Sci 1993; 685:237–247.

55. Iltzsch MH, el Kouni MH, Cha S. Kinetic studies of thymidine phosphorylase from mouse liver. Biochemistry 1985; 24:6799–6807.

56. Moghaddam A, Bicknell R. Expression of platelet-derived endothelial cell growth factor in *Escherichia coli* and confirmation of its thymidine phosphorylase activity. Biochemistry 1992; 31:12141–12146.

57. Sumizawa T, Furukawa T, Haraguchi M, et al. Thymidine phosphorylase activity associated with platelet-derived endothelial cell growth factor. J Biochem 1993; 114:9–14.

58. Finnis C, Dodsworth N, Pollitt CE, et al. Thymidine phosphorylase activity of platelet-derived endothelial cell growth factor is responsible for endothelial cell mitogenicity. Eur J Biochem 1993; 212:201–210.

59. Eda H, Fujimoto K, Watanabe SI, et al. Cytokines induce thymidine phosphorylase expression in tumor cells and make them more susceptible to 5′-deoxy-5-fluorouridine. Cancer Chemother Pharmacol 1993; 32:333–338.

60. Trams EG, Lauter CJ. Adenosine deaminase in cultured brain cells. Biochem J 1975; 152:681–687.

61. Franco R, Canela EI, Bozal J. Heterogeneous localization of some purine enzymes in subcellular fractions of rat brain and cerebellum. Neurochem Res 1986; 11:423–435.

62. Franco R, Arran JM, Colomer D, et al. Association of adenosine deaminase with the plasma membrane of erythrocytes and platelets. J Histochem Cytochem 1990; 38:653–658.

63. Kameoka J, Tanaka T, Nojima Y, et al. Direct association of adenosine deaminase with a T cell activation antigen, CD26. Science 1993; 261:466–469.

64. Sakamoto J, Watanabe T, Teramukai S, et al. Distribution of adenosine deaminase binding protein in normal and malignant tissues of the gastrointestinal tract studied by monoclonal antibodies. J Surg Oncol 1993; 52:124–134.

65. Agarwal RP, Parks RE. A possible association between the nucleoside transport system of human erythrocytes and adenosine deaminase. Biochem Pharmacol 1975; 24:547–550.

66. Geiger JD, Nagy JI. Heterogeneous distribution of adenosine transport sites labelled by [^{3}H]nitrobenzylthioinosine in rat brain: an autoradiographic and membrane binding study. Brain Res Bull 1984; 13:657–666.

67. Centelles JJ, Franco R. Is adenosine deaminase involved in adenosine transport? Med Hypotheses 1990; 33:245–250.

68. Che M, Nishida T, Gatmaitan Z, et al. A nucleoside transporter is functionally linked to ectonucleotidases in rat liver canalicular membrane. J Biol Chem 1992; 267:9684–9688.

69. Lin S-H. Localization of the ecto-ATPase (ecto-nucleotidase) in the rat hepatocyte plasma membrane. J Biol Chem 1989; 264:14403–14407.

70. Centelles JJ, Cascante M, Canela EJ, et al. A model for adenosine transport and metabolism. Biochem J 1992; 287:461–472.

71. Newby AC. Adenosine and the concept of "retaliatory metabolites." Trends Biochem Sci 1984; 9:42–44.

72. Drury AN, Szent-Györgyi A. The physiological activity of adenine compounds with special reference to their action upon the mammalian heart. J Physiol (Lond) 1929; 68:213–237.

73. Sattin A, Rall TW. The effect of adenosine and adenine nucleotides on the cyclic adenosine 3′,5′-phosphate content of guinea pig cerebral cortex slices. Mol Pharmacol 1970; 6:13–23.

74. Tagawa H, Vander AJ. Effects of adenosine compounds on renal function and renin secretion in dogs. Circ Res 1970; 26:327–338.

75. Burnstock G. Purinergic nerves. Pharmacol Rev 1972; 24:509–581.

76. Burnstock, G. A basis for distinguishing two types of purinergic receptor. In: Bolis L, Straub RCO, eds. Cell Membrane Receptors for Drugs and Hormones: A Multidisciplinary Approach. New York: Raven Press, 1978:107–118.

77. Jacobson KA, Daly JW, Manganiello V. Purines in Cellular Signalling: Targets for New Drugs. New York: Springer Verlag, 1990.

78. Stone, T. Adenosine in the Nervous System. London: Academic Press, 1991.

79. Phillis JW. Adenosine and Adenine Nucleotides as Regulators of Cellular Function. Boca Raton, FL: CRC Press, 1991.

80. Inscho EW, Mitchell KD, Navar LG. Extracellular ATP in the regulation of renal microvascular function. FASEB J 1994; 8:319–328.

81. Fredholm BB, Abbracchio M, Burnstock G, et al. VI. Nomenclature and classification of purinoceptors. Pharmacol Rev 1994; 46:143–156.

82. Daly JW. Adenosine receptors: targets for future drugs. J Med Chem 1982; 25:19–207.

83. Jacobson KA. Molecular probes for adenosine receptors. In: Jacobson KA, Daly JW, Manganiello V, eds. Purines in Cellular Signalling: Targets for New Drugs. New York: Springer Verlag, 1990:100–125.

84. Churchill PC, Ellis VR. Pharmacological characterization of the renovascular P$_2$ purinergic receptors. J Pharmacol Exp Ther 1993; 265:334–338.

85. Jacobson KA, Fischer B, Maillard M, et al. Novel molecular probes for ATP receptors. Drug Dev Res 1994; 34:281.

86. Olsson RA, Pearson JD. Cardiovascular purinoceptors. Physiol Rev 1990; 70:761–845.

87. Stiles GL. Adenosine receptors. J Biol Chem 1992; 267:6451–6454.

88. Olah ME, Stiles GL. Adenosine receptors. Annu Rev Physiol 1992; 54:211–225.

89. Collis MG, Hourani SM. Adenosine receptor subtypes. Trends Pharmacol Sci 1993; 14:360–366.

90. Tucker AL, Linden J. Cloned receptors and cardiovascular responses to adenosine. Cardiovasc Res 1993; 27:62–67.

91. Libert F, Parmentier M, Lefort A, et al. Selective amplification and cloning of four new members of the G protein-coupled receptor family. Science 1989; 244:569–572.

92. Maenhaut C, Van Sande J, Libert F, et al. *RDC8* codes for an adenosine A_2 receptor with physiological constitutive activity. Biochem Biophys Res Commun 1990; 173:1169–1178.

93. Mahan LC, McVittie LD, Smyk-Randall EM, et al. Cloning and expression of an A_1 adenosine receptor from rat brain. Mol Pharmacol 1991; 40:1–7.

94. Reppert SM, Weaver DR, Stehle JH, et al. Molecular cloning and characterization of a rat A_1-receptor that is widely expressed in brain and spinal cord. Mol Endocrinol 1991; 5:1037–1048.

95. Townsend-Nicholson A, Shine J. Molecular cloning and characterisation of a human brain A_1 adenosine receptor cDNA. Mol Brain Res 1992: 16:365–370.

96. Rivkees SA, Reppert SM. *RFL9* encodes an A_{2b}-adenosine receptor. Mol Endocrinol 1992; 6:1598–1604.

97. Pierce KD, Furlong TJ, Selbie LA, et al. Molecular cloning and expression of an adenosine A_{2b} receptor from human brain. Biochem Biophys Res Commun 1992; 187:86–93.

98. Zhou QY, Li C, Olah ME, et al. Molecular cloning and characterization of an adenosine receptor: the A_3 adenosine receptor. Proc Natl Acad Sci USA 1992; 89:7432–7436.

99. Olah ME, Ren H, Ostrowski J, et al. Cloning, expression, and characterization of the unique bovine A_1 adenosine receptor. Studies on the ligand binding site by site-directed mutagenesis. J Biol Chem 1992; 267:10764–10770.

100. Tucker AL, Linden J, Robeva AS, et al. Cloning and expression of a bovine adenosine A_1 receptor cDNA. FEBS Lett 1992; 297:107–111.

101. Salvatore CA, Jacobson MA, Taylor HE, et al. Molecular cloning and characterization of the human A_3 adenosine receptor. Proc Natl Acad Sci USA 1993; 90:10365–10369.

102. Sajjadi FG, Firestein GS. cDNA cloning and sequence analysis of the human A_3 adenosine receptor. Biochim Biophys Acta 1993; 1179:105–107.

103. Yakel JL, Warren RA, Reppert SM, et al. Functional expression of adenosine A_{2b} receptor in *Xenopus* oocytes. Mol Pharmacol 1993; 43:277–280.

104. Lustig KD, Shiau AK, Brake AJ, et al. Expression cloning of an ATP

receptor from mouse neuroblastoma cells. Proc Natl Acad Sci USA 1993; 90:5113–5117.

105. Webb, TE, Simon J, Krishek BJ, et al. Cloning and functional expression of a brain G-protein-coupled ATP receptor. FEBS Lett 1993; 324:219–225.

106. Erb L, Lustig KD, Sullivan DM, et al. Functional expression and photoaffinity labeling of a cloned P_{2U} purinergic receptor. Proc Natl Acad Sci USA 1993; 90:10449–10453.

107. Parr CE, Sullivan DM, Paradiso AM, et al. Cloning and expression of a human P_{2U} nucleotide receptor, a target for cystic fibrosis pharmacotherapy. Drug Dev Res 1994; 31:305.

108. Gödecke S, Schrader J. Cloning and expression analysis of the rat ATP receptor. Drug Dev Res 1994; 31:273.

109. Jacobson MA. Cloning and expression of human adenosine receptor subtypes. Drug Dev Res 1994; 31:281.

110. Meghji P, Rubio R, Berne RM. Intracellular adenosine formation and its carrier-mediated release in cultured embryonic chick heart cells. Life Sci 1988; 43:1851–1859.

111. Frick GP, Lowenstein JM. Studies of 5′-nucleotidase in the perfused rat heart, including measurements of the enzyme in perfused skeletal muscle and liver. J Biol Chem 1976; 251:6372–6378.

112. Sweeney MI, White TD, Sawynok J. Morphine-evoked release of adenosine from the spinal cord occurs via a nucleoside carrier with differential sensitivity to dipyridamole and nitrobenzylthioinosine. Brain Res 1993; 614:301–307.

113. Gu JG, Parkinson F, Gieger JD. L-Adenosine release from rat brain synaptosomes: a novel system for determination of bidirectional transport of purine nucleosides. Drug Dev Res 1994; 31:275.

114. Van Belle H. Nucleoside transport inhibition: a therapeutic approach to cardioprotection via adenosine? Cardiovasc Res 1993; 27:68–76.

115. Gottesman MM, Pastan I. Biochemistry of multidrug resistance. Annu Rev Biochem 1993; 62:385–427.

116. Abraham EH, Prat AG, Gerweck L, et al. The multi-drug resistance (*mdr1*) gene functions as an ATP channel. Proc Natl Acad Sci USA 1993; 90:312–316.

117. Abraham EH. P-Glycoprotein serves as a transporter of cellular ATP. Drug Dev Res 1994; 31:241.

118. Deckert J, Morgan PF, Marangos PJ. Adenosine uptake site heterogeneity in the mammalian CNS? Uptake inhibitors as probes and potential neuropharmaceuticals. Life Sci 1988; 42:1331–1345.

119. Marangos PJ, Von Lubitz D, Daval JL, et al. Adenosine: its relevance to the treatment of brain ischemia and trauma. In: Meldrum BS, Williams M, eds. Current and Future Trends in Anticonvulsant, Anxiety, and Stroke Therapy. New York: Wiley–Liss, 1990:331–349.

120. Parkinson FE, Fredholm BB. Effects of propentofylline on adenosine A_1 and A_2 receptors and nitrobenzylthioinosine-sensitive nucleoside transport-

ers: a quantitative autoradiographical analysis. Eur J Pharmacol 1991; 202:361–366.

121. Wainwright, CL, Parratt, JR, Van Belle H. The antiarrhythmic effects of the nucleoside transporter inhibitor, R75231, in anaesthetized pigs. Br J Pharmacol 1993; 109:592–599.

122. Abd-Elfattah AS, Ding M, Dyke CM, et al. Protection of the stunned myocardium. Selective nucleoside transport blocker administered after 20 minutes of ischemia augments recovery of ventricular function. Circulation 1993; 88:336–343.

123. Périgaud CG, Gosselin G, Imbach J-L. Nucleoside analogues as chemotherapeutic agents: a review. Nucleosides Nucleotides 1992; 11:903–945.

124. Handschumacher RE, Cheng YC. Purine and pyrimidine antimetabolites. In: Holland JF, Frei E III, Bast RC Jr, et al, eds. Cancer Medicine. Philadelphia: Lea & Febiger, 1993:712–732.

125. De Clercq E. Antivirals for the treatment of herpesvirus infections. J Antimicrob Chemother 1993; 32:121–132.

126. De Clercq E. Antiviral agents: characteristic activity spectrum depending on the molecular target with which they interact. Adv Virus Res 1993; 42:1–55.

127. Bean B. Antiviral therapy: current concepts and practices. Clin Microbiol Rev 1992; 5:146–182.

128. Morse GD, Shelton MJ, O'Donnel AM. Comparative pharmacokinetics of antiviral nucleoside analogues. Clin Pharmacokinet 1993; 24:101–123.

129. Bryson HM, Sorkin EM. Cladribine. A review of its pharmacodynamic and pharmacokinetic properties and therapeutic potential in haematological malignancies. Drugs 1993; 46:872–894.

130. Jaiyesimmi IA, Kantarjian HM, Estey EH. Advances in therapy for hairy cell leukemia. A review. Cancer 1993; 72:5–16.

131. Plunkett W, Gandhi V, Huang P, et al. Fludarabine: pharmacokinetics, mechanisms of action, and rationales for combination therapies. Semin Oncol 1993; 20:2–12.

132. Ross, SR, McTavish D, Faulds D. Fludarabine. A review of its pharmacological properties and therapeutic potential in malignancy. Drugs 1993; 45:737–759.

133. Mayer RJ. Chemotherapy for metastatic colorectal cancer. Cancer 1992; 70:1414–1424.

134. Chu E, Johnston PG, Takimoto CH, et al. Antimetabolites. Cancer Chemother Biol Response Modif 1993; 14:1–25.

135. Shelton MJ, O'Donnell AM, Morse GD. Didanosine. Ann Pharmacother 1992; 26:660–670.

136. Yarchoan R, Pluda JM, Perno CF, et al. Antiretroviral therapy of human immunodeficiency virus infection: current strategies and challenges for the future. Blood 1991; 87:859–884.

137. Clumeck N. Current use of anti-HIV drugs in AIDS. J Antimicrob Chemother 1993; 32:133–138.

138. Kamali F. Clinical pharmacology of zidovudine and other 2′,3′-dideoxynucleoside analogues. Clin Invest 1993; 71:392–405.

139. McLeod GX, Hammer SM. Zidovudine: five years later. Ann Intern Med 1992; 117:487–501.

140. Cohen A, Ullman B, Martin DW. Characterization of a mutant mouse lymphoma cell with deficient transport of purine and pyrimidine nucleosides. J Biol Chem 1979; 254:112–116.

141. Cass CE, Kolassa N, Uehara Y, et al. Absence of binding sites for the transport inhibitor nitrobenzylthioinosine on nucleoside transport deficient mouse lymphoma cells. Biochim Biophys Acta 1981; 649:769–777.

142. Cohen A, Leung C, Thompson E. Characterization of mouse lymphoma cells with altered nucleoside transport. J Cell Physiol 1985; 123:431–434.

143. Sobrero AR, Moir RD, Bertino JR, et al. Defective facilitated diffusion of nucleosides, a primary mechanism of resistance to 5-fluoro-2′-deoxyuridine in the HCT-8 human carcinoma line. Cancer Res 1985; 45:3155–3160.

144. Vijayalakshmi D, Dagnino L, Belt JA, et al. L1210/B23.1 cells express equilibrative inhibitor-sensitive nucleoside transport activity and lack two parental nucleoside transport activities. J Biol Chem 1992; 267:16951–16956.

145. Warnick CT, Muzik H, Paterson ARP. Interference with nucleoside transport in mouse lymphoma cells proliferating in culture. Cancer Res 1972; 32:2017–2022.

146. Paterson ARP, Yang S, Lau EY, et al. Low specificity of the nucleoside transport mechanism of RPMI 6410 cells. Mol Pharmacol 1979; 16:900–908.

147. Cass CE, King KM, Montano JT, et al. A comparison of the abilities of nitrobenzylthioinosine, dilazep, and dipyridamole to protect human hematopoietic cells from 7-deazaadenosine (tubercidin). Cancer Res 1992; 52:5879–5886.

148. Stein WD. Transport and Diffusion Across Cell Membranes. New York: Academic Press, 1986.

149. Vijayalakshmi D, Belt JA. Sodium-dependent nucleoside transport in mouse intestinal epithelial cells. Two transport systems with differing substrate specificities. J Biol Chem 1988; 263:19419–19423.

150. Crawford CR, Ng CYC, Belt JA. Isolation and characterization of an L1210 cell line retaining the sodium-dependent carrier *cif* as its sole nucleoside transport activity. J Biol Chem 1990; 265:13730–13734.

151. Dagnino L, Bennett LJ, Paterson ARP. Substrate specificity, kinetics, and stoichiometry of sodium-dependent adenosine transport in L1210/AM mouse leukemia cells. J Biol Chem 1991; 266:6312–6317.

152. Williams TC, Jarvis SM. Multiple sodium-dependent nucleoside transport systems in bovine renal brush-border membrane vesicles. Biochem J 1991; 274:27–33.

153. Huang Q-Q, Harvey CM, Paterson ARP, et al. Functional expression of Na$^+$-dependent nucleoside transport systems of rat intestine in isolated oocytes of *Xenopus laevis*. Demonstration that rat jejunum expresses the purine-selective system N1 (*cif*) and a second, novel system N3 having

broad specificity for purine and pyrimidine nucleosides. J Biol Chem 1993; 268:20613–20619.

154. Wu X, Yuan G, CM Brett, et al. Sodium-dependent nucleoside transport in choroid plexus from rabbit. Evidence for a single transporter for purine and pyrimidine nucleosides. J Biol Chem 1992; 267:8813–8818.

155. Gutierrez MM, Brett CM, Ott RJ, et al. Nucleoside transport in brush border membrane vesicles from human kidney. Biochim Biophys Acta 1992; 1105:1–9.

156. Gutierrez MM, Giacomini KM. Substrate selectivity, potential sensitivity and stoichiometry of Na^+–nucleoside transport in brush border membrane vesicles from human kidney. Biochim Biophys Acta 1993; 1149:202–208.

157. Paterson ARP, Gati WP, Vijayalakshmi D, et al. Inhibitor-sensitive, Na^+-linked transport of nucleoside analogs in leukemia cells from patients. Proc Am Assoc Cancer Res 1993; 34:14.

158. Crawford CR, Ng CYC, Noel D, et al. Nucleoside transport in L1210 murine leukemia cells. J Biol Chem 1990; 265:9732–9736.

159. Hogue DL, Hodgson, KC, Cass CE. 1990. Effects of inhibition of N-linked glycosylation by tunicamycin on nucleoside transport polypeptides of L1210 leukemia cells. Biochem Cell Biol 1990; 68:199–209.

160. Oliver JM, Paterson ARP. Nucleoside transport. I. A mediated process in human erythrocytes. Can J Biochem 1971; 49:262–270.

161. Cass CE, Paterson ARP. Mediated transport of nucleosides in human erythrocytes. Accelerative exchange diffusion of uridine and thymidine and specificity toward pyrimidine nucleosides as permeants. J Biol Chem 1972; 247:3314–3320.

162. Cass CE, Paterson ARP. Mediated transport of nucleosides in human erythrocytes. Specificity toward purine nucleosides as permeants. Biochim Biophys Acta 1973; 291:734–746.

163. Plagemann PGW, Marz R, Erbe J. Transport and countertransport of thymidine in ATP depleted and thymidine kinase-deficient Novikoff rat hepatoma and mouse L cells: evidence for a high K_m facilitated diffusion system with wide nucleoside specificity. J Cell Physiol 1975; 89:1–18.

164. Cabantchik ZI, Ginsburg H. Transport of uridine in human red blood cells—demonstration of a simple carrier-mediated process. J Gen Physiol 1977; 69:75–96.

165. Boleti H. Nucleoside Transport in K562 Leukemia Cells. M.Sc. dissertation. University of Alberta, Edmonton, Alberta, Canada, 1991.

166. Cass CE, Gaudette LA, Paterson ARP. Mediated transport of nucleosides in human erythrocytes. Specific binding of the inhibitor nitrobenzylthioinosine to nucleoside transport sites in the erythrocyte membrane. Biochim Biophys Acta 1974; 345:1–10.

167. Cass CE, Paterson ARP. Nitrobenzylthioinosine binding sites in the erythrocyte membrane. Biochim Biophys Acta 1976; 419:285–294.

168. Jarvis SM, Young JD. Nucleoside transport in human and sheep erythrocytes—evidence that nitrobenzylthioinosine binds specifically to functional nucleoside-transport sites. Biochem J 1980; 190:377–383.

169. Dahlig-Harley E, Eilam Y, Paterson ARP, et al. Binding of nitrobenzylthio-inosine to high-affinity sites on the nucleoside transport mechanism of HeLa cells. Biochem J 1981; 200:295–305.

170. Belt JA. Nitrobenzylthioinosine-insensitive uridine transport in human lymphoblastoid and murine leukemia cells. Biochem Biophys Res Commun 1983; 110:417–423.

171. Belt JA. Heterogeneity of nucleoside transport in mammalian cells. Two types of transport activity in L1210 and other cultured neoplastic cells. Mol Pharmacol 1983; 24:479–484.

172. Belt JA, Noel LD. Nucleoside transport in Walker 256 rat carcinosarcoma and S49 mouse lymphoma cells. Biochem J 1985; 232:681–688.

173. Plagemann PGW, Wohlhueter RM. Nitrobenzylthioinosine-sensitive and -resistant nucleoside transport in normal and transformed rat cells. Biochim Biophys Acta 1985; 816:387–395.

174. Jarvis SM, Young JD. Nucleoside transport in rat erythrocytes: two components with differences in sensitivity to inhibition by nitrobenzylthioinosine and p-chloromercuriphenyl sulfonate. J Membr Biol 1986; 93:1–10.

175. Belt JA, Noel LD. Isolation and characterization of a mutant of L1210 murine leukemia deficient in nitrobenzylthioinosine-insensitive nucleoside transport. J Biol Chem 1988; 263:13819–13822.

176. Fincham DA, Wolowyk MW, Young JD. Nucleoside uptake by red blood cells from a primitive vertebrate, the Pacific hagfish (*Eptatretus stouti*), is mediated by a nitrobenzylthioinosine-insensitive transport system. Biochim Biophys Acta 1991; 1069:123–126.

177. Jarvis SM, McBride D, Young JD. Erythrocyte nucleoside transport: asymmetrical binding of nitrobenzylthioinosine to nucleoside permeation sites. J Physiol 1982; 324:31–46.

178. Agbanyo FR, Paterson ARP, Cass CE. External location of sites on pig erythrocytes that bind nitrobenzylthioinosine. Mol Pharmacol 1988; 33:332–337.

179. Paterson ARP, Lau EY, Dahlig E, et al. A common basis for inhibition of nucleoside transport by dipyridamole and nitrobenzylthioinosine. Mol Pharmacol 1980; 18:4044–4052.

180. Harley ER, Cass CE, Paterson ARP. Initial rate kinetics of the transport of adenosine and 4-amino-7-(β-D-ribofuranosyl)pyrrolo-[2,3-*d*]pyrimidine (tubercidin) in cultured cells. Cancer Res 1982; 42:1289–1295.

181. Paterson ARP, Harley ER, Cass CE. Inward fluxes of adenosine in erythrocytes and cultured cells measured by a quenched flow method. Biochem J 1984; 244:1001–1008.

182. Woffendin C, Plagemann PG. Nucleoside transporter of pig erythrocytes. Kinetic properties, isolation and reaction with nitrobenzylthioinosine and dipyridamole. Biochim Biophys Acta 1987; 903:18–30.

183. Dagnino L, Paterson ARP. Sodium-dependent and equilibrative nucleoside transport systems in L1210 mouse leukemia cells: effect of inhibitors of equilibrative systems on the content and retention of nucleosides. Cancer Res 1990; 50:6549–6553.

184. Plagemann PGW, Wohlhueter RM. Nucleoside transport in cultured mammalian cells. Multiple forms with different sensitivity to inhibition by nitrobenzylthioinosine or hypoxanthine. Biochim Biophys Acta 1984; 773:39–52.

185. Plagemann PG, Woffendin C. Species differences in sensitivity of nucleoside transport in erythrocytes and cultured cells to inhibition by nitrobenzylthioinosine, dipyridamole, dilazep and lidoflazine. Biochim Biophys Acta 1988; 969:1–8.

186. Hammond JR. Comparative pharmacology of the nitrobenzylthioguanosine-sensitive and -resistant nucleoside transport mechanisms of Ehrlich ascites tumor cells. J Pharmacol Exp Ther 1991; 259:799–807.

187. Jones KW, Hammond JR. Heterogeneity of [^{3}H]dipyridamole binding to CNS membranes: correlation with [^{3}H]nitrobenzylthioinosine binding and [^{3}H]uridine influx studies. Neurochemistry 1992; 59:1363–1371.

188. Boleti H, Cass CE. Nitrobenzylthioinosine-insensitive nucleoside transport processes of K562 cells. Proc Am Assoc Cancer Res 1992; 33:18.

189. Plagemann PGW, Aran JM, Woffendin C. Na$^+$-dependent, active and Na$^+$-independent, facilitated transport of formycin B in mouse spleen lymphocytes. Biochim Biophys Acta 1990; 1022:93–102.

190. Darnowski JW, Holdridge C, Handschumacher RE. Concentrative uridine transport by murine splenocytes: kinetics, substrate specificity, and sodium dependency. Cancer Res 1987; 47:2614–2619.

191. Baer HP, Moorji AA. Sodium-dependent and inhibitor-insensitive uptake of adenosine by mouse peritoneal exudate cells. Biochim Biophys Acta 1990; 1026:241–247.

192. Plagemann PGW, Aran JM. Characterization of Na$^+$-dependent, active nucleoside transport in rat and mouse peritoneal macrophages, a mouse macrophage cell line and normal rat kidney cells. Biochim Biophys Acta 1990; 1028:289–298.

193. Dagnino L, Bennett LL Jr, Paterson ARP. Sodium-dependent nucleoside transport in mouse leukemia L1210 cells. J Biol Chem 1991; 266:6308–6311.

194. Plagemann PGW. Na$^+$-dependent, active nucleoside transport in S49 mouse lymphoma cells and loss in AE$_1$ mutant deficient in facilitated nucleoside transport. J Cell Biochem 1991; 46:54–59.

195. Franco R, Centelles JJ, Kinne RKH. Further characterization of adenosine transport in renal brush-border membranes. Biochim Biophys Acta 1990; 1024:241–248.

196. Le Hir M. Evidence for separate carriers for purine nucleosides and for pyrmidine nucleosides in the renal brush border membrane. Renal Physiol Biochem 1990; 13:154–161.

197. Le Hir M, Dubach UC. Sodium gradient-energized concentrative transport of adenosine in renal brush border vesicles. Pflugers Arch 1984; 401:58–63.

198. Lee CW, Cheeseman CI, Jarvis SM. Transport characteristics of renal brush border Na$^+$- and K$^+$-dependent uridine carriers. Am J Physiol 1990; 258:F1203–F1210.

199. Plagemann PG. Na^+-dependent, concentrative nucleoside transport in rat macrophages. Specificity for natural nucleosides and nucleoside analogs, including dideoxynucleosides, and comparison of nucleoside transport in rat, mouse and human macrophages. Biochem Pharmacol 1991; 42:247–252.
200. Crawford CR, Belt JA. Sodium-dependent, concentrative nucleoside transport in Walker 256 rat carcinosarcoma cells. Biochem Biophys Res Commun 1991; 715:846–851.
201. Spector R, Huntoon S. Deoxycytidine transport and metabolism in choroid plexus. J Neurochem 1983; 40:1474–1480.
202. Spector R. Nucleoside transport in choroid plexus: mechanism and specificity. Arch Biochem Biophys 1982; 216:693–703.
203. Spector R, Huntoon S. Specificity and sodium dependence of the active nucleoside transport system in choroid plexus. J Neurochem 1984; 42:1048–1052.
204. Betcher SL, Forrest JN Jr, Knickelbein RG, Dobbins JW. Sodium–adenosine cotransport in brush-border membranes from rabbit ileum. Am J Physiol 1990; 259:G504–G510.
205. Roden M, Paterson ARP, Turnheim K. Sodium-dependent nucleoside transport in rabbit intestinal epithelium. Gastroenterology 1991; 100:1553–1562.
206. Jarvis SM. Characterization of sodium-dependent nucleoside transport in rabbit intestinal brush-border membrane vesicles. Biochim Biophys Acta 1989; 979:132–138.
207. Williams TC, Doherty AJ, Griffith DA, et al. Characterization of sodium-dependent and sodium-independent nucleoside transport systems in rabbit brush-border and basolateral plasma-membrane vesicles from the renal outer cortex. Biochem J 1989; 264:223–231.
208. Schwenk M, Hegazy E, Lopez Del Pino V. Uridine uptake by isolated intestinal epithelial cells of guinea pig. Biochim Biophys Acta 1984; 805:370–374.
209. Lee CW, Sokoloski JA, Sartorelli AC, et al. Induction of the differentiation of HL-60 cells by phorbol 12-myristate 13-acetate activates a Na^+-dependent uridine-transport system. Biochem J 1991; 274:85–90.
210. Belt JA, Harper E, Byl J, et al. Na^+-dependent nucleoside transport in human myeloid leukemic cell lines and freshly isolated myeloblasts. Proc Am Assoc Cancer Res 1992; 33:20.
211. Jakobs EW, Paterson ARP. Sodium-dependent, concentrative nucleoside transport in cultured intestinal epithelial cells. Biophys Res Commun 1986; 140:1028–1035.
212. Jakobs ES, Van Os-Corby DJ, Paterson ARP. Expression of sodium-linked nucleoside transport activity in monolayer cultures of IEC-6 intestinal epithelial cells. J Biol Chem 1990; 265:22210–22216.
213. Fleming SA, Rawlins DB, Robins MJ. Photochemistry of the nucleoside membrane transport inhibitor 6-[(4-nitrobenzyl)thio]-9-(β-D-ribofuranosyl)purine. Tetrahedron Lett 1990; 31:4995–4998.
214. Young JD, Jarvis SM, Robins MJ, et al. Photoaffinity labelling of the human

erythrocyte nucleoside transporter by N^6-(p-azidobenzyl)adenosine and nitrobenzylthioinosine. J Biol Chem 1983; 258:2202–2208.

215. Jarvis SM, Young JD. Extraction and partial purification of the nucleoside-transport system from human erythrocytes based on the assay of nitrobenzylthioinosine-binding activity. Biochem J 1981; 194:331–339.

216. Wu JR, Kwong FYP, Jarvis SM, et al. Identification of the erythrocyte nucleoside transporter as a band 4.5 polypeptide. J Biol Chem 1983; 258:13745–13751.

217. Wu JW, Jarvis SM, Young JD. The human erythrocyte nucleoside and glucose transporters are both band 4.5 membrane polypeptides. Biochem J 1983; 214:995–997.

218. Good AH, Craik JD, Jarvis SM, et al. Characterization of monoclonal antibodies that recognize band 4.5 polypeptides associated with nucleoside transport in pig erythrocytes. Biochem J 1987; 244:749–755.

219. Kwong FY, Tse C-M, Jarvis SM, et al. Purification and reconstitution studies of the nucleoside transporter from pig erythrocytes. Biochim Biophys Acta 1987; 904:105–116.

220. Craik JD, Good H, Gottschalk R, et al. Identification of glucose and nucleoside transport proteins in neonatal pig erythrocytes using monoclonal antibodies against band 4.5 polypeptides of adult human and pig erythrocytes. Biochem Cell Biol 1988; 66:839–852.

221. Agbanyo FR, Vijayalakshmi D, Craik JD, et al. SAENTA, a novel ligand with high affinity for polypeptides associated with nucleoside transport: partial purification of the nitrobenzylthioinosine-binding protein of pig erythrocytes by affinity chromatography. Biochem J 1990; 270:605–614.

222. Shi MM, Wu JR, Lee C, et al. Nucleoside transport: photoaffinity labelling of high-affinity nitrobenzylthioinosine binding sites in rat and guinea pig lung. Biochem Biophys Res Commun 1984; 118:594–600.

223. Young JD, Jarvis SM, Belt JA, et al. Identification of the nucleoside transporter in cultured mouse lymphoma cells. Photoaffinity labeling of plasma membrane-enriched fractions from nucleoside transport-competent (S49) and nucleoside transport-deficient (AE$_1$) cells with [^{3}H]nitrobenzylthioinosine. J Biol Chem 1984; 259:8363–8365.

224. Crawford CR, Ng CYC, Ullman B, et al. Identification and reconstitution of the nucleoside transporter of CEM human leukemia cells. Biochim Biophys Acta 1990; 1024:289–297.

225. Boleti H, Cass CE. Nucleoside transport in K562 human erythroleukemia cells. Int J Purine Pyrimidine Res 1991; 2:35.

226. Boumah CE, Hogue, DL, Cass CE. Expression of high levels of nitrobenzylthioinosine-sensitive nucleoside transport in cultured human choriocarcinoma (BeWo) cells. Biochem J 1992; 288:987–996.

227. Jarvis SM, Hammond JR, Paterson ARP, et al. Species differences in nucleoside transport. A study of uridine transport and nitrobenzylthioinosine binding by mammalian erythrocytes. Biochem J 1982; 208:83–88.

228. Smith CL, Pilarski LM, Egerton ML, et al. Nucleoside transport and prolif-

erative rate in human thymocytes and lymphocytes. Blood 1989; 74:2038–2042.

229. Baldwin SA. Mammalian passive glucose transporters: members of a ubiquitous family of active and passive transport proteins. Biochim Biophys Acta 1993; 1154:17–49.

230. Henderson PFJ. The 12-transmembrane helix transporters. Curr Opin Cell Biol 1993; 5:708–721.

231. Kwong FYP, Baldwin SA, Scudder PR, et al. Erythrocyte nucleoside and sugar transport. Biochem J 1986; 240:349–356.

232. Jhun, BH, Rampal AL, Berenski CJ, et al. Chromatographic characterization of nitrobenzylthioinosine binding proteins in band 4.5 of human erythrocytes: purification of a 40 kDa truncated nucleoside transporter. Biochim Biophys Acta 1990; 1028:251–260.

233. Jhun BH, Berenski CJ, Craik JD, et al. Glucose and nucleoside transporters of human erythrocytes: effects of detergents on immunoreadsorption of a membrane protein to its monoclonal antibody. Biochim Biophys Acta 1991; 1061:149–155.

234. Ziedler RB, Lee P, Kim HD. Kinetics of 3-*O*-methyl glucose transport in red blood cells of newborn pigs. J Gen Physiol 1976; 67:67–80.

235. Watts RP, Brendel K, Luthra MG, et al. Inosine from liver as a possible energy source for pig red blood cells. Life Sci 1979; 25:1577–1582.

236. Wu JS, Young JD. Photoaffinity labelling of nucleoside transport proteins in plasma membranes isolated from rat and guinea pig liver. Biochem J 1984; 220:499–506.

237. Kwan KF, Jarvis SM. Photoaffinity labeling of adenosine transporter in cardiac membranes with nitrobenzylthioinosine. Am J Physiol 1984; 246:H710–H715.

238. Gati WP, Belt JA, Jakobs ES, et al. Photoaffinity labelling of a nitrobenzylthioinosine-binding polypeptide from cultured Novikoff hepatoma cells. Biochem J 1986; 236:665–670.

239. Kwong FY, Fincham HE, Davies A, et al. Mammalian nitrobenzylthioinosine-sensitive nucleoside transport proteins. Immunological evidence that transporters differing in size and inhibitor specificity share sequence homology. J Biol Chem 1992; 267:21954–21960.

240. Kwong FYP, Wu J-S R, Shi WM, et al. Enzymic cleavage as a probe of the molecular structures of mammalian equilibrative nucleoside transporters. J Biol Chem 1993; 268:22127–22134.

241. Jarvis SM, Young JD. Nucleoside transport in rat erythrocytes: two components with differences in sensitivity to inhibition by nitrobenzylthioinosine and *p*-chloromercuriphenyl sulfonate. J Membr Biol 1986; 93:1–10.

242. Baldwin SA, Beaumont N, Barros LF, et al. Antibodies as probes of nitrobenzylthioinosine-sensitive nucleoside transporters. Drug Dev Res 1994; 31:245.

243. Barros LF, Beaumont N, Jarvis SM, et al. Immunological detection of nucleoside transporters in human placental trophoblast brush-border plasma

membranes and placental capillary endothelial cells. J Physiol (Lond) 1992; 452:348P.

244.   Barros LP, Bustamante JC, Yudilevich DL, et al. Adenosine transport and nitrobenzylthioinosine binding in human placental membrane vesicles from brush-border and basal sides of the trophoblast. J Membr Biol 1991; 119:151–161.

245.   Wiley JS, Brockleband AM, Snook MB, et al. SAENTA-x_2-fluorescein: a fluorescent probe for the equilibrative, inhibitor-sensitive nucleoside transporter. Biochem J 1991; 273:667–672.

246.   Jamieson GP, Brocklebank AM, Snook MB, et al. Flow cytometric quantitation of nucleoside transporter sites on human leukemic cells. Cytometry 1993; 14:32–38.

247.   Buolamwini JK, Craik JD, Wiley JS, et al. Conjugates of fluorescein and SAENTA (5′-5-(2-aminoethyl)-N^6-(4-nitrobenzyl)-5′-thioadenosine): flow cytometry probes for the *es* nucleoside transporter elements of the plasma membrane. Nucleosides Nucleosides 1994; 13:737–751.

248.   Boumah CE, Harvey CM, Paterson ARP, et al. Candidate cDNA clones encoding the nitrobenzylthioinosine-sensitive transporter of nucleosides in cultured human choriocarcinoma (BeWo) cells. Biochem Cell Biol 71:Axvi.

249.   Boumah CE, Harvey CM, Paterson ARP, et al. Functional expression of the nitrobenzylthioinosine-sensitive nucleoside transporter of human choriocarcinoma (BeWo) cells in isolated oocytes of *Xenopus laevis*. Biochem J 1994; 299:769–773.

250.   Pajor AM. Molecular cloning and expression of SNST1, a renal sodium/nucleoside cotransporter. Drug Dev Res 1994; 31:305.

251.   Wright EM, Hirayama B, Hazama A, et al. The sodium/glucose cotransporter (SGLT1). Soc Gen Physiol Ser 1993; 48:229–241.

252.   Hediger MA, Turk E, Wright EM. Homology of the human intestinal Na$^+$/glucose and *Escherichia coli* Na$^+$/proline cotransporters. Proc Natl Acad Sci USA 1989; 86:5748–5752.

253.   Ohta T, Isselbacher KJ, Rhoads DB. Regulation of glucose transporters in LLC-PKC$_1$ cells: effects of D-glucose and monosaccharides. Mol Cell Biol 1990; 10:6491–6499.

254.   Kwon HM, Hanuchi A, Uchida S, et al. Cloning of the cDNA for a Na$^+$/*myo*-inositol cotransporter, a hypertonicity stress protein. J Biol Chem 1992; 267:6297–6301.

255.   Nako T, Yamato I, Anraku Y. Nucleotide sequence of *putP1*, the proline carrier gene of *Escherichia coli* K12. Mol Gen Genet 1987; 208:70–75.

256.   Jackowski S, Alix J-H. Cloning sequence and expression of the pantothenate permease (*panF*) gene of *Escherichia coli*. J Bacteriol 1990; 172:3842–3848.

257.   Hediger MA, Coady MJ, Ikeda TS, et al. Expression cloning and cDNA sequencing of the Na$^+$/glucose co-transporter. Nature 1987; 330-379–381.

258.   Lubbert H, Hoffman BJ, Snutch TP, et al. cDNA cloning of a serotinin 5-HT$_{1C}$ receptor by electrophysiological assays of mRNA-injected *Xenopus* oocytes. Proc Natl Acad Sci USA 1987; 84:4332–4336.

259. Masu Y, Nakayama K, Tamaki H, et al. cDNA cloning of bovine substance-K receptor through oocyte expression system. Nature 1987; 329:836–838.

260. Noma Y, Sideras P, Naito T, et al. Cloning of cDNA encoding the murine IgG$_1$ induction factor by a novel strategy using SP6 promoter. Nature 1986; 319:640–646.

261. Jarvis SM, Griffith DA. Expression of the rabbit intestinal N2 Na$^+$/nucleoside transporter in *Xenopus laevis* oocytes. Biochem J 1991; 278:605–607.

262. Terasaki T, Kadowaki A, Higashida H, et al. Expression of the Na$^+$ dependent uridine transport system of rabbit small intestine: studies with mRNA-injected *Xenopus laevis* oocytes. Biol Pharm Bull 1993; 16:493–496.

263. Munch-Petersen A, Mygind B. Transport of nucleic acid precursors. In: Munch-Petersen A, ed. Metabolism of Nucleotides, Nucleosides and Nucleobases in Microorganisms. London: Academic Press, 1983:259–305.

264. Yao SYM, Huang QQ, Ritzel MWL, et al. Cloning and functional expression of a Na$^+$-dependent nucleoside transporter protein from rat jejunum that is not a member of any of the known transporter families. Biochem Cell Biol 1993; 71:Axv.

265. Domin BA, Mahony WB, Zimmerman TP. Purine nucleobase transport in human erythrocytes. Reinvestigation with a novel ''inhibitor-stop'' assay. J Biol Chem 1988; 263:9276–9284.

266. Mahony WB, Domin BA, McConnell RT, et al. Acyclovir transport into human erythrocytes. J Biol Chem 1988; 263:9285–9291.

267. Domin BA, Mahony WB, Zimmerman TP. Desciclovir permeation of the human erythrocyte membrane by nonfacilitated diffusion. Biochem Pharmacol 1991; 42:147–152.

268. Mahony WB, Domin BA, Zimmerman TP. Ganciclovir permeation of the human erythrocyte membrane. Biochem Pharmacol 1991; 41:263–271.

269. Gati WP, Paterson AR, Tyrrell DL, et al. Nucleobase transporter-mediated permeation of 2′,3′-dideoxyguanosine in human erythrocytes and human T-lymphoblastoid CCRF-CEM cells. J Biol Chem 1992; 267:22272–22276.

270. Mahony WB, Domin BA, Daluge SM, et al. Enantiomeric selectivity of carbovir transport. J Biol Chem 1992; 267:19792–19797.

271. Domin BA, Mahony WB, Zimmerman TP. Transport of 5-fluorouracil and uracil into human erythrocytes. Biochem Pharmacol 1993; 46:503–510.

272. Domin BA, Mahony WB, Zimmerman TP. Membrane permeation mechanisms of 2′,3′-dideoxynucleosides. Biochem Pharmacol 1993; 46:725–729.

273. King KE, Cass CE. Membrane transport of 2-chloro-2′-deoxyadenosine and 2-chloro-2′-arabinofluoro-2′-deoxyadenosine is required for cytotoxicity. Biochem Cell Biol 1993; 71:Axvii.

274. King KE, Cass CE. Membrane transport of 2-chloro-2′-deoxyadenosine is required for cytotoxicity. Proc Am Assoc Cancer Res 1994; 35:577.

275. Plagemann PGW, Marz R, Wohlhueter RM. Transport and metabolism of deoxycytidine and 1-β-D-arabinofuranosylcytosine into cultured Novikoff rat hepatoma cells, relationship to phosphorylation, and regulation of triphosphate synthesis. Cancer Res 1978; 38:978–989.

276. Wiley JW, Jones SP, Sawyer WH, et al. Cytosine arabinoside influx and nucleoside transport sites in acute leukemia. J Clin Invest 1982; 69:479–489.

277. Wiley JS, Taupin J, Jamieson GP, et al. Cytosine arabinoside transport and metabolism in acute leukemias and T cell lymphoblastic lymphoma. J Clin Invest 1985; 75:632–642.

278. Jamieson GP, Snook MB, Bradley TR, et al. Transport and metabolism of 1-β-D-arabinofuranosylcytosine in human ovarian adenocarcinoma cells. Cancer Res 1989; 49:309–313.

279. Wright SE, Hines LH, White JC. Effects of the lipophilic anticancer drug teniposide (VM-26) on membrane transport. Chem Biol Interact 1990; 75:31–48.

280. Sirotnak FM, Chello PL, Dorick DM, et al. Specificity of systems mediating transport of adenosine, 9-β-D-arabinofuranosyl-2-fluoroadenine, and other purine nucleoside analogues in L1210 cells. Cancer Res 1983; 43:104–109.

281. Sirotnak FM, Barrueco JR. Membrane transport and the antineoplastic action of nucleoside analogues. Cancer Metastasis Rev 1987; 6:459–480.

282. Barrueco JR, Jacobsen DM, Chang CH, et al. Proposed mechanism of therapeutic selectivity for 9-β-D-arabinofuranosyl-2-fluoroadenine against murine leukemia based upon lower capacities for transport and phosphorylation in proliferative intestinal epithelium compared to tumor cells. Cancer Res 1987; 47:700–706.

283. Wiley JS, Smith CL, Jamieson GP. Transport of 2′-deoxycoformycin in human leukemic and lymphoma cells. Biochem Pharmacol 1991; 42:708–710.

284. Bowen D, Diasio RB, Goldman ID. Distinguishing between membrane transport and intracellular metabolism of fluorodeoxyuridine in Ehrlich ascites tumor cells by application of kinetic and high performance liquid chromatographic techniques. J Biol Chem 1979; 254:5333–5339.

285. Gati WP, Knaus EE, Wiebe LI. Interaction of 2′-halogeno-2′-deoxyuridines with the human erythrocyte nucleoside transport mechanism. Mol Pharmacol 1982; 23:146–152.

286. Ullman B, Coons T, Rockwell S, et al. Genetic analysis of 2′,3′-dideoxycytidine incorporation into cultured human T lymphoblasts. J Biol Chem 1988; 263:12391–12396.

287. Plagemann PG, Woffendin C. Dideoxycytidine permeation and salvage by mouse leukemia cells and human erythrocytes. Biochem Pharmacol 1989; 38:3469–3475.

288. Ullman B. Dideoxycytidine metabolism in wild type and mutant CEM cells deficient in nucleoside transport or deoxycytidine kinase. J Physiol (Lond) 1989; 601:416–421.

289. Cass CE, Paterson ARP. Inhibition by nitrobenzylthioinosine of uptake of adenosine, 2′-deoxyadenosine and 9-β-D-arabinofuranosyladenine by human and mouse erythrocytes. Biochem Pharmacol 1975; 24:1989–1993.

290. Zimmerman TP, Mahony WB, Prus KL. 3′-Azido-3′-deoxythymidine. An

unusual nucleoside analogue that permeates the membrane of human erythrocytes and lymphocytes by nonfacilitated diffusion. J Biol Chem 1987; 262:5748–5754.

291. Domin BA, Mahony WB, Zimmerman TP. 2′,3′-Dideoxythymidine permeation of the human erythrocyte membrane by nonfacilitated diffusion. Biochem Biophys Res Commun 1988; 825–831.

292. Plagemann PGW, Woffendin C. Permeation and salvage of dideoxyadenosine in mammalian cells. Mol Pharmacol 1989; 36:185–192.

293. August EM, Birks EM, Prusoff WH. 3′-Deoxythymidin-2′-ene permeation of human lymphocyte H9 cells by nonfacilitated diffusion. Mol Pharmacol 1991; 39:246–249.

294. Magnani M, Bianchi M, Rossi L, et al. 2′,3′-Dideoxycytidine permeation of the human erythrocyte membrane. Biochem Int 1989; 19:227–234.

295. Chan TCK, Shaffer L, Redmond R, et al. Permeation and metabolism of anti-HIV and endogenous nucleosides in human immune effector cells. Biochem Pharmacol 1993; 46:273–278.

296. Plagemann PGW, Woffendin C, Puziss MB, et al. Purine and pyrimidine transport and permeation in human erythrocytes. Biochim Biophys Acta 1987; 905:17–29.

297. Gati WP, Dagnino L, Paterson ARP. Enantiomeric selectivity of adenosine transport systems in mouse erythrocytes and L1210 cells. Biochem J 1989; 263:957–960.

298. Belt JA, Welch AD. Transport of uridine and 6-azauridine in human lymphoblastoid cells (specificity for the uncharged 6-azauridine molecule). Mol Pharmacol 1982; 23:153–158.

299. Dahlig-Harley E, Paterson ARP, Robins MJ, et al. Transport of uridine and 3-deazauridine in cultured lymphoblastoid cells. Cancer Res 1984; 44:161–165.

300. Viswanadhan VN, Ghose AK, Weinstein JN. Mapping the binding site of the nucleoside transporter protein: a 3D-QSAR study. Biochim Biophys Acta 1990; 1039:356–366.

301. Chen SF, Cleveland JS, Hollman AB, et al. Changes in nucleoside transport of HL-60 human promyelocytic cells during N,N-dimethylformamide induced differentiation. Cancer Res 1986; 46:3449–3455.

302. Sokoloski JA, Lee CW, Handschumacher RE, et al. Effects of uridine on the growth and differentiation of HL-60 leukemia cells. Leuk Res 1991; 15:1051–1058.

303. Sokoloski JA, Sartorelli AC, Handschumacher RE, et al. Inhibition by pertussis toxin of the activation of Na^+-dependent uridine transport in dimethyl-sulphoxide-induced HL-60 leukaemia cells. Biochem J 1991; 280:515–519.

304. Goh L-B, Sokoloski JA, Sartorelli AC, et al. Enhancement of pertussis-toxin-sensitive Na^+-dependent uridine transporter activity in HL-60 granulocytes by N-formylmethionyl-leucyl-phenylalanine. Biochem J 1993; 294:693–697.

305. Meckling-Gill KA, Guilbert L, Cass CE. CSF-1 stimulates nucleoside transport in S1 macrophages. J Cell Physiol 1993; 155:530–538.
306. Meckling-Gill KA, Cass CE. Effects of v-*fps* transformation on nucleoside transport in rat-2 fibroblasts. Biochem J 1992; 282:147–154.
307. Tsiftsoglou AS, Gerogatsos JG. Metabolism of nucleosides by isolated liver mitochondria. Biochim Biophys Acta 1972; 262:239–246.
308. Lee LS, Cheng YC. Human deoxythymidine kinase. I. Purification and general properties of the cytoplasmic and mitochondrial isozymes derived from blast cells of acute myelocytic leukemia. J Biol Chem 1976; 251:2600–2604.
309. Lee LS, Cheng YC. Human deoxythymidine kinase II: substrate specificity and kinetic behaviour of the cytoplasmic and mitochondrial isozymes derived from blast cells of acute myelocytic leukemia. Biochemistry 1976; 15:3686–3690.
310. Cheng YC, Domin B, Lee LS. Human deoxycytidine kinase. Purification and characterization of the cytoplasmic and mitochondrial isozymes derived from blast cells of acute myelocytic leukemia patients. Biochim Biophys Acta 1977; 481:481–492.
311. Lewis RA, Link L. Phosphorylation of arabinosylguanine by a mitochondrial enzyme of bovine liver. Biochem Pharmacol 1989; 38:2001–2006.
312. Lewis RA, Link L, Chen W. Degradation of purine nucleosides by mitochondrial enzymes of bovine liver. Adv Exp Med Biol 1989; 253A:353–357.
313. Ziegler M, Dubiel W, Pimenov AM, et al. The catabolism of endogenous adenine nucleotides in rat liver mitochondria. Mol Cell Biochem 1990; 93:7–12.
314. Lewis RA, Haag RK. Purine nucleoside phosphorylase of bovine liver mitochondria. Adv Exp Med Biol 1991; 309B:181–184.
315. Lindley ER, Pisoni RL. Demonstration of adenosine deaminase activity in human fibroblast lysosomes. Biochem J 1993; 290:457–462.
316. Pisoni RL, Thoene JG. Detection and characterization of a nucleoside transport system in human fibroblast lysosomes. J Biol Chem 1989; 264:4850–4856.
317. Pisoni RL, Thoene JG. The transport systems of mammalian lysosomes. Biochim Biophys Acta 1991; 1071:351–373.
318. Mitra RS, Berstein IA. Thymidine incorporation into deoxyribonucleic acid by isolated rat mitochondria. J Biol Chem 1970; 245:1255–1260.
319. Watkins LF, Lewis RA. The metabolism of deoxyguanosine in mitochondria. Characterization of the uptake process. Mol Cell Biochem 1987; 77:71–77.
320. Hogue D, Ellison M, Cass CE. A method for identification of a thymidine transport protein by functional expression in yeast. J Gen Physiol 1992; 100:42a.
321. Hirschberg CB, Snider MD. Topography of glycosylation in the rough endoplasmic reticulum and Golgi apparatus. Annu Rev Biochem 1987; 56:63–87.
322. Capasso JM, Keenan TW, Abeijon C, et al. Mechanism of phosphorylation in the lumen of the Golgi apparatus. J Biol Chem 1989; 264:5233–5240.

323. Arnaudo E, Dalakas M, Shanske S, et al. Depletion of muscle mitochondrial DNA in AIDS patients with zidovudine-induced myopathy. Lancet 1991; 337:508–510.

324. Chalmers AC, Greco CM, Miller RG. Prognosis in AZT myopathy. Neurology 1991; 41:1181–1184.

325. Mhiri C, Baudrimont M, Bonne G, et al. Zidovudine myopathy: a distinctive disorder associated with mitochondrial dysfunction. Ann Neurol 1991; 29:606–614.

326. Peters BS, Winer J, Landon DN, et al. Mitochondrial myopathy associated with chronic zidovudine therapy in AIDS. Q J Med 1993; 86:5–15.

327. Dubinsky RM, Yarchoan R, Dalakas M, et al. Reversible axonal neuropathy from the treatment of AIDS and related disorders with 2′,3′-dideoxycytidine (ddC). Muscle Nerve 1989; 12:856–860.

328. Parker WB, Cheng YC. Mitochondrial toxicity of antiviral nucleoside analogs. J NIH Res 1994; 6:57–61.

329. Chen CH, Cheng YC. Delayed cytotoxicity and selective loss of mitochondrial DNA in cells treated with the anti-human immunodeficiency virus compound 2′,3′-dideoxycytidine. J Biol Chem 1989; 264:11934–11937.

330. Chen CH, Vazquez Padua M, Cheng YC. Effect of anti-human immunodeficiency virus nucleoside analogs on mitochondrial DNA and its implication for delayed toxicity. Mol Pharmacol 1991; 39:625–628.

331. Chen CH, Cheng YC. The role of cytoplasmic deoxycytidine kinase in the mitochondrial effects of the antihuman immunodeficiency virus compound, 2′,3′-dideoxycytidine. J Biol Chem 1992; 267:2856–2859.

332. Herzberg NH, Zorn I, Zwart R, et al. Major growth reduction and minor decrease in mitochondrial enzyme activity in cultured human muscle cells after exposure to zidovudine. Muscle Nerve 1992; 15:706–710.

333. Wang H, Fliegel L, Cass CE, et al. Nucleoside analogues increase the proportion of mutant mitochondrial DNA in heteroplasmic Kearns-Sayre syndrome fibroblasts. Biochem Cell Biol 1993; 71:Axxxi.

334. Simpson MV, Chin CD, Keilbaugh SA, et al. Studies on the inhibition of mitochondrial DNA replication by 3′-azido-3′-deoxythymidine and other dideoxynucleoside analogs which inhibit HIV-1 replication. Biochem Pharmacol 1989; 38:1033–1036.

335. Berk AJ, Clayton DA. A genetically distinct thymidine kinase in mammalian mitochondria. Exclusive labeling of mitochondrial deoxyribonucleic acid. J Biol Chem 1973; 248:2722–2729.

336. Klingenberg M. Molecular aspects of the adenine nucleotide carrier from mitochondria. Arch Biochem Biophys 1989; 270:1–14.

337. Klingenberg M. Structure–function of the ADP/ATP carrier. Biochem Soc Trans 1992; 20:547–50.

338. Vickers M, Hogue D, Ellison M, et al. Evidence of a functional role for the mitochondrial ND4 protein. Biochem Cell Biol 1993; 71:Axxi.

339. Walker JE. The NADH:ubiquinone oxidoreductase (complex I) of respiratory chains. Q Rev Biophys 1992; 25:253–324.

16

Mechanisms of Receptor-Mediated Folate and Antifolate Membrane Transport in Cancer Chemotherapy

Larry H. Matherly
Michigan Cancer Foundation, Detroit, Michigan

I. INTRODUCTION

Membrane transport is essential to the maintenance of metabolic homeostasis. In certain circumstances, complex mechanisms have evolved to optimize delivery of essential metabolites to intracellular compartments to meet demands for cell replication. Transport is commonly mediated by specific receptors that exhibit specificity for substrate binding and plasma membrane translocation. Transport, within this context, can involve facilitated diffusion, an equilibrating process that requires no expenditure of energy, or active uptake, an energy-requiring process by which a transport substrate accumulates against a chemical gradient or electrochemical potential gradient (see Chap. 4). Regardless of the transport mechanism involved, the intracellular substrate concentration ultimately achieved in vivo is the net result of rates of plasma clearance, and the relative activities of opposing membrane transport fluxes (e.g., drug uptake and efflux).

For chemotherapeutic drugs used to treat cancer, membrane transport is an important event in their antitumor activity, since most agents achieve their effects at intracellular loci. Indeed, for many agents, antitumor activities are limited by the failure of sufficient concentrations of drugs to reach critical intracellular targets. For no class of chemotherapeutic drugs more than the antifolates has carrier-mediated membrane transport been as thoroughly studied. Laboratory investigations have now progressed beyond the basic descriptions of radioactive folate and antifolate surface receptor binding, or simple measurements of radioactive drug influx and efflux, to sophisticated biochemical and molecular analyses of the membrane transport systems that mediate these processes. For many years, influx of classical antifolates, such as methotrexate, was considered to involve a single, active transport process; however, more recent literature suggests potentially important roles for alternative systems in folate and antifolate uptake. It may be possible to exploit the unique specificities of these separate uptake processes in different tissues or tumors in the design of antifolate inhibitors as therapeutic agents. Likewise, as the detailed characteristics of the membrane pumps that mediate antifolate efflux are clarified, it may be possible to modulate drug retention in tumor cells through the use of specific efflux "blockers."

Several excellent reviews on the biology of folate and antifolate membrane transport have appeared (1–4). In this chapter, I will expand on these by focusing on the molecular properties of the major receptor-mediated transport systems most relevant to antifolate therapeutics and cancer chemotherapy. I hope to integrate the currently accepted models for folate and antifolate membrane transport with the pharmacology of these compounds, the regulation of these processes, and the possibilities for drug design based on the unique specificities of different transport systems. Finally, I will address the relevance of variations in membrane transport among tumors or tissues to clinical response during therapy with antifolates and the development of chemotherapeutic drug resistance. I hope that my perspective on this exciting and important research area will foster creative insight into future research possibilities, and further prompt the rational development of new folate analogues as therapeutic agents, or alternative treatment strategies with antifolates based on their capacities for membrane transport.

II. BIOCHEMICAL RATIONALE BEHIND FOLATE ANTAGONISTS AS THERAPEUTIC AGENTS

A. Overview of Folate Metabolism

The cofactors related to folic acid are essential to cell survival, because these derivatives participate in a variety of carbon transfer reactions leading to the biosynthesis of purine nucleotides, thymidylate, serine, and methionine (Fig. 1). The parent vitamin, folic acid, is of little physiological importance, because it is the fully reduced (i.e., tetrahydrofolate) cofactor forms that are absorbed in the intestine, circulate in plasma, and facilitate

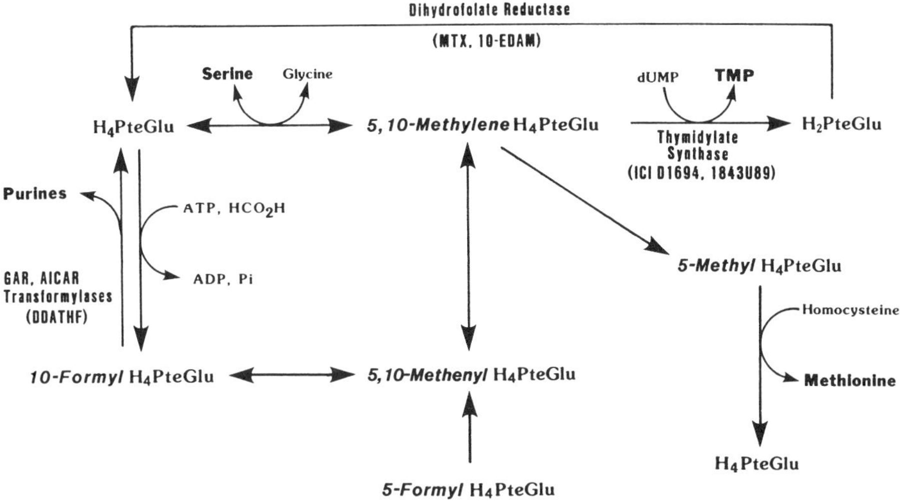

Figure 1 Interconversion and biosynthetic utilization of the natural folates. The enzyme targets for assorted antifolate inhibitors (in parentheses) are indicated. Abbreviations: AICAR, aminoimidazolecarboxamide ribonucleotide; DDATHF, 5,10-dideaza-5,6,7,8-tetrahydrofolate; 10-EDAM, 10-ethyl-10-deazaaminopterin; GAR, glycinamide ribonucleotide; H_2PteGlu, dihydrofolate; H_4PteGlu, tetrahydrofolate; MTX, methotrexate. (From Ref. 11.)

anabolic one-carbon transfer. Folates are predominantly found within cells as polyglutamates, characterized by the presence of additional (generally two to eight) γ-linked glutamyl residues (5,6). The glutamate condensation reaction, catalyzed by folylpolyglutamate synthetase (EC 6.3.2.17), confers enhanced cellular retention of folate derivatives (7,8) and increased rates of carbon transfer over monoglutamyl folates (5,6).

Carbon transfer from tetrahydrofolate polyglutamates to nucleotide or amino acid precursors involves one-carbon units attached at the 5- or 10-position of the cofactor, at the oxidation levels of formaldehyde, formate, or methanol. As a result of carbon transfer during de novo serine, methionine, and purine nucleotide syntheses, unsubstituted tetrahydrofolate is generated (see Fig. 1). The latter reassociates with endogenous one-carbon units from serine and formate to form metabolically interconvertible 5,10-methylenetetrahydrofolate and 10-formyltetrahydrofolate, respectively (see Fig. 1). By contrast, during the synthesis of thymidylate, carbon transfer from 5,10-methylenetetrahydrofolate is accompanied by an *oxidation* of the reduced folate to dihydrofolate, a relatively inert cofactor form, with limited metabolic options. Dihydrofolate is reduced back to tetrahydrofolate in an NADPH-dependent reaction catalyzed by dihydrofolate reductase.

B. Dihydrofolate Reductase as an Intracellular Target for Antifolates

Dihydrofolate reductase is critical to cell replication, since if this enzyme is inhibited or absent altogether, the continued generation of dihydrofolate during thymidylate biosynthesis eventually depletes cellular 5,10-methylenetetrahydrofolate pools (see Fig. 1); likewise, other tetrahydrofolate forms, following their conversion to 5,10-methylenetetrahydrofolate, are depleted. Although somewhat oversimplified (e.g., see Refs. 9–11), the "depletion" of this net tetrahydrofolate pool (including both unsubstituted and carbon-substituted forms), which accompanies decreased rates of dihydrofolate reductase catalysis, effects a slowing of folate-dependent biosynthetic pathways for DNA, RNA, and protein precursors.

As with most of the clinically important anticancer agents, when the first synthetic antifolate, aminopterin, was introduced into the clinic over 45 years ago (12), little was understood of how this agent achieved its antitumor effects. Despite its greater antitumor activity, aminopterin was subsequently replaced by methotrexate because the considerable host toxicity accompanying its use compromised its therapeutic efficacy (13). Although the primary target for both aminopterin and methotrexate was identified as dihydrofolate reductase, as early as 1958 (14), many of the details relating to its mechanism of action, in particular, the basis for its therapeutic selectivity, have emerged only in recent years. Today, methotrexate is the only antifolate to receive widespread clinical use for cancer, and it is an essential component of multidrug regimens for treating acute lymphocytic leukemia, choriocarcinoma, non-Hodgkin's lymphoma, osteosarcoma, breast cancer, and head and neck cancer (15).

Methotrexate binding to dihydrofolate reductase is kinetically complex and involves an initial rapid formation of a methotrexate–NADPH–dihydrofolate reductase ternary complex that undergoes a slow isomerization (16,17). The net result of this two-step process is a K_i for ternary complex formation on the order of 10^{-10} M (18). In spite of the low dissociability of this ternary complex, *within cells* the metabolic effects of methotrexate treatment are readily reversible as extracellular drug concentrations fall (19–22). This surprising observation strongly suggested that the relationship between methotrexate binding to dihydrofolate reductase and the suppression of tetrahydrofolate-dependent biosynthetic processes within cells was much more complicated than predicted from experiments in cell-free systems.

It is now established that to maintain the complete suppression of dihydrofolate reductase in cells, substantial levels of methotrexate *in excess* of that bound to dihydrofolate reductase are necessary (19–23). In the absence of this free, or unbound intracellular drug fraction, the metabolic effects of enzyme-bound methotrexate on tetrahydrofolate cofactor pools and folate-dependent reactions are readily reversed as the intracellular drug declines accompanying the disappearance of extracellular methotrexate.

This reversibility of the metabolic effects of dihydrofolate reductase inhibition within cells is based on the requirement for only a small fraction of the total enzyme to provide adequate levels of tetrahydrofolate cofactors for macromolecular biosynthesis and cell replication (20,21,23–25). Moreover, at low methotrexate concentrations, intracellular dihydrofolate polyglutamates, which accumulate from 5,10-methylenetetrahydrofolate polyglutamates during the biosynthesis of thymidylate when dihydrofolate reductase is inhibited (see Fig. 1), directly compete with methotrexate for binding to dihydrofolate reductase. This competition occurs because extremely high intracellular levels of dihydrofolate polyglutamates under these conditions compensate for the large disparity in the binding affinities for this substrate and the antifolate inhibitor. Competition continues until sufficient enzyme-bound methotrexate is displaced and catalytic activity reactivated to restore tetrahydrofolate pools from the accumulated dihydrofolate (20–24). Whereas in cultured cells, as little as 5% of the dihydrofolate reductase activity is estimated to be sufficient to sustain tetrahydrofolate-dependent biosynthetic processes (20,21,23–25), a somewhat larger fraction may be necessary in human tumors in vivo because of their lower dihydrofolate reductase contents (26).

In any event, the critical role of membrane transport is to generate sufficient unbound (i.e., in excess of intracellular dihydrofolate reductase) intracellular methotrexate to sustain maximal enzyme inhibition, even in the presence of elevated dihydrofolate polyglutamates. However, with the recognition that methotrexate and related antifolates, such as the natural folates, were substrates for polyglutamylation, another role of membrane transport was identified: namely, to generate sufficient intracellular antifolate substrate for the synthesis of these conjugated drug forms.

C. The Role of Polyglutamylation in Methotrexate Pharmacology

There are important pharmacological ramifications of the metabolism of methotrexate to its polyglutamyl forms. (1) Methotrexate polyglutamates are at least equivalent to monoglutamyl methotrexate as inhibitors of dihydrofolate reductase within cells. Increased affinities of methotrexate polyglutamates for dihydrofolate reductase have occasionally been reported (27,28); however, small differences between binding constants, on the order of 10^{-10} M, are unlikely to significantly alter drug sensitivities (23). (2) Similar to the natural folylpolyglutamates, methotrexate polyglutamates are retained within cells over monoglutamyl methotrexate, to an extent that directly correlates with polyglutamate chain length (29–35). The net effect of this increased retention is a sustained inhibition of dihydrofolate reductase and folate-dependent biosynthetic reactions long after extracellular methotrexate has declined to low levels (36). In this fashion, polyglutamylation effectively converts methotrexate from a rapidly reversible inhibitor of dihydrofolate reductase to a much more slowly reversible inhibitor. (3) The accumulation of methotrexate polyglutamates within cells appears to be a selective determinant of cytotoxicity, since high levels of these metabolites are generally synthesized in tumors that are drug-sensitive (36,37). Conversely, low levels of methotrexate polyglutamates have been reported for methotrexate-insensitive tumors (37) and for drug-limiting host tissues (bone marrow, gastrointestinal epithelium; 36,38–40). For cells or tissues that accumulate sufficient methotrexate polyglutamates, dihydrofolate reductase is inhibited, regardless of the changes in the extracellular drug concentration. (4) Polyglutamyl forms of methotrexate are far better inhibitors of key "distal" enzyme targets, including thymidylate synthase (41), aminoimidazolecarboxamide ribonucleotide (AICAR) transformylase (42), and glycinamide ribonucleotide (GAR) transformylase (43). The importance of these inhibitions to the antitumor effects of methotrexate, in general, is uncertain, since it is not obvious how they could further augment drug activity when dihydrofolate reductase is already inhibited and the tetrahydrofolate pool depleted. Still, they could limit the biosynthetic utilization of tetrahydrofolate cofactors during leucovorin "rescue" (44,45). The biochemistry and pharmacology of methotrexate polyglutamylation, including its relation to leucovorin rescue, has been previously reviewed (45).

D. The Development of a New Generation of Classic Antifolates

The recognition of membrane transport and polyglutamylation as key determinants in methotrexate antitumor activity led to the rational synthesis of numerous folate analogues. The idea was to identify agents with greater activity toward malignant disease, including solid tumors, reduced host toxicities, or increased activity against methotrexate-resistant tumors, based on improved uptake or capacities to be polyglutamylated. Interestingly, aminopterin, another early dihydrofolate reductase inhibitor (Fig. 2), is transported more efficiently than methotrexate (46) and is one of the better antifolate substrates for folylpolyglutamate synthetase (47–49). The net effect is a significantly increased accumulation of polyglutamyl forms of aminopterin over methotrexate in drug-sensitive tumors (50,51). However, its use in vivo is generally accompanied by unacceptable levels of host toxicity (13), demonstrating that these characteristics alone do not make a better drug. With the aim of circumventing methotrexate resistance, the focus of drug design has been on enzyme targets other than dihydrofolate reductase, including thymidylate synthase and GAR transformylase, or alternative modes of cellular uptake. Several of these "new-generation" antifolates are described in the following sections. Their chemical structures are depicted in Figure 2. Nonclassic, lipid-soluble antifolate inhibitors are discussed in Section VII.D.

1. 10-Ethyl-10-Deazaaminopterin (Edatrexate; 10-Edam)

10-Edam is a dihydrofolate reductase inhibitor that was developed on the basis of its high substrate activity for membrane transport and folylpolyglutamate synthetase catalysis in murine tumors (52). 10-Edam was considerably more active than methotrexate against several murine ascites and solid tumors in vivo (52,53); moreover, 10-Edam was highly active against a series of human tumor xenographs, including mammary, small-cell lung, and colon carcinomas (52,54). 10-Edam is equivalent to methotrexate as an inhibitor of mammalian dihydrofolate reductase, but is a better substrate for membrane transport and polyglutamylation (49,51,52,55). Interestingly, both membrane transport and polyglutamylation of 10-Edam are markedly increased in murine tumor cells relative to proliferative normal cells (49,52,55), suggesting a pharmacological basis for its considerable in vivo antitumor selectivity. 10-Edam has completed Phase I clinical trials (56); likewise, the results of several Phase II trials have also been reported (57,58).

2. CB3717, ICI 198583, and ICI D1694

Partly as a means of circumventing methotrexate resistance resulting from increased or structurally altered dihydrofolate reductase, a series of quinazoline analogues of folic acid were synthesized as inhibitors of thymidylate synthase. The prototype, CB3717 (N^{10}-propargyl-5,8-dideazafolate) (Fig. 2), is a potent competitive inhibitor of thymidylate synthase ($K_i = 4.9$ nM for the human enzyme) (59). Inhibition could be increased approximately 100-fold accompanying its polyglutamylation (60,61), and following this metabolism in L1210 cells, the pharmacological effects of CB3717 in vitro were sustained at least 24 h (61). Whereas CB3717 was active against

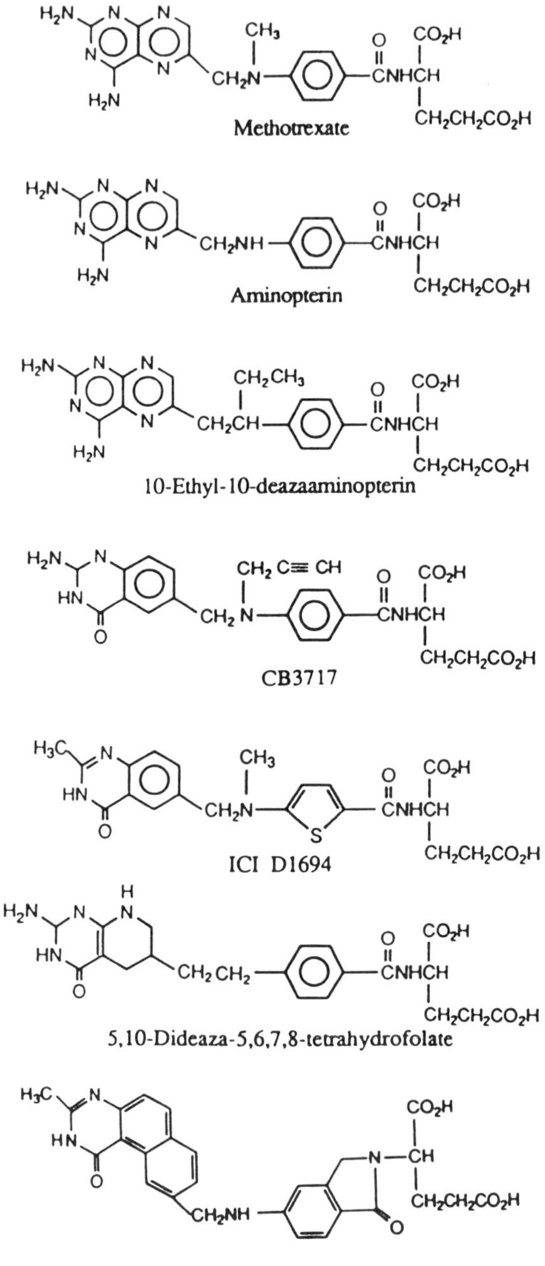

Figure 2 Structures of ''classical'' antifolates.

both methotrexate-sensitive and methotrexate-resistant tumor cells in vitro (59,61,62), it generally required high concentrations because of its poor membrane transport. Likewise, CB3717 exhibited antitumor activity in humans, including breast, ovary, and liver tumors (63–66); however, its poor solubility properties resulted in dose-limiting hepatic and renal toxicities (66).

A systematic search was undertaken for more water-soluble quinazoline inhibitors of thymidylate synthase with improved transport characteristics and high levels of substrate activity for folylpolyglutamate synthetase. One derivative, ICI 198583, the 2-desamino-2-methyl analogue of CB3717, was 40-fold more cytotoxic than the parent drug (67). This was followed by ICI D1694 [N-(5-[N-(3,4-dihydro-2-methyl-4-oxoquinazolin-6-ylmethyl)-N-methylamino]-2-thenoyl)-L-glutamic acid; see Fig. 2], a prototype for a series of 2-desamino-2-methyl-N^{10}-quinazolines in which the p-aminobenzoate was replaced by a thiophene or thiazole ring (68). ICI D1694 is approximately 500-fold more active against cultured cells than CB3717, despite its 20-fold decreased inhibitory potency toward thymidylate synthase (68). This results from its high levels of membrane transport (68), its excellent substrate activity for folylpolyglutamate synthetase (approx. 200-fold greater than CB3717; 69), and the significantly increased inhibitory potencies of its polyglutamyl forms for thymidylate synthase (K_i = 1 nM for tetraglutamyl ICI D1694; 70). A high therapeutic index was demonstrated for ICI D1694 in various xenograph models, including lung, colon, gastric, and ovarian carcinomas, and, unlike CB1717, no significant renal or hepatic toxicities were apparent (71–73). ICI D1694 has completed Phase I testing (74) and is currently in Phase II clinical trials.

3. *1843U89*

A 3-methyl-substituted benzoquinazoline folate analogue, 1843U89 [(S)-2-(5(((1,2-dihydro-3-methyl-1-oxobenzo(F)quinolin-9-yl)methyl)amino) 1-oxo-2-isoindolinyl) glutaric acid; see Fig. 2], was developed during the course of a systematic search for lipid-soluble inhibitors of thymidylate synthase (75). Its considerable pharmacological activity against cultured human tumor cells appears to result from its excellent membrane transport activity and highly potent noncompetitive inhibition of thymidylate synthase (K_i = 90 pM; 75). It is interesting that the inhibitory effects of 1843U89 toward thymidylate synthase were not appreciably increased for its major polyglutamyl product, 1843U89-diglutamate, over monoglutamyl 1843U89 (76); however, polyglutamylation was still important to drug activity, as methotrexate-resistant cell lines with impaired capacities for polyglutamylation were, likewise, resistant to 1843U89 (77). 1843U89 is intriguing because of its high specificity toward human over that toward murine tumor cells in culture, a difference attributable to variations in membrane transport (75; see Sec. VII.C.1). The destruction of WiDr human colon carcinoma spheroids with 1843U89 in the presence of physiological concentrations of thymidine (0.1 μM) suggests its potential solid tumor activity, as well (78). Early in vivo studies with the human thymidine kinase-deficient colon carcinoma line, GC_3TK^-, grown subcutaneously or under the renal capsule, indicated a marked antitumor response with 1843U89 (75).

4. 5,10-Dideaza-5,6,7,8-tetrahydrofolate

5,10-Dideaza-5,6,7,8-tetrahydrofolate (DDATHF) is an analogue of tetrahydrofolic acid, with carbon instead of nitrogen at positions 5 and 10 (79–82), modifications that render it incapable of participating in one-carbon transfer and interconversion or isomerization reactions typical of these cofactors. DDATHF binds poorly to dihydrofolate reductase and thymidylate synthase, but derives its antitumor effects by inhibiting GAR transformylase (EC 2.1.2.1.)(Fig. 1), the first folate-dependent step in de novo purine biosynthesis (81–83). The net effect is a depletion of intracellular pools of adenosine triphosphate (ATP) and guanosine triphosphate (GTP) (84). DDATHF can exist in two stereospecific configurations centered at the asymmetric 6-carbon (the 6R diastereomer is known as lometrexol). Both stereoisomers are among the best-known substrates for mammalian folylpolyglutamate synthetases (82,85) and are excellent substrates for the system that mediates methotrexate and tetrahydrofolate cofactor influx (86,87), as well as high-affinity folate-binding membrane receptors (86,88,89) (Sec. VII.C). The growth inhibitory effects of DDATHF toward CCRF-CEM and L1210 cells in culture likely results from the accumulation of DDATHF polyglutamates, which are highly retained within cells (87,90) and are up to 100-fold more inhibitory than the underivatized antifolate toward GAR transformylase (83). Although DDATHF circumvents dihydrofolate reductase-based resistance, it likewise is active toward transport-impaired tumors in vitro (see Sec. VII.C.4)(Refs. 87,88,91). On the basis of preclinical data that show its activity against murine solid tumors and human tumor xenographs (92), several clinical studies have been initiated. The results of a number of Phase I studies of DDATHF toxicity and therapeutic activity have been described (93–95). In one recent report, DDATHF showed an unusual pattern of toxicity, with thrombocytopenia as the major dose-limiting toxicity (93).

III. CHARACTERISTICS OF THE CLASSICAL REDUCED FOLATE MEMBRANE CARRIER

A. Transport Properties

An active, carrier-mediated transport process for natural folates and certain analogues, termed the "classical" carrier or reduced folate carrier (RFC), has been described in an extraordinary array of murine and human tumor cells, including leukemias, sarcomas, hepatomas, and carcinomas of the ovary, lung, and breast (reviewed in Ref. 96). The functional characteristics of this system are nearly invariant from tissue to tissue or species to species, with a few exceptions noted later. The RFC-mediated uptake is saturable at low (i.e., 1–5) micromolar concentrations for most substrates (1,3,96); however, its overall capacity is quite low (estimated as three cycles per minute per carrier site for L1210 cells), compared with other nutrient (nucleoside, amino acid) transporters (96). Furthermore, transport is pH- and temperature-dependent, sodium-independent, and sensitive to inhibition by sulfhydryl-reactive agents and folate analogues (1,3,96–98).

Although the physiological substrate for RFC-transport is believed to be (6R)5-methyltetrahydrofolate, it is of interest that (6S)5-methyltetrahydrofolate is also an excellent transport substrate (99,100). However, transport of 5-formyltetrahydrofolate is highly stereospecific for the (6S) isomer (101), implying that (6R)5-formyltetrahydrofolate in preparations of calcium leucovorin [(6R,S)5-formyltetrahydrofolate)] is pharmacologically inert. Several antifolates are also excellent substrates for the transporter, including aminopterin (46,52), 10-Edam (46,52), methotrexate (46,96,97), ICI D1694 (68,102), ICI 198583 (67,102,103), 1843U89 (75), and both (6R) and (6S) stereoisomers of DDATHF (86,87).

Methotrexate has been extensively used to investigate the kinetics of RFC transport because of the commercial availability of its radioactive form and its chemical stability. Furthermore, the metabolism of methotrexate is restricted to its limited polyglutamylation and is minimal under transport-permissive conditions over the short time intervals during which initial influx rates are generally measured. An additional advantage of methotrexate over the natural folates for studying membrane transport is that methotrexate binds virtually instantaneously to dihydrofolate reductase after entering cells, so that accurate measurements of *unidirectional* influx are possible at short exposure times (3,97,98). Only when dihydrofolate reductase is completely bound with methotrexate (generally after several minutes at micromolar concentrations of extracellular methotrexate), does antifolate efflux commence (3,97,98). As the intracellular methotrexate approaches its steady-state level, rates of drug influx and efflux approach equality.

Since methotrexate is a divalent anion at physiological pH and is also substrate for a separate, high-capacity efflux pump (see Sec. V), at all but the lowest drug concentrations, the intracellular concentration of unbound, osmotically active antifolate at steady state is less than the extracellular level (3,97,98). In fact, uphill transport into negatively charged cells is often not apparent unless comparisons are made between the concentration ratios of osmotically active intracellular to extracellular methotrexate actually achieved and those predicted for an equilibrating system by the Nernst equation from considerations of membrane potentials (3,97,98).

Transport by the RFC appears to involve a physical translocation of the carrier protein within the membrane because, under certain conditions, efflux of intracellular transport substrates is directly coupled to methotrexate influx. Hence, methotrexate influx is accelerated, or "trans-stimulated," in cells preloaded with reduced folates that are also transport substrates (98,104). The enhanced rate of methotrexate influx in L1210 cells trans-stimulated by preloading with 5-formyltetrahydrofolate is associated with an increased influx V_{max}, with no significant change in the influx K_t (104). This effect presumably reflects the binding of folate cofactors at the inner membrane surface, followed by a more rapid reorientation of loaded versus unloaded carrier toward the external membrane surface (104). However, trans-stimulation of radiolabeled methotrexate influx into cells preloaded with unlabeled methotrexate was not observed under identical experimental conditions, nor was methotrexate efflux stimulated by high levels of extracellular reduced folates (98,104).

B. The Role of Anions in RFC Transport

An assortment of inorganic anions, likewise, enhance the influx of methotrexate into plasma membrane vesicles (105) and intact L1210 cells (98,106–109). Hence, replacing extracellular physiological anions with nonanionic HEPES–sucrose buffers results in a highly concentrative uptake of methotrexate (110). This, in part, reflects the decreased competition for substrate binding to RFC in anion-free buffers, since methotrexate influx is competitively inhibited by assorted inorganic anions (chloride, bicarbonate, and phosphate) in physiological buffers (98,105,106,110) and the K_t values for methotrexate influx are reduced nearly tenfold in the absence of anions (110). Although no influx V_{max} effects were reported in these experiments with L1210 cells (110), in other studies with membrane vesicles transloaded with sulfate or phosphate anions, the influx V_{max} for methotrexate was increased twofold (105).

The rate of methotrexate efflux from L1210 cells is inhibited in anion-free buffers without glucose and, in contrast with experiments performed with physiological anion-containing buffers, can be stimulated by both inorganic and organic anions (i.e., folic acid, 5-formyltetrahydrofolate, AMP, ADP, thiamine pyrophosphate, phosphate, sulfate, and chloride; 106,107,111). Efflux under these conditions involves the RFC, and the anion concentrations required for half-maximal stimulation of efflux are similar to their K_i values for inhibition of influx.

Taken together, these results suggest that the presence of large electrochemical anion gradients accelerate the movement of the RFC protein across the membrane. In this fashion, the extrusion of intracellular anions, in particular phosphate or adenine nucleotides (98,106,107,111), into the extracellular medium and down a concentration gradient could conceivably serve as the driving force for methotrexate uptake by the RFC and provide the energy source for concentrating methotrexate within cells (98,106–109). However, the demonstration that the presence of sodium chloride markedly decreases the trans-stimulation of methotrexate influx by phosphate and sulfate in plasma membrane vesicles (105) raises doubts about the physiological importance of this mechanism.

C. Biochemical Properties of the RFC

1. Receptor Binding and Affinity Inhibitors as Specific Probes for the RFC

Compared with the extensive literature documenting dihydrofolate reductase as a target for methotrexate and related analogues, characterization of the RFC has focused primarily on its transport kinetics, whereas the biochemical characterization of the carrier protein itself has been limited. This is because the RFC transport system is generally present in low levels in most cultured mammalian cells and, for many years, there were no effective radioactive or fluorescent probes for specifically tagging the membrane carrier.

To circumvent the problems resulting from low carrier expression, Sirotnak et al. devised a novel strategy to select L1210 cell lines that up-regulate the expression of the reduced folate transporter (112,113). Selection was based on the concept of carrier-mediated folate uptake as rate-limiting to cofactor utilization in rapidly growing cells, and involved growing cultures in folic acid-free medium containing growth-restricting concentrations of $(6R,S)$5-formyltetrahydrofolate, conditions under which only variants with increased transport capacities for reduced folates were capable of sustained growth. L1210 lines with 3- to 40-fold increased RFC levels were obtained by this approach (112,113). Identical methods were extended to the selection of transport–up-regulated human tumor cells, including CCRF-CEM (114), K562 (115), and HL60 (116) lines. Interestingly, this approach was also used to isolate L1210 cell variants that express increased levels of the high-affinity membrane folate-binding receptor (117–119; also Sec. V.A).

Binding of 5-methyl[^{3}H]tetrahydrofolate, [^{3}H]methotrexate, or [^{3}H]aminopterin to surface RFCs at 0°C in intact cells provides an overall estimate of carrier levels (86,112,119,121–123). Reduced folate carrier values of 2.2 and 5.8 pmols/10^7 cells have been reported for L1210 and K562 cells, respectively (122,123). However, this complex is freely dissociable and, therefore, unsuitable for monitoring the transport protein following its detergent release from plasma membranes. Several agents were identified that showed potential for generating stable, *covalent* complexes with the RFC protein, including 8-azidoadenosine-5′-monophosphate (124), 4,4′-diisothiocyanostilbene-2,2′-disulfonate (125), carbodiimide-activated antifolates (126), 3,3′-dithiobissulfosuccinimidyl propionate (127), N-hydroxysuccinimide (NHS) methotrexate ester (128,129), and N^α-(4-amino-4-deoxy-10-methylpteroyl)-N^ϵ-(4-azido-5-salicylyl)-L-lysine (APA-ASA-Lys) (130–132). All of these agents irreversibly inhibited [^{3}H]methotrexate influx into cultured cells; however, only NHS-methotrexate and APA-ASA-Lys exhibited the sensitivity and specificity to be adapted for radioaffinity labeling the RFC protein.

N-Hydroxysuccinimide-[^{3}H]methotrexate and NHS-[^{3}H]aminopterin have been extensively used for radiolabeling the carrier (113,115, 120,122,128), since they are easily synthesized and exhibit a high specificity for the transporter in both cultured murine and human cells. Hence, inhibition of methotrexate influx parallels the covalent incorporation of an ^{3}H-labeled antifolate into L1210 plasma membranes (128). In L1210 cells, incorporation involves a 42- to 48-kDa plasma membrane polypeptide, detectable on sodium dodecyl sulfate (SDS) gels (116,120,122) or by gel filtration in the presence of 0.1% SDS (113); the level of radioaffinity inhibitor incorporation is suppressed by unlabeled transport substrates to a degree that closely approximates their affinities for the carrier protein (113,128). In human tumor cells, the radioaffinity-labeled carrier migrates on SDS gels as a higher relative molecular mass (M_r; i.e., 79- to 99-kDa) species (115,116,123; see Sec. III.C.2). Recently, fluorescein (133) and biotin (134) derivatives of methotrexate were covalently attached to the 43-kDa L1210 transporter by their activated NHS esters. Following labeling of L1210 cells with biotinylated methotrexate, Fan et al. used a streptavidin affinity resin to purify a putative affinity-labeled transport protein to apparent homogeneity (134).

The reactive form(s) of these NHS-activated antifolate esters have not been identified, but presumably represents either NHS α- or γ-antifolate esters. Likewise, the stable covalent adduct(s) generated between the membrane carrier and these radiolabeled affinity inhibitors have not been characterized.

APA-^{125}I-ASA-Lys is an radioiodinated derivative (at the 5-salicylyl position) of APA-ASA-Lys. This compound is a photoaffinity ligand originally developed for covalently modifying dihydrofolate reductase (135) and, more recently, the RFC protein from L1210 (130–132) and CCRF-CEM cells (130). Activation of a reactive nitrene in APA-^{125}I-ASA-Lys by ultraviolet irradiation effects a covalent modification of proteins to which it binds. The advantages of APA-^{125}I-ASA-Lys over NHS-[^{3}H]methotrexate include its increased specificity for methotrexate-binding proteins, resulting from its decreased reactivity in the absence of ultraviolet irradiation, and its greater sensitivity, associated with the incorporation of the ^{125}I radionuclide.

In addition, because of its limited chemical reactivity under subdued light, APA-^{125}I-ASA-Lys is uniquely useful for pulse–chase experiments that examine time-dependent reversible associations between this folate analogue and membrane or intracellular proteins to which it binds (130,132). Whereas incorporation from APA-^{125}I-ASA-Lys into L1210 or CCRF-CEM cells membrane proteins appears to involve the same RFC components labeled with NHS-[^{3}H]methotrexate (M_r of 46–48 and 80–85 kDa, respectively), additional 38-kDa and 21-kDa cytosolic proteins were labeled when cells were irradiated at various times following the addition of APA-^{125}I-ASA-Lys (130,132). The 21-kDa protein is, presumably, dihydrofolate reductase, and it was suggested that the 38-kDa species is an uncharacterized cytosolic or peripheral membrane protein that, in some fashion, "shuttles" folates to intracellular enzymes following their internalization by the RFC (130,132).

2. Structure and Function of the RFC: Preparation of Antiserum to a Putative Component of the Human RFC and Isolation of a Putative cDNA to the Murine RFC

The 42- to 48-kDa RFC protein from L1210 murine leukemia cells was considered the structural and functional prototype of the mammalian RFC until the demonstration that cultured human tumor cells (i.e., K562, CCRF-CEM, HL-60, and KB) synthesized distinctly different RFC isoforms (115,116,123,130,136). As with L1210 cells, the human transporter could be radiolabeled with NHS-[^{3}H]methotrexate (115) or aminopterin (116), or APA-^{125}I-ASA-Lys (130). Incorporation involved an anomalously broad, high molecular weight band on SDS gels (range 75–99 kDa) and could be abolished by unlabeled methotrexate or 5-formyltetrahydrofolate (115,116,130). For K562 cells, the molecular size of the NHS-[^{3}H]methotrexate-labeled transporter was dependent on the gel system used for analysis and ranged from 75 to 86 kDa on 3–17% gradient gels, and from 85 to 99 kDa on a 7.5% gel system (115).

Many of these characteristics reflect the glycosylation of the human RFC (115,130). Hence, the electrophoretic migration of affinity-labeled RFC is altered by digestion with endoglycosidases, including *endo*-β-galactosidase (Fig. 3; 117), *N*-glycanase (123,130), and *O*-glycanase/neuraminidase (123). Likewise, a NHS-[^{3}H]methotrexate-labeled protein from transport–up-regulated K562 cells, presumably identical to RFC and des-

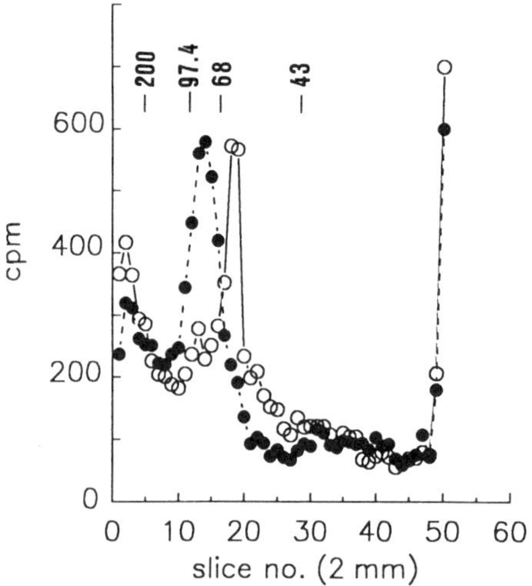

Figure 3 Radioaffinity labeling of the RFC protein with NHS-[^{3}H]methotrexate. Transport–up-regulated K562 cells (K562.4CF) were treated with 700 nM NHS-[^{3}H]methotrexate. Membranes were prepared and proteins solubilized with 1% 3-[(3-cholamidopropyl)dimethylamino]-1-propanesulfonate (CHAPS). Equal portions were incubated for 4 h at 37°C in the presence and absence of endo-β-galactosidase. The digests were electrophoresed on a 7.5% polyacrylamide gel in the presence of SDS; the gel was sliced into 2-mm segments, and the radioactivity extracted and counted. Closed circles, no treatment; open circles, *endo*-β-galactosidase-treated samples. The migration positions of known molecular weight standards are indicated. (From Ref. 115.)

ignated GP-MTX, bound to selected lectins (as the agarose-immobilized derivatives), including wheat germ agglutinin and *Ricinus communis* agglutinin I (123). On this basis, sufficient radioaffinity-labeled GP-MTX was purified from detergent-solubilized K562 plasma membranes by *R. communis* agglutinin I-agarose chromatography and preparative electrophoresis to immunize rabbits (123). The resulting antiserum was highly specific for a single membrane glycoprotein (median molecular weight, 99 kDa), of which the expression for a series of K562 subclones approximates their capacities for methotrexate uptake (Fig. 4).

It has been suggested that differences in the levels of glycosylation may contribute to the disparity in the apparent sizes of homologous RFC proteins from human and murine cells (115), since cultured L1210 and CCRF-CEM cells show virtually identical binding specificities and transport kinetics for most folate and antifolate substrates, yet only the human isoform seems to be glycosylated (134). Moreover, transport efficiency in

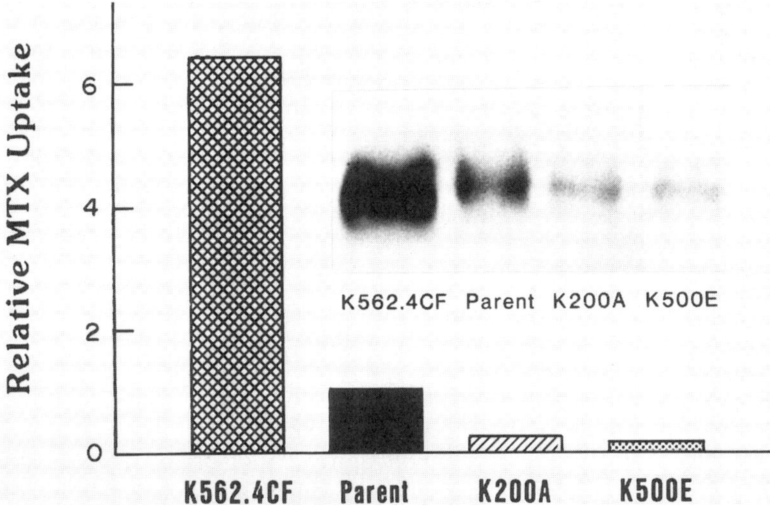

Figure 4 Correlation between levels of immunoreactive GP-MTXs and [³H]methotrexate uptake in parent, transport–up-regulated (K562.4CF), and transport-impaired (K200A, K500E) K562 sublines. Uptake of [³H]methotrexate (0.5 μM) was assayed over 420. In the inset are the results of immunoblot analysis of plasma membrane proteins. Fifty micrograms of protein were electrophoresed on 4–10% gels, electrophoretically transferred to Immobilon membranes for probing with GP-MTX-specific antiserum; immunoreactive complexes were detected with ^{125}I-Protein A and autoradiography. On this gel system, GP-MTX migrated as a 99-kDa band.

CCRF-CEM cells is minimally affected by tunicamycin exposures (1–2 μg/ml), which result in major inhibitions of N-glycosylation (66–82%) and reductions in the GP-MTX molecular size (approx. 30–41%; 137). However, these systems also differ in ways unrelated to their degrees of glycosylation, since the murine and human carriers can be distinguished in their rates of membrane translocation (116), immunoreactivities with GP-MTX-specific antiserum (Matherly L H, unpublished data) and, at least for one substrate (1843U89), membrane transport (75).

Tetrahydrofolate cofactor and methotrexate transport activity can be restored in transport-impaired Chinese hamster ovary cells (Pro-4MTX^{RII}-Oua^{R}2-4) on transfection with total DNA from drug-sensitive human or hamster cells (138) or a Chinese hamster ovary genomic cosmid library (139). More recently, Dixon et al. used expression cloning to isolate a cDNA, reportedly for the L1210 RFC, that could restore methotrexate transport activity and methotrexate sensitivity in transport-impaired ZR-75-1 cells (140); the homologous clone from a Chinese hamster ovary cell cDNA expression library restored MTX transport and binding activity in transport-impaired Chinese hamster ovary cells (141). The disparity between the M_r of the cDNA-encoded peptide (58 kDa) and radioaffinity-labeled murine RFC (42–48 kDa) raises doubts about whether these transporters are actually the same. This question will undoubtedly be resolved as the functional and structural properties of these proteins are further compared.

3. Regulation of RFC-Mediated Uptake

Variations in RFC transport between different tumors can arise at multiple levels, including RFC gene copy or gene expression, that manifest as increased or decreased carrier numbers. Alternatively, changes in uptake may result from effects on substrate binding or rates of carrier translocation. These may involve direct binding of small-molecule effectors to the transporter or, perhaps, posttranslational modifications of the carrier. All of these elements may be relevant to the up-regulation or down-regulation of RFCs in cultured mammalian cells and, likewise, the expression of impaired RFC transport in methotrexate-resistant tumors (see Sec. VII).

The ability to up-regulate RFC activity by culturing cells in low physiological or subphysiological concentrations of reduced folates strongly suggests that transport is subject to regulation by endogenous folates or folate-dependent metabolites (112–116). For up-regulated L1210 (3- to 40-fold; 112,113) or HL-60 cells (four- to fivefold; 116), elevated capacities for ^{3}H-antifolate transport closely correlate with increased specific surface binding of [^{3}H]aminopterin at 0°C, or labeling with NHS-[^{3}H]aminopterin. This implies that the transport effect results from the increased synthesis of RFC proteins. In one L1210 line, with 40-fold elevated transport, a gene amplification cytogenetic abnormality (i.e., homogeneously staining region) in chromosome 10 was identified (142). For an up-regulated HL-60 subline, decreased levels of [^{3}H]methotrexate influx and NHS-[^{3}H]aminopterin labeling accompanied the induction of terminal differentiation by cytodifferentiation agents (116).

A somewhat different phenotype is exemplified by K562 (designated K562.4CF) (115) or CCRF-CEM (designated CEM-7A; 114, 130) sublines with up-regulated RFC transport. In these lines, an "activation" of the RFC uptake process was apparent, since the increases in methotrexate transport (approximately 6- and 90-fold, respectively) were disproportionate to the levels of RFC–protein (increased 3- and 30-fold, respectively). Furthermore, elevated uptake was sustained only as long as the cells were maintained in the low 5-formyltetrahydrofolate concentrations used for selection (0.4 and 0.25 nM, respectively), and marked decreases in influx rates (three to sevenfold) were observed at higher physiological folate concentrations (10 and 25 nM, respectively). Notably, these folate-dependent variations in transport were *not* accompanied by corresponding changes in radioaffinity-labeled RFCs (114).

The demonstration that physiological concentrations of reduced folates suppressed transport in vitro, implies that an analogous regulation of RFC function may occur in vivo and that certain transport-up-regulated phenotypes may involve an enhanced sensitivity of these regulatory mechanisms that results in increased rates of carrier translocation. The inhibitory effects of added folates on RFC activity may involve direct binding of particular folate polyglutamate forms to the RFC at the inner membrane surface, or it may be mediated indirectly by folate-dependent products (i.e., nucleotides). In support of the latter possibility are data that show that folate-dependent down-regulation of [^{3}H]methotrexate transport in CEM-7A cells is abolished by pretreatment with methotrexate or trimetrexate (114,130), and that an analogous suppression of up-regulated methotrexate transport occurs on exposure to nontoxic concentrations of adenosine (130).

Although the effects of adenosine on transport may reflect a putative phosphorylation of RFC, attempts to confirm this possibility yielded conflicting results (130). Hence, elevated concentrations of cAMP were associated with decreased methotrexate uptake in cultured L1210 cells (143,144); however, in Ehrlich tumor cells these correlations could be temporally dissociated from the transport effect (145). Whereas 9-Br-cAMP has no effect on [^{3}H]methotrexate influx in CEM-7A cells (130), in phytohemagglutinin-stimulated lymphocytes (146) or K562.4CF cells (L. H. Matherly, unpublished observation) dibutyryl cAMP pretreatment inhibits methotrexate transport. Although recent studies suggest that impaired RFC-mediated transport in cisplatin-resistant L1210 cells involves decreased tyrosine phosphorylation of membrane proteins (147), it is not certain that this modification actually involves the RFC.

IV. MECHANISMS FOR FOLATE AND ANTIFOLATE MEMBRANE TRANSPORT UNRELATED TO THE CLASSIC RFC SYSTEM

Folic acid influx is partly mediated by the RFC, as described in the foregoing; however, the poor affinity of folic acid for this carrier system (20 to 50-fold less than methotrexate) raises doubts about how this nonphysiological cofactor form penetrates mammalian cell membranes. This question might be academic, if it was not that most tissue culture media contain folic acid as the only source of folates for cell growth. Furthermore, there is considerable interest in the basis by which methotrexate-resistant tumor cells in vitro continue to replicate at high levels in the presence of folic acid when RFC-mediated influx is inoperative (148,149). Identical mechanisms may serve to salvage exogenous physiological folate cofactors (i.e., 5-methyltetrahydrofolate) in vivo while continuing to exclude methotrexate.

In recent years, three transport processes, separate from RFC, have been suggested to facilitate folic acid uptake into tumor cells. These include (1) a family of high-affinity membrane folate-binding proteins (FBPs), characterized by extremely tight binding of folic acid and 5-methyltetrahydrofolate, relative to 5-formyltetrahydrofolate and methotrexate (2,4); (2) a largely uncharacterized system that exhibits high-influx capacities and low affinities for folic acid, reduced folates, and antifolates (150); and (3) a minor, pH- and energy-dependent transport system that has now been documented only for cultured L1210 cells (151). A multiplicity of additional uptake routes for folates and antifolates have been described in particular tissues (i.e., liver and intestine) and are reviewed elsewhere (152–154).

A. High-Affinity Membrane Folate-Binding Proteins as Mechanisms of Folate and Antifolate Uptake

The FBPs are a family of membrane-localized (mFBPs) and soluble (sFBPs) high-affinity folate binders that have been described in several cultured cell lines (KB, MA104, L1210, CCRF-CEM) (117–119, 155–158), tissues (placenta, proximal kidney tubules, and choroid plexus; 159–161), and extracellular fluids (tissue culture medium, milk, serum, and umbilical cord serum; 162–166). Recent studies indicate that FBPs are also expressed in certain human ovarian carcinomas, both in vitro and in vivo (167,168). In some cases (e.g., placenta or KB cells), sFBPs that accumulate extracellularly have been found to arise from the membrane-localized forms (169–173).

Although high-affinity FBPs proteins were first described in the late 1960s (174,175), it was not until nearly a decade later that their importance as modes of folate cofactor uptake began to be seriously considered. The term "binding proteins" is unfortunate, since it fails to convey any role of these membrane receptors in folate and antifolate transport. Rather, it reflects the early confusion about their biological function. Indeed, because of their extraordinary affinities for folic acid and 5-methyltetrahydrofolate, compared with other folate transporters (see later discussion), it was originally suggested that FBPs function in folate cofactor storage or retention, rather than membrane transport (155).

The association of mFBPs with folate transport arose from (1) pulse–chase studies in KB or MA104 cells that showed that binding of [^{3}H]folic acid and 5-methyl [^{3}H]tetrahydrofolate initially involved an acid-dissociable or trypsin-sensitive particulate membrane fraction before internalization into an acid-insensitive (intracellular) compartment (156,176,177); (2) the demonstration that anti-FBP antibodies could inhibit uptake of 5-methyl [^{3}H]tetrahydrofolate (177) or [^{3}H]methotrexate (178) into KB cells, or 5-methyl [^{3}H]tetrahydrofolate binding to MA104 cells (156); (3) the inhibition of mFBP-mediated [^{3}H]methotrexate uptake in KB cells by NHS-methotrexate (178); (4) the induction of megaloblastic morphological changes and reduction in intracellular folates in cultured human bone marrow cells treated with FBP-specific antiserum (179); and (5) the selection of L1210 (117–119) or CCRF-CEM (158) sublines in low medium folates, or the isolation of transformants following transfection with mFBP cDNAs (173,180–183), for which elevated mFBP levels accompanied increased surface binding and accumulation of radiolabeled folate substrates.

Elevated mFBP expression, in general, confers increased capacities for growth in low levels of folates (173). Moreover, mFBP-cDNA transfected NIH/3T3 cells grown in nude mice produced tumors with a threefold greater mean volume than mock transfected NIH/3T3 cells (173), suggesting that, as least for this in vivo model, mFBP expression confers a growth advantage.

1. Analysis of mFBP Structures

Relative to the RFC in mammalian cells, studies of the biochemical and molecular characteristics of the FBP family are far advanced. Progress for the latter has been undoubtedly facilitated by the availability of cultured cells (i.e., KB, MA104) and tissues (placenta) that synthesize high levels of FBPs. For instances in which FBPs are "shed" from plasma membranes, abundant amounts of FBPs can be isolated from extracellular fluids (i.e., tissue culture media; 166,173,184). In addition, mFBPs retain their high affinities for folic acid on solubilization with nonionic detergents, facilitating their affinity purification on columns of folic acid–Sepharose (166,184).

Both soluble and particulate FBPs from a variety of sources are homologous in their substrate-binding affinities (166), glycosylation (166), and amino acid compositions (185). Likewise, amino-terminal sequence data for the particulate and soluble binders from KB cells are identical (185). Although sFBPs are generally derived from membrane-bound congeners (170), mFBPs are much more hydrophobic and bind up to three times their M_r in Triton X-100 micelles (162,166,185). This property appears, at least in part, to derive from the presence of covalently bound fatty acids on mFBPs (181,185,186).

Human FBP cDNAs were isolated with antisense oligonucleotides or specific antibodies from cDNA libraries prepared from KB nasopharyngeal epidermoid carcinoma (187,188), two colon carcinomas (CaCo-2 and HT-29; 167,181), human placenta (189,190), and two ovarian carcinomas (SKOV3 and IGROV2; 167,191). From all sources, FBP cDNAs were obtained that encoded an *identical polypeptide* (termed FBP1 for the following discussion; 167,181,187–191); however, in placenta, additional FBP isoforms (termed FBP2 and FBP3) were isolated (189,190). From the cDNA sequences, FBP2 and FBP3 are, respectively, 68 and 77% homologous to FBP1 (189,190). FBP3 is highly homologous to FBP2, but contains a unique 5' terminus, and minor differences within the open-reading frame and at the exon I and II junction (190). A preliminary report describes an additional mFBP isoform from variant CCRF-CEM cells. Interestingly, this form shows limited immunoreactivity (approx. 10%) with mFBP1 or mFBP2 antisera, and also significant differences in its amino acid composition and mode of membrane anchoring from either mFBP1 or mFBP2 isoforms (192). The cDNA for this mFBP isoform from CCRF-CEM cells has not been described.

It is notable that the FBP1 cDNAs from different sources are highly heterogeneous in both their 5'- and 3'-noncoding regions (167). This variability presumably reflects alternative splicing of mRNA precursors and may be associated with tissue-specific stabilities or translational activities of these mFBP transcripts (167). Although murine FBPs have not yet been purified, two FBP cDNAs with close similarities to human FBP1 and FBP2 were isolated from L1210 cDNA libraries by hybridization with oligonucleotides corresponding to regions of the human FBPs (117). The murine FBP1 homologue was overexpressed in L1210 cells adapted to growth-limiting concentrations of 5-formyltetrahydrofolate (117).

The FBP cDNAs from both murine and human libraries encode polypeptides of 251–257 amino acids, including signal peptides of 16–25 amino acids (117,167,181,187–191). The putative signal sequences in the different FBPs are dissimilar and may serve to target distinct isoforms to particular membrane locales (189). After cleavage of the signal peptides, the sequence data predict polypeptide molecular weights of 28–30 kDa (117,167,181,187–191) and three (mFBP1; 117,167,181,187–189,191) or two (mFBP2 and mFBP3; 117,189,190) N-glycosylation sites. Although all cDNA sequences predict only a *single* stretch of apolar amino acids at the carboxyl-terminus that could anchor the folate receptors into plasma membranes, no vicinal hydrophilic segments, typical of transmembrane domains, are apparent (117,167,181,187–191).

Although it is generally recognized that the soluble binders are derived from the membrane-localized forms (169–172), it is difficult to reconcile the findings of Luhrs et al. (185,186) with those of Elwood et al. (166,169) on the structural relationships between these proteins and the mode of mFBP membrane anchoring. Whereas Elwood et al. (166) reported a greater apparent M_r and a larger number of hydrophobic amino acids for the mFBP versus sFBP from KB cells, Luhrs et al. (185), using the same line, reported no differences in either amino acid contents or molecular weights for these forms. Moreover, Elwood et al. reported that up to 31 amino acids are removed from the intact KB mFBP by a membrane-associated, Mg^{+2}-dependent protease to release an sFBP (169); however, Luhrs and Slomiany (186) demonstrated the presence of covalently bound fatty acids on mFBPs and their attachment to plasma membranes by glycosylphosphatidylinositol anchors. Several laboratories have also provided data on an assortment of cells or tissues (KB, MA104, placenta) that indicate that the hydrophobic mFBP carboxyl-terminus is a signal for addition of a glycosylphosphatidylinositol anchor (181,191,193,194). Glycosylphosphatidylinositol attachment generally involves the cleavage of the carboxyl-terminal end of the nascent protein and the formation of an amide bond between the new carboxyl-terminal amino acid and the ethanolamine of the glycosylphosphatidylinositol moiety (195).

These distinct modes of membrane attachment may reflect the presence of separate cell populations (4), since different mechanisms of membrane anchoring have, likewise, been reported for another glycosylphosphatidylinositol-linked protein (human CD16 receptor; 196). Alternatively, the posttranslational modification of mFBP may be unusual in that there is no cleavage of the carboxyl-terminal sequence associated with attachment of the glycosylphosphatidylinositol anchor (169), or the cleavage of the nascent polypeptide, and addition of the glycosylphosphatidylinositol anchor occurs near the carboxyl-terminus of the unprocessed protein, and just proximal to the site of metalloprotease hydrolysis (194).

2. Mechanisms of mFBP Uptake

Assays of FBPs in tissues or cultured cells have generally involved measurements of high-affinity surface [³H]folic acid binding in situ, or [³H]folic acid binding to purified or crude mFBP preparations incubated with nanomolar concentrations of [³H]folic acid. The folic acid K_ds so calculated are relatively uniform for different preparations, and range from 0.07 to 0.77 nM (121,156,159,162,166). Binding affinities for assorted (anti)-folates are often measured relative to folic acid, as their capacities to compete for FBP binding with [³H]folic acid and are expressed as K_is or IC$_{50}$s (88,89,102,103,118,155,156,197). Affinities for folic acid generally exceed those for 5-methyltetrahydrofolate by five- to tenfold; however, relative affinities for 5-formyltetrahydrofolate and methotrexate are more varied and range from 5- to 1000-fold, and 33- to 3600-fold, respectively, lower than for folic acid. Whereas other 4-aminoantifolates, likewise, show low affinities for mFBPs (i.e., 10-Edam binds 33- to 125-fold less avidly than folic acid), the affinities of 4-*oxo*-antifolates (ICID1694 or DDATHF) approximate those of folic acid (88,102,103,118,158). The variations of mFBP-binding affinities for a particular (anti)folate may partly reflect changes in substrate specificities for different mFBP isoforms (189,190).

The characteristic high-affinity binding of folic acid and 5-methyltetrahydrofolate relative to 5-formyltetrahydrofolate and methotrexate clearly identified mFBPs as distinct from the RFC system, which had previously been reported to mediate methotrexate transport into tumor cells. Moreover, for none of the published mFBP cDNA sequences could more than a single transmembrane peptide be unambiguously identified—a seemingly improbable result if mFBPs functioned as *integral* membrane carriers that repeatedly traversed the plasma membrane while mediating folate cofactor uptake from the outer to the inner membrane surface.

Rather, primarily from studies with a line of immortalized monkey kidney epithelial cells, MA104, a picture has emerged of a slowly cycling membrane receptor that binds folic acid with a high affinity at the outer membrane surface and undergoes endocytosis by a novel uncoated pit pathway ("potocytosis";198,199). The rate for mFBP-mediated influx by this mechanism has been estimated as less than *one turnover per mFBP per hour* (2), far slower than RFC transport (see Sec. II), but apparently still adequate to supply exogenous folic acid or 5-methyltetrahydrofolate for replicating cells. For KB cells, a cell line characterized by particularly elevated levels of mFBPs, it was calculated that one-tenth of a transport cycle per binding site per cell doubling is enough to provide sufficient exogenous folic acid for growth (4).

Folate uptake by MA104 cells has been shown by quantitative immuno-cytochemistry as involving cholesterol-dependent mFBP clusters (750 mFBPs per cluster), associated with non–clathrin-coated invaginated regions of the plasma membrane, or caveolae (198–200). During folate uptake, these caveolae transiently invaginate and reseal, while maintaining their plasma membrane attachment. No receptor is detectable in endosomes or lysosomes. Since substrate internalization is sensitive to weak acids or other endosomal disruptive agents (176), it was further proposed that transient acidification effects a release of the mFBP-bound folates, which enter into the cytoplasm by diffusion of their protonated forms, or, alternatively, by an unknown anion transporter (199). In either event, the resulting "apo-mFBPs" that remain associated with the caveolar membranes are recycled back to the cell surface to participate in another transport cycle. The extent of dissociation of the internalized cofactor is greater for 5-methyltetrahydrofolate than folic acid (177), perhaps reflecting differences in substrate-binding affinities for mFBPs, or in the capacities for metabolism (polyglutamylation) by intracellular folate-dependent enzymes.

It has not been confirmed whether this mechanism is operative in other cells or tissues that express mFBPs. Indeed, mFBPs may serve different roles in different tissues since, in tumor cells, mFBPs mediate intracellular folate uptake; however, in normal epithelial cells, such as the kidney and choroid plexus, they presumably scavenge folates and transport these derivatives to specific tissue spaces. The placental mFBP isoforms may facilitate the transfer of folate cofactors across the placental barrier from the maternal to the fetal circulation. Interestingly, in KB cells, mFBPs were also detected in membranes surrounding organelles (155), implying that they are relevant to cellular folate metabolism. Separate roles in disparate cells or tissues may account for the existence of multiple mFBP isoforms with different affinities for assorted folates and antifolates (89) (see Sec. IV.A.1).

In light of the results with MA104 cells, it is of particular interest that mFBPs in rat kidney proximal tubule brush-border membranes exhibit similar binding specificities to mFBP1 (161); however, no obvious clustering of mFBPs was demonstrable by immunocytochemistry (201). Moreover, mFBPs were transferred from endocytic invaginations *into endocytic vacuoles* during transport, followed by their recycling back to the luminal plasma membrane (presumably, as apo-mFBPs) through dense apical tubules (201).

It has been suggested that RFCs in MA104 cells may operate in tandem with mFBPs in mediating uptake across the caveolar membranes (199,202); however, evidence in support of this mechanism is largely indirect (i.e., differential inhibition by probenecid of 5-methyl [^{3}H]-tetrahydrofolate binding versus internalization). Indeed, there is no indication that mFBP and RFC function are obligatorily coupled, since mFBP uptake is clearly operative in a CCRF-CEM line with defective RFC transport (158), and many cells exhibit high levels of RFC uptake in the absence of detectable mFBPs.

A related question involves the presence of an RFC uptake component in cells that have been reported to use mFBPs as a primary mode of folate uptake. For instance, in KB cells, RFCs are detectable by radioaffinity labeling (136) or immunoblotting (203) and likely contribute to their sensitivities to 4-aminoantifolates (methotrexate, 10-ethyl-10-deazaaminopterin), particularly in the presence of folic acid (136). However, for KB sublines grown in low, subphysiological folate concentrations, the overproduction of mFBPs may effectively mask the RFC uptake component, even though the catalytic turnover rate for the latter is far greater. This may explain the reports of impaired methotrexate transport caused by reduced levels of mFBPs in certain KB sublines (204); likewise, the increased methotrexate sensitivities of certain mFBP cDNA transformants (183), but not others (180), may correlate with the extent to which mFBPs are overexpressed.

3. Regulation of mFBP Expression and Function

It has been suggested that the lack of detectable FBPs in most cultured mammalian cells is simply due to a repression of their biosynthesis over time, a consequence of high, nonphysiological concentrations of folates in standard tissue culture media (118,158,176,205–207). In support of this hypothesis, several laboratories selected mFBP-overproducing L1210 (117–119) or CCRF-CEM (158) lines in subphysiological folate concentrations, conditions not unlike those used to isolate RFC–up-regulated sublines of L1210 (112,113), K562 (115), or CCRF-CEM (114) cells. Even in cells with constitutively high levels of mFBP expression (i.e., KB or MA104), mFBP levels can still be up- or down-regulated by variations in the concentrations of exogenous folate cofactors (156,188,205,206).

Detection of FBPs in these studies has often relied on assays of [^{3}H]folic acid binding and is subject to interference by endogenous bound folates, unless the latter are sufficiently "stripped" with acidic buffers (156). In KB cells, grown in limiting folates over several months, increased [^{3}H]folic acid binding correlates with increased immunoreactive mFBP receptors (208) and transcripts (188,206). For mFBP–up-regulated KB cells, grown under folate-restrictive conditions, no differences in mFBP1 gene organization, methylation, or transcription rates were associated with the increased mFBP1 transcript and receptor levels (206). Rather, the data were best explained by changes in mFBP mRNA stabilities, although other factors relating to nuclear mRNA transport and splicing could not be excluded. It is unclear how changes in exogenous folate levels would translate into effects on mRNA stabilities. In a similar fashion, alterations in intracellular folate pools or metabolism may result in *decreased* mFBP and transcript levels in a number of KB sublines (204,205,208). Whereas sFPBs are generated from mFBPs (170—173), it is not established whether this shedding of surface receptors represents a regulatory response to particular physiological effectors.

In contrast with this dynamic regulation of mFBP expression in KB cells, for a folate-deficient L1210 line, the insertion of a retrovirus-like sequence (i.e., intracisternal A particle or IAP) into the 5'-regulatory region of the FBP gene was associated with *constitutive* expression of elevated mFBP transcripts and receptors (117,209). Elevated mFBP expression in these cells appeared to involve a novel transcript, with greater stability or increased mFBP transcription from a cryptic IAP promoter near the IAP–FBP junction (209). Campbell et al. (167) mapped the mFBP locus to chromosome 11q13.3-q13.5, near INT2, the human homologue of the mouse mammary tumor virus integration site. Long-terminal repeat (LTR)-mediated activation could similarly facilitate enhanced expression of mFBP gene(s) in certain human tumors (i.e., ovarian carcinomas) by virtue of their juxtaposition (209).

From RNAse protection and Northern blotting assays, both mFBP1 and mFBP3 transcripts are independently and variously expressed in assorted human fetal and adult tissues, apparently from independent genes (190). Although mFBP1 and mFBP3 expression is clearly unrelated to fetal development, mFBP2 expression appears to be confined to placenta, consistent with its role as a fetal-specific mFBP isoform (190); mFBP2 seems to be encoded by an independent gene from either mFBP1 or mFBP3 (190).

Membrane folate-binding proteins may also be subject to posttranslational controls. Hence, in KB cells, the mFBP receptor is phosphorylated (210); the functional significance of this modification is uncertain. Although the presence of high mannose oligosaccharides is not required for ligand-binding activity, their addition during the processing of the nascent polypeptide is essential to the development of a functionally active ligand-binding site (211).

Interestingly, polyglutamylation of methotrexate *increases* the apparent binding affinities of the antifolate to FBPs for KB cells, since identical

K_ds were calculated for hexaglutamyl methotrexate and 5-methyltetrahydrofolate monoglutamate (i.e., 3 nM; 166). Although methotrexate polyglutamate–mFBP complexes were identified in folate-restricted KB lines (178,205), their relevance to the regulation of mFBP function is not established.

B. Additional Non-RFC Uptake Systems for Folate and Antifolate Transport

Although folic acid appears to be partially accumulated in tumor cells by the RFC and, in certain tissues, mFBPs, the question of still other transport routes remains controversial (150,212,213). This is partly due to differences in experimental conditions for assaying these transport fluxes, since in anion-free buffers without an energy source, the multiplicity in folic acid uptake seen in the presence of physiological anions is not observed (150). Rather, the markedly increased RFC flux under these conditions virtually obscures any contribution from putative additional influx systems.

The existence of a separate "low-affinity" system for [3H]folic acid influx in mammalian cells with a 20-fold higher transport capacity than the RFC has been well documented (149,150,214–219). Additional evidence for a transport system separate from RFC includes (1) the demonstration in L1210 cells or plasma membranes of large differences in the inhibition of methotrexate versus folic acid by organic mercurials (214) or the stilbenes, 4,4'-diisothiocyano-2,2'-disulfonic acid stilbene (DIDS) and 4-acetamido-4'-isothiocyano stilbene-2,2'-disulfonic acid (SITS; 216); (2) the absence of [3H]folic acid trans-stimulation in L1210 plasma membrane vesicles preloaded with 5-methyl- or 5-formyltetrahydrofolate (216); (3) major discrepancies between K_i values for assorted folate inhibitors (methotrexate, folic acid, (*d*)- and (*l*)5-methyltetrahydrohomofolate) of [3H]methotrexate versus [3H]folic acid influx (150); and (4) the lack of impaired folic acid influx in methotrexate-resistant tumor cells with defective methotrexate and reduced folate uptake (149,150,218,219) and, likewise, the unimpeded capacities of RFC-impaired cells to grow in folic acid (148,149).

In wild-type and transport-impaired L1210 cells, Henderson and Strauss (151) described a minor, energy-dependent, and saturable system that can be activated fivefold at pH 6.8. This system was undetectable in CCRF-CEM cells. Although the system showed specificities for folic acid, methotrexate, and 5-formyltetrahydrofolate as transport substrates, 5-methyltetrahydrofolate was not a substrate, even though it inhibited [3H]folic acid uptake (151).

V. MECHANISMS OF METHOTREXATE EFFLUX

The free intracellular methotrexate concentration in excess of that bound to dihydrofolate reductase is critical to the sustained suppression of enzymatic activity within tumor cells and is determined by relative rates of both drug influx and efflux (see Sec. II.B). Our understanding of the complex relationships between these opposing membrane fluxes has clearly evolved since the original suggestion by Hakala (220) that increased net methotrexate accumulation in S180 cells incubated with 2,4-dinitrophenol involved an inhibition of energy-dependent drug efflux. The mechanism of methotrexate efflux remains controversial (221,222), partly because murine and human tumor cells contain multiple routes for drug exit, including RFC, and because their relative contributions are dependent on the experimental conditions used to assay transport. These separate efflux pathways have been dissected from their differential responses to various inhibitors, including NHS-methotrexate, prostaglandin A_1, vincristine, reserpine, verapamil, bromosulfophthalein, and probenecid (109,221–227), their different pH optima (226), and their sensitivities to perturbations in cellular energy status (221,223,228–230). For instance, in the absence of an energy substrate, or in the presence of an energy inhibitor (i.e., azide, oligomycin, or 2,4-dinitrophenol), ATP levels in L1210 cells are depleted, and virtually all of the outward flux of drug involves the bidirectional RFC and can be inhibited by NHS-methotrexate (109,221,223). By contrast, in ATP-replete L1210 cells, total methotrexate efflux is markedly stimulated over this basal level (up to threefold; 221,223). Under these conditions, routes that are largely undetected in energy-depleted L1210 cells now constitute most of drug efflux (estimated as 70–90% of the total) and can be inhibited by probenecid, bromosulfophthalein, and verapamil (221–224). The contributions of these separate efflux components may differ in other cell lines (109). It has been reported that energy-dependent methotrexate efflux separate from RFC in L1210 cells is actually composed of multiple (at least two) separate systems, characterized by differences in their sensitivities to certain of these inhibitors (222–228).

Regardless of whether a single energy-dependent outward flux, or additional minor systems are also involved, the critical point is that, in energetically competent cells in physiological media, the vast majority of the intracellular methotrexate is pumped out by systems unrelated to the membrane carriers that mediate drug influx. Hence, methotrexate efflux is virtually unaffected by elevated or impaired RFC influx (86,112–116,232,233). Moreover, these opposing fluxes exhibit different responses to transport inhibitors or other biochemical perturbations (109,221–225,229–231). For instance, in the presence of energy poisons

(229,230) or in the absence of glucose (231), methotrexate efflux is preferentially blocked and only minor effects on RFC influx are observed; moreover, a number of agents (verapamil, bromosulfophthalein, vinca alkaloids, teniposide (VM-26), etoposide (VP-16), reserpine, quinidine) (109,221–225,234), including some used clinically, also block methotrexate efflux. It is interesting that methotrexate efflux is inhibited by bromosulfophthalein in the *trans* (outer membrane) orientation only, whereas probenecid requires both *cis* (inner) and *trans* inhibitor, and verapamil only *cis* inhibitor (221). Although the underlying bases for these differences are unclear, these findings strongly suggest that the efflux pump is mobile within its membrane milieu and is capable of interacting with ligands on both the inner and outer membrane surfaces. Moreover, these results suggest that pharmacological intervention at the level of efflux carrier to promote enhanced net antifolate accumulation by tumor cells may ultimately be possible. Jolivet et al. (235) reported that methotrexate resistance in a ZR-75-1 breast carcinoma line could be partially reversed by probenecid—apparently through a selective blockade of methotrexate efflux.

Until recently, descriptions of methotrexate efflux relied exclusively on kinetic analyses of first-order efflux rates from methotrexate-preloaded cells. Although general concepts relating to substrate specificities and kinetics and the energetics of efflux were attainable by this approach, further characterization of the catalytic properties of the efflux pump(s) was limited.

Recently, Schlemmer and Sirotnak (236) developed an elegant approach for assaying carrier-mediated methotrexate efflux with inside-out plasma membrane vesicles, prepared from L1210 cells deficient in carrier-mediated methotrexate influx. A low-affinity ($K_m = 46\ \mu M$) and high-capacity ($V_{max} = 106\ \text{pmol mg}^{-1}\ \text{min}^{-1}$) methotrexate efflux process was identified with an inhibitor profile identical with the energy-dependent efflux in intact cells, and with a requirement for ATP that could partially be satisfied by CTP and GTP. No transport occurred with vesicles incubated with a nonhydrolyzable ATP analogue, adenosine-5'-O-(3-thiotriphosphate), in lieu of ATP. Moreover, since both this analogue and orthovanadate inhibited transport in the presence of catalytic amounts of ATP, ATP hydrolysis must be absolutely required for efflux by this system, and the energy-dependent efflux pump for methotrexate is probably an ATPase.

The natural substrate for this energy-dependent efflux system has not been established; however, it is interesting that this carrier shows an unusual lack of substrate specificity. Hence, structurally diverse organic anions, such as cholate and cAMP, appear to share a common carrier with methotrexate, folic acid, assorted reduced cofactors, (6S)DDATHF, and ICI D1694 (226,227,228,236–238). Another antifolate, CB3717, is not transported (237), suggesting that it may be possible to design antifolates with increased cellular accumulation resulting from their poor transport activity by the major efflux carrier. Of course, the antitumor effectiveness of CB3717 is so compromised by its poor cellular uptake and toxic side effects (see Sec. II.D.2) that its activity as an efflux substrate is largely irrelevant.

Of special interest are data that indicate that both methotrexate and its di-, tri-, and pentaglutamyl forms are equipotent competitive inhibitors of [^{3}H]methotrexate transport in inside-out vesicles (K_i = 43–48 μM; 239); for radiolabeled methotrexate mono- and diglutamate substrates, equivalent transport activities were measured. These data are intriguing, since they seem to contradict the dogma that the extent of cellular retention for mono- versus polyglutamyl forms of methotrexate reflects their differing affinities for the major energy-dependent efflux pump.

From the preceding discussion of energy-dependent methotrexate efflux, it appears that this system and P-glycoprotein in multidrug-resistant cells (240) (see Chap. 17) share a number of common features: (1) both are ATPases, requiring an obligatory ATP hydrolysis, coupled to transport; (2) both show highly relaxed substrate specificities, P-glycoprotein toward cationic and hydrophobic molecules, and the methotrexate efflux pump toward an assortment of organic anions; (3) both P-glycoprotein and the methotrexate efflux pump are inhibited by verapamil, quinidine, and reserpine. Taken together, these data suggest that P-glycoprotein and the methotrexate efflux pump are separate but, perhaps, related members of the ATP-binding cassette superfamily of membrane transporters (241). Vincristine, a substrate for P-glycoprotein, also inhibits energy-dependent methotrexate efflux; however, this effect likely involves the disruption of microtubules (225), rather than its direct binding to the efflux carrier.

VI. THE ROLE OF MEMBRANE TRANSPORT IN THE CLINICAL PHARMACOLOGY OF THE ANTIFOLATES

A. Pharmacokinetic Considerations

Various pharmacokinetic considerations must be incorporated into our transport-based analysis of antifolate therapeutics relating to the in vivo pharmacology of these agents. These concern drug binding to plasma proteins, the extent of liver detoxification, and rates of renal clearance.

Following methotrexate IV infusion, its elimination follows a biexponential curve over 72 h, with an initial fast elimination ($t_{1/2}$ = 2.3 h) during the first 24 h, followed by a slower elimination ($t_{1/2}$ = 15.2 h) during the subsequent 48 h (242). Hence, for tumor cells with RFC-mediated methotrexate influx and energy-dependent efflux, the rates of plasma drug clearance are considerably slower than the flux rates across plasma membranes. Moreover, the extracellular drug level in plasma following infusion exceeds that within tumor cells (1). Although this partly reflects methotrexate bound to serum proteins (approximately 50%; 242), even if only unbound plasma methotrexate is considered, the intracellular methotrexate concentration is still less than the extracellular concentration because of the high-capacity efflux pump and the electrical restrictions on net antifolate transport (see Secs. III.A and V).

Because the rates of transport are rapid compared with plasma clearance, the intracellular antifolate remains at a continuous, albeit slowly, decreasing, steady-state concentration that parallels the loss of plasma methotrexate (1). This will be true for antifolate inhibitors other than methotrexate with similar rates of clearance, or other folate transport systems, *as long as the rates of influx and efflux exceed those for plasma drug clearance*. However, for much slower-uptake mechanisms (i.e., mFBPs), transport could potentially become rate-limiting, particularly during the "fast" elimination phase. In either event, the absolute steady-state levels of free intracellular antifolate are determined by the respective transport capacities for these different membrane systems and can vary considerably from tumor to tumor or tissue to tissue. Since multiple transport systems (i.e., mFBPs and RFCs) are likely to coexist within a single tumor cell or tissue, the net drug level achieved will be a composite of these separate drug fluxes.

For methotrexate, it is the level of free intracellular antifolate, determined by the plasma concentration and the kinetics of membrane transport, that is essential to achieving suppression of dihydrofolate reductase activity and tetrahydrofolate-dependent processes (see Sec. II.B). This results from the competition between methotrexate and dihydrofolate at dihydrofolate reductase and the requirement for free "monoglutamyl" drug for maximal enzyme inhibition; however, transport is also critical to the synthesis of methotrexate polyglutamates, required for sustained drug activity as plasma methotrexate levels decline.

Methotrexate polyglutamylation is slow relative to membrane transport and binding to dihydrofolate reductase (30,33). Because of the high K_m for methotrexate binding to folylpolyglutamate synthetase (47,48), the levels of methotrexate polyglutamates formed are generally low unless considerable unbound intracellular methotrexate is generated. Not surprisingly, this transport limitation on polyglutamylation becomes more acute for drug-resistant tumor cells characterized by impaired methotrexate influx and the generation of little or no free methotrexate substrate in excess of that bound to dihydrofolate reductase (29,87,243,244). Hence, regardless of the transport processes involved in mediating drug influx and efflux, the formation of methotrexate polyglutamate derivatives is limited by the kinetic properties of these systems. Obviously, these considerations may not necessarily apply to antifolates, such as DDATHF, that are far better substrates than methotrexate for mammalian folylpolyglutamate synthetase (see Sec. VII.B.4).

An additional element in the in vivo activity of antifolates, such as methotrexate, involves its hydroxylation at the 7-position of the pteridine. Although hydroxylation has also been reported for antifolates other than methotrexate (i.e., aminopterin; 2,6-dichloromethotrexate; 10-Edam; 56,245,246), it has not been established whether some of the newer inhibitors (i.e., DDATHF, ICI D1694, 1843U89) are also metabolized in this fashion.

High levels of 7-hydroxymethotrexate have been described in humans following the administration of moderate to high doses of methotrexate. Following infusion of high doses of methotrexate in osteosarcoma patients, 7-hydroxymethotrexate concentrations exceeded those for methotrexate within 3 h, owing to its slower clearance (up to 11 times slower than methotrexate) (247). When methotrexate plasma levels had declined to approximately 0.1 μM, the plasma concentration of 7-hydroxymethotrexate was still 17–190 times higher. Elevated concentrations of 7-hydroxymethotrexate have been implicated in both acute nephrotoxicity (248) and hepatotoxicity (249) accompanying high-dose methotrexate therapy.

Because of its reduced affinity for dihydrofolate reductase (6700-fold less than for methotrexate; 250), 7-hydroxymethotrexate is far less toxic than methotrexate toward cultured mammalian cells (251). Although other potential cellular targets for 7-hydroxymethotrexate have been suggested, including thymidylate synthase and AICAR transformylase (252), their pharmacological significance is debatable (see following discussion). 7-Hydroxymethotrexate directly competes with methotrexate and reduced folates for transport by the RFC (K_t two- to four-fold greater than methotrexate) (46,253) and, thus, could conceivably influence the antitumor activity of methotrexate. However, this is unlikely to be of major importance, since as little as 10% of the plasma 7-hydroxymethotrexate is readily available for transport (i.e., as much as 90% of 7-hydroxymethotrexate is bound to plasma protein) (254); furthermore, 7-hydroxymethotrexate levels are maximal only after plasma methotrexate has begun to fall (247) and intracellular monoglutamyl methotrexate and methotrexate polyglutamates have already presumably accumulated to high levels in drug-sensitive tumor cells. Likewise, the effects of any direct inhibition of intracellular folate-dependent enzyme targets should be minimal because dihydrofolate reductase would already be inhibited by methotrexate or by its polyglutamyl derivatives, and folate-dependent metabolic processes would be suppressed by the time that any significant 7-hydroxymethotrexate had accumulated.

However, 7-hydroxymethotrexate could profoundly influence the effectiveness of leucovorin rescue following methotrexate administration, since the reduced folate is administered at a time when plasma concentrations of 7-hydroxymethotrexate are high. Interference with RFC transport of reduced folates by 7-hydroxymethotrexate (255) would decrease the levels of exogenous tetrahydrofolates available for one-carbon–dependent processes and limit the competitive interactions at dihydrofolate reductase between metabolites of leucovorin and methotrexate that are key to the rescue phenomenon (44,45,256).

B. Distribution of RFCs Versus mFBPs in Human Tumors and Tissues

Most experiments of mFBP structure and function have involved cells and tissues that inherently overproduce this system or have been selected for increased mFBPs that allow growth in subphysiological concentrations of folate cofactors (117–119,155,156,158,159). Whereas FBP transcripts (FBP1 and FBP3) are independently expressed in an assortment of human fetal and adult tissues (190), there is limited information on the actual levels of mFBP receptors in normal tissues and human malignancies; therefore, it is not obvious to what extent the conclusions from experiments with cell lines can be generalized in vivo.

Monoclonal antibodies (MOv18 and MOv19) to epitopes of a glycosylphosphatidylinositol-anchored, 38-kDa ovarian carcinoma glycoprotein, identified as mFBP, were obtained (257) and were reported to detect varying levels of mFBP epitopes in a range of normal tissues by immunohistochemistry or Western blotting (i.e., choroid plexus, fallopian tube, uterus, epididymis, breast acini, submandibular salivary, kidney proximal tubules, lung alveolar lining, bronchial glands, vas deferens, ovary, thyroid, pancreas, and the trophoblastic cells of the placenta; 168,258). Moreover, MOv18 and MOv19 appeared to detect mFBPs in biopsy materials from ovarian and renal carcinomas, as well as primary brain tumors (257–259). Conversely, liver, spleen, myocardium, myometrium, adrenal, cerebrum, cerebellum, spinal cord, thymus, testis, and small intestine, all failed to express MOv19-reactive epitopes (258).

Table 1 Immunohistochemical Detection of GP-MTX in Assorted Human Primary Tumors and Tissues[a]

Tissue or tumor	n	Intensity
Adrenal	5	1–3
Brain	5	0
Heart	5	0
Kidney	5	1
L. intestine	3	1
Liver	5	1–2
Lung	5	0
Ovary	5	0
Pancreas	5	1
Prostate	5	2–3
S. intestine	1	1
Spleen	5	1
Stomach	5	1
Testis	5	1–2
Thyroid	5	1
Uterus	5	1
Acute lymphocytic leukemia	10	2
Astrocytoma	2	1–2
Breast	4	1–3
Carcinoid	3	1
Colon	2	1–2
Epithelial carcinoma	1	0
Ewing's carcinoma	2	0
Gastric carcinoma	2	1–2
Hepatocellular	2	1–3
Hodgkin's lymphoma	13	0
Leiomyoma	2	0
Lung	2	1–2
Lymphoma	3	1–2
Mal. fibrous histiocytoma	1	0
Melanoma	4	2–3
Mesothelioma	2	1
Ovarian–colon	2	1–2
Pancreatic carcinoma	2	0–1
Prostatic carcinoma	2	1–2
Renal	2	1
Rhabdomyosarcoma	2	0–1
Thyroid	2	1
Undifferentiated carcinoma	4	1–2

[a] Formalin-fixed and paraffin-imbedded tissues and tumors were treated with GP-MTX-specific antiserum, followed by avidin–biotin–immunoperoxidase reagents. GP-MTX expression in methanol-fixed ALL blasts (five T-cell, five B-cell) was detected by indirect immunofluorescence with GP-MTX-specific antiserum and antirabbit FITC-labeled secondary antibody. Sections were scored using a scale of 0 (no reactivity) to 3 (darkest). n, number of sections scored.

A more limited distribution of mFBPs, compared with RFCs, was suggested by analogous experiments with specific antisera raised to mFBP1 and GP-MTX, a glycosylated RFC component (203). In contrast with the high levels of expression of immunoreactive GP-MTX in cell lines (K562, CCRF-CEM, KB, SKOV3) and a broad range of tissues and primary tumors (from cytospun cells or multitissue paraffin blocks prepared by Dr. Hector Battifora) (see Ref. 260), mFBPs were detected in only the KB epidermoid carcinoma and SKOV3 ovarian carcinoma lines (even after formalin fixation and paraffin-embedding). The results for the GP-MTX distribution among assorted tissues and primary tumors are summarized in Table 1.

Although it is difficult to reconcile these different conclusions on mFBP expression among independent studies, the results of the latter report, nonetheless, strongly argue that mFBP expression in human tissues and tumors is more restricted and considerably lower than RFC expression. In spite of data that show that mFBPs mediate methotrexate uptake in mFBP-overproducing lines (178,205), it is doubtful that this system plays a major role in methotrexate uptake in vivo, even for tissues or tumors that express these receptors. This is because of the low levels of mFBPs and the direct-binding competition between methotrexate and physiological concentrations (i.e., 20–50 nM) of 5-methyltetrahydrofolate. This route could be of greater importance for antifolate substrates (i.e., ICI D1694 and DDATHF) that bind more avidly to mFBPs than does methotrexate. However, since RFCs are probably present in many tissues that express mFBPs, the high capacity RFC flux would be likely to overshadow the mFBP-uptake component.

VII. MEMBRANE TRANSPORT AND METHOTREXATE RESISTANCE

A. General Considerations

It is apparent from the foregoing discussion that membrane transport of methotrexate and related agents into tumor cells is paramount to their chemotherapeutic effectiveness, since the intracellular antifolate level achieved is an important determinant of direct drug binding to enzyme targets (i.e., dihydrofolate reductase). Moreover, transport is critical to the metabolism of antifolates to polyglutamyl forms required for drug retention and, for certain analogues (DDATHF and ICI D1694), high-affinity binding to enzyme targets. Hence, it is not surprising that impaired membrane transport is a frequently observed mode of antifolate resistance. Resistance generally involves the RFC and, for methotrexate, impaired influx has been reported in cultured murine (120,122,232,261–265) and human (123,244,266–268) tumor cells, as well as murine tumor cells derived in vivo during methotrexate chemotherapy (233). Recent experiments with a fluorescent analogue of methotrexate (PT430), in combination with flow cytometry, detected impaired methotrexate transport accompanying clinical resistance in acute lymphocytic leukemia patients (269). Whereas there have been occasional reports of increased rates of drug efflux in methotrexate-resistant mammalian cells (122,270), these are rare and unlikely to be of general importance.

Although high-affinity mFBPs have also been implicated in the uptake of folates and several "new generation" antifolates by some mammalian cells and tissues (86,88,102,103,118,207) and decreased mFBP levels were recently described in methotrexate-resistant KB cells (204), their roles in in vivo antifolate pharmacology, in general, and methotrexate resistance, in particular, are uncertain. Nonetheless, it is of interest that methotrexate-resistant CCRF-CEM and L1210 cells with impaired RFC function synthesize mFBPs in response to low, nanomolar concentrations of medium folates (117,121,158). An analogous mechanism might provide for the accumulation of endogenous tetrahydrofolates in transport-impaired tumors in vivo.

The interrelations amongst antifolate uptake, binding to intracellular targets, and polyglutamate synthesis are often complicated. Furthermore, for methotrexate, resistance is rarely attributed to a single mechanism, since increased levels of dihydrofolate reductase (120,233,265,271,272), kinetically altered dihydrofolate reductase (265,273–275), or diminished methotrexate polyglutamate synthesis (29,243,244,265,276–279) may accompany impaired methotrexate influx.

The relative importance of these various mechanisms of methotrexate resistance have not been firmly established. Nonetheless, a few generalizations can be made. (1) Both impaired transport and increased dihydrofolate reductase were recorded in methotrexate-resistant mouse leukemia cells following methotrexate chemotherapy in vivo (233). (2) When cells are selected by stepwise increases in methotrexate, alterations in transport accompany low levels of resistance and generally precede elevated levels of dihydrofolate reductase (267,280). This suggests that impaired transport is the first line of defense in tumor cells presented with cytotoxic concentrations of antifolate. (3) At high levels of methotrexate resistance, dihydrofolate reductase almost always predominates (280); however, it is often accompanied by impaired transport and polyglutamate synthesis (244,265,267).

For tumor cells with increased dihydrofolate reductase and normal levels of membrane transport, a greater amount of free intracellular methotrexate is necessary to achieve maximal enzyme suppression than in cells with normal enzyme levels. This results because the percentage of total dihydrofolate reductase necessary to sustain maximal tetrahydrofolate synthesis is decreased, so that a higher level of active site inhibition by methotrexate is required to maximally suppress one-carbon metabolism. Since it is the combination of the administered drug dose and the activity of the membrane transport system that ultimately determines the steady-state methotrexate level required for enzyme saturation, an equivalent effect would result in cells with normal dihydrofolate reductase and decreased drug influx.

Impaired methotrexate transport that renders cells insensitive to conventional doses of drug should, at least in part, be circumvented by increasing the level of extracellular antifolate to force the drug into the cell by a carrier with a reduced affinity, or by increasing entry by passive diffusion. Similar logic applies to the use of high-dose methotrexate (generally with leucovorin rescue) in the treatment of solid tumors. In either case, as extracellular methotrexate is continually increased, a point is eventually reached at which greater drug doses effect a negligible change in the intracellular antifolate concentration. This is because of the saturability of the influx carrier, the electrical restrictions on net antifolate accumulation, and the presence of a high-capacity, energy-dependent efflux system. Hence, it is apparent how relatively small increases in cellular dihydrofolate reductase, or seemingly minor decreases in methotrexate influx, rapidly result in a requirement for a steady-state intracellular drug level that clinically is unattainable.

Numerous reports of polyglutamylation-based methotrexate resistance have appeared (29,243,244,265,276–279). Interpretation of these phenotypes is sometimes nearly impossible, since high levels of methotrexate substrate are necessary to support polyglutamate synthesis within cells, and decreased drug influx results in corresponding changes in both monoglutamyl and polyglutamyl methotrexate. This is further confounded by the inability of investigators to measure significant differences in folylpolyglutamate synthetase catalytic activities in cell-free extracts from wild-type and polyglutamylation-deficient cells (243,265). Although findings of polyglutamylation-based resistance accompanying impaired drug influx must be interpreted with caution, a few reports have described cell lines with decreased methotrexate polyglutamylation independent of transport alterations (277–279).

B. Mechanisms of Impaired Methotrexate Membrane Transport

Membrane transport alterations resulting in methotrexate resistance can manifest as reduced rates of carrier translocation (decreased $V_{\max}$), or of decreased affinities for transport substrates (increased K_t), or both (120,122,123,233). RFC deletions were suggested from the loss of radioaffinity labeling or surface [³H]methotrexate binding in methotrexate-resistant cells in culture (113,128,131,133,262). Alternatively, drug-resistant cells synthesize "defective" RFCs, since nonfunctional carriers in transport-impaired L1210 or CCRF-CEM cells could be identified by radioaffinity labeling with NHS-[³H]methotrexate or surface binding with [³H]methotrexate (86,120,122). Although defective RFCs were also described in transport-impaired L1210 (designated R81) cells by Western analysis with antiserum to placental mFBPs (131), it is uncertain whether the membrane proteins identified in these experiments were actually RFCs. Other studies have suggested that altered expression of membrane proteins seemingly unrelated to the transport carrier may contribute to the transport-impaired phenotype. Hence, decreased levels of immunoreactive SQM1 protein were implicated in the impaired transport of methotrexate and cisplatin in a series of human squamous carcinoma lines (281), and an overproduced 190-kDa membrane glycoprotein was identified in 100-fold methotrexate-resistant L1210 cells (122).

Given the availability of specific antiserum to a component of the human RFC (GP-MTX; see Sec. III.C.2), we recently began a systematic investigation into the causal elements involved in impaired methotrexate membrane transport in drug-resistant human tumor lines derived from K562 erythroleukemia (K200A, K500E;123), CCRF-CEM T-cell leukemia (CEM/MTX;123), and ZR-75-1 breast carcinoma cells (ZR-MTX®). Two apparently distinct mechanisms of impaired influx were identified in these variants by Western blotting. (1) At low levels of methotrexate resistance (33- and 70-fold, respectively, for K200A and K500E sublines), decreased rates of carrier translocation were associated with reduced GP-MTX levels (see Fig. 4). (2) At higher levels of methotrexate resistance (243-fold for CEM/MTX), a decreased translocation rate and reduced affinity for methotrexate accompanied GP-MTX structural alterations, as reflected in an increased electrophoretic mobility on SDS gels for the transport-defective GP-MTX isoform (Fig. 5). The structural alterations in the CEM/MTX GP-MTX isoform appeared to be independent of carrier glycosylation (see Fig. 5) (123) and was accompanied by significant changes in the binding of a wide variety of transport substrates (87).

A structurally altered GP-MTX isoform was, likewise, identified by Western blotting in 1000-fold methotrexate-resistant ZR-75-1 breast carcinoma cells (M. F. Pinard, L. H. Matherly, J. Jolivet, manuscript submitted). Whereas immunoreactive GP-MTX was detected on the surface of both wild-type and methotrexate-resistant ZR-75-1 cells by confocal laser microscopy, only the wild type was capable of internalizing γ-fluorescein

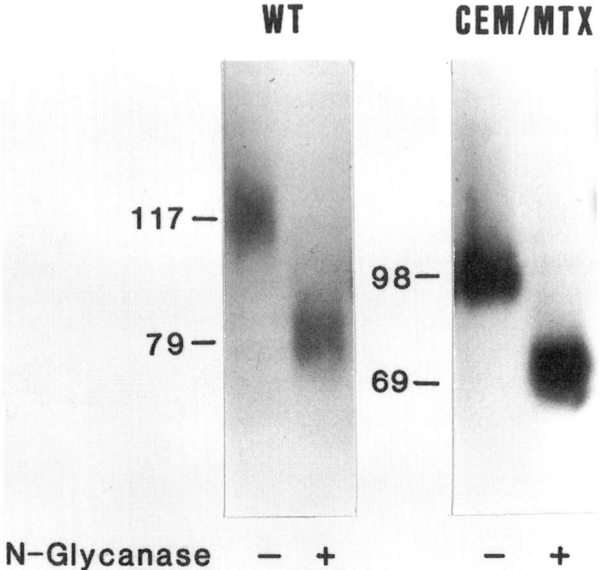

Figure 5 GP-MTX isoforms in wild-type and transport-impaired CCRF-CEM cells. Plasma membranes from wild-type CCRF-CEM (designated WT) and transport-impaired cells (CEM/MTX) were solubilized in 15 mM sodium phosphate, pH 7.2, containing 1.25% N-octylglucoside and 0.2 mM PMSF. Untreated and N-glycanase-digested samples were electrophoresed on 4–10% gradient gels, electrophoretically transferred to Immobilon P, for treatment with GP-MTX-specific antiserum and ^{125}I-Protein A. Immunoreactive complexes were detected by autoradiography. The M_rs of the GP-MTX isoforms are indicated.

methotrexate during short exposures (282), consistent with the presence of an inoperative RFC.

C. Structure–Function Considerations of Antifolate Membrane Transport: Relevance to the Design of Alternative Antifolates

It is essential that considerations of transport specificities be included in any strategy for the design of antifolate inhibitors as chemotherapeutic agents. Over the years, many potent inhibitors of intracellular folate-dependent targets have been described that exhibited abysmal levels of pharmacological activity in tissue culture or in vivo owing to their poor cellular uptake. Partly because of its longevity as a recognized mode of folate and antifolate transport, the substrate specificities for RFC-mediated transport have been reasonably well characterized. More recently, interest has focused on the therapeutic exploitation of mFBPs, since these receptors exhibit a somewhat different spectrum of (anti)folate specificities from the RFCs. Only a limited number of radiolabeled antifolates have been prepared and are available for direct measurements of membrane transport. Consequently, many studies have relied on cytotoxicity determinations in the presence of competing folates, or on assays of competitive inhibition of RFC-mediated [³H]methotrexate influx or [³H]folic acid binding to mFBPs as indirect measures of relative uptake activity.

1. RFC-Mediated Transport

Differences in membrane transport for various RFC substrates generally reflect changes in binding affinities (i.e., K_t), rather than rates of carrier translocation (i.e., V_{max}). The 4-aminopteridine structure is critical to RFC binding, since folic acid binds 50- to 100-fold less avidly than does aminopterin, methotrexate, or related structures (46,87,102,103,112,115, 150,207). However, reduction of the pteridine ring, as in 5-methyl- and 5-formyltetrahydrofolate, restores high-affinity binding for 4-oxo,2-amino-antifolate substrates to levels approximating the 2,4-diamino antifolates (K_t = 1–5 μM). DDATHF is a tetrahydrofolate analogue that differs by carbon-for-nitrogen substitutions at positions 5 and 10 and, likewise, is an excellent substrate for RFC transport (K_t = 0.7–1.5 μM; 86, 87). Transport is 2.3-fold more efficient for (6R)DDATHF over its (6S)-stereoisomer (86). Although equivalent substrate activity for the (6S)- and (6R)-stereo-isomers of 5-methyltetrahydrofolates were reported for the murine RFC (99,100), transport was highly stereospecific for (6S)5-formyltetrahydrofolate (101).

The bridge N-10 is also an important determinant of RFC-mediated uptake; however, the effects of alkylation of the 10-position differ depending on whether an N-10 (as in aminopterin) or C-10 (i.e., 10-deazaamino-pterin) is involved (46,52). Hence, 10-deazaaminopterin and its 10-ethyl-substituted analogue are comparable transport substrates, whereas aminopterin is approximately four- to fivefold more active than methotrexate (46,52). Finally, substitution at the 7-position (as in 7-hydroxy-methotrexate) causes only a slight (two- to fourfold) reduction in transport efficiency (46,253).

The quinazoline thymidylate synthase inhibitor, CB3717, is a poor substrate for RFC uptake, compared with its 2-desamino-2-methyl- (ICI 198583) and N^{10}-methylthiophene (ICI D1694) analogues (approx. 30-fold difference; 102,103,207). The 3-methylbenzoquinazoline analogue, 1843U89, is the tightest-binding substrate for the human RFC yet reported (75,87). In MOLT 4 human lymphocytic leukemia cells, 1843U89 is characterized by a K_t of 0.33 μM and a V_{max}/K_t of 20.3 (75). These constants are, respectively, 12-fold less and 80-fold greater than the corresponding values for RFC transport of 1843U89 in murine L1210 cells (75). Moreover, these differences likely account for the greater antitumor activities of 1843U89 against human versus murine tumors in vitro (ranging from 102- to 1325-fold for different tumors) (75) and, presumably, reflect the disparate structures of these homologous transport systems from different species (see Sec. III.C.2).

2. mFBP Uptake

Substrate activity for mFBPs also correlates with binding affinity. Whereas the 2-amino, 4-oxo structures exemplified by folic acid and CB3717 are poor RFC substrates, these are among the tightest-binding substrates for mFBPs (102,103,207). Likewise, ICI 198583, ICI D1694, and DDATHF are excellent substrates for mFBPs (30–80% as efficient as folic acid) (86,88,89,102,103,207). Modification of N-3 (i.e., 3-deaza ICI-198583) or replacement of the 4-oxo group by 4-H (i.e., 4-deoxy ICI-198583) of ICI 198583 decreases the apparent binding affinities 333- and 16-fold, respectively; the effects of modifications involving the quinazoline and heterocyclic benzoyl rings or the glutamate side chain of ICI 198583 were minimal (102).

Recent studies focused on the relative specificities of the human mFBP1 versus mFBP2 isoforms (89). Hence, mFBP1 exhibited 2- to 100-fold greater affinities over mFBP2 for folic acid, methotrexate, and the (6S)- and (6R)-stereoisomers of 5-methyl- and 5-formyltetrahydrofolate, and DDATHF. Furthermore, mFBP1 preferentially bound the physiological (6S)-diastereomers of 5-formyl- and 5-methyltetrahydrofolate, whereas mFBP2 bound the unnatural (6R)-isomers with greater affinities. By contrast, the stereospecificity for the (6S)- over the (6R)DDATHF stereoisomer for either the mFBP1 or mFBP2 isoforms was much reduced (89). Similar findings were recently reported by Brigle et al. (283) for the murine homologues of mFBP1 and mFBP2.

3. Relevance of mFBP and RFC-Mediated Transport to Drug Selectivity and Resistance

The demonstration of even slightly distinct substrate specificities for RFC versus mFBP binding suggests the potential of targeting antifolate inhibitors to specific tissues or tumors based on their expression of a particular uptake system. This model is based on a notion that a *single predominant transport system* is expressed in a certain tissue or tumor type; however, it is certain that multiple influx and efflux systems coexist, although a differential up- or down-regulation in response to external stimuli may significantly alter their relative proportions. Hence, the concept of antifolate selectivity that is predicated primarily on the expression of a particular mode of membrane uptake seems unlikely. Rather, selective antifolate activity is likely a composite of multiple parameters, including transport, polyglutamylation, and intracellular binding. For tumors or tissues with *both* mFBPs and RFCs, the relative magnitudes of the respective membrane fluxes for agents that use both systems will be determined by the extracellular drug levels, since only mFBPs will be maximally active at even the lowest (i.e., nanomolar) concentrations. However, the selectivity afforded by an already-saturated mFBP uptake component will be lost at higher (micromolar) drug concentrations, which favor an increased contribution from the RFC flux.

Methotrexate-resistant CCRF-CEM and L1210 lines with defective RFCs have been described with high levels of mFBP expression when cultured in subphysiological concentrations of folates (117,158). If an analogous phenotype occurs in vivo, it may be possible to circumvent methotrexate resistance with antifolate substrates (CB3717, ICI D1694, ICI 198583, or DDATHF) for mFBPs. In addition, since these drugs all inhibit enzyme targets other than dihydrofolate reductase (i.e., thymidylate synthase or GAR transformylase), they can circumvent methotrexate resistance resulting from elevated or structurally altered dihydrofolate reductase. However, since polyglutamylation is essential to the pharmacological effects of all these antifolates, cross-resistance would likely be observed for tumors with defective polyglutamylation.

4. *The Anomaly of DDATHF: The Basis for the Disparate Antitumor Activities of* (6R) *DDATHF and Methotrexate Toward Methotrexate-Resistant Tumor Cells with Severely Impaired Antifolate Membrane Transport*

As described earlier (see Sec. VI.A), in part due to its high K_m for mammalian folylpolyglutamate synthetase, membrane transport of methotrexate is limiting to methotrexate polyglutamate accumulation. However, for antifolates that are significantly better folylpolyglutamate synthetase substrates than methotrexate, a very different relationship between transport and polyglutamate synthesis is possible (87).

For instance, methotrexate-resistant CCRF-CEM cells (CEM/MTX) polyglutamylate the GAR transformylase inhibitor, DDATHF, so extensively that even severe impairment in RFC-mediated drug uptake (95–97%) is effectively circumvented (87). In experiments with nominal concentrations (2 μM) of [^{14}C]DDATHF, over short exposure times (i.e., 10 min), virtually all of the intracellular drug is polyglutamylated. This suggests that for this excellent folylpolyglutamate synthetase substrate (approx. 60-fold better than methotrexate) (82,85), *transport is rate-limiting to its metabolism*. The net result is nearly equivalent accumulations in both wild-type and transport-impaired CCRF-CEM cells of highly retained long chain length DDATHF polyglutamyl forms. This occurs in spite of very large differences in intracellular levels of monoglutamyl substrate, and results in an impressive lack of cross-resistance for DDATHF (3.6-fold) compared with other antifolate inhibitors (162- to 300-fold, including methotrexate, aminopterin, 10-Edam, ICI D1694, and 1843U89). An analogous effect to that seen with DDATHF might occur with other antifolates that are polyglutamylated to high levels, for other transport-impaired cells with adequate levels of drug uptake to sustain polyglutamate synthesis, and for which folylpolyglutamate synthesis is not limiting.

D. The Role of Lipid-Soluble Antifolates in Antifolate Therapeutics

1. General Considerations

As the search continues for improved antifolate therapeutics, the concept of completely removing the charge on the antifolate molecule periodically resurfaces. The significance of this modification relates to the elimination of the requirement for receptor-mediated drug uptake altogether, since an uncharged antifolate should be able to readily diffuse across plasma membranes. These nonclassic antifolates should, likewise, penetrate the blood–brain barrier, permitting access to tumors within the central nervous system, as well as solid tumors. Moreover, these inhibitors circumvent antifolate resistance owing to impaired RFC uptake (62,120).

This mechanistic approach to drug design, typified by the prototype, metoprine (DDMP; 2,4-diamino-5-(3′,4′-dichlorophenyl)-6-methyl pyrimidine) (284), is among the first to significantly affect the field of antifolate therapeutics. Second-generation lipid-soluble antifolates include trimetrexate (2,4-diamino-5-methyl-6-(3,4,5-trimethoxyanilino)methyl quinazoline) (285–287) and piritrexim (BW301; 3,4-diamino-6-(2,5-dimethoxybenzyl)-5-methylpyrido[2,3-*d*]pyrimidine) (288,289). All of these agents were developed as potent inhibitors of dihydrofolate reductase, albeit generally less so than for methotrexate. However, they generally exhibit greater in vitro cytotoxicity.

For trimetrexate, uptake occurs in direct proportion to the extracellular drug concentration (290,291) and, presumably, involves simple diffusion, although evidence for a facilitated diffusion has been described (290). In part because of a large nonspecific binding component (290,291), high levels of antifolate are accumulated within cells, far in excess of that achieved at comparable extracellular concentrations of methotrexate.

Even after efflux into drug-free medium, the total level of cellular antifolate (mostly nonspecific) still exceeds the dihydrofolate reductase-binding capacity by a large margin (290,291). Hence, correlations between pharmacological activities and *total* or *nonexchangeable* antifolate accumulations, analogous to methotrexate, are impossible to establish for these agents. Although these lipid-soluble antifolates circumvent resistance associated with defective methotrexate membrane transport in vitro, methotrexate-resistant strains that overproduce dihydrofolate reductase are generally cross-resistant to these drugs (62). Another notable feature of these nonclassic inhibitors is the absence of the structural determinants necessary for binding and polyglutamylation by folylpolyglutamate synthetase. Consequently, these agents should be active against resistant tumors with "defective" polyglutamylation, albeit at the expense of a less-sustained, in vivo activity and the therapeutic selectivity afforded by polyglutamylation.

The use of lipid-soluble antifolates in combination with leucovorin has been promoted as a means of targeting antifolate activity toward methotrexate-resistant tumors with impaired RFC transport, since these tumors, likewise, would be incapable of transporting tetrahydrofolate cofactors circulating in plasma or generated from exogenous leucovorin (292). Conversely, susceptible host tissues with normal transport activity should accumulate sufficient levels of tetrahydrofolates to circumvent the effects of the antifolate. Interestingly, tumors expressing mFBPs in the absence of RFCs are collaterally sensitive to trimetrexate and are essentially unaffected by the provision of leucovorin (293).

Trimetrexate and piritrexim exhibit impressive in vitro activity against a variety of murine and human cell lines, and in vivo activity against several murine transplanted tumors (285,286,288,289,294,295). Although clinical trials have indicated responses in assorted tumors, notably colon, head and neck, breast, sarcoma, and lung cancers, and malignant melanoma (295–303), the considerable promise offered by this approach to antifolate drug design has yet to be realized.

2. The Role of Membrane Transport Alterations in the Resistance to Nonclassic Antifolates

Although trimetrexate and related agents presumably diffuse bidirectionally across plasma membranes, membrane transport alterations still play a significant role in the resistance to these lipid-soluble inhibitors. For instance, WI-L2 human lymphoblastoid cells, highly resistant to trimetrexate (62-fold), metoprine (68-fold), and piritrexim (96-fold), were reported with a 50% decreased rate of [^{14}C]trimetrexate influx and net drug accumulation (290). Moreover, resistance to lipid-soluble antifolates is commonly a component of the multidrug-resistant phenotype, in which mammalian cells are treated or selected with a single chemotherapeutic agent can acquire resistance to a wide range of lipid-soluble or cationic drugs with no or limited structural or functional similarities (i.e., anthracyclines, vinca alkaloids, epidophyllotoxins, dactinomycin, and colchicine; see Chap. 17). Resistance is widely associated with the overproduction of the highly glycosylated ATP-dependent drug efflux pump, P-glycoprotein, increased transcriptional rates of the gene(s) that encodes P-glycoprotein and, occasionally, amplification of the P-glycoprotein genes (240). Hence, Klohs et al. (304), Assaraf et al. (305), and Arkin et al. (306) all demonstrated collateral resistance to lipid-soluble antifolates in multidrug-resistant tumor lines. In trimetrexate-resistant breast and ovarian carcinoma lines, resistance was reversible by quinidine or verapamil, suggesting direct competition for antifolate binding to P-glycoprotein (305).

Of particular interest were experiments that examined the changes in dihydrofolate reductase versus P-glycoprotein expression, accompanying the stepwise selection of trimetrexate resistance (307). Hence, low levels of trimetrexate resistance in Chinese hamster ovary cells were associated only with increased expression of dihydrofolate reductase; at higher resistance levels, the multidrug-resistant gene was amplified and the overproduction of P-glycoprotein resulted in widespread resistance, not only to lipid-soluble antifolates, but also to doxorubicin (Adriamycin), dactinomycin (actinomycin D), vinca alkaloids, etoposide, and colchicine (307). It is notable that low levels of piritrexim resistance involved an unknown mechanism, independent of either dihydrofolate reductase or P-glycoprotein. An analogous mode of piritrexim resistance was recently described in a patient with head and neck cancer in a Phase II trial with oral piritrexim (308). At higher levels of piritrexim resistance, dihydrofolate reductase was amplified; however, increased P-glycoprotein was still not observed (307). Hence, the use of nonclassic antifolates, such as trimetrexate, may circumvent transport-mediated resistance to methotrexate; however, these agents may themselves select for increased levels of dihydrofolate reductase or the multidrug-resistant phenotype.

VIII. CONCLUSIONS AND PERSPECTIVES

This chapter attempts to provide an overview of the role of membrane transport in the pharmacology of the antifolate therapeutics currently used for treating cancer. The modern era of cancer chemotherapy was ushered in over 40 years ago with the introduction of these agents for the clinical management of acute lymphocytic leukemia—long before the molecular bases for their antitumor effects and therapeutic selectivities were established. In the intervening years, the clinical use of methotrexate has expanded considerably, as has our understanding of the biochemistry and molecular biology of the cellular processes involved in the antitumor activity and therapeutic selectivity of this and related agents. These relate to the interactions of diverse antifolates with intracellular enzyme targets, their metabolism to polyglutamyl conjugates and 7-hydroxyl catabolite, the selectivity of leucovorin rescue, and development of drug resistance. As described in this review, membrane transport is critical to virtually all facets of antifolate activity.

The present picture of membrane transport involves a level of complexity unimaginable as recently as 1985. Not only have non-RFC transport systems been identified and extensively characterized, but distinct folate receptor isoforms have been described that exhibit unique patterns of tissue expression and substrate-binding specificities from each other and also the classic RFC system. Although the development of specific probes of RFC structure and function has permitted new insights into mechanisms of transport-based methotrexate resistance, a host of previously unrecognized vagaries relating to RFC transport have surfaced. These include its regulation by folates and purine nucleosides, the possible involvement of multiple membrane protein components, and the identification of structural and functional differences between the murine and human RFC homologues.

Even though major insight has been gained over the past decade into the structure, function, and genetics of the family of mFBP receptors, we are only marginally closer to understanding the physiological and pharmacological roles of these proteins in diverse tissues and cells. Hence, investigations have, by necessity, employed in vitro cell models that overexpress mFBPs to the exclusion of other systems; however, there is virtually no indication of whether the principles gleaned from many of these experiments are in any way predictive of in vivo events, during which elements, including endogenous competing folate substrates and lower expression levels, all come into play. Moreover, although cDNAs for at least three mFBP isoforms have been isolated and sequenced, their functional and regulatory significance is uncertain.

Furthermore, the detection of multiple transport systems in a single cell or tissue type, coupled with the wide distribution of the RFC system among assorted tumors and normal tissues, strongly suggest that expression of a particular uptake mode is unlikely, by itself, to confer significant therapeutic selectivity to antifolate inhibitors. Rather, drug selectivity is undoubtedly a function of a host of pharmacokinetic and pharmacodynamic parameters, including plasma clearance, metabolism, and enzyme binding, as well as transport.

Although the vast literature relating to antifolate inhibitors has, by necessity, focused on studies of radiolabeled methotrexate transport, it is essential to recognize that many of the key concepts concerning the interrelations between transport, enzyme binding, and polyglutamylation for methotrexate may not always apply to certain of the newer agents. This is aptly illustrated by the GAR transformylase inhibitor, DDATHF, for which increased substrate activity for folylpolyglutamate synthetase effectively circumvents limitations on drug accumulation imposed by the RFC transport system in transport-impaired tumors.

As structural determinants for folate and antifolate transport become clearer, approaches to drug design must incorporate constraints dictated by the requirements for binding by different influx and efflux systems. The design of antifolate inhibitors with greater cellular retention based on their increased affinities for one or more uptake systems or their lack of substrate activity for the major drug efflux pump, may ultimately be possible. Moreover, studies should focus on identifying specific blockers of one or more efflux systems to promote increased net antifolate uptake. Even if approaches for effectively blocking a particular efflux process are developed, the presence of more than one separate efflux pump may obviate any detectable benefits achieved. Within the context of the complications imposed by the development of multidrug resistance or alternative modes of resistance, it is important to reassess whether the use of lipid-soluble antifolate therapeutics truly represents a viable strategy for penetrating tumor sanctuaries or for treating solid or methotrexate-resistant tumors.

Finally, a major goal of research into the biology of antifolate transport processes involves the understanding of transport-based resistance. Although a methotrexate-binding component of the human RFC has been isolated, and specific antiserum to this protein has identified possible causal elements in this mode of resistance, it will be critical to further explore these issues once cDNA cloning and expression of the human RFC has been finalized. The molecular characterization of RFC transport in this fashion will better facilitate the detection of transport-based antifolate resistance in cancer patients, including the identification of specific markers, the expression of which correlate with response to therapy.

ACKNOWLEDGMENTS

I would like to thank Dr. So Wong for her critical reading of the text and Ms. Daryel Taliaferro for assistance in preparing this review. This work was supported by grant CA53535 from the National Cancer Institute, National Institutes of Health, and a Scholar Award from the Leukemia Society of America, Inc.

APPENDIX: ABBREVIATIONS

AICAR	aminoimidazolecarboxamide ribonucleotide
APA-ASA-Lys	N^{α}-(4-amino-4-deoxy-10-methylpteroyl)-N^{ϵ}-(4-azido-5-salicylyl)-L-lysine
CB3717	N^{10}-propargyl-5,8-dideazafolate
DDATHF	5,10-dideaza-5,6,7,8-tetrahydrofolate
DIDS	4,4′-diisothiocyano-2,2′-disulfonic acid stilbene
10-Edam	10-ethyl-10-deazaaminopterin
GAR	glycinamide ribonucleotide
GP-MTX	a glycosylated RFC component, as defined in the text
ICI 198583	2-desamino-2-methyl-N^{10}-propargyl-5,8-dideazafolate
ICID1694	N-(5-[N-(3,4-dihydro-2-methyl-4-oxoquinazolin-6-ylmethyl)-N-methylamino]-2-thenoyl)-L-glutamic acid
IAP	intracisternal A particle
K_t	Michaelis–Menten constant for transport
LTR	long-terminal repeat
mFBP1–3	membrane folate-binding protein isoforms 1 to 3, as defined in the text
NHS	N-hydroxysuccinimide
RFC	reduced folate carrier
SDS	sodium dodecyl sulfate
SITS	4′-acetamide-4′-isothiocyanostilbene-2,2′-disulfonic acid
1843U89	(S)-2-(5((((1,2-dihydro-3-methyl-1-oxobenzo(F) quinolin-9-yl) methyl)amino)-1-oxo-2-isoindolinyl) glutaric acid.

REFERENCES

1. Goldman ID, Matherly LH. The cellular pharmacology of methotrexate. Pharmacol Ther 1985; 28:77–100.
2. Henderson GB. Folate binding proteins. Annu Rev Nutr 1990; 10:319–335.
3. Sirotnak FM. Correlates of folate analog transport, pharmacokinetics, and selective antitumor action. Pharmacol Ther 1980; 8:71–103.
4. Antony AC. The biological chemistry of folate receptors. Blood 1992; 79:2807–2820.
5. McGuire JJ, Coward JK. Pteroylpolyglutamates. Biosynthesis, degradation, and function. In: Blakley RL, Benkovic SJ, eds. Chemistry and Biochemistry of Folates. New York: John Wiley & Sons, 1984:135–190.
6. Shane B. Folylpolyglutamate synthesis and role in the regulation of one-carbon metabolism. Vitam Horm 1989; 45:263–335.
7. Foo SK, Shane B. Regulation of folylpoly-γ-glutamate synthesis in mamma-

lian cells. In vivo and in vitro synthesis of pteroylpoly-γ-glutamates by Chinese hamster ovary cells. J Biol Chem 1982; 257:13587–13592.

8. McBurney MW, Whitmore GF. Isolation and biochemical characterization of folate deficient mutants of Chinese hamster cells. Cell 1974; 2:173–182.

9. Seither RL, Trent DF, Mikulecky DC, Rape TJ, Goldman ID. Folate pool interconversions and inhibition of biosynthetic processes after exposure of L1210 cells to antifolates. Experimental and network thermodynamic analyses of the role of dihydrofolate polyglutamates in antifolate action in cells. J Biol Chem 1989; 264:17016–17023.

10. Seither RL, Trent DF, Mikulecky DC, Rape TJ, Goldman ID. Effect of direct suppression of thymidylate synthase at the 5,10-methylene tetrahydrofolate binding site on the interconversion of tetrahydrofolate cofactors to dihydrofolate by antifolates: influence of degree of dihydrofolate inhibition. J Biol Chem 1991; 266:4112–4118.

11. Matherly LH, Muench SP. Evidence for a localized conversion of endogenous tetrahydrofolate cofactors to dihydrofolate as an important element in antifolate action in murine leukemia cells. Biochem Pharmacol 1990; 39:2005–2014.

12. Farber S, Diamond LK, Mercer RD, Sylvester RF, Wolff JA. Temporary remissions in acute leukemia in children produced by the folic acid antagonist 4-aminopteroylglutamic acid (aminopterin). N Engl J Med 1978; 238:787–793.

13. Goldin A, Venditti JM, Humphreys SR, Dennis D, Mantel N, Greenhouse SW. A quantitative comparison of the antileukemic effectiveness of two folic acid antagonists in mice. JNCI 1955; 15:1657–1664.

14. Osborne MJ, Freeman M, Huennekens FM. Inhibition of dihydrofolate reductase by aminopterin and amethopterin. Proc Soc Exp Biol Med 1958; 97:429–431.

15. Jolivet J, Cowan KH, Curt GA, Clendeninn NJ, Chabner BA. The pharmacology and clinical use of methotrexate. N Engl J Med 1983; 309:1094–1104.

16. Cha S. Tight binding inhibitors. I. Kinetic behavior. Biochem Pharmacol 1975; 24:2177–2185.

17. Williams JW, Dugglby RG, Cutler R, Morrison JF. The inhibition of dihydrofolate reductase by folate analogues: structural requirements for slow and tight binding inhibition. Biochem Pharmacol 1980; 29:589–595.

18. Blakley RL. Dihydrofolate reductase. In: Blakley RL, Benkovic SJ, eds. Chemistry and Biochemistry of Folates. New York: John Wiley & Sons, 1984:191–253.

19. Goldman ID. The mechanism of action of methotrexate. I. Interaction with a low affinity intracellular site required for maximum inhibition of deoxyribonucleic acid synthesis in L-cell mouse fibroblasts. Mol Pharmacol 1974; 10:257–274.

20. White JC. Reversal of methotrexate binding to dihydrofolate reductase by dihydrofolate. Studies with purified enzyme and computer modeling using network thermodynamics. J Biol Chem 1979; 254:10889–10895.

21. White JC, Goldman ID. Mechanism of action of methotrexate. IV. Free intracellular methotrexate required to suppress dihydrofolate reduction to tetrahydrofolate by Ehrlich ascites tumor cells in vitro. Mol Pharmacol 1976; 12:711–719.

22. White JC, Loftfield S, Goldman ID. The mechanism of action of methotrexate. IV. Requirement of free intracellular methotrexate for maximal suppression of ^{14}C-formate incorporation into nucleic acids and proteins. Mol Pharmacol 1975; 11:287–297.

23. Jackson RC, Harrap KR. Studies with a mathematical model of folate metabolism. Arch Biochem Biophys 1973; 158:827–841.

24. Jackson RC, Niethammer D, Hart LI. Reactivation of dihydrofolate reductase inhibited by methotrexate or aminopterin. Arch Biochem Biophys 1977; 182:646–656.

25. White JC, Goldman ID. Methotrexate resistance in a L1210 cell line resulting from increased dihydrofolate reductase, decreased thymidylate synthetase activity, and normal membrane transport: computer simulations based on network thermodynamics. J Biol Chem 1981; 256:5722–5727.

26. Kamen B, Nylen P, Whitehead V, Abelson H, Dolnick B, Peterson D. Lack of dihydrofolate reductase in human tumor and leukemia cells in vivo. Cancer Drug Deliv 1985; 2:133–138.

27. Drake JC, Allegra CJ, Baram J, Kaufman BT, Chabner BA. Effects on dihydrofolate reductase of methotrexate metabolites and intracellular folates formed following methotrexate exposure of human breast cancer cells. Biochem Pharmacol 1987; 36:2416–2418.

28. Kumar P, Kisliuk RL, Gaumont Y, Freisheim JH, Nair M.G. Inhibition of human dihydrofolate reductase by antifolyl polyglutamates. Biochem Pharmacol 1989; 38:541–543.

29. Curt GA, Jolivet J, Bailey BD, Carney DN, Chabner BA. Synthesis and retention of methotrexate polyglutamates by human small cell lung cancer. Biochem Pharmacol 1984; 33:1682–1685.

30. Fry DW, Yalowich JC, Goldman ID. Rapid formation of poly-γ-glutamyl derivatives of methotrexate and their association with dihydrofolate reductase as assessed by high pressure liquid chromatography in Ehrlich ascites tumor cells. J Biol Chem 1982; 257:1890–1896.

31. Galivan J. Evidence for the cytotoxic activity of polyglutamate derivatives of methotrexate. Mol Pharmacol 1980; 17:105–110.

32. Galivan J, Nimec Z. Effects of folinic acid on hepatoma cells containing methotrexate polyglutamates. Cancer Res 1983; 43:551–555.

33. Jolivet J, Schilsky RL, Bailey BD, Drake JC, Chabner BA. Synthesis, retention, and biological activity of methotrexate polyglutamates in cultured human breast cancer cells. J Clin Invest 1982; 70:351–360.

34. McGuire JJ, Mini E, Hsieh P, Bertino JJ. Role of methotrexate polyglutamates in methotrexate and sequential methotrexate-5-fluorouracil mediated cell kill. Cancer Res 1985; 45:6395–6400.

35. Rosenblatt DS, Whitehead VM, Vera N, Pottier A, DuPont M, Vuchich MJ.

Prolonged inhibition of DNA synthesis associated with the accumulation of methotrexate polyglutamates in cultured human cells. Mol Pharmacol 1978; 14:1143–1147.

36. Fabre I, Fabre G, Goldman ID. Selectivity of glycine, adenosine, and thymidine protection of granulocytic progenitor cells versus tumor cells against methotrexate cytotoxicity in vitro. Correlation with the formation of methotrexate polyglutamates. Cancer Res 1984; 44:3190–3195.

37. Fabre G, Fabre I, Matherly LH, Goldman ID. Polyglutamylation of methotrexate as a key element in drug cytotoxicity and selectivity: formation of 7-hydroxymethotrexate polyglutamyl derivatives within tumor cells. In: Goldman ID, ed. Proceedings of the Second Workshop on Folyl and Antifolyl Polyglutamates. New York: Praeger Publishers, 1985:125–151.

38. Fry DW, Anderson LA, Borst M, Goldman ID. Analysis of the role of membrane transport and polyglutamylation of methotrexate in gut and the Ehrlich tumor in vivo as factors in drug sensitivity and selectivity. Cancer Res 1983; 43:1087–1092.

39. Koizumi S, Curt GA, Fine RL, Griffin JD, Chabner BA. Formation of methotrexate polyglutamates in purified myeloid precursor cells from normal human bone marrow. J Clin Invest 1985; 75:1008–1014.

40. Poser RG, Sirotnak FM, Chello PL. Differential synthesis of methotrexate polyglutamates in normal proliferative and neoplastic mouse tissues in vivo. Cancer Res 1981; 41:4441–4446.

41. Allegra CJ, Chabner BA, Drake JC, Lutz R, Rodbard D, Jolivet J. Enhanced inhibition of thymidylate synthase by methotrexate polyglutamates. J Biol Chem 1985; 260:9720–9726.

42. Allegra CJ, Drake J, Jolivet J, Chabner BA. Inhibition of phosphoribosyl aminoimidazolecarboxamide transformylase by methotrexate and dihydrofolate acid polyglutamates. Proc Natl Acad Sci USA 1985; 82:4881–4885.

43. Allegra CJ, Drake JC, Jolivet J, Chabner BA. Inhibition of folate-dependent enzymes by methotrexate polyglutamates. In: Goldman ID, ed. Proceedings of the Second Workshop on Folyl and Antifolyl Polyglutamates. New York: Praeger Publishers, 1985:348–359.

44. Matherly LH, Barlowe CK, Phillips VM, Goldman ID. The effects of 4-amino antifolates on 5-formyltetrahydrofolate metabolism in L1210 cells. A biochemical basis for the selectivity of leucovorin rescue. J Biol Chem 1987; 262:710–717.

45. Matherly LH, Seither RL, Goldman ID. Metabolism of the diamino antifolates: biosynthesis and pharmacology of the 7-hydroxyl and polyglutamyl metabolites of methotrexate and related antifolates. Pharmacol Ther 1987; 35:27–56.

46. Moccio DM, Sirotnak FM, Samuels LL, Ahmed A, Yagoda A, DeGraw JI, Piper JR. Similar specificity of membrane transport for folate analogues and their metabolites by murine and human tumor cells: a clinically directed laboratory study. Cancer Res 1984; 44:352–357.

47. George S, Cichowicz DJ, Shane B. Mammalian folylpoly-γ-glutamate synthetase. 3. Specificity for folate analogues. Biochemistry 1987; 26:522–529.

48. Moran RG, Colman PD, Rosowsky A, Forsch RA, Chan KK. Structural features of 4-amino antifolates required for substrate activity with mammalian folylpolyglutamate synthetase. Mol Pharmacol 1985; 27:156–166.

49. Rumberger BG, Barrueco JR, Sirotnak FM. Differing specificities for 4-aminofolate analogues, of folylpolyglutamyl synthetase from tumors and proliferative intestinal epithelium of the mouse with significance for selective antitumor action. Cancer Res 1990; 50:4639–4643.

50. Matherly LH, Voss MK, Anderson LA, Fry DW, Goldman ID. Enhanced polyglutamylation of aminopterin relative to methotrexate in the Ehrlich ascites tumor cell in vitro. Cancer Res 1985; 45:1073–1078.

51. Samuels LL, Moccio DM, Sirotnak FM. Similar differential for total polyglutamylation and cytotoxicity among various folate analogues in human and murine tumor cells in vitro. Cancer Res 1985; 45:1488–1495.

52. Sirotnak FM, Schmid FA, Samuels LL, DeGraw JI. 10-Ethyl-10-deazaaminopterin: structural design and biochemical, pharmacologic, and antitumor properties. NCI Monogr 1987; 5:127–131.

53. Sirotnak FM, DeGraw JI, Moccio DM, Samuels LL, Goutas LJ. New folate analogs of the 10-deazaaminopterin series. Further evidence for markedly increased antitumor efficacy compared to methotrexate in ascitic and solid murine tumor models. Cancer Chemother Pharmacol 1984; 12:26–30.

54. Schmid FA, Sirotnak FM, Otter GM, DeGraw JI. New folate analogs of the 10-deazaaminopterin series. Markedly increased activity of the 10-ethyl analog compared to the parent compound and methotrexate against some human tumor xenographs in nude mice. Cancer Treat Rep 1985; 69:551–553.

55. Sirotnak FM, DeGraw JI, Moccio DM, Samuels LL, Goutas, LJ. New folate analogs of the 10-deaza-aminopterin series. Basis for structural design and biochemical and pharmacologic properties. Cancer Chemother Pharmacol 1984; 12:18–25.

56. Kris MF, Kinahan JJ, Gralla RJ, Fanucchi MP, Wertheim MS, O'Connell JP, Marks LD, Williams L, Farag F, Young CW, Sirotnak FM. Phase I trial and clinical pharmacological evaluation of 10-ethyl-10-deazaaminopterin in adult patients with advanced cancer. Cancer Res 1988; 48:5573–5579.

57. Kemeny N, Israel K, O'Hehir M. Phase II trial of 10-Edam in patients with advanced colorectal carcinoma. Am J Clin Oncol 1990; 13:42–44.

58. Shum KY, Kris, MG, Gralla RJ, Burhe MT, Marks LD, Heelan RT. Phase II study of 10-ethyl-10-deazaaminopterin in patients with stage III and IV non-small cell lung cancer. J Clin Oncol 1988; 6:446–450.

59. Jackson RC, Jackman AL, Calvert AH. Biochemical effects of a quinazoline inhibitor of thymidylate synthetase N-(4-(N-((2-amino-4-hydroxy-6-quinazolinyl)methyl)prop-2-ynylamino)benzoyl)-L-glutamic acid (CB3717), on human lymphoblastoid cells. Biochem Pharmacol 1983; 32:3783–3790.

60. Cheng YC, Dutschman GE, Starnes MC, Fisher, MH, Nanavathi NT, Nair MG. Activity of the new antifolate, N^{10}-propargyl-5,8-dideazafolate and its polyglutamates against human dihydrofolate reductase, human thymidylate synthetase, and KB cells containing different levels of dihydrofolate reductase. Cancer Res 1985; 45:598–600.

61. Sikora E, Jackman AL, Newell DR, Calvert AH. Formation and retention and biological activity of N^{10}-propargyl-5,8-dideazafolic acid (CB3717) polyglutamates in L1210 cells in vitro. Biochem Pharmacol 1988; 37:4047–4054.

62. Diddens H, Niethammer D, Jackson RC. Patterns of cross resistance to the antifolate drugs trimetrexate, metoprine, homofolate, and CB3717 in human lymphoma and osteosarcoma cells resistant to methotrexate. Cancer Res 1983; 43:5286–5292.

63. Calvert AH, Alison DL, Harland SJ, Robinson BA, Jackman AL, Jones TR, Newell DR, Siddik ZH, Wiltshaw E, McElwain TJ, Smith ID, Harrap, KR. A Phase 1 evaluation of the quinazoline antifolate thymidylate synthase inhibitor N^{10}-propargyl-5,8-dideazafolic acid, CB3717. J Clin Oncol 1986; 4:1245–1252.

64. Bassendine MF, Curtin NJ, Loose H, Harris AL, James OFW. Indication of remission in hepatocellular carcinoma with a new thymidylate synthase inhibitor, CB3717: a Phase II study. J Hepatol 1987; 4:349–356.

65. Cantwell BMJ, Macaulay V, Harris AL, Kaye SB, Smith IE, Milstead RAV, Calvert AH. Phase II study of the antifolate N^{10}-propargyl-5,8-dideazafolic acid (CB3717) in advanced breast cancer. Eur J Cancer Clin Oncol 1988; 24:733–736.

66. Calvert AH, Newell DR, Jackman AL, Gumbrell LA, Sikora E, Grzelakowska-Sztabert B, Bishop JAM, Judson IR, Harland SJ, Harrap KR. Recent preclinical and clinical studies with the thymidylate synthase inhibitor N^{10}-propargyl-5,8-dideazafolic acid (CB3717). NCI Monogr 1987; 5:213–218.

67. Jackman AL, Newell DR, Gibson W, Jodrell DI, Taylor GA, Bishop JA, Hughes LR, Calvert AH. The biochemical pharmacology of the thymidylate synthase inhibitor, 2-desamino-2-methyl-N^{10}-propargyl-5,8-dideazafolic acid (ICI 198583). Biochem Pharmacol 1991; 42:1885–1895.

68. Jackman AL, Taylor GA, Gibson W, Kimbell R, Brown M, Calvert AH, Judson IR, Hughes LR. ICI D1694, a quinazoline antifolate thymidylate synthase inhibitor that is a potent inhibitor of L1210 cell growth in vitro and in vivo: a new agent for clinical study. Cancer Res 1991; 51:5579–5586.

69. Jackman AL, Marsham PR, Moran RG, Kimbell R, O'Connor BM, Hughes LR, Calvert AH. Thymidylate synthase inhibitors: the in vitro activity of a series of heterocyclic benzoyl ring modified 2-desamino-2-methyl-N^{10}-substituted-5,8-dideazafolates. Adv Enzyme Regul 1991; 31:13–27.

70. Ward WHJ, Kimbell R, Jackman AL. Kinetic characteristics of ICI D1694: a quinazoline antifolate which inhibits thymidylate synthase. Biochem Pharmacol 1992; 43:2029–2031.

71. Stephens TC, Valcaccia BE, Sheader ML, Hughes IR, Jackman AL. The thymidylate synthase (TS) inhibitor ICI D1694 is superior to CB3717, 5-fluorouracil (5-FU) and methotrexate (MTX) against a panel of human tumor xenographs. Proc Am Assoc Cancer Res 1991; 32:328.

72. Stephens TC, Calvete JA, Janes D, Waterman SE, Valcaccia BE, Hughes LR, Calvert, AH. Antitumor activity of a new thymidylate synthase (TS) inhibitor, D1694. Proc Am Assoc Cancer Res 1990; 31:342.

73. Jodrell DI, Newell DR, Morgan SE, Clinton S, Bensted JDM, Hughes LR, Calvert AH. The renal effects of N^{10}-propargyl-5,8-dideazafolic acid (CB3717) and a nonnephrotoxic analogue ICI D1694, in mice. Br J Cancer 1991; 64:833–838.

74. Clarke S, Ward J, Planting A, Spiers J, Smith R, Verweij J, Judson I. Phase I trial of ICI D1694: a novel thymidylate synthase inhibitor. Proc Am Assoc Cancer Res 1992; 33:406.

75. Duch DS, Banks S, Dev IK, Dickerson SH, Ferone R, Heath LS, Humphreys J, Knick V, Pendergast W, Singer S, Smith GK, Waters K, Wilson HR. Biochemical and cellular pharmacology of 1843U89, a novel benzoquinazoline inhibitor of thymidylate synthase. Cancer Res 1993; 53:810–818.

76. Ferone R, Hanlon MH, Waters KA, Dev IK. Influence of intracellular polyglutamation on the cytotoxicity of the thymidylate synthase inhibitor 1843U89. Proc Am Assoc Cancer Res 1993; 34:274.

77. Humphreys J, Smith G, Waters K, Duch D. Antitumor activity of the novel thymidylate synthase inhibitor 1843U89 in cells resistant to antifolates by multiple mechanisms. Proc Am Assoc Cancer Res 1993; 34:273.

78. Banks SD, Waters KA, Barret, LL, Smith GK. Destruction of WiDr multicellular tumor spheroids with novel thymidylate synthase inhibitor at physiological thymidine concentrations. Proc Am Assoc Cancer Res 1992; 33:407.

79. Taylor EC, Harrington PJ, Fletcher SR, Beardsley GP, Moran RG. Synthesis of the antileukemia agents 5,10-dideazaaminopterin and 5,10-dideaza-5,6,7,8-tetrahydroaminopterin. J Med Chem 1985; 28:914–921.

80. Boschelli DH, Webber S, Whiteley JM, Oronsky AL, Kerwar, SS. Synthesis and biological properties of 5,10-dideaza-5,6,7,8-tetrahydrofolic acid. Arch Biochem Biophys 1988; 265:43–49.

81. Beardsley GP, Moroson BA, Taylor EC, Moran RG. A new folate antimetabolite, 5,10-dideaza-5,6,7,8-tetrahydrofolate, is a potent inhibitor of de novo purine synthesis. J Biol Chem 1989; 264:328–333.

82. Moran RG, Baldwin SW, Taylor EC, Shih C. The $6S$- and $6R$-diastereomers of 5,10-dideaza-5,6,7,8-tetrahydrofolate are equiactive inhibitors of de novo purine synthesis. J Biol Chem 1989; 264:21047–21051.

83. Baldwin SW, Tse A, Gossett LS, Taylor EC, Rosowsky A, Shih C, Moran RG. Structural features of 5,10-dideaza-5,6,7,8-tetrahydrofolate that determine inhibition of mammalian glycinamide ribonucleotide formyltransferase. Biochemistry 1991; 30:1997–2006.

84. Pizzorno G, Moroson BA, Cashmore AR, Beardsley GP. 5,10-Dideaza-5,6,7,8-tetrahydrofolic acid effects on nucleotide metabolism in CCRF-CEM human T-lymphoblast leukemia cells. Cancer Res 1991; 51:2291–2295.

85. Moran RG, Colman PD, Rosowsky A. Structural requirements for the activity of antifolates as substrates for mammalian folylpolyglutamate synthetase. NCI Monogr 1987; 5:133–138.

86. Pizzorno G, Cashmore AR, Moroson BA, Cross AD, Smith AK, Marling

Cason M, Kamen BA, Beardsley GP. 5,10-Dideazatetrahydrofolic acid (DDATHF) transport in CCRF-CEM and MA104 cell lines. J Biol Chem 1993; 268:1017–1023.

87. Matherly LH, Angeles SM, McGuire JJ. Determinants of the disparate antitumor activities of (6R)-5,10-dideaza-5,6,7,8-tetrahydrofolate and methotrexate toward human lymphoblastic leukemia cells, characterized by severely impaired antifolate membrane transport. Biochem Pharmacol 1993; 46:2185–2195.

88. Jansen G, Westerhof GR, Kathmann I, Rijksen G, Schornagel JH. Growth inhibitory effects of 5,10-dideazatetrahydrofolic acid on variant murine L1210 and human CCRF-CEM leukemia cells with different membrane transport characteristics for (anti)folate compounds. Cancer Chem Pharmacol 1991; 28:115–117.

89. Wang X, Shen F, Freisheim JH, Gentry LE, Ratnam M. Differential stereospecificities and affinities of folate receptor isoforms for folate compounds and antifolates. Biochem Pharmacol 1992; 44:1898–1901.

90. Pizzorno G, Sokoloski JA, Cashmore AR, Moroson BA, Cross AD, Beardsley GP. Intracellular metabolism of 5,10-dideazatetrahydrofolic acid in human leukemia cell lines. Mol Pharmacol 1991; 39:85–89.

91. Sirotnak FM, Otter GM, Piper JR, DeGraw JI. Analogs of tetrahydrofolate directed at folate-dependent purine biosynthetic enzymes. Characteristics of mediated entry and transport-related resistance in L1210 cells for 5,10-dideazatetrahydrofolate and two 10-alkyl derivatives. Biochem Pharmacol 1988; 37:4775–4777.

92. Beardsley GP, Taylor EC, Grindey GB, Moran RG. Deaza derivatives of tetrahydrofolic acid. A new class of folate antimetabolite. In: Cooper BA, Whitehead VM, eds. Chemistry and Biology of Pteridines. Berlin: Walter de Gruyter & Co, 1986:953–957.

93. Ray MS, Muggia FM, Leichman CG, Grunberg SM, Nelson RL, Dyke RW, Moran RG. Phase I study of (6R)-5,10-dideazatetrahydrofolate: a folate antimetabolite inhibitory to de novo purine biosynthesis. JNCI 1993; 85:1154–1159.

94. Nelson R, Butler F, Dugan W, Davis-Lung C, Stone M, Dyke R. Phase I clinical trial of LY264618 (dideazatetrahydrofolic acid; DDATHF). Proc Am Soc Clin Oncol 1990; 9:293.

95. Young CW, Currie VE, Muindi JF, Saltz LB, Pisters KMW, Esposito AJ, Dyke RW. Improved clinical tolerance of lometrexol with oral folic acid. Proc Am Assoc Cancer Res 1992; 33:406.

96. Sirotnak FM. Obligate genetic expression in tumor cells of a fetal membrane property mediating "folate" transport: biological significance and implications of improved therapy of human cancer. Cancer Res 1985; 45:3992–4000.

97. Goldman ID, Lichtenstein NS, Oliverio VT. Carrier-mediated transport of the folic acid analogue, methotrexate, in the L1210 leukemia cell. J Biol Chem 1968; 243:5007–5017.

98. Goldman ID. The characteristics of the membrane transport of amethopterin and the naturally occurring folates. Ann NY Acad Sci 1971; 186:400–422.

99. White JC, Bailey BD, Goldman ID. Lack of stereospecificity at carbon 6 of methyltetrahydrofolate transport in Ehrlich ascites tumor cells. J Biol Chem 1978; 253:242–245.

100. Chello PL, Sirotnak FM, Wong E, Kisliuk RL, Gaumont Y, Combepine G. Further studies of stereospecificity at carbon 6 for membrane transport of tetrahydrofolates: diastereoisomers of 5-methyltetrahydrofolates as competitive inhibitors of transport of methotrexate in L1210 cells. Biochem Pharmacol 1982; 31:1527–1530.

101. Sirotnak FM, Chello PL, Moccio D, Kisliuk RL, Combepine G, Gaumont Y, Montgomery JA. Stereospecificity at carbon 6 of formyltetrahydrofolate as a competitive inhibitor of transport and cytotoxicity of methotrexate in vitro. Biochem Pharmacol 1979; 28:2993–2997.

102. Jansen G, Westerhof GR, Schornagel JH, Jackman AL, Boyle FT. The reduced folate/methotrexate carrier and a membrane-associated folate binding protein as transport routes for novel antifolates: structure-activity relationships. In: Ayling JE, Nair MG, Baugh CM, eds. Chemistry and Biology of Pteridines and Folates. New York: Plenum Press, 1993:767–770.

103. Jansen G, Schornagel JH, Westerhof, GR, Rijksen G, Newell DR, Jackman AL. Multiple membrane transport systems for the uptake of folate-based thymidylate synthase inhibitors. Cancer Res 1990; 50:7544–7548.

104. Goldman ID. A model system for the study of heteroexchange diffusion: methotrexate–folate interactions in L1210 and Ehrlich ascites tumor cells. Biochim Biophys Acta 1971; 233:624–633.

105. Yang CH, Sirotnak FM, Dembo M. Interaction between anions and reduced folate/methotrexate transport system in L1210 cell plasma membrane vesicles: directional symmetry and anion specificity for differential mobility of loaded and unloaded carrier. J Membr Biol 1984; 79:285–292.

106. Henderson GB, Zevely EM. Anion exchange mechanism for transport of methotrexate in L1210 cells. Biochem Biophys Res Commun 1981; 99:163–169.

107. Henderson GB, Zevely EM. Structural requirements for anion substrates of the methotrexate transport system in L1210 cells. Arch Biochem Biophys 1983; 221:438–446.

108. Henderson GB, Zevely EM. Intracellular phosphate and its possible role as an exchange anion for active transport of methotrexate in L1210 cells. Biochem Biophys Res Commun 1982; 104:474–482.

109. Henderson GB, Tsuji JM, Kumar HP. Characterization of the individual transport routes that mediate the influx and efflux of methotrexate in CCRF-CEM human lymphoblastic cells. Cancer Res 1986; 46:1633–1638.

110. Henderson GB, Zevely EM. Use of non-physiological buffer systems in the analysis of methotrexate transport in L1210 cells. Biochem Int 1983; 6:507–515.

111. Henderson GB, Zevely EM. Transport of methotrexate in L1210 cells: effect of ions on the rate and extent of uptake. Arch Biochem Biophys 1980; 200:149–155.

112. Sirotnak FM, Moccio DM, Yang C-H. A novel class of genetic variants of the L1210 cell up-regulated for folate analogue transport inward. Isolation, characterization, and degree of metabolic instability of the system. J Biol Chem 1984; 259:13139–13144.

113. Yang CH, Sirotnak FM, Mines LS. Further studies on a novel class of genetic variants of the L1210 cell with increased folate analogue transport inward. Transport properties of a new variant, evidence for increased level of a specific transport protein, and its partial characterization following affinity labeling. J Biol Chem 1988; 263:9703–9709.

114. Jansen G, Westerhof GR, Jarmuszewski MJA, Kathmann I, Rijksen G, Schornagel JH. Methotrexate transport in variant human CCRF-CEM leukemia cells with elevated levels of the reduced folate carrier. Selective effect on carrier-mediated transport of physiological concentrations of reduced folates. J Biol Chem 1990; 265:18272–18277.

115. Matherly LH, Czajkowski CA, Angeles SM. Identification of a highly glycosylated methotrexate membrane carrier in K562 erythroleukemia cells up-regulated for tetrahydrofolate cofactor and methotrexate transport. Cancer Res 1991; 51:3420–3426.

116. Yang C-H, Pain J, Sirotnak FM. Alteration of folate analogue transport inward after induced maturation of HL-60 leukemia cells: molecular properties of the transporter in an overproducing variant and evidence for down-regulation of its synthesis in maturating cells. J Biol Chem 1992; 267:6628–6634.

117. Brigle KE, Westin EH, Houghton MT, Goldman ID. Characterization of two cDNAs encoding folate-binding proteins from L1210 murine leukemia cells: increased expression associated with a genomic rearrangement. J Biol Chem. 1991; 266:17243–17249.

118. Jansen G, Kathmann I, Rademaker BC, Braakhuis BJM, Westerhof GR, Rijksen G, Schornagel JH. Expression of a folate binding protein in L1210 cells grown in low folate medium. Cancer Res 1989; 49:1959–1963.

119. Henderson GB, Grzelakowska-Sztabert B, Zevely EM, Huennekens FM. Binding properties of the 5-methyl tetrahydrofolate/methotrexate transport system in L1210 cells. Arch Biochem Biophys 1980; 202:144–149.

120. Schuetz JD, Matherly LH, Westin EH, Goldman ID. Evidence for a functional defect in the translocation of the methotrexate transport carrier in a methotrexate resistant murine L1210 leukemia cell line. J Biol Chem 1988; 263:9840–9847.

121. Henderson GB, Tsuji JM, Kumar HP. Mediated uptake of folate by a high affinity folate binding protein in sublines of L1210 cells adapted to low concentrations of folate. J Membr Biol 1988; 101:247–258.

122. Schuetz JD, Westin EH, Matherly LH, Pincus R, Swerdlow PS, Goldman ID. Membrane protein changes in an L1210 leukemia cell line with a translo-

cation defect in the methotrexate-tetrahydrofolate cofactor transport carrier. J Biol Chem 1989; 264:16261–16267.

123. Matherly LH, Angeles SM, Czajkowski CA. Characterization of transport-mediated methotrexate resistance in human tumor cells with antibodies to the membrane carrier for methotrexate and tetrahydrofolate cofactors. J Biol Chem 1992; 267:23253–23260.

124. Henderson GB, Zevely EM, Huennekens FM. Photoinactivation of the methotrexate transport system of L1210 cells by 8-azidoadenosine 5'-monophosphate. J Biol Chem 1979; 254:9973–9975.

125. Henderson GB, Zevely EM. Functional correlations between the methotrexate and general anion transport systems in L1210 cells. Biochem Int 1982; 4:493–502.

126. Henderson GB, Zevely EM, Huennekens FM. Irreversible inactivation of the methotrexate transport system of L1210 cells by carbodiimide-activated substrates. J Biol Chem 1980; 255:4829–4833.

127. Jansen G, Westerhof GR, Rijksen G, Schornagel JH. Interaction of N-hydroxy(sulfo)succinimide active esters with the reduced folate/methotrexate transport system from human leukemic CCRF-CEM cells. Biochim Biophys Acta 1989; 985:266–270.

128. Henderson GB, Zevely EM. Affinity labeling of the 5-methyltetrahydrofolate/methotrexate transport protein of L1210 cells by treatment with an N-hydroxysuccinimide ester of [^{3}H]methotrexate. J Biol Chem 1984; 259:4558–4562.

129. Henderson GB, Montague-Wilkie B. Irreversible inhibitors of methotrexate transport in L1210 cells. Characteristics of inhibition by an N-hydroxysuccinimide ester of methotrexate. Biochim Biophys Acta 1983; 735:123–130.

130. Freisheim JH, Ratnam M, McAlinden TP, Prasad KMR, Williams FE, Westerhof GR, Schornagel JH, Jansen G. Molecular events in the membrane transport of methotrexate in human CCRF-CEM leukemia cell lines. Adv Enzyme Regul 1992; 32:17–31.

131. Price EM, Freisheim JH. Photoaffinity analogues of methotrexate as folate antagonist binding probes. 2. Transport studies, photoaffinity labeling, and identification of the membrane carrier protein for methotrexate from murine L1210 cells. Biochemistry 1987; 26:4757–4763.

132. Price EM, Ratnam M, Rodeman KM, Freisheim JH. Characterization of the methotrexate transport pathway in murine L1210 leukemia cells: involvement of a membrane receptor and a cytosolic protein. Biochemistry 1988; 27:7853–7858.

133. Fan J, Pope LE, Vitols KS, Huennekens FM. Affinity labeling of folate transport proteins with the N-hydroxysuccinimide ester of the γ-isomer of fluorescein–methotrexate. Biochemistry 1991; 30:4573–4580.

134. Fan J, Vitols KS, Huennekens FM. Biotin derivatives of methotrexate and folate. Synthesis and utilization for affinity purification of two membrane-associated folate transporters from L1210 cells. J Biol Chem 1991; 266:14862–14865.

135. Price EM, Sams L, Harpring KM, Kempton RJ, Freisheim JH. Photoaffinity analogues of methotrexate as probes for dihydrofolate reductase structure and function. Biochem Pharmacol 1986; 35:4341–4343.

136. Westerhof GR, Schornagel JH, Rijnboutt S, Pinedo HM, Jansen G. Identification of a reduced folate/methotrexate carrier in human KB-cells expressing high levels of membrane associated folate binding protein. In: Ayling JE, Nair MG, Baugh CM, eds Chemistry and Biology of Pteridines and Folates. New York: Plenum Press, 1993:771–774.

137. Matherly LH, Angeles SM. Role of N-glycosylation in the structure and function of the methotrexate membrane transporter from CCRF-CEM human lymphoblastic leukemia cells. Biochem Pharmacol 1994; 47: 1094–1098.

138. Underhill TM, Flintoff WF. Complementation of a methotrexate uptake defect in Chinese hamster ovary cells by DNA-mediated gene transfer. Mol Cell Biol 1989; 9:1754–1758.

139. Underhill M, Williams FMR, Murray RC, Flintoff WF. Molecular cloning of a gene involved in methotrexate uptake by DNA-mediated gene transfer. J Cell Mol Genet 1992; 18:337–349.

140. Dixon KH, Lampher BC, Chiu J, Kelley K, Cowan KH. A novel cDNA restores reduced folate carrier activity and methotrexate sensitivity to transport-deficient cells. J Biol Chem 1994; 269:17–20.

141. Williams FMR, Murray RC, Underhill TM, Flintoff WF. Isolation of a hamster cDNA clone coding for a function involved in methotrexate uptake. J Biol Chem 1994; 269:5810–5816.

142. Mines LS, Yang CH, Spengler BA, Biedler JL, Sirotnak FM. A gene amplification-associated cytogenetic abnormality in an L1210 cell variant overproducing the folate transporter. Proc Am Assoc Cancer Res 1988; 29: 289.

143. Henderson GB, Schrecker AW, Smith C, Gordon M, Zevely EM, Vitols KS, Huennekens FM. Transport of methotrexate and other folate compounds: components, mechanism and regulation by cyclic nucleotides. Adv Enzyme Regul 1977; 15:141–151.

144. Henderson GB, Zevely EM, Huennekens FM. Cyclic adenosine 3′:5′-monophosphate and methotrexate transport in L1210 cells. Cancer Res 1978; 38:859–861.

145. White JC, Carchman RA, Fry DW, Goldman ID. Relationship between membrane transport of methotrexate and endogenous cyclic adenosine 3′:5′-monophosphate in the Ehrlich ascites tumor. Cancer Res 1980; 40:2400–2404.

146. Hoffbrand AJ, Tripp E, Catovsky D, Das KC. Transport of methotrexate into normal haemopoietic cells and into leukemic cells and its effects on DNA synthesis. Br J Haematol 1973; 25:497–511.

147. Xuan YZ, Bhushan A, Hacker MP, Tritton TR. Tyrosine phosphorylation of a membrane protein (P66) may play an important role in methotrexate transport. Proc Am Assoc Cancer Res 1993; 34:353.

148. Sirotnak FM, Goutas LJ, Mines LS. Extent of the requirement for folate

transport by L1210 cells for growth and leukemogenesis in vivo. Cancer Res 1985; 45:4732–4734.

149. Pincus R, Schuetz J, Seither R, Westin E, Goldman ID. Minimal change in transport and growth requirement for folic acid in an L1210 leukemia cell line with markedly impaired transport of methotrexate. Proc Am Assoc Cancer Res 1988; 29:283.

150. Sirotnak FM, Goutas LJ, Jacobsen DM, Mines LS, Barrueco JR, Gaumont Y, Kisliuk RL. Carrier-mediated transport of folate compounds in L1210 cells. Initial rate kinetics and extent of duality of entry routes for folic acid and diastereomers of 5-methyltetrahydrohomofolate in the presence of physiological anions. Biochem Pharmacol 1987; 36:1659–1667.

151. Henderson GB, Strauss BP. Characteristics of a novel transport system for folate compounds in wild-type and methotrexate-resistant L1210 cells. Cancer Res 1990; 50:1709–1714.

152. Horne DW. Transport of folates and antifolates in liver. Proc Soc Exp Biol Med 1993; 202:385–391.

153. Zimmerman J. Methotrexate transport in the human intestine. Evidence for heterogeneity. Biochem Pharmacol 1992; 43:2377–2383.

154. Selhub J, Dhar GJ, Rosenberg IH. Gastrointestinal absorption of folates and antifolates. In: Goldman ID, ed. Membrane Transport of Antineoplastic Agents. New York: Pergamon Press, 1986:147–168.

155. McHugh M, Cheng YC. Demonstration of a high affinity folate binder in human cell membranes and its characterization in cultured human KB cells. J Biol Chem 1979; 254:11312–11318.

156. Kamen BA, Capdevila A. Receptor-mediated folate accumulation is regulated by the cellular folate content. Proc Natl Acad Sci USA 1986; 83:5983–5987.

157. Henderson GB, Strauss BP. Growth inhibition by homofolate in tumor cells utilizing a high affinity folate binding protein as a means for folate internalization. Biochem Pharmacol 1990; 39:2019–2025.

158. Jansen G, Westerhof GR, Kathmann I, Rademaker BC, Rijksen G, Schornagel JH. Identification of a membrane-associated folate binding protein in human leukemic CCRF-CEM cells with transport-related methotrexate resistance. Cancer Res 1989; 49:2455–2459.

159. Antony AC, Utley C, Van Horne KC, Kolhouse JF. Isolation and characterization of a folate receptor from human placenta. J Biol Chem 1981; 256:9684–9692.

160. Suleiman AS, Spector R. Purification and characterization of a folate binding protein from porcine choroid plexus. Arch Biochem Biophys 1981; 208:87–94.

161. Selhub J, Franklin WA. The folate binding protein of rat kidney: purification, properties, and cellular distribution. J Biol Chem 1984; 259:6601–6606.

162. Antony AC, Utley CS, Marcell PD, Kolhouse JF. Isolation, characterization, and comparison of solubilized particulate and soluble folate binding proteins from human milk. J Biol Chem 1982; 257:10081–10089.

163. Svendsen I, Hansen SI, Holm J, Lyngbye J. Amino acid sequence homology

between human and bovine low molecular weight folate binding protein isolated from milk. Carlsberg Res Commun 1982; 47:371–376.

164. Waxman S, Schreiber C. Characteristics of folic acid binding protein in folate-deficient serum. Blood 1973; 42:291–301.

165. Kamen BA, Caston DJ. Purification of folate binding factor in normal umbilical cord serum. Proc Natl Acad Sci USA 1975; 72:4261–4264.

166. Elwood PC, Kane MA, Portillo RM, Kolhouse JF. The isolation, characterization, and comparison of the membrane-associated and soluble folate-binding proteins from human KB cells. J Biol Chem 1986; 261:15416–15423.

167. Campbell IG, Jones TA, Foulkes WD, Trowsdale J. Folate-binding protein is a marker for ovarian cancer. Cancer Res 1991; 51:5329–5338.

168. Weitman SD, Weinberg AG, Coney LR, Zurawski VR, Jennings DS, Kamen BA. Cellular localization of the folate receptor: potential role in drug toxicity and folate homeostasis. Cancer Res 1992; 52:6708–6711.

169. Elwood PC, Deutsch JC, Kolhouse JF. The conversion of the human membrane-associated folate binding protein (folate receptor) to the soluble folate binding protein by a membrane-associated metalloprotease. J Biol Chem 1991; 266:2346–2353.

170. Kane MA, Elwood PC, Portillo RM, Antony AC, Kolhouse, JF. The interrelationship of the soluble and membrane-associated folate-binding proteins in human KB cells. J Biol Chem 1986; 261:15625–15631.

171. Antony AC, Verma RS. Hydrophobic erythrocyte folate binding proteins are converted to hydrophilic forms by trypsin in vitro. Biochim Biophys Acta 1989; 979:62–68.

172. Antony AC, Verma RS, Unune AR, LaRosa JA. Identification of a Mg^{2+}-dependent protease in human placenta which cleaves hydrophobic folate-binding proteins to hydrophilic forms. J Biol Chem 1989; 264:1911–1914.

173. Bottero F, Tomassetti A, Canevari S, Miotti S, Menard S, Colnaghi MI. Gene transfection and expression of the ovarian carcinoma marker folate binding protein on NIH/3T3 cells increases cell growth in vitro and in vivo. Cancer Res 1993; 53:5791–5796.

174. Ghitis J. The folate binding in milk. Am J Clin Nutr 1967; 20:1–4.

175. Rothenberg SP. A macromolecular factor in some leukemic cells which binds folic acid. Proc Soc Exp Biol Med 1970; 133:428–432.

176. Kamen BA, Wang MT, Streckfuss AJ, Peryea X, Anderson RGW. Delivery of folates to the cytoplasm of MA104 cells is mediated by a surface membrane receptor that recycles. J Biol Chem 1988; 263:13602–13609.

177. Antony AC, Kane MA, Portillo RM, Elwood PC, Kolhouse, JF. Studies of the role of a particulate folate-binding protein in the uptake of 5-methyltetrahydrofolate by cultured human KB cells. J Biol Chem 1985; 260:14911–14917.

178. Deutsch JC, Elwood PC, Portillo RM, Macey MG, Kolhouse JF. Role of the membrane-associated folate binding protein (folate receptor) in methotrexate transport in human KB cells. Arch Biochem Biophys 1989; 274:327–337.

179. Antony AC, Bruno E, Briddel RA, Brandt JE, Verma RS, Hoffman R.

Effect of perturbation of specific folate receptors during in vitro erythropoiesis. J Clin Invest 1987; 80:1617–1623.

180. Dixon KH, Mulligan T, Chung KN, Elwood PC, Cowan KH. Effects of folate receptor expression following stable transfection into wild type and methotrexate transport deficient ZR-75-1 human breast cancer cells. J Biol Chem 1992; 267:24140–24147.

181. Lacey SW, Sanders JM, Rothberg KG, Anderson RGW, Kamen BA. Complementary DNA for the folate binding protein correctly predicts anchoring to the membrane glycosyl-phosphatidylinositol. J Clin Invest 1989; 84:715–720.

182. Luhrs CA, Raskin CA, Durbin R, Wu B, Sadasivan E, McAllister W, Rothenberg SP. Transfection of glycosylated phosphatidylinositol-anchored folate-binding protein complementary DNA provides cells with the ability to survive in low folate medium. J Clin Invest 1992; 90:840–847.

183. Chung KN, Saikawa Y, Paik TH, Dixon KH, Mulligan T, Cowan KH, Elwood PC. Stable transfectants of human MCF-7 breast cancer cells with increased levels of human folate receptor exhibit an increased sensitivity to antifolates. J Clin Invest 1993; 91:1289–1294.

184. Luhrs CA, Sadasivan E, da Costa M, Rothenberg SP. The isolation and properties of multiple forms of folate binding proteins in cultured KB cells. Arch Biochem Biophys 1986; 250:94–105.

185. Luhrs CA, Pitiranggon P, daCosta M, Rothenberg SP, Slomiany BL, Brink L, Tous GI, Stein S. Purified membrane and soluble folate binding proteins from cultured KB cells have similar amino acid compositions and molecular weights but differ in fatty acid acylation. Proc Natl Acad Sci USA 1987; 84:6546–6549.

186. Luhrs CA, Slomiany BL. A human membrane-associated folate binding protein is anchored by a glycosyl-phosphatidylinositol tail. J Biol Chem 1989; 264:21446–21449.

187. Elwood PC. Molecular cloning and characterization of the human folate binding protein cDNA from placenta and malignant tissue culture (KB) cells. J Biol Chem 1989; 264:14893–14901.

188. Sadasivan E, Rothenberg SP. The complete amino acid sequence of a human folate binding protein from KB cells determined from the cDNA. J Biol Chem 1989; 264:5806–5811.

189. Ratnam M, Marquardt H, Duhring JL, Freisheim JH. Homologous membrane folate binding proteins in human placenta: cloning and sequence of a cDNA. Biochemistry 1989; 28:8249–8254.

190. Page ST, Owen WC, Price K, Elwood PC. Expression of the human placental folate receptor transcript is regulated in human tissues. Organization and full nucleotide sequence of the gene. J Mol Biol 1993; 229:1175–1183.

191. Coney LR, Tomassetti A, Carayannopoulos L, Frasca V, Kamen BA, Colnaghi MI, Zurawski VR. Cloning of a tumor associated antigen: MOv18 and MOv19 antibodies recognize a folate-binding protein. Cancer Res 1991; 51:6125–6132.

192. Westerhof GR, Wang X, Schornagel JH, Freisheim JH, Jansen G, Ratnam

M. Purification and characterization of a novel membrane-folate receptor from variant CCRF-CEM human leukemic cells. Proc Am Assoc Cancer Res 1992; 33:1.

193. Tomassetti A, Coney LR, Canevari S, Miotti S, Facheris P, Zurawski VR, Colnaghi MI. Isolation and biochemical characterization of the soluble and membrane forms of folate binding protein expressed in the ovarian carcinoma cell line IGROV1. FEBS Lett 1993; 317:143–146.

194. Verma RS, Gullapalli S, Antony AC. Evidence that the hydrophobicity of isolated, in situ, and de novo-synthesized native human placental folate receptors is a function of glycosylphosphatidylinosol anchoring to membranes. J Biol Chem 1992; 267:4119–4127.

195. Englund PT. The structure and biosynthesis of glycosyl phosphatidyl protein anchors. Annu Rev Biochem 1993; 62:121–138.

196. Lanier LL, Cwirla S, Yu G, Testi R, Phillips JH. Membrane anchoring of a human IgG Fc receptor (CD16) determined by a single amino acid. Science 1989; 246:1611–1613.

197. Selhub J, Franklin WA. The folate binding protein of rat kidney. Purification, properties and cellular distribution. J Biol Chem 1984; 259:6601–6606.

198. Anderson RGW, Kamen BA, Rothberg KG, Lacey SW. Potocytosis: sequestration and transport of small molecules by caveolae. Science 1992; 255:410–411.

199. Rothberg KG, Ying Y, Kolhouse JF, Kamen BA, Anderson RGW. The glycophospholipid-linked folate receptor internalizes folate without entering the clathrin-coated pit endocytic pathway. J Cell Biol 1990; 110:637–649.

200. Chang W-J, Rothberg KG, Kamen BA, Anderson RGW. Lowering the cholesterol content of MA104 cells inhibits receptor-mediated transport of folate. J Cell Biol 1992; 118:63–69.

201. Birn H, Selhub J, Christensen EI. Internalization and intracellular transport of folate-binding protein in rat kidney proximal tubule. Am J Physiol 1993; 264:C302–C310.

202. Kamen B, Smith AK, Anderson RGW. The folate receptor works in tandem with a probenecid-sensitive carrier in MA104 cells in vitro. J Clin Invest 1991; 87:1442–1449.

203. Matherly LH, Wong SC, Angeles SM, Taub JW, Smith GK. Distribution of the reduced folate carrier versus the high affinity membrane folate binding protein in human tumors and tissues. Proc Am Assoc Cancer Res 1994; 35:307.

204. Saikawa Y, Knight CB, Saikawa T, Page ST, Chabner BA, Elwood PC. Decreased expression of the human folate receptor mediates transport-defective methotrexate resistance in KB cells. J Biol Chem 1993; 268:5293–5301.

205. Kane MA, Portillo RM, Elwood PC, Antony AC, Kolhouse JF. The influence of extracellular folate concentration on methotrexate uptake by human KB cells. Partial characterization of a membrane associated methotrexate binding protein. J Biol Chem 1986; 261:44–49.

206. Hsueh C-T, Dolnick BJ. Altered folate-binding mRNA stability in KB cells grown in folate-deficient medium. Biochem Pharmacol 1993; 45:2537–2545.

207. Westerhof GR, Jansen G, van Emmerik N, Kathmann I, Rijksen G, Jackman AL, Schornagel JH. Membrane transport of natural folates and antifolate compounds in murine L1210 leukemia cells: role of carrier- and receptor-mediated transport systems. Cancer Res 1991; 51:5507–5513.

208. Kane MA, Elwood PC, Portillo RM, Antony AC, Najfeld V, Finley A, Waxman S, Kolhouse JF. Influence on immunoreactive folate-binding proteins of extracellular folate concentration in cultured human cells. J Clin Invest 1988; 81:1398–1406.

209. Brigle KE, Westin EH, Houghton MT, Goldman ID. Insertion of an intracisternal A particle within the 5'-regulatory region of a gene encoding folate-binding protein in L1210 leukemia cells in response to low folate selection: association with increased protein expression. J Biol Chem 1992; 267:22351–22355.

210. Knight CB, Chabner BA, Elwood PC. Studies of the phosphorylation of the membrane associated folate-binding protein in human nasopharyngeal carcinoma (KB) cells. Blood 1988; 72:91a.

211. Luhrs CA. The role of glycosylation in the biosynthesis and acquisition of ligand-binding activity of the folate-binding protein in cultured KB cells. Blood 1991; 77:1171–1180.

212. Henderson GB, Suresh MR, Vitols KS, Huennekens FM. Transport of folate compounds in L1210 cells: kinetic evidence that folate influx proceeds via the high affinity transport system for 5-methyltetrahydrofolate and methotrexate. Cancer Res 1986; 46:1639–1643.

213. Henderson GB, Tsuji JM, Kumar HP. Transport of folate compounds by leukemic cells. Evidence for a single influx carrier for methotrexate, 5-methyl tetrahydrofolate, and folate in CCRF-CEM human lymphoblasts. Biochem Pharmacol 1987; 36:3007–3014.

214. Rader JI, Niethammer D, Huennekens FM. Effects of sulfhydryl inhibitors upon transport of folate compounds in L1210 cells. Biochem Pharmacol 1974; 23:2057–2059.

215. Goldman ID. Membrane transport of methotrexate (NSC-740) and other folate compounds: relevance to rescue protocols. Cancer Chemother Rep 1975; 6:63–72.

216. Yang CH, Dembo M, Sirotnak FM. Relationships between carrier-mediated transport of folate compounds by L1210 leukemia cells: evidence for multiplicity of entry routes with different kinetic properties expressed in plasma membrane vesicles. J Membr Biol 1983; 75:11–20.

217. Yang CH, Peterson RHF, Sirotnak FM, Chello PL. Folate analog transport by plasma membrane vesicles isolated from L1210 leukemia cells. J Biol Chem 1979; 254:1402–1407.

218. Jackson RC, Niethammer D, Huennekens FM. Enzymic and transport mechanisms of amethopterin resistance in 11210 mouse leukemia cells. Cancer Biochem Biophys 1975; 1:151–155.

219. Niethammer D, Jackson RC. Changes of molecular properties associated with the development of resistance against methotrexate in human lymphoblastoid cells. Eur J Cancer 1975; 11:845–854.

220. Hakala MT. On the nature of permeability of sarcoma-180 cells to amethopterin in vitro. Biochim Biophys Acta 1965; 102:210–225.

221. Sirotnak FM, O'Leary DF. The issues of transport multiplicity and energetics pertaining to methotrexate efflux in L1210 cells addressed by an analysis of *cis* and *trans* effects of inhibitors. Cancer Res 1991; 51:1412–1417.

222. Henderson GB. Separation and inhibitor specificity of a second unidirectional efflux route for methotrexate in L1210 cells. Biochim Biophys Acta 1992; 1110:137–143.

223. Henderson GB, Zevely EM. Transport routes utilized by L1210 cells for the influx and efflux of methotrexate. J Biol Chem 1984; 259:1526–1531.

224. Henderson GB, Zevely EM. Inhibitory effects of probenecid on the individual transport routes which mediate the influx and efflux of methotrexate in L1210 cells. Biochem Pharmacol 1985; 34:1725–1729.

225. Henderson GB, Tsuji JM. Identification of the bromosulfophthalein-sensitive efflux route for methotrexate as the site of action of vincristine in the vincristine-dependent enhancement of methotrexate uptake in L1210 cells. Cancer Res 1988; 48:5995–6001.

226. Henderson GB, Tsuji JM. Identification of cholate as a shared substrate for the unidirectional efflux systems for methotrexate in L1210 mouse cells. Biochim Biophys Acta 1990; 1051:60–70.

227. Henderson GB, Tsuji JM. Methotrexate efflux in L1210 cells. Kinetic and specificity properties of the efflux system sensitive to bromosulfophthalein and its possible identity with a system which mediates the efflux of 3',5'-cyclic AMP. J Biol Chem 1987; 262:13571–13578.

228. Henderson GB, Hughes TR. Altered expression of unidirectional extrusion routes for methotrexate and cholate in an efflux variant of L1210 cells. Biochim Biophys Acta 1993; 1152:91–98.

229. Goldman ID. Transport energetics of the folic acid analogue methotrexate, in L1210 leukemia cells. Enhanced accumulation by metabolic inhibitors. J Biol Chem 1969; 244:3779–3785.

230. Fry DW, White JC, Goldman ID. Effects of 2,4-dinitrophenol and other metabolic inhibitors on the bidirectional carrier fluxes, net transport, and intracellular binding of methotrexate in Ehrlich ascites tumor cells. Cancer Res 1980; 40:3669–3673.

231. Dembo M, Sirotnak FM, Moccio DM. Effects of metabolic deprivation on methotrexate transport in L1210 leukemia cells: further evidence for separate influx and efflux systems with different energetic requirements. J Membr Biol 1984; 78:9–17.

232. Hill BT, Bailey BD, White CJ, Goldman ID. Characteristics of transport of 4-amino antifolates and folate compounds by two lines of L5178Y lymphoblasts, one with impaired transport of methotrexate. Cancer Res 1979; 39:2440–2446.

233. Sirotnak FM, Moccio DM, Kelleher LE, Goutas LJ. Relative frequency and

kinetic properties of transport-defective phenotypes among methotrexate resistant L1210 clonal cell lines derived in vivo. Cancer Res 1981; 41:4447–4452.

234. Yalowich JC, Fry DW, Goldman ID. VM-26 and VP-16-213 induced augmentation of methotrexate uptake and intracellular levels of polyglutamyl derivatives in Ehrlich ascites tumor cells in vitro. Cancer Res 1982; 42:3648–3653.

235. Jolivet J, Gravel S, Pinard MF, Bertrand R. Probenecid reverses methotrexate resistance in a human breast cancer cell line. Proc Am Assoc Cancer Res 1989; 30:475.

236. Schlemmer SR, Sirotnak FM. Energy dependent efflux of methotrexate in L1210 leukemia cells. Evidence for a role of an ATPase obtained from inside-out plasma membrane vesicles. J Biol Chem 1992; 267:14746–14752.

237. Schlemmer SR, Sirotnak FM. Specificity of ATP-dependent efflux in L1210 cells for folates, their analogues, and polyglutamates. Proc Am Assoc Cancer Res 1993; 34:276.

238. Henderson GB, Strauss BP. Evidence for cAMP and cholate extrusion in C6 rat glioma cells by a common anion efflux pump. J Biol Chem 1991; 266:1641–1645.

239. Schlemmer SR, Sirotnak FM. Retentiveness of methotrexate polyglutamates in cultured L1210 cells. Evidence against a role for mediated plasma membrane transport outward. Biochem Pharmacol 1993; 45:1261–1266.

240. Gottesman MM, Pastan I. Biochemistry of multidrug resistance mediated by the multidrug transporter. Annu Rev Biochem 1993; 62:385–427.

241. Hyde SC, Emsley P, Hartshorn MJ, Mimmack MM, Gileadi U, Pearce SR, Gallagher MP, Gill DR, Hubbard RE, Higgins CF. Structural model of ATP-binding proteins associated with cystic fibrosis, multidrug resistance, and bacterial transport. Nature 1990; 346:362–365.

242. Paxton JW. The protein binding and elimination of methotrexate after intravenous infusions in cancer patients. Clin Exp Pharmacol Physiol 1982; 9:225–234.

243. Cowan KH, Jolivet J. A methotrexate resistant human breast cancer cell line with multiple defects, including diminished formation of methotrexate polyglutamates. J Biol Chem 1984; 259:10793–10800.

244. Frei E, Rosowsky A, Wright JE, Cucchi CA, Lippke JA, Ervin TJ, Jolivet J, Haseltine WA. Development of methotrexate resistance in a human squamous cell carcinoma of the head and neck in culture. Proc Natl Acad Sci USA 1984; 81:2873–2877.

245. Johns DG, Iannotti AT, Sartorelli AC. Enzymatic oxidation of methotrexate and aminopterin. Life Sci 1964; 3:1383–1388.

246. Fabre G, Seither RL, Goldman ID. Hydroxylation of 4-amino antifolates by partially purified aldehyde oxidase from rabbit liver. Biochem Pharmacol 1986; 35:1325–1330.

247. Breihaupt H, Kuenzlen E. Pharmacokinetics of methotrexate and 7-hydroxymethotrexate following infusions of high dose methotrexate. Cancer Treat Rep 1982; 66:1733–1741.

248. Jacobs SA, Stoller RG, Chabner BA, Johns DG. 7-Hydroxymethotrexate as a urinary metabolite in human subjects and rhesus monkeys receiving high dose methotrexate. J Clin Invest 1976; 57:534–538.

249. Bremnes RM, Slordal L, Wist E, Aarbakke J. Dose-dependent pharmacokinetics of methotrexate and 7-hydroxymethotrexate in the rat in vivo. Cancer Res 1989; 49:6359–6364.

250. Drake JC, Allegra CJ, Baram J, Kaufman BT, Chabner BA. Effects on dihydrofolate reductase of methotrexate metabolites and intracellular folates formed during methotrexate exposure of human breast cancer cells. Biochem Pharmacol 1987; 36:2416–2418.

251. Fabre G, Goldman ID. Formation of 7-hydroxymethotrexate polyglutamyl derivatives of methotrexate and 7-hydroxymethotrexate in human chronic myelogenous lymphoblastic leukemia cells. Cancer Res 1985; 45:80–85.

252. Sholar PW, Baram J, Seither R, Allegra CJ. Inhibition of folate-dependent enzymes by 7-OH-methotrexate. Biochem Pharmacol 1988; 37:3531–3534.

253. Fabre G, Matherly LH, Fabre I, Cano JP, Goldman ID. Interactions between 7-hydroxymethotrexate and methotrexate at the cellular level in the Ehrlich tumor in vitro. Cancer Res 1984; 44:970–975.

254. Slordal L, Sager G, Huseby NE, Aarbakke J. Distribution of 7-hydroxymethotrexate in human blood. J Pharm Pharmacol 1988; 40:50–52.

255. Payet B, Fabre I, Fabre G, Cano JP. Interactions between 7-hydroxymethotrexate and folinic acid in RAJI cells, in vitro. Cancer Lett 1988; 39:45–58.

256. Matherly LH, Barlowe CK, Goldman ID. Antifolate polyglutamylation and competitive drug displacement at dihydrofolate reductase as important elements in leucovorin rescue in L1210 cells. Cancer Res 1986; 46:588–593.

257. Miotti S, Canevari S, Menard S, Mezzanzanica D, Porro G, Pupa SM, Regazzoni M, Tagliabue E, Colnaghi MI. Characterization of human ovarian carcinoma-associated antigens defined by novel monoclonal antibodies with tumor-restricted specificity. Int J Cancer 1987; 39:297–303.

258. Weitman SD, Lark RH, Coney LR, Fort DW, Frasca V, Zurawski VR, Kamen BA. Distribution of the folate receptor GP38 in normal and malignant cell lines and tissues. Cancer Res 1992; 52:3396–3401.

259. Vegglan R, Fasolato S, Menard S, Minucci D, Pizzetti P, Regazzoni M, Tagliabue E, Colnaghi MI. Immunohistochemical reactivity of a monoclonal antibody prepared against human ovarian carcinoma on normal and pathological female genital tissues. Tumori 1989; 75:510–513.

260. Battifora H, Mehta P. Methods in laboratory investigation. The checkerboard tissue block. An improved multitissue control block. Lab Invest 1990; 63:722–724.

261. Fischer GA. Defective transport of amethopterin (methotrexate) as a mechanism of resistance to the antimetabolite in L5178Y leukemic cells. Biochem Pharmacol 1962; 11:1233–1237.

262. Flintoff WF, Nagainis CR. Transport of methotrexate in Chinese hamster ovary cells: a mutant defective in methotrexate uptake and cell binding. Arch Biochem Biophys 1983; 223:433–440.

263. McCormick JI, Susten SS, Freisheim JH. Characterization of the methotrexate transport defect in a resistant L1210 lymphoma cell line. Arch Biochem Biophys 1981; 212:311–318.

264. Galivan J. Transport and metabolism of methotrexate in normal and resistant cultured rat hepatoma cells. Cancer Res 1978; 39:735–743.

265. Assaraf YG, Feder JN, Sharma RC, Wright JE, Rosowsky A, Shane B, Schimke RT. Characterization of the coexisting multiple mechanisms of methotrexate resistance in mouse 3T6 R50 fibroblasts. J Biol Chem 1992; 267:5776–5784.

266. Rosowsky A, Lazarus H, Yuan GC, Beltz WR, Mangini L, Abelson HT, Modest EJ, Frei E. Effects of methotrexate esters and other lipophilic antifolates on methotrexate resistant human leukemic lymphoblasts. Biochem Pharmacol 1980; 29:648–652.

267. Ohnuma T, Lo RJ, Scanlon KJ, Kamen BA, Ohnoshi T, Wolman SR, Holland JF. Evolution of methotrexate resistance of human acute lymphoblastic leukemia cells in vitro. Cancer Res 1985; 45:1815–1822.

268. Pinard MF, Matherly LH, Jolivet J. Methotrexate resistance associated with a unique combination of influx and efflux defects. Cell Pharmacol 1993; 1:43–47.

269. Trippett T, Schlemmer S, Elisseyeff Y, Goker E, Wachter M, Steinherz P, Tan C, Berman E, Wright JE, Rosowsky A, Schweitzer B, Bertino JR. Defective transport as a mechanism of acquired resistance to methotrexate in patients with acute lymphocytic leukemia. Blood 1992; 80:1158–1162.

270. Wright JE, Rosowsky A, Cucchi CA, Flatow J, Frei E. Methotrexate and γ-*tert*-butyl methotrexate transport in CEM and CEM/MTX human leukemic lymphoblasts. Biochem Pharmacol 1993; 46:871–876.

271. Biedler JL, Albrecht AM, Hutchinson DJ, Spengler BA. Drug response, dihydrofolate reductase, and cytogenetics of amethopterin resistant Chinese hamster cells in vitro. Cancer Res 1972; 32:153–161.

272. Schimke RT. Gene amplification, drug resistance, and cancer. Cancer Res 1984; 44:1735–1742.

273. Flintoff WF, Essani K. Methotrexate resistant Chinese hamster ovary cells contain a dihydrofolate reductase with an altered affinity for methotrexate. Biochemistry 1990; 19:4321–4327.

274. Goldie JH, Krystal G, Hartley D, Gudauskas G, Dedhar S. A methotrexate insensitive variant of folate reductase present in two lines of methotrexate-resistant L5178Y cells. Eur J Cancer 1980; 16:1539–1546.

275. Melera PW, Lewis JA, Biedler JL, Hession C. Antifolate resistant Chinese hamster cells. Evidence for dihydrofolate reductase gene amplification amongst independently derived sublines overproducing different dihydrofolate reductases J Biol Chem 1980; 255:7014–7028.

276. Wright JE, Rosowsky A, Waxman DJ, Trites D, Cucchi CA, Flatow J, Frei E. Metabolism of methotrexate and γ-*tert*-butyl methotrexate by human leukemic cells in culture and by hepatic aldehyde oxidase in vitro. Biochem Pharmacol 1987; 36:2209–2217.

277. Pizzorno G, Chang YM, McGuire JJ, Bertino JR. Inherent resistance

of human squamous carcinoma cell lines to methotrexate as a result of decreased polyglutamylation of this drug. Cancer Res 1989; 49:5275–5280.

278. Pizzorno G, Mini E, Coronnello M, McGuire JJ, Moroson BA, Cashmore AR, Dreyer RN, Lin JT, Mazzei T, Periti P, Bertino JR. Impaired polyglutamylation of methotrexate as a cause of resistance in CCRF-CEM cells after short-term, high-dose treatment with this drug. Cancer Res 1988; 48:2149–2155.

279. McCloskey DE, McGuire JJ, Russell CA, Rowan BG, Bertino JR, Pizzorno G, Mini E. Decreased folylpolyglutamate synthetase activity as a mechanism of methotrexate resistance in CCRF-CEM human leukemia sublines. J Biol Chem 1991; 266:6181–6187.

280. Assaraf YG, Schimke RT. Identification of methotrexate transport deficiency in mammalian cells using fluoresceinated methotrexate and flow cytometry. Proc Natl Acad Sci USA 1987; 84:7154–7158.

281. Bernal SD, Speak JA, Boeheim K, Dreyfuss AI, Wright JE, Teicher BA, Rosowsky A, Tsao SW, Wong YC. Reduced membrane protein associated with resistance of human squamous carcinoma cells to methotrexate and *cis*-platinum. Mol Cell Biochem 1990; 95:61–70.

282. Pinard MF, Jolivet J. Confocal laser scanning analysis of fluorescein-methotrexate uptake by human breast cancer cells. Proc Am Assoc Cancer Res 1993; 34:278.

283. Brigle KE, Spinella MJ, Westin EH, and Goldman ID. Increased expression and characterization of two distinct folate binding proteins in murine erythroleukemia cells. Biochem Pharmacol 1994; 47:337–345.

284. Hill BT, Price LA. DDMP [2,4,-diamino-5-(3′,4′-dichlorophenyl)methylpyrimidine]. Cancer Treat Rev 1970; 7:95–112.

285. Jackson RC, Fry DW, Boritzki TJ, Besserer JA, Leopold WR, Sloan BJ, Elslager ET. Biochemical pharmacology of the lipophilic antifolate, trimetrexate. Adv Enzyme Regul 1984; 22:187–222.

286. O'Dwyer PJ, DeLap RJ, King SA, Grillo-Lopez AJ, Hoth, DF, Leyland-Jones B, Trimetrexate: clinical development of a nonclassical antifolates. NCI Monogr 1987; 5:105–109.

287. Lin JT, Bertino JR. Update on trimetrexate, a folate antagonist with antineoplastic and antiprotozoal properties. Cancer Invest 1991; 9:159–172.

288. Duch D, Edelstein MP, Bowers SW, Nichol CA. Biochemical and chemotherapeutic studies on 2,4-diamino-6-(2,5-dimethoxybenzyl)-5-methylpyrido[2,3-*d*]pyrimidine (BW301U), a novel lipid-soluble inhibitor of dihydrofolate reductase. Cancer Res 1982; 42:3987–3994.

289. Sigel CW, Macklin AW, Woolley JL, Johnson NW, Collier MA, Blum MR, Clendeninn NJ, Everitt BJM, Grebe G, Mackars A, Foss RG, Duch DS, Bowers SW, Nichol CA. Preclinical biochemical pharmacology and toxicology of piritrexim, a lipophilic inhibitor of dihydrofolate reductase. NCI Monogr 1987; 5:111–120.

290. Fry DW, Besserer JA. Characterization of trimetrexate transport in human lymphoblastoid cells and development of impaired influx as a mechanism of resistance to lipophilic antifolates. Cancer Res 1988; 48:6986–6991.

291. Kamen BA, Eibl B, Cashmore A, Bertino JR. Uptake and efficacy of trimetrexate (TMQ, 2,4-diamino-5-methyl- 6-[(3,4,5-trimethoxyanilino)methyl]-quinazoline), a non-classical antifolate, in methotrexate resistant leukemia cells in vitro. Biochem Pharmacol 1984; 33:1697–1699.

292. Sirotnak FM, Moccio DM, Goutas LJ, Kelleher LE, Montgomery JA. Biochemical correlates of responsiveness and collateral sensitivity of some methotrexate resistant murine tumors to the lipophilic antifolate, metoprine. Cancer Res 1982; 42:924–928.

293. Van Der Veer LJ, Westerhof GR, Rijksen G, Schornagel JH, Jansen G. Cytotoxicity of methotrexate and trimetrexate and its reversal by folinic acid in human leukemic CCRF-CEM cells with carrier-mediated and receptor-mediated folate uptake. Leuk Res 1989; 13:981–987.

294. Bertino JR, Sawicki WL, Moroson BA, Cashmore AR, Elslager EF. 2,4-Diamino-5-methyl-6-[(3,4,5-trimethoxyanilino)methyl]quinazoline (TMQ), a potent nonclassical folate antagonist inhibitor: I. Effect on dihydrofolate reductase and growth of rodent tumors in vitro and in vivo. Biochem Pharmacol 1979; 28:1983–1987.

295. O'Dwyer PJ, Shoemaker DD, Plowman J, Cradock J, Grill-Lopez A, Leyland-Jones, B. Trimetrexate: a new antifolate entering clinical trials. Invest New Drugs 1985; 3:71–75.

296. Robert F. Trimetrexate as a single agent in patients with advanced head and neck cancer. Semin Oncol 1988; 15:17–21.

297. Licht JD, Gonin R, Antman KH. Phase II trial of trimetrexate in patients with advanced soft-tissue sarcoma. Cancer Chemother Pharmacol 1991; 28:223–225.

298. Maroun J. Clinical response to trimetrexate as sole therapy for nonsmall cell lung cancer. Semin Oncol 1988; 15(suppl 2):17–21.

299. Leiby JM. Trimetrexate: a phase 2 study in previously treated patients with metastatic breast cancer. Semin Oncol 1988; 15:27–31.

300. Laszlo J, Brenckman WD, Morgan E, Clendeninn NJ, Williams T, Currie V, Young C. Initial clinical studies with piritrexim. NCI Monogr 1987; 5:121–125.

301. Kris MG, Gralla RJ, Burke MT, Berkowitz LD, Marks LD, Kelssen DP, Heelan RT. Phase II trial of oral piritrexim (BW301U) in patients with stage III non-small cell lung cancer. Cancer Treat Rep 1987; 71:763–764.

302. Uen WC, Huang AT, Clendeninn NJ, Craig J, Spaulding M. Phase II piritrexim study in squamous head and neck cancer. Proc Am Assoc Cancer Res 1988; 29:208.

303. Feun LG, Gonzalez R, Savaraj N, Hanlon J, Collier M, Robinson WA, Clendennin NJ. Phase II study of piritrexim in metastatic melanoma using intermittent low-dose administration. J Clin Oncol 1991; 9:464–467.

304. Klohs WD, Steinkampf RW, Besserer JA, Fry DW. Cross resistance of pleiotropically drug resistant P388 leukemia cells to the lipophilic antifolates trimetrexate and BW301W. Cancer Lett 1986; 31:253–260.

305. Assaraf YG, Molina A, Schimke RT. Cross-resistance to the lipid-soluble antifolate trimetrexate in human carcinoma cells with the multidrug-resistant phenotype. JNCI 1989; 81:290–294.

306. Arkin H, Ohnuma T, Kamen BA, Holland JF, Vallbhajosula S. Multidrug resistance in a human cell line selected for resistance to trimetrexate. Cancer Res 1989; 49:6556–6561.
307. Assaraf YG, Molina A, Schimke RT. Sequential amplification of dihydrofolate reductase and multidrug resistance genes in Chinese hamster ovary cells selected for stepwise resistance to the lipid soluble antifolate, trimetrexate. J Biol Chem 1989; 264:18326–18334.
308. Cvitkovic E, Domenge C, Gandia D. Case report of acquired piritrexim resistance and collateral methotrexate sensitivity in recurrent squamous cell carcinoma of the head and neck. JNCI 1993; 85:1248.

17

Cellular and Biochemical Aspects of Multidrug Resistance

Suresh V. Ambudkar
*The Johns Hopkins University School of Medicine,
Baltimore, Maryland*

Ira Pastan and Michael M. Gottesman
*National Cancer Institute, National Institutes of Health,
Bethesda, Maryland*

I. INTRODUCTION

A. Overview of the Multidrug Resistance Phenomenon

A variety of cancer cells in vivo exhibit resistance to multiple cytotoxic agents. This phenomenon is called multidrug resistance, and the salient feature of this phenotype is that the cells, when exposed to a single class of anticancer agents, develop cross-resistance to several other chemically unrelated agents (1–4). A majority of metastatic cancers are intrinsically resistant to chemotherapy (see Chap. 2). Others initially respond to treatment, but eventually acquire resistance to the drugs being used in the treatment and to other drugs. Numerous multidrug-resistant human and rodent tumor cell lines have been derived that provide in vitro models for the study of the acquired drug resistance (5,6). There may be several mechanisms involved in the development of resistance to multiple drugs, including drug detoxification and alterations in drug targets (reviewed in Ref. 7). However, the best-characterized mechanism of multidrug resistance is one leading to decreased accumulation of cytotoxic drugs in cells and results from overexpression of an energy-dependent drug transport system. A variety of compounds (Table 1) to which cancer cells develop

Table 1 Agents That Interact with P-Glycoprotein

Anticancer drugs
    Vinca alkaloids (vinblastine, vincristine)
    Anthracyclines (daunorubicin, doxorubicin)
    Epipodophyllotoxins (etoposide, teniposide)
    Antibiotics (dactinomycin; actinomycin D)
    Mitomycin
    Taxol
    Topotecan
Other cytotoxic agents
    Colchicine
    Emetine
    Gramicidin D
    N-Acetyl-leucyl-leucyl-norleucine (ALLN)
    Podophyllotoxin
    Puromycin
    Valinomycin
Agents that reverse multidrug resistance
    Calcium channel blockers (verapamil, dihydropyridines, azidopine)
    Antiarrhythmics (quinidine, quinine)
    Antihypertensives (reserpine, yohimbine)
    Antibiotics (hydrophobic cephalosporins)
    Diterpenes (forskolin)
    Detergents (Tween-80, Triton X-100)
    Immunosuppressants (cyclosporine A, FK506)
    Lipophilic cations (tetraphenylphosphonium)
    Steroid hormones (progesterone)

Source: Adapted from Ref. 1.

cross-resistance are known to interact with this transport system. Although these agents have little in common structurally, they are hydrophobic (i.e., preferentially soluble in lipid) and usually exhibit a tendency to be positively charged at neutral pH. The list in Table 1 also includes noncytotoxic compounds that reverse the multidrug-resistance phenotype. Some of these reversing agents (e.g., verapamil) appear to be substrates transported by the system that handles cytotoxic drugs, whereas others (e.g., cyclosporine A and progesterone) appear to compete only for binding to the transporter itself.

Ling and co-workers, in the early 1970s, observed the increased expression of a 170-kDa plasma membrane phosphoglycoprotein termed P-glycoprotein (P denotes altered permeability; Pgp, also called P170, or the multidrug transporter) in multidrug-resistant Chinese hamster cells (8). P-glycoprotein is encoded by the *MDR1* gene in humans and by *mdr1a* and *mdr1b* genes in rodents (9,10). In many multidrug-resistant cells, including human KB carcinoma cells, the levels of Pgp and its mRNA are directly proportional to the degree of resistance (2,4,11), suggesting that the expression of this protein is the major means by which these cells become drug-resistant. Transfection experiments have demonstrated that expression of the mouse or the human *mdr* cDNAs in drug-sensitive cells is sufficient to confer the drug-resistance phenotype (1,2,4). Recently, Cole and co-workers (12) have observed increased expression of a 190-kDa membrane protein, termed multidrug resistance-associated protein (MRP), in a doxorubicin-resistant small-cell lung cancer cell line, H69AR, that displays the multidrug-resistance phenotype, but does not overexpress Pgp. The *MRP* gene has been cloned, and the overall predicted structural organization of the protein is similar to Pgp (12). It is believed that, similar to Pgp, MRP functions as an ATP-dependent transporter for anticancer drugs. This review will focus on recent data on the cellular, molecular biological, and biochemical aspects of Pgp (throughout this chapter, the *MDR1* gene product will be referred to either as Pgp or the multidrug transporter). Chapter 18, which follows, deals with modulation of multidrug resistance.

II. CHARACTERIZATION OF THE MULTIDRUG-RESISTANCE GENE FAMILY

A. Isolation of the *MDR1* Gene

The presence of homogeneously staining regions of chromosomes, as well as minute and double-minute chromosomes, was observed in multidrug-resistant cells. This suggested that some of the genes were amplified in the resistant cells and, indeed, this phenomenon facilitated the isolation of *mdr* genes. By using techniques such as "in-gel renaturation," differential cDNA libraries, and Pgp-specific monoclonal antibodies, *mdr* cDNAs were isolated from human, mouse, and Chinese hamster cells, respectively (reviewed in Refs. 1,2). The human and hamster *mdr* genes are also referred to as *pgy* and *pgp*, respectively.

B. Mammalian *MDR* Gene Family

The mammalian *mdr* gene family is composed of two highly homologous members in humans and three members in rodents (13). The human *MDR1* and *MDR2* genes encode proteins that are about 76% identical in their amino acid sequence, but only the *MDR1* gene confers drug resistance. Similarly, mouse *mdr1a* and *mdr1b* (also called *mdr3* and *mdr1*, respectively) and their hamster homologues, *pgp1* and *pgp2*, code for proteins that are more than 80% identical in amino acid sequence with human Pgp, the *MDR1* gene product. These mouse and hamster genes also confer multidrug resistance. The *mdr* genes are genetically linked and, in humans, they are localized on chromosome 7 near q21.1 (3). Recent work with *mdr2* knock-out mice indicates that the *mdr2* gene product is essential for phosphatidylcholine to be secreted into bile (14). In addition, an *MDR1–MDR2* chimeric protein containing *MDR2* ATP-binding folds is functional as an ATP-dependent drug efflux pump (15; Germann UA, Wu P, Currier SJ, Aksentijevich I, Pastan I, Gottesman MM, unpublished data), strongly suggesting that the MDR2 protein can function as an ATP-dependent pump. Genes that are either homologues of, or related to, *mdr* genes have been found in yeast, protozoan parasites, worms (*Caenorhabditis elegans*), *Drosophila*, marine sponges, and plants (reviewed in Refs.

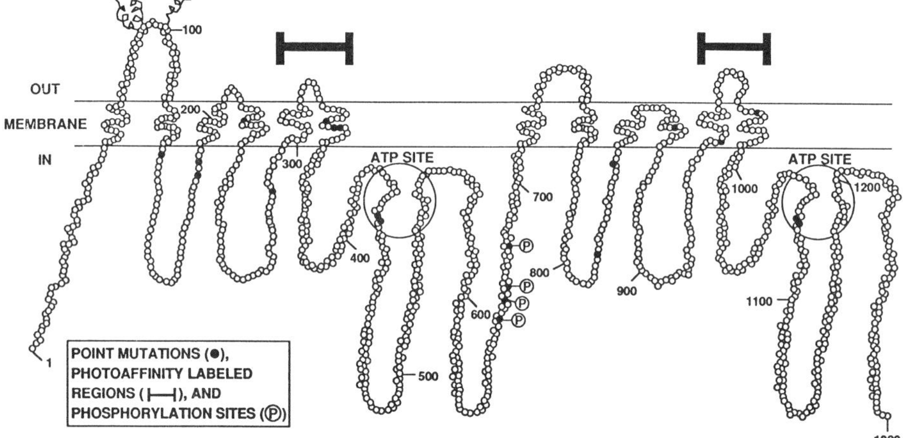

Figure 1 Two-dimensional model of human P-glycoprotein based on hydropathy analysis of the amino acid sequence (9). The ATP sites (nucleotide-binding folds) are circled and the putative *N*-linked glycosylation sites are indicated by wiggly lines. The bars above the model show the regions labeled with photoaffinity analogues. Darkened circles represent amino acid residues, except for those in the ATP sites, in which mutations have been shown to affect drug transport specificity. The mutations in the amino acid residues in the 6th and 11th transmembrane domains were originally described in Chinese hamster and mouse Pgp, respectively. Serine residues at positions 661, 667, 671, and 683 have been shown in vitro to be phosphorylated either by protein kinase C or by protein kinase A (65,66). (Adapted from Ref. 1.)

1,16,17). Although most of these gene products are not yet well characterized, many of them are associated with the development of drug resistance.

The human *MDR1* cDNA encodes an 1280-amino acid protein. Hydropathy profiling of the deduced amino acid sequences has led to a secondary structure model of Pgp (Fig. 1), which contains 12 putative transmembrane segments with two ATP (nucleotide)-binding domains on the cytoplasmic surface of the membrane (2,9). Each half of the protein contains a hydrophobic region, with six transmembrane helices and a large hydrophilic region with one ATP-binding fold. Although the NH_2-terminal half of the molecule exhibits 43% sequence identity with the COOH-terminal half, the lack of homologous introns suggests that the two halves of the molecule might have either evolved independently or undergone a major rearrangement of introns after a duplication event (18). Among the human and rodent Pgps, the ATP-binding domains and the first, second, fourth, and fifth intracytoplasmic loops are most conserved, whereas the NH_2- and COOH-termini, first extracellular loop, and the linker region connecting both halves of the molecule are the least homologous regions.

C. Superfamily of ABC Transporters

Because of considerable similarities in the predicted overall topology and the presence of homologous ATP-binding domains, Pgp belongs to the ATP-binding cassette (ABC) superfamily of transporters (reviewed in Refs. 16,17). The most conserved regions in the ATP-binding domain are the Walker motifs A and B, the center region, and the "linker peptide" (also called Walker C motif) -LSGGXRhXhXhA (X, any amino acid; h, hydrophobic) preceding the Walker B region (19,20). Although the Walker A and B regions are present in other ATP-binding proteins, the center region and the linker peptide are found only in ABC transporters. The linker-dodecapeptide appears to be a signature of these transporters, and it has been suggested that this region may be responsible for coupling the ATP hydrolysis-dependent conformational changes to the drug-transport process, likely through the interaction with the membrane domains of the transporters (20). The ABC superfamily, also known as the solute ATPases or traffic ATPases (16,17), now includes more than 50 members (20,21). The eukaryotic members of this family include Pgp (also a protozoan pfMDR, which is associated with chloroquine resistance in *Plasmodium falciparum* (see Chap. 13); CFTR, the cystic fibrosis transmembrane conductance regulator; STE6, the yeast **a** mating factor transporter; RING-4, HAM1, and HAM2 [also known as Tap-1 and Tap-2 (transporters associated with antigen presentation)]; the human and mouse MHC-linked transporters and peroxisomal proteins, such as PMP70 and the adrenoleukodystrophy protein (ALDP) (22). The prokaryotic members include binding protein-dependent permeases for amino acids (e.g., histidine permease (19), ions and sugars, and proteins involved in the export of toxins (HylB, LktB) and glycans (ChvA, NdvA) (for a complete list of these transporters see Refs. 17,20,21). Thus, the substrates transported by members of this superfamily include ions, solutes, peptides, proteins, lipids, and cytotoxic natural product drugs.

III. TOPOLOGY OF THE MULTIDRUG TRANSPORTER

The secondary structure model with 12 transmembrane helices of Pgp proposed by our group (see Fig. 1) is supported by epitope localization for both monoclonal (23,24) and polyclonal antibodies (25), and is similar to that of several secondary transporters, including bacterial lactose permease, the topology of which has been confirmed by *PhoA* (alkaline phosphatase) fusions. Recently, alternative models have been proposed that are based on (1) coupled in vitro translation and translocation of full-length or truncated forms of mouse Pgp into canine pancreatic microsomal membranes (26,27), and (2) expression of human Pgp in frog oocytes (28). From in vitro studies, Ling and co-workers proposed that the third and tenth transmembrane domains might be exposed in the cytoplasm, whereas the fifth and eighth might be extracellular. By this model, in addition to glycosylation sites in the first extracellular loop, another site on the second extracellular loop, between the fourth and fifth transmembrane domain, is also glycosylated. Skach and colleagues have proposed yet another model with ten transmembrane domains, and here, the eighth and ninth domains are extracellular and the truncated or full-length molecules are glycosylated on Asn-809, which is located in the loop between the eighth and ninth domains. Several observations strongly suggest that Pgp molecules with either eight or ten transmembrane domains might be formed as a result of a defective biogenesis process, and that such molecules may not be functional under normal physiological conditions: (1) Pgps with alternative structures (i.e., with eight or ten transmembrane domains) have not yet been demonstrated on cell surfaces of mammalian cells. (2) Treatment of Pgp, purified from human multidrug-resistant KB-V1 cells, with trypsin results in the cleavage of the protein in the linker region, generating 110- and 55-kDa fragments corresponding to NH_2- and COOH-termini, respectively. This COOH-terminal fragment, which contains the 7th through 12th transmembrane helices and an ATP-binding domain, is not glycosylated, indicating that Asn-809 is not used for glycosylation in these cells (Ambudkar SV, Zhang J, Lelong I, Cardarelli CO, Pastan I, Gottesman MM, unpublished data). (3) Mutant Pgp molecules lacking all the glycosylation sites located in the first extracellular loop are not glycosylated, but do appear at the cell surface, although with decreased efficiency (29). Thus, in these mutants other potential glycosylation sites, including one in the second extracellular loop or Asn-809 in the COOH-terminal region, are not used (see Sec. IV.C). (4) The functional integrity of Pgp molecules with alternative structures remains to be assessed. The availability in large quantity of homogenous Pgp molecules with alternative structures will help resolve these issues. Similarly, antibodies directed against regions that are predicted to be on opposite sides of the plasma membrane by these three models will be useful in determining the predominant form of topology of Pgp in mammalian cells.

IV. STRUCTURE–FUNCTION STUDIES

During recent years, considerable attention has been focused on the structure–function analysis of Pgp. The intriguing question is how a membrane protein, a product of a single gene, can handle a wide variety of cytotoxic drugs, as well as other hydrophobic agents (see Table 1). The analysis and mapping of various structural domains of Pgp that are associated with substrate recognition, and with coupling the ATP utilization site(s) with the substrate binding and translocation processes, will be required to understand the mechanism of the transporter. A combination of biochemical, genetic, and molecular biological approaches has been employed to resolve these issues. This section summarizes the recent data on mutational analysis of Pgp, labeling of substrate binding sites on Pgp with photoaffinity analogues, and the role of posttranslational modifications in the function of Pgp.

A. Analysis of Mutations

Several naturally occurring and genetically engineered point mutations have been described that affect the substrate specificity of Pgp. These mutations, as illustrated in Figure 1, are scattered throughout the Pgp molecule, suggesting that the substrate recognition site(s) have a complex structure. The first well-characterized point mutation in Pgp was described in human KB carcinoma cells that were selected in high levels of colchicine. In this mutant, substitution of Gly-185 by valine in the intracellular loop near the third transmembrane segment (see Fig. 1) resulted in increased resistance to colchicine and etoposide, but decreased resistance to vinblastine and dactinomycin (actinomycin D) (30–32). Whether this mutation affects the initial drug-binding step, or the subsequent drug release from the transporter, is still an open question (reviewed in Ref. 1). Another spontaneously selected mutation has been described by Melera's group, in Chinese hamster cells selected for a high degree of resistance to dactinomycin (33). In the mutant Pgp, two adjacent amino acids were changed, glycine to alanine and alanine to proline at positions 338 and 339 in the transmembrane domain 6. These mutations appear to increase the level of relative resistance to dactinomycin. Gros and co-workers changed Ser-941 to phenylalanine within transmembrane domain 11 of mouse *mdr1* (34). This mutation drastically decreased the resistance to certain drugs (doxorubicin and colchicine), while increasing resistance to others (dactinomycin). These substitutions (Ser-941 to phenylalanine and Ser-939 to phenylalanine in mouse *mdr1* and *mdr3*, respectively) also reduce the capacity of reversing agents, such as verapamil and progesterone, to modulate Pgp activity (35,36). Interestingly, the Val-185 as well as the Phe-939 mutation also drastically affect the ability of human *MDR1* or mouse *mdr3* to complement the activity of yeast **a**-mating factor transporter, *STE6*, suggesting that these mutations affect not only the specificity for cytotoxic drugs, but also for hydrophobic peptides (37,38).

Loo and Clarke (39) have employed a site-directed mutagenesis approach to change 13 proline residues, located in the putative transmembrane domains, to alanine in the human kidney Pgp. Similarly, they also changed 31 phenylalanine residues in the putative transmembrane regions to alanine and 20 glycine residues in the predicted cytoplasmic loops to valine (40,41). The mutant cDNAs were transfected in mouse NIH 3T3 cells to assess their ability to confer drug resistance. Mutations of either Pro-223 in the fourth transmembrane domain or Pro-866 in the tenth transmembrane segment significantly altered the ability of mutant proteins to confer resistance to colchicine, doxorubicin, or dactinomycin. However, these mutant Pgps conferred resistance to vinblastine to the same degree as the wild-type protein. Thus, these proline residues in transmembrane domains 4 and 10, which occupy the same positions when NH_2- and COOH-terminal halves are aligned, may play important roles in substrate recognition. Analysis of mutant Pgps with replacement of phenylalanines in the membrane segments by alanine revealed that mutation of either Phe-335 in transmembrane domain 6, or Phe-978 in transmembrane domain 12, substantially altered the drug-resistance profile of transfected cells. The mutant Phe-335 to alanine protein conferred increased resistance to colchicine and doxorubicin, whereas mutant Phe-978 to alanine conferred little or no resistance to these drugs. Mutation of Gly-141, 187, 288, 812, or 830 to valine also altered the drug resistance profiles. These mutations resulted in increased resistance to colchicine and doxorubicin, without affecting the relative resistance to vinblastine. Since the mutations just described are spread across the entire molecule, it is not clear whether the observed effects are due to alteration in substrate recognition site(s), or are mainly a secondary effect of alteration in the three-dimensional conformation of the protein.

Mutations have also been engineered in the highly conserved sequences of the Walker A motifs of both NH_2- and COOH-terminal ATP-binding domains (42). The substitution of a glycine with an alanine at positions 431 or 1073 or of a lysine with arginine at positions 432 or 1074 (see Fig. 1) in the mouse *mdr1* gene reduced the ability of Pgp to confer drug resistance to transfected cells. However, photoaffinity labeling of mutant Pgps with 8-azido-ATP was not affected, indicating that a step subsequent to ATP-binding is impaired. In addition to point mutations, several studies have been carried out on deletions, insertions, substitutions, and chimeric *MDR1–MDR2* proteins. Because of space limitations, these will not be discussed here (see Ref. 1).

B. Drug Binding and Photoaffinity Labeling

Studies on binding of isotopically labeled cytotoxic agents (vinblastine) or a reversing agent (verapamil) to the isolated plasma membranes of drug-resistant cells provided the initial biochemical evidence for the involvement of Pgp in the development of multidrug-resistance phenomena (43). Currently, numerous radiolabeled photoaffinity substrates and substrate analogues are available that specifically bind to Pgp. These include vinblastine, verapamil, colchicine, iodomycin, azidopine, azidoprazosin, cyclosporine, and forskolin (44,45). Photoaffinity labeling of Pgp with these agents is specific, since it can be inhibited by an excess amount of cytotoxic drugs or reversing agents. The photoaffinity-labeling approach has been used to identify the region(s) on the Pgp molecule that are involved in the substrate recognition or transport. By proteolytic digestion and cyanogen bromide cleavage, [³H]azidopine-labeled fragments of human Pgp have been identified using antibodies specific to various regions of the molecule (46). Both the NH_2- and COOH-regions are labeled equally; one of these sites is located in the region around transmembrane domains 5 and 6, and the other is near transmembrane domains 11 and 12 (see Fig. 1). Recently, by using iodoazidoprazosin and iodoforskolin analogues for photolabeling, the labeled regions have been localized to the fifth or sixth transmembrane segment or the region immediately following the sixth transmembrane segment and a region within the 12th transmembrane segment or the cytoplasmic region immediately following the 12th segment (47,48). The specific amino acids labeled with these photoaffinity agents have not yet been identified. However, these findings, together with the observation that labeling of both halves of Pgp is inhibited equally by vinblastine (49), strongly suggest that the two halves of the molecule together form a single transport pore or channel.

C. Post-Translational Modifications

1. Glycosylation

The mammalian Pgps are heavily N-glycosylated, mainly with oligosaccharides of the complex type. The exact chemical structure of the polysaccharide moiety has not yet been determined. The following observations suggest that N-glycosylation may not be essential for the functional activity of Pgp: (1) inhibition of N-glycosylation with tunicamycin treatment does not affect drug resistance of multidrug-resistant cells (50); (2) multidrug-resistant sublines can be selected from N-glycosylation-defective, lectin-resistant mutants (51); (3) transfectants expressing mutant human Pgp lacking all three potential N-glycosylation sites in the first extracellular loop (see Fig. 1) still display drug resistance patterns similar to those expressing wild-type, N-glycosylated Pgp (29); and (4) recombinant Pgps produced in heterologous expression systems, such as Sf9 (insect) cells and yeast in which no significant glycosylation can be observed, exhibit either drug-stimulated ATPase activity or ATP-dependent drug transport (52–54; Ni B, Pastan I, Gottesman MM, unpublished data). It is possible that N-glycosylation may be involved to some extent in routing or sorting Pgp to the cell surface, since mutants lacking glycosylation sites in the first extracellular loop show reduced expression at the cell surface, or N-glycosylation may stabilize the protein in the plasma membrane (29).

2. Phosphorylation

There is considerable evidence to suggest that protein kinases may be involved in the expression and function of Pgp and multidrug resistance (for additional details see Chap. 18). Several groups have reported an increase in kinase activities or increased phosphorylation of Pgp in multidrug-resistant cells (55–59). Elevated levels of protein kinase C (PKC) are associated with increased multidrug resistance of some, but not all, multidrug-resistant cells (56,57,60). Glazer's group (61,62) has shown that transfection of a plasmid expressing functional PKC-α, but not PKC-γ, is associated with an increase in multidrug resistance in BC-19 cells. This indicates that the regulation of Pgp is dependent on specific isoform(s) of PKC. However, it is possible that, in these transfected cells, PKC-α may have an indirect effect on Pgp, such as by increasing mRNA (63). Bates et al. (64) have demonstrated that the inhibition of PKC with calphostin

C or staurosporine, or by prolonged treatment with the phorbol ester 12-O-tetradecanoylphorbal-13-acetate (TPA), led to decreased phosphorylation of Pgp, and these treatments also affected the action of certain antagonists, but a direct effect of phosphorylation has not been shown.

The specific serine residues in human Pgp phosphorylated in vitro by PKC have been identified (65). Serine residues 661, 667, and 671 are phosphorylated by PKC, whereas Ser-683 is phosphorylated by PKA. These residues are clustered in the linker region located between the two halves of Pgp (see Fig. 1). Similarly, in mouse *mdr1b* gene-encoded Pgp, Ser-669 and Ser-681 are phosphorylated by PKC and PKA, respectively (66). This region (amino acids 629–687), encoded by exon 16, contains 38% charged residues and has been called a "mini R domain," as it is analogous to the R domain of CFTR protein (67). The R domain of CFTR contains several PKA and PKC consensus phosphorylation sites, and this region is implicated in the regulation of CFTR function (68). Recently, we have purified a novel 55- to 60-kDa membrane-associated kinase from human multidrug-resistant KB-V1 cells that predominantly phosphorylates Pgp. The kinase can function either in the presence of Mg^{2+} or Mn^{2+} and is inhibited by a calcium concentration greater than 1 mM. This kinase, referred to as "V-1 kinase," does not phosphorylate histone or peptide-substrates of PKC or PKA, and is inhibited only by staurosporine (Ambudkar SV, Park G, Cardarelli CO, Pastan I, Gottesman MM, unpublished data). Analysis of the amino acid sequence of the purified V-1 kinase will facilitate the determination of its identity. The conclusive evidence of a direct role of PKC-, PKA- or V-1 kinase-mediated phosphorylation in regulating the activity of Pgp remains to be demonstrated by using pure Pgp functionally reconstituted into phospholipid vesicles.

V. IN VITRO ANALYSIS OF THE MULTIDRUG TRANSPORTER-ASSOCIATED ACTIVITIES

The hallmark of multidrug-resistant cells is decreased accumulation of cytotoxic drugs in these cells when compared with sensitive cells. This decreased accumulation can be either due to a decrease in drug influx, an increase in drug efflux, or a combination of both. The energy-dependent drug efflux process can be studied in plasma membrane vesicles with inside-out orientation, as drug will be transported into the lumen of vesicles, resulting in accumulation against the concentration gradient of the drug. Plasma membrane vesicles, as well as phospholipid vesicles reconstituted with partially or homogeneously purified Pgp, have been used to demonstrate that Pgp functions as an ATP-dependent transporter. Additionally, the ATPase activity of Pgp stimulated by its substrates has also been characterized. These recent advances are summarized below.

A. Drug Transport by Membrane Vesicles and Reconstituted Proteoliposomes

Plasma membrane vesicles of mixed orientation prepared from multidrug-resistant human KB-V1 cells transport [³H]vinblastine, but similar preparations from drug-sensitive KB-3-1 cells fail to do so (69). Accumulation of the drug in inside-out vesicles is ATP-dependent, sensitive to osmolarity, and appears to occur against a concentration gradient. Among various nucleotides tested as a source of energy, only GTP, and to some extent ITP, supported vinblastine transport in vesicles, whereas CTP, UTP, ADP, and AMP were ineffective (70). AMP-PNP, a nonhydrolyzable ATP analogue, competitively inhibits ATP-driven, vinblastine transport, whereas vanadate, a P-type ATPase inhibitor, is a noncompetitive inhibitor. Drugs to which multidrug-resistant cell lines are resistant inhibit transport to various degrees in a competitive manner (71), suggesting that Pgp may have a single or small number of overlapping binding sites. Verapamil and quinidine, which are potent reversing agents, also inhibit transport competitively in the vesicle system. Doige and Sharom (72) have characterized ATP-dependent [³H]colchicine transport in inside-out membrane vesicles prepared from the multidrug-resistant Chinese hamster ovary cell line, CH^R C5. As just noted for vinblastine transport, colchicine transport was also inhibited by vanadate and by other Pgp substrates, such as vinblastine and verapamil. In general, the hydrophobic nature of Pgp substrates leads to increased nonspecific binding and, consequently, it has been difficult to carry out detailed kinetic analysis of inhibition by various substrates in the plasma membrane vesicle system.

Sharom and co-workers partially purified Pgp from CH^R C5 cell (see foregoing) by using CHAPS detergent and subsequently reconstituted the protein into phospholipid vesicles (73). In these proteoliposomes, about 50% of Pgp molecules are reconstituted with an inside-out orientation. These proteoliposomes catalyze ATP-dependent [³H]colchicine transport that is osmotically sensitive and is also inhibited by vinblastine, verapamil, or daunomycin. We have obtained over 90% pure Pgp by conventional chromatographic procedures on octylglucoside-solubilized plasma membrane proteins of KB-V1 cells. Purified Pgp was reconstituted into proteoliposomes by detergent dialysis, followed by Sephadex G-50 column chromatography. In these proteoliposomes, more than 90% of Pgp is reconstituted with inside-out orientation. Such proteoliposomes display ATP-dependent saturable [³H]vinblastine accumulation that is blocked by vanadate, indicating that ATP hydrolysis is required for the drug uptake. Additionally, the vinblastine transport is inhibited by verapamil and doxorubicin, but not by camptothecin, which is not a substrate for Pgp (Ambudkar SV, Zhang J, Lelong I, Park G, Cardarelli CO, Pastan I, Gottesman MM, unpublished data). These studies with purified Pgp provide compelling evidence that Pgp, the *MDR1* gene product, functions as a multidrug transporter. The detailed kinetic analysis of the drug transport process as well as the stoichiometry of ATP hydrolysis and vinblastine transport have not yet been determined.

B. Drug-Dependent ATPase Activity in Membranes and Reconstituted System

Almost 20 years ago Dano observed that treatment with azide resulted in accumulation of anticancer drugs in multidrug-resistant cells, suggesting the involvement of an ATP-driven process (74). Mutational analysis of conserved residues in the ATP-binding sites (see Sec. IV.A) further strengthened this view. However, the Pgp-associated ATPase activity has only recently been biochemically characterized. Crude membranes of Sf9 (insect) cells infected with baculovirus–*MDR1* exhibit high levels of vinblastine- or verapamil-stimulated ATPase activity (3–5 μmol/min per milligram of Pgp) (53). Although some of the recombinant Pgp is associated with the plasma membranes of Sf9 cells, most of the protein is retained in intracellular vesicles, which can be separated from other membranes by centrifugation of the postnuclear lysate at 5000 g. Both the plasma and intracellular membrane fractions exhibit similar drug-stimulated Pgp–ATPase activity. However, the octylglucoside-solubilized protein from these membranes elutes at different salt concentrations during anion-exchange chromatography (Ambudkar SV, Germann U, Pastan I, Gottesman MM, unpublished data). This heterogeneity may be due to the differences in the posttranslational modifications of Pgp and also in lipid composition of these membranes. The ATPase activity of Pgp in plasma membranes from highly drug-resistant Chinese hamster ovary cell lines, which overexpress Pgp so that it constitutes 5–30% by weight of total plasma membrane protein, has been characterized (75,76). These cells were selected for resistance to colchicine at very high concentrations (5–30 μg/ml), and this might result in overexpression of various *mdr* genes (i.e., *mdr1*, *mdr3*, and *mdr2*) (see Sec. II.B). Thus, the observed ATPase activities may be due to Pgps encoded by one or more *mdr* genes.

We have partially purified Pgp from human multidrug-resistant KB-V1 cells that overexpress only *MDR1* (Schoenlein PV, Gottesman MM, unpublished data) and reconstituted it into artificial membrane vesicles prepared from a lipid mixture of *Escherichia coli* bulk phospholipid, phosphatidylcholine, phosphatidylserine, and cholesterol (77). The Pgp is predominantly reconstituted into proteoliposomes in an inside-out orientation (>90%), and the ATPase activity was stimulated only by drugs that are known to be its substrates. Camptothecin, the hydrophobic anticancer drug that is not a substrate for Pgp, does not stimulate ATPase activity (Fig. 2). Although the basal ATPase activity of Pgp is preserved in the detergent solution, the stimulation by cytotoxic drug–substrates (vinblastine) or reversing agents (verapamil) is not. The lack of effect of these agents may be due to an interaction of hydrophobic detergent with the drug–substrate-binding site(s) on Pgp. Alternatively, the conformation of soluble Pgp may not be suitable for substrate-induced activation. The requirement of a membrane environment for the substrate-induced stimulation has also been reported for other members of the superfamily of ABC transporters (78,79), and it is quite possible that this property will turn out to be the diagnostic feature of these transporters.

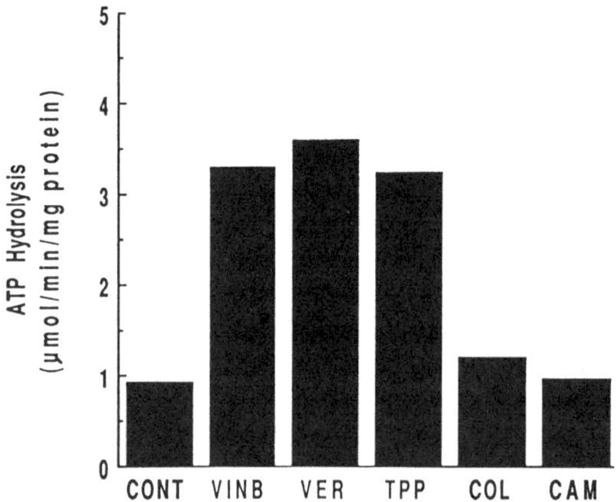

Figure 2   Effect of various drugs on ATPase activity of reconstituted P-glycoprotein. The partially purified human P-glycoprotein was reconstituted into proteoliposomes by detergent–dilution procedure and the ATPase activity in the presence and absence of 100 μM vanadate was measured (77). CONT, control (dimethyl sulfoxide-treated); VINB, 20 μM vinblastine; VER, 100 μM verapamil; TPP, 100 μM tetraphenylphosphonium bromide; COL, 100 μM colchicine; CAM, 100 μM camptothecin. Only the vanadate-sensitive activities are shown. [Adapted from Ref. 77 and Ambudkar SV, Lelong I, Zhang J, Pastan I, Gottesman MM, unpublished data.]

The interaction of substrate–drugs with Pgp leads to increase in the maximal velocity of ATPase activity, without affecting the apparent K_m for ATP (300 μM; 77). The vinblastine-stimulated ATPase activity of purified Pgp in proteoliposomes ranges from 5 to 25 μmol/min per milligram of protein, depending on the method of reconstitution, confirming our earlier work with the partially purified protein showing that this is a high-capacity pump similar to other ion-transporting ATPases (Ambudkar SV, Zhang J, Lelong I, Park G, Cardarelli CO, Pastan I, Gottesman MM, unpublished data). Several cytotoxic drugs, such as vinblastine, doxorubicin, daunomycin, and dactinomycin, stimulate the ATPase activity in a dose-dependent manner. However, colchicine is only marginally effective as a stimulator of Pgp–ATPase activity, even in Chinese hamster cells, which are selected in high concentrations of this drug (see Fig. 2; 75,76). The reason for this discrepancy is not now known. In addition to ATP, 2'-dATP, 8-azido-ATP, and 2-azido-ATP are also good substrates for Pgp–ATPase (80).

Vanadate is a potent inhibitor of ATPase activity as well as the drug transport activity. The mechanism of vanadate inhibition of Pgp is not yet clear. Sulfhydryl reagents, such as N-ethylmaleimide, also inhibit the Pgp–ATPase activity, and Mg–ATP protects from such inactivation (80). This suggests that the sulfhydryl groups may be located within the catalytic site. The analysis of primary structure indicates that the cysteine residue in the Walker A region of both ATP-binding domains is conserved in all mammalian Pgps encoded either by *MDR1* or *MDR2* genes and also in some of the other ABC transporters (9,10,16,17,20). It is possible that NH_2- and COOH-terminal ATP domains are linked by a disulfide bond. Directed mutagenesis of these cysteines will help elucidate their role in Pgp function. Although it is known that the ATP-binding domain alone (see Fig. 1) is sufficient for ATP binding, it is unclear whether other parts of the molecule, such as the transmembrane region(s), are also required for ATP hydrolysis. The availability of large quantities of pure ATP-binding domains by overexpression in a heterologous expression system may help resolve some of these issues. Similarly, the nature of the interaction between the NH_2- and COOH-terminal nucleotide-binding domains is not yet known.

VI. MECHANISM OF ACTION OF THE MULTIDRUG TRANSPORTER

The detailed mechanism by which Pgp regulates intracellular drug levels below a toxic threshold in multidrug-resistant cells is not yet completely understood. The physiological, pharmacological, and cell biological aspects of drug transport experiments with multidrug-resistant cells suggest that decreased drug influx or increased drug efflux, or a combination of both, could account for the maintenance of drugs at low levels in the cytoplasm. The compounds that interact with Pgp (see Table 1), because of their hydrophobic nature, partition into and out of membrane in a rapid equilibrium, but move more slowly through the membrane bilayer. The kinetic analysis of drug uptake and efflux data (32), and other experimental evidence (see later) supports the hypothesis that drugs are directly removed from the plasma membrane. Hydrophobic peptides (e.g., gramicidin D, valinomycin, or N-acetyl-leucyl-leucyl-norleucine) to which multiresistant cells are cross-resistant are thought to accumulate mainly in the plasma membrane of drug-sensitive cells that do not express Pgp (81). A fluorescent dye, rhodamine 123, which is a substrate for Pgp, is distributed predominantly in an aqueous environment in multidrug-resistant cells, suggesting that the drug has been cleared from the plasma membrane (82,83). These conclusions are also supported by the labeling of Pgp in multidrug-resistant cells with iodinated naphthalene azide after photoactivation in the presence of doxorubicin (84).

According to our current model (see Fig. 3 in Ref. 1), drug efflux by Pgp results from the extraction of drugs that partition into the plasma membrane from either the extracellular medium or the cytoplasm. In addition, drugs from the cytoplasm may be directly expelled by Pgp. This implies that the drug recognition or binding site(s) may be accessible from the aqueous cytoplasmic side as well as from the nonpolar interior of the membrane. Another important feature of our model is that both halves of single or multiple molecules of Pgp cooperate to form a pore or channel through which drugs are expelled, at the expense of energy derived from the hydrolysis of ATP. This proposal is consistent with data from mutational analysis, photoaffinity analysis, and inhibitor studies already described (see Secs. IV.A and B). For the initial drug binding, however, our model still allows multiple interaction sites that may differ for various substrates. It is unknown how the energy from ATP hydrolysis is coupled to drug transport. Similarly, the broad substrate specificity of Pgp is another major unresolved issue. The mechanism of action of Pgp is not yet confirmed, and the model discussed here represents only one of several suggested working hypotheses. The description of other models and relevant aspects have been reviewed elsewhere (1–4,7,21,85–87).

VII. MULTIDRUG TRANSPORTER: IS IT ALSO AN ANION CHANNEL?

The biochemical studies discussed in the foregoing clearly demonstrate that Pgp functions as an ATP-driven pump for the extrusion of a variety of hydrophobic compounds. Work by Higgins and co-workers suggests that Pgp may also function as an anion channel. These workers observed that human *MDR1*-transfected NIH 3T3 cells exhibit chloride channel activity that is activated by hyposmotic swelling. The volume-regulated chloride channel activity requires the binding of ATP, but not its hydrolysis, and it is blocked by drugs that are known to interact with Pgp (88,89). Another ABC transporter, CFTR, functions as a chloride channel that is activated by protein kinase A-dependent phosphorylation (67,68). Although the idea that Pgp may be bifunctional and act as both a drug transporter and as an anion channel is very attractive, the latter function is still controversial. Two groups have recently reported that they failed to observe Pgp-associated volume-regulated chloride channel activity in a variety of multidrug-resistant cell lines (90,91). Similarly, we failed to detect chloride channel activity in the presence of ATP when purified Pgp was incorporated into a planar phospholipid bilayer. P-glycoprotein phosphorylated by protein kinase C before its incorporation into the bilayer also failed to exhibit the chloride conductance activity (Ambudkar SV, Chanturiya AN, Zimmerberg J, Pastan I, Gottesman MM, unpublished data). Although it is quite possible that Pgp can function as a modulator of chloride channel activity associated with volume regulation, definite proof for such role will require coreconstitution of Pgp and channel protein in phospholipid vesicles.

A recent report also suggests that Pgp may function as an ATP channel (92). Release of ATP into extracellular medium was proportional to the Pgp amount in highly drug-resistant Chinese hamster ovary and human lung tumor cell lines. The measurement of single-channel current requires the presence of nonphysiological concentrations (100 mM) of ATP on both sides of the excised patch. Further work is required to determine whether Pgp functions as an ATP channel, or whether expression of Pgp results in activation of already existing channels. The physiological significance of such activity is now unclear.

ACKNOWLEDGMENTS

We thank Joyce Sharrar for the help with preparation of the figures. SVA was supported in part by the American Cancer Society research grant, BE-157.

REFERENCES

1. Gottesman MM, Pastan I. Biochemistry of multidrug resistance mediated by the multidrug transporter. Annu Rev Biochem 1993; 62:385–427.

2.   Gottesman MM, Pastan I. The multidrug-transporter: a double-edged sword. J Biol Chem 1988; 263:12163–12166.
3.   Roninson IB. Molecular and Cellular Biology of Multidrug Resistance in Tumor Cells. New York: Plenum Press, 1991.
4.   Endicott JA, Ling V. The biochemistry of P-glycoprotein-mediated multidrug-resistance. Annu Rev Biochem 1989; 58:137–171.
5.   Beck WT, Danks MK. Characteristics of multidrug resistance in human tumor cells. In: Roninson IB, ed. Molecular and Cellular Biology of Multidrug Resistance in Tumor Cells. New York: Plenum Publishing, 1991:3–46.
6.   Sugimoto Y, Tsuruo T. Development of multidrug resistance in rodent cell lines. In: Roninson IB, ed. Molecular and Cellular Biology of Multidrug Resistance in Tumor Cells. New York: Plenum Publishing, 1991:57–70.
7.   Simon SM, Schindler M. Cell biological mechanisms of multidrug resistance in tumors. Proc Natl Acad Sci USA 1994; 91:3497–3504.
8.   Juliano RL, Ling V. A surface glycoprotein modulating drug permeability in Chinese hamster ovary cell mutants. Biochim Biophys Acta 1976; 455:152–162.
9.   Chen C-J, Chin CE, Ueda K, Clark DP, Pastan I, Gottesman MM, Roninson IB. Internal duplication and homology with bacterial transport proteins in the *mdr1* (P-glycoprotein) gene from multidrug-resistant gene from human cells. Cell 1986; 47:381–389.
10. Gros P, Croop J, Housman DE. Mammalian multidrug resistance gene: complete cDNA sequence indicates strong homology to bacterial transport proteins. Cell 1986; 47:371–380.
11. Ueda K, Cornwell MM, Gottesman MM, Pastan I, Roninson IB, Ling V, Riordan JR. The *mdr1* gene, responsible for multidrug-resistance, codes for P-glycoprotein. Biochem Biophys Res Commun 1986; 141:956–962.
12. Cole SPC, Bhardwaj G, Gerlach JH, Mackie JE, Grant CE, Almquist KC, Stewart AJ, Kurz EU, Duncan AMV, Deeley RG. Overexpression of a transporter gene in a multidrug-resistant human lung cancer cell line. Science 1992; 258:1650–1654.
13. Ng WF, Sarangi F, Zastawny RL, Veinot-Drebot L, Ling V. Identification of members of the P-glycoprotein multigene family. Mol Cell Biol 1989; 9:1224–1232.
14. Smit JJM, Schinkel AH, OudeElferink RPJ, Groen AK, Wagenaar E, van Deemter L, Mol CAM, Ottenhoff R, van der Lugt NMT, van Roon MA, van der Valk MA, Offerhaus GJA, Berns, AJM, Borst P. Homozygous disruption of the murine *mdr2* P-glycoprotein gene leads to a complete absence of phospholipid from bile and to liver disease. Cell 1993; 75:451–462.
15. Dhir R, Gros P. Functional analysis of chimeric proteins constructed by exchanging homologous domains of 2 P-glycoproteins conferring distinct drug resistance profiles. Biochemistry 1992; 31:6103–6110.
16. Doige CA, Ames GFL. ATP-dependent transport systems in bacteria and humans—relevance to cystic fibrosis and multidrug resistance. Annu Rev Microbiol 1993; 47:291–319.

17. Higgins CF. ABC transporters—from microorganisms to man. Annu Rev Cell Biol 1992; 8:67–113.

18. Chen C-J, Clark D, Ueda K, Pastan I, Gottesman MM, Roninson IB. Genomic organization of the human multidrug resistance (*MDR1*) gene and origin of P-glycoproteins. J Biol Chem 1990; 265:506–514.

19. Shyamala V, Baichwald V, Gant TW, Beall E, Ames GF-L. Structure–function analysis of the histidine permease and comparison with the cystic fibrosis mutations. J Biol Chem 1991; 266:18714–18719.

20. Hyde SC, Emsley P, Hartshorn MJ, Mimmack MM, Gilleardi U, Pearce SR, Gallagher MP, Gill DR, Hubbard RE, Higgins CF. Structural model of ATP-binding proteins associated with cystic fibrosis, multidrug resistance and bacterial transport. Nature 1990; 346:362–3365.

21. Childs S, Ling V. The MDR superfamily of genes and its biological implications. In: DeVita VT, Hellman S, Rosenberg SA, eds. Important Advances in Oncology. Philadelphia: JB Lippincott, 1994:21–36.

22. Mosser J, Douar A-M, Sarde C-O, Kioschis P, Feil R, Moser H, Poustka A-M, Mandel J-L, Aubourg P. Putative X-linked adrenoleukodystrophy gene shares unexpected homology with ABC transporters. Nature 1993; 361:726–730.

23. Schinkel AH, Arceci RJ, Smit JJM, Wagenaar E, Baas F, Dolle M, Tsuruo T, Mechetner EB, Roninson IB, Borst P. Binding properties of monoclonal antibodies recognizing external epitopes of the human MDR1 P-glycoprotein. Int J Cancer 1993; 55:478–484.

24. Georges E, Tsuruo T, Ling V. Topology of P-glycoprotein as determined by epitope mapping of MRK-16 monoclonal antibody. J Biol Chem 1993; 268:1792–1798.

25. Yoshimura A, Kuwazuru Y, Sumizawa T, Ichikawa M, Ikeda S-I, Uda T, Akiyama S-I. Cytoplasmic orientation and two-domain structure of the multidrug transporter, P-glycoprotein, demonstrated with sequence-specific antibodies. J Biol Chem 1989; 264:16282–16291.

26. Zhang JT, Ling V. Study of membrane orientation and glycosylated extracellular loops of mouse P-glycoprotein by in vitro translation. J Biol Chem 1991; 266:18224–18232.

27. Zhang JT, Duthie M, Ling V. Membrane topology of the N-terminal half of the hamster P-glycoprotein molecule. J Biol Chem 1993; 268:15101–15110.

28. Skach WR, Calayag MC, Lingappa VR. Evidence for an alternate model of human P-glycoprotein structure and biogenesis. J Biol Chem 1993; 268:6903–6908.

29. Schinkel AH, Kemp S, Dolle M, Rudenko G, Wagenaar E. *N*-Glycosylation and deletion mutants of the human MDR1 P-glycoprotein. J Biol Chem 1993; 268:7474–7481.

30. Choi K, Chen C-J, Kriegler M, Roninson IB. An altered pattern of cross-resistance in multidrug-resistant human cells results from spontaneous mutations in the *mdr1* (P-glycoprotein) gene. Cell 1989; 53:519–529.

31. Safa AR, Stern RK, Agresti M, Tamai I, Mehta ND, Roninson IB. Molecular basis of preferential resistance to colchicine in multidrug-resistant human

cells conferred by Gly to Val-185 substitution in P-glycoprotein. Proc Natl Acad Sci USA 1990; 87:7225–7229.

32. Stein WD, Cardarelli CO, Pastan I, Gottesman MM. Kinetic evidence suggesting that the multidrug transporter differentially handles influx and efflux of its substrates. Mol Pharmacol 1994; 45:763–772.

33. Devine SE, Ling V, Melera PW. Amino acid substitutions in the 6th transmembrane domain of P-glycoprotein alter multidrug resistance. Proc Natl Acad Sci USA 1992; 89:4564–4568.

34. Gros P, Dhir R, Croop J, Talbot F. A single amino acid substitution strongly modulates the activity and substrate specificity of the mouse *mdr1* and *mdr3* drug efflux pumps. Proc Natl Acad Sci USA 1991; 88:7289–7293.

35. Kajiji S, Talbot F, Grizzuti K, Andykephillips VV, Agresti M, Safa AR, Gros P. Functional analysis of P-glycoprotein mutants identifies predicted transmembrane domain-11 as a putative drug binding site. Biochemistry 1993; 32:4185–4194.

36. Dhir R, Grizzuti K, Kajiji S, Gros P. Modulatory effects on substrate specificity of independent mutations at the serine (939/941) position in predicted transmembrane domain-11 of P-glycoproteins. Biochemistry 1993; 32:9492–9499.

37. Raymond M, Gros P, Whiteway M, Thomas DY. Functional complementation of yeast *ste6* by a mammalian multidrug resistance *mdr* gene. Science 1992; 256:232–234.

38. Kuchler K, Thorner J. Functional expression of human *mdr1* in the yeast *Saccharomyces cerevisiae*. Proc Natl Acad Sci USA 1992; 89:2302–2306.

39. Loo TW, Clarke DM. Functional consequences of proline mutations in the predicted transmembrane domain of P-glycoprotein. J Biol Chem 1993; 268:3143–3149.

40. Loo TW, Clarke DM. Functional consequences of phenylalanine mutations in the predicted transmembrane domain of P-glycoprotein. J Biol Chem 1993; 268:19965–19972.

41. Loo TW, Clarke DM. Functional consequences of glycine mutations in the predicted cytoplasmic loops of P-glycoprotein. J Biol Chem 1994; 269:7243–7248.

42. Azzaria M, Schurr E, Gros P. Discrete mutations introduced in the predicted nucleotide-binding sites of the *mdr1* gene abolish its ability to confer multidrug resistance. Mol Cell Biol 1989; 9:5289–5297.

43. Cornwell MM, Gottesman MM, Pastan I. Increased vinblastine binding to membrane vesicles from multidrug resistant KB cells. J Biol Chem 1986; 262:7921–7928.

44. Beck WT, Qian X-D. Photoaffinity substrates for P-glycoprotein. Biochem Pharmacol 1992; 43:89–93.

45. Safa AR. Photoaffinity labeling of P-glycoprotein in multidrug resistant cells. Cancer Invest 1993; 11:46–56.

46. Bruggemann EP, Germann UA, Gottesman MM, Pastan I. Two different regions of P-glycoprotein are photolabeled by azidopine. J Biol Chem 1989; 264:15483–15488.

47. Greenberger LM. Major photoaffinity drug labeling sites for iodoaryl azido-prazosin in P-glycoprotein are within, or immediately C-terminal to, transmembrane domain-6 and domain-12. J Biol Chem 1993; 268:11417–11425.

48. Morris DI, Greenberger LM, Bruggemann EP, Cardarelli CO, Gottesman MM, Pastan I, Seamon KB. Localization of the labeling sites of forskolin to both halves of P-glycoprotein: similarity of the sites labeled by forskolin and prazosin. Mol Pharmacol 1994; 46:329–337.

49. Bruggemann EP, Currier SJ, Gottesman MM, Pastan I. Characterization of the azidopine and vinblastine binding site of P-glycoprotein. J Biol Chem 1992; 267:21020–21026.

50. Beck WT, Cirtain MC. Continued expression of vinca alkaloid resistance by CCRF-CEM cells after treatment with tunicamycin or pronase. Cancer Res 1982; 42:184–189.

51. Ling V, Kartner N, Sudo T, Siminovitch L, Riordan JR. The multidrug-resistance phenotype in Chinese hamster ovary cells. Cancer Treat Rep 1983; 67:869–874.

52. Germann UA, Willingham MC, Pastan I, Gottesman MM. Expression of the human multidrug transporter in insect cells by a recombinant baculovirus. Biochemistry 1990; 29:2295–2303.

53. Sarkadi B, Price EM, Boucher RC, Germann UA, Scarborough GA. Expression of the human multidrug resistance cDNA in insect cells generates a high activity drug-stimulated membrane ATPase. J Biol Chem 1992; 267:4854–4858.

54. Ruetz S, Raymond M, Gros P. Functional expression of P-glycoprotein encoded by the mouse *mdr3* gene in yeast cells. Proc Natl Acad Sci USA 1993; 90:11588–11592.

55. Mellado W, Horwitz SB. Phosphorylation of the multidrug resistance associated glycoprotein. Biochemistry 1987; 26:6900–6904.

56. Hamada H, Hagiwara K-I, Nakajima T, Tsuruo T. Phosphorylation of the M_r 170,000 to 180,000 glycoprotein specific to multidrug-resistant tumor cells: effects of verapamil, trifluoperazine, and phorbol esters. Cancer Res 1987; 47:2860–2865.

57. Fine RL, Patel J, Chabner BA. Phorbol esters induce multidrug resistance in human breast cancer cells. Proc Natl Acad Sci USA 1988; 85:582–586.

58. Richert ND, Aldwin L, Nitecki D, Gottesman MM, Pastan I. Stability and covalent modification of P-glycoprotein in multidrug-resistant KB cells. Biochemistry 1988; 27:7607–7613.

59. Epand RM, Stafford AR. Protein kinases and multidrug resistance. Cancer J 1993; 6:154–158.

60. Chambers TC, McAvoy EM, Jacobs JW, Eilon G. Protein kinase C phosphorylates P-glycoprotein in multidrug resistant human KB carcinoma cells. J Biol Chem 1990; 265:7679–7686.

61. Ahmad S, Trepel JB, Ohno S, Suzuki K, Tsuruo T, Glazer RI. Role of protein kinase-C in the modulation of multidrug resistance—expression of the atypical gamma-isoform of protein kinase-C does not confer increased resistance to doxorubicin. Mol Pharmacol 1992; 42:1004–1009.

62. Ahmad S, Glazer RI. Expression of the antisense cDNA for protein kinase-C-alpha attenuates resistance in doxorubicin-resistant MCF-7 breast carcinoma cells. Mol Pharmacol 1992; 43:858–862.

63. Chaudhary PM, Roninson IB. Activation of MDR1 (P-glycoprotein) gene expression in human cells by protein kinase-C agonists. Oncol Res 1992; 4:281–290.

64. Bates SE, Lee JS, Dickstein B, Spolyar M, Fojo AT. Differential modulation of P-glycoprotein transport by protein kinase inhibition. Biochemistry 1993; 32:9156–9164.

65. Chambers TC, Pohl J, Raynor RL, Kuo JF. Identification of specific sites in human P-glycoprotein phosphorylated by protein kinase-C. J Biol Chem 1993; 268:4592–4595.

66. Orr GA, Han EK-H, Browne PC, Nieves E, O'Connor BM, Yang C-P, Horowitz SB. Identification of the major phosphorylation domain of murine *mdr1b* P-glycoprotein. J Biol Chem 1993; 268:25054–25062.

67. Riordan JR, Rommens JM, Kerem BS, Alon N, Rozmahel R, Grzelczak A, Aielenski J, Lok S, Plavsic N, Chou J-I, Drumm ML, Iannuzzi MC, Collins FS, Tsui L-C. Identification of the cystic fibrosis gene: cloning and characterization of complementary DNA. Science 1989; 245:1066–1073.

68. Riordan JR. The cystic fibrosis transmembrane conductance regulator. Annu Rev Physiol 1993; 55:609–630.

69. Horio M, Gottesman MM, Pastan I. ATP-dependent transport of vinblastine in vesicles from human multidrug-resistant cells. Proc Natl Acad Sci USA 1988; 85:3580–3584.

70. Lelong IH, Padmanabhan R, Lovelace E, Pastan I, Gottesman MM. ATP and GTP as alternative energy sources for vinblastine transport by P-170 in KB-V1 plasma membrane vesicles. FEBS Lett 1992; 304:256–260.

71. Horio M, Lovelace E, Pastan I, Gottesman MM. Agents which reverse multidrug-resistance are inhibitors of ^{3}H-vinblastine transport by isolated vesicles. Biochim Biophys Acta 1991; 1061:106–111.

72. Doige CA, Sharom FJ. Transport properties of P-glycoprotein in plasma membrane vesicles from multidrug-resistant Chinese hamster ovary cells. Biochim Biophys Acta 1992; 1109:161–171.

73. Sharom FJ, Yu X, Doige CA. Functional reconstitution of drug transport and ATPase activity in proteoliposomes containing partially purified P-glycoprotein. J Biol Chem 1993; 268:24197–24202.

74. Dano K. Active outward transport of daunorubicin in resistant Ehrlich ascites tumor cells. Biochim Biophys Acta 1973; 323:466–483.

75. Doige CA, Yu XH, Sharom FJ. ATPase activity of partially purified P-glycoprotein from multidrug-resistant Chinese hamster ovary cells. Biochim Biophys Acta 1992; 1109:149–160.

76. Al-Shawi MK, Senior AE. Characterization of the adenosine triphosphatase activity of Chinese hamster P-glycoprotein. J Biol Chem 1993; 268:4197–4206.

77. Ambudkar SV, Lelong IH, Zhang J, Cardarelli CO, Gottesman MM, Pastan

I. Partial purification and reconstitution of the human multidrug resistance pump: characterization of the drug-stimulatable ATP hydrolysis. Proc Natl Acad Sci USA 1992; 89:8472–8476.

78. Davidson AL, Shuman HA, Nikaido H. Mechanism of maltose transport in *Escherichia coli*: transmembrane signaling by periplasmic binding proteins. Proc Natl Acad Sci USA 1992; 89:2360–2364.

79. Bishop L, Agbayani R, Ambudkar SV, Maloney PC, Ames GF-L. Reconstitution of a bacterial periplasmic permease in proteoliposomes and demonstration of ATP hydrolysis concomitant with transport. Proc Natl Acad Sci USA 1989; 86:6953–6957.

80. Al-Shawi MK, Urbatsch IL, Senior AE. Covalent inhibitors of P-glycoprotein ATPase activity. J Biol Chem 1994; 269:8986–8992.

81. Sharma RC, Inoue S, Roitelman J, Schimke RT, Simoni RD. Peptide transport by the multidrug resistance pump. J Biol Chem 1992; 267:5731–5734.

82. Kessel D. Exploring multidrug resistance by using rhodamine 123. Cancer Commun 1989; 1:145–149.

83. Neyfakh AA, Serpinska AS, Chervonsky AV, Apasov SG, Kazarov AR. Multi-drug resistance phenotype of a subpopulation of T-lymphocytes without drug selection. Exp Cell Res 1989; 185:496–505.

84. Raviv Y, Pollard HB, Bruggemann EP, Pastan I, Gottesman MM. Photosensitized labeling of a functional multidrug transporter in living drug-resistant tumor cells. J Biol Chem 1990; 265:3975–3980.

85. Higgins CF, Gottesman MM. Is the multidrug transporter a flippase? Trends Pharmacol Sci 1992; 17:18–21.

86. Michelson S, Slate D. A mathematical model of the P-glycoprotein pump as a mediator of multidrug resistance. Bull Math Biol 1992; 54:1023–1038.

87. Roninson IB. The role of the *MDR1* (P-glycoprotein) gene in multidrug resistance in vitro and in vivo. Biochem Pharmacol 1992; 43:95–102.

88. Valverde MA, Díaz M, Sepúlveda FV, Gill DR, Hyde SC, Higgins CF. Volume-regulated chloride channels associated with the human multidrug resistance P-glycoprotein. Nature 1992; 355:830–833.

89. Gill DR, Hyde SC, Higgins CF, Valverde MA, Mintenig GM, Sepúlveda FV. Separation of drug transport and chloride channel functions of the human multidrug resistance P-glycoprotein. Cell 1992; 71:23–32.

90. Rasola A, Galietta LJV, Gruenert DC, Romeo G. Volume-sensitive chloride currents in 4 epithelial cell lines are not directly correlated to the expression of the *MDR-1* gene. J Biol Chem 1994; 269:1432–1436.

91. Wang XY, Wall DM, Parkin JD, Zalcberg JR, Kemm RE. P-glycoprotein expression in classical multi-drug resistant leukemia cells does not correlate with enhanced chloride channel activity. Clin Exp Pharmacol Physiol 1994; 21:101–108.

92. Abraham EH, Prat AG, Gerweck L, Seneveratne T, Arceci RJ, Kramer R, Guidotti G, Cantiello HF. The multidrug resistance (*mdr1*) gene product functions as an ATP channel. Proc Natl Acad Sci USA 1993; 90:312–316.

18

Modulation of Multidrug Resistance in Tumor Cells

Mikihiko Naito and Takashi Tsuruo
The University of Tokyo, Tokyo, Japan

I. INTRODUCTION

Resistance of tumors to a variety of chemotherapeutic agents presents a major problem in cancer treatment (see Chap. 2). Simultaneous resistance to such agents as doxorubicin (Adriamycin; ADM), *Vinca* alkaloids, and dactinomycin (actinomycin D) can be acquired by tumor cells after treatment with a single drug (1). The gene responsible for multidrug resistance (MDR), termed *mdr1*, encodes a particular type of membrane glycoprotein (P-glycoprotein) that pumps out various cytotoxic drugs from the cell (2). The P-glycoprotein binds anticancer drugs (3,4) and is an ATPase (5,6) localized at the plasma membrane of resistant cells (7). Transfection of *mdr1* gene confers MDR to sensitive cells (8–10).

The amount of P-glycoprotein expressed in cells has been measured in tumor samples and was elevated in intrinsically drug-resistant cancers of the colon, kidney, and adrenal glands, as well as in some tumors that acquired drug resistance during chemotherapy (11–15). The expression of *MDR1* gene in tumors correlates well with the clinical drug resistance (16,17). In addition to tumor cells, the P-glycoprotein is also expressed in various normal tissues, such as adrenal, gravid uterus, kidney, liver, colon, and capillary endothelium in brain (18–24). P-glycoprotein expressed in such normal tissues could have physiological functions specific to the tissues.

Because P-glycoprotein appears to be involved in both acquired and intrinsic drug resistance in human cancer, the selective killing of tumor cells expressing P-glycoprotein could be very important for cancer therapy, although the side effects on normal cells expressing P-glycoprotein must be considered carefully. In an effort to circumvent MDR of tumor cells and devise effective treatments for human drug-resistant cancers, several approaches have been developed. These include (1) application of new antitumor agents; (2) application of chemosensitizing agents; and (3) application of monoclonal antibodies against P-glycoprotein. In this chapter, these therapeutic approaches are described and discussed.

II. ANTITUMOR DRUGS ACTIVE AGAINST MDR TUMORS

Enormous efforts have been made in many laboratories to search for effective agents against MDR tumor cells. Recently, several new antitumor drugs were reported to be effective against MDR tumor cells. 3'-Deamino-3'-morpholino-13-deoxo-10-hydroxycarminomycin (MX2; Fig. 1) may be a candidate antitumor agent active against MDR tumor cells (25). MX2 induced the same level of myelosuppression as doxorubicin at the same doses. The subacute cardiotoxicity, however, was much weaker than that of doxorubicin.

Antitumor activities of MX2 were examined with various experimental murine tumors and human tumor xenografts. MX2 showed an activity superior to that of doxorubicin against L1210 leukemia, Lewis lung carcinoma, and colon adenocarcinomas 26 and 38 (25). This drug also showed an activity comparable with doxorubicin against human tumor xenografts. It was effective against P388/ADM, P388/ACR (amsacrine-resistant), and P388/MMC (mitomycin-resistant) cells in vitro (Fig. 2) and in vivo (Fig. 3). A maximum percentage increase in life span of about 90% was obtained in P388/ADM-bearing mice (see Fig. 3). MX2 seems to be a unique anthracycline antibiotic active on drug-sensitive as well as MDR murine and human cells. The drug is in Phase II clinical studies in Japan.

To elucidate the mechanism whereby MX2 overcomes MDR, the cellular pharmacology of MX2 was examined in human myelogenous leukemia K562 and its doxorubicin-resistant subline K562/ADM (26). Both K562 and K562/ADM cells accumulated MX2 more rapidly than doxorubicin, and the intracellular accumulation of MX2 attained a steady state in both cell lines within 30 min of incubation at 37°C. The amount of MX2 that accumulated in K562/ADM at a steady state was only 1.3 times lower than that in K562, whereas the steady-state concentration of ADM in cells resistant to doxorubicin (K562/ADM) was 8.3 times lower than that in

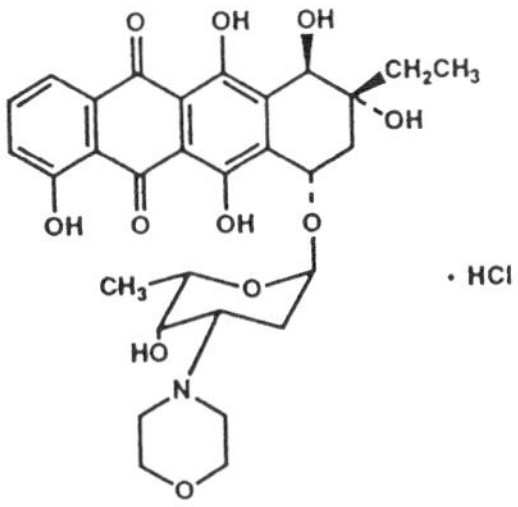

MX2

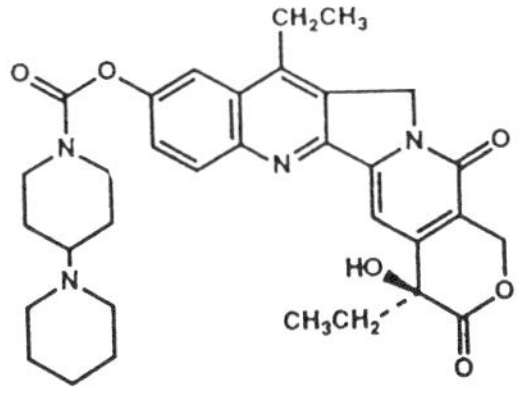

CPT-11

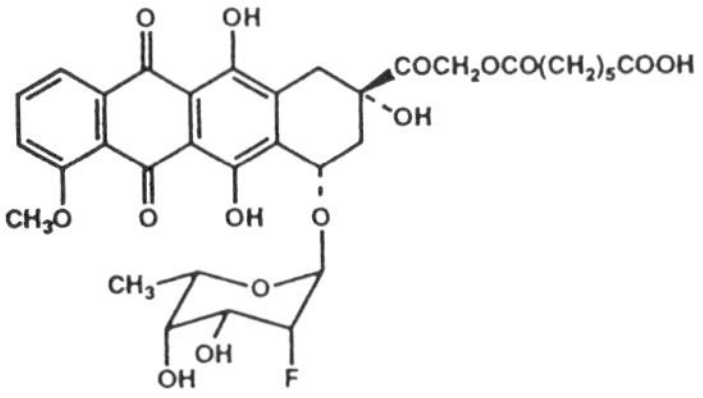

ME2303

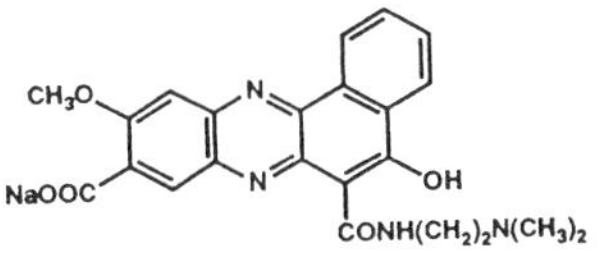

NC-190

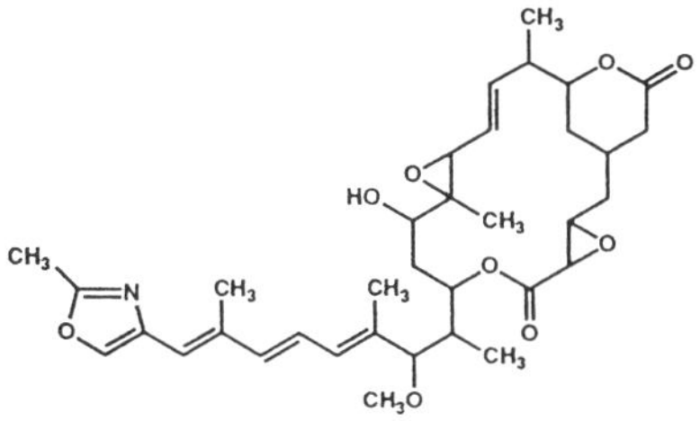

Rhizoxin

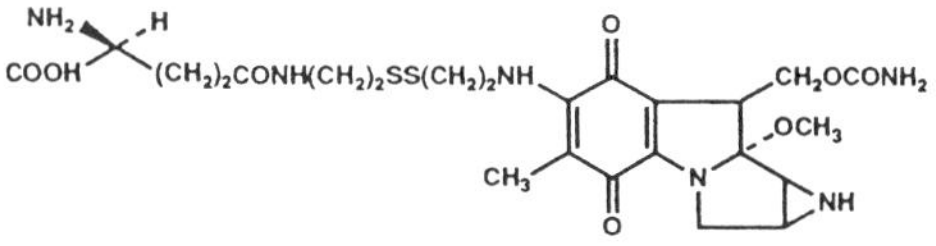

KW2149

Figure 1 Structure of new drugs effective against MDR tumor cells.

K562. MX2 effectively inhibited ATP/Mg^{2+}-dependent [^{3}H]vincristine (VCR) binding to K562/ADM membrane preparations, indicating that MX2 could be transported outside the cell by P-glycoprotein. The high intracellular accumulation and retention of MX2 in K562/ADM through the rapid influx of the drug into the cells may be one of the reasons why

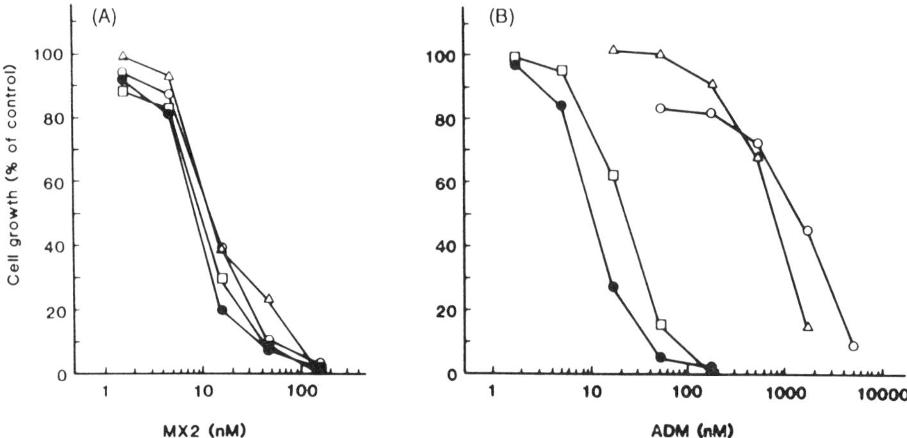

Figure 2 Growth-inhibitory effects of (A) MX2 and (B) doxorubicin (ADM) on drug-sensitive and drug-resistant P388 leukemia. P388 (●), and P388 leukemia lines resistant to ADM (○), ansacrine (ACR; △), and mitomycin (MMC; □) were seeded at 2×10^4 cells in 2 ml of growth medium and treated with the indicated concentrations of (A) MX2 or (B) ADM for 72 h. Points are means of triplicate determinations.

MX2 circumvents pleiotropic drug resistance, although it could have an affinity to P-glycoprotein.

Other interesting compounds are ME2303 and rhizoxin (see Fig. 1). ME2303, a new fluorine-containing anthracycline derivative, showed excellent antitumor activity against various experimental tumor models, including L1210 leukemia, P388 leukemia, colon adenocarcinomas 26 and 38, Lewis lung carcinoma, B16 melanoma, M5076 sarcoma, and various human tumor xenografts (27,28). ME2303 was effective against human and murine MDR cells in vitro. For example, K562/ADM was only 2.8-fold more resistant to ME2303 than K562, whereas the cells were 200-fold more resistant to doxorubicin. ME2303 was also more effective than doxorubicin against human leukemia CCRF-CEM resistant to vinblastine, human ovarian carcinoma A2780 resistant to doxorubicin, human epidermoid carcinoma KB cells resistant to colchicine, P388/ADM, and P388/VCR. The therapeutic effects were obtained in vivo against P388/ADM and, more remarkably, P388/VCR. ME2303 is an interesting potential antitumor agent in Phase I clinical studies in Japan.

Rhizoxin is a new 16-membered macrolide, isolated from the plant pathogenic fungus *Rhizopus chinensis* Rh-2 (29). Among ansa macrolides,

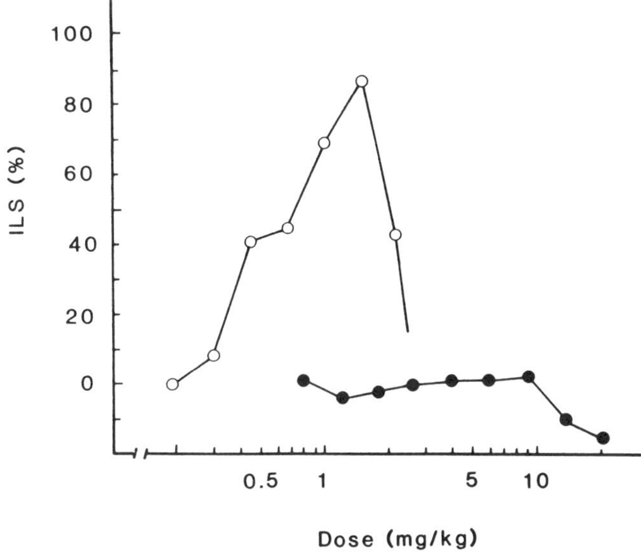

Figure 3 Antitumor activity of MX2 and doxorubicin (ADM) against ADM-resistant P388 leukemia measured as increased life span (ILS). One million P388/ADM cells were inoculated i.p. in female CD2F$_1$ mice (six mice per group) on day 0. MX2 (○) or ADM (●) was administered i.v. on days 1, 5, and 9. Median survival time of the control group was 9.1 days.

maytansine has previously been developed, but this compound was disappointing in clinical trials. Rhizoxin inhibits mitosis of tumor cells in a manner similar to that of vinca alkaloids (i.e., at the level of tubulin), as revealed by morphological studies and flow cytometric analyses. Rhizoxin showed chemotherapeutic effects similar to vincristine against L1210 and P388 leukemia-bearing mice. The drug is also effective against B16 melanoma inoculated intraperitoneally or subcutaneously. Interestingly, rhizoxin, in contrast with maytansine, was effective against human and murine tumor cells resistant to vincristine and doxorubicin in vitro and in vivo. A maximum 60% increase in life span was obtained in mice inoculated with P388/VCR. We are now developing derivatives of rhizoxin to achieve antitumor activity against experimental solid tumors. These compounds, including rhizoxin itself, seem to merit consideration for further development as new chemotherapeutic agents.

A new derivative of camptothecin (CPT-11; see Fig. 1) is another interesting compound. The drug showed a chemotherapeutic effect superior to vincristine and doxorubicin in P388 leukemia-bearing mice, and was also effective in P388/VCR- and P388/ADM-bearing mice (30). Significantly, the survival advantages in mice with resistant tumors by CPT-11 were almost equal to those with parental P388 leukemia. CPT-11 was effective against human tumor cells, especially various MDR human tumor lines. CPT-11 should be considered for further development (now in Phase II clinical studies in Japan) as a new chemotherapeutic agent potentially effective against MDR tumors.

A benzophenazine derivative (N-β-dimethylaminoethyl-9-carboxy-5-hydroxy-10-methoxybenzo[a]phenazine-6-carboxamide; NC-190) (see Fig. 1), was effective against MDR human and mouse tumor cells in vitro and in vivo (31). When P388/VCR-bearing mice were treated with an optimal dose of NC-190, four of six mice were cured. The compound also showed chemotherapeutic effect against P388/ADM-bearing mice and was effective against various MDR human and murine tumor cells in vitro. The accumulation of NC-190 in K562/ADM cells was slightly lower than that observed in parental K562 cells. The compound did not efficiently inhibit the binding of vincristine to the plasma membrane of resistant cells, indicating that NC-190 has little affinity for P-glycoprotein. NC-190 inhibited the activity of DNA topoisomerase II, resulting in effectiveness against various MDR tumor cells.

Finally, KW-2149 (see Fig. 1), 7-N-[2[[2-(γ-glutamylamino)ethyl]di-thio]ethyl]mitomycin, is an effective compound against MDR tumors. It showed a marked effect against intraperitoneally inoculated P388 leukemia and subcutaneously implanted colon adenocarcinoma 38 (32). The activity of KW-2149 against human tumor xenografts was similar to that of mitomycin. KW-2149 was effective against gastric adenocarcinomas and non–small-cell lung carcinomas. KW-2149 was more effective against a subline of P388 leukemia resistant to mitomycin in vitro as well as in vivo (33). The activation mechanism of KW-2149 seems to be different from that of mitomycin: it could be chemically activated by cellular thiol molecules, such as glutathione (34), whereas mitomycin needs particular enzymes to be activated. The difference in the activation mechanism may account for the effectiveness of KW-2149 on various drug-resistant tumors (34).

III. ASSAY SYSTEMS FOR MODULATORS OF MDR

A. In Vitro Systems

Because P-glycoprotein plays a central role in the mechanism of MDR, therapeutic approaches targeting P-glycoprotein would be interesting to study. If a modulator can inhibit the efflux of antitumor agents from MDR tumor cells caused by P-glycoprotein, it would restore the sensitivity of the cells to the antitumor agents.

Currently, several MDR tumor cells lines have been developed and are used to evaluate new antitumor drugs and modulators. These cell lines include human leukemia K562, resistant to vincristine (K562/VCR) (35) and to doxorubicin (K562/ADM; 36), human ovarian cancer A2780 resistant to doxorubicin (2780AD) (37), and a series of resistant variants of human epidermoid carcinoma KB cells (38). Murine leukemia P388 and its resistant sublines against various drugs (39) are also often used.

The sensitivity of cells to antitumor drugs is evaluated by treating cells with graded concentrations of the drugs then counting cell numbers or colonies. The effective concentrations of the drugs needed to inhibit cell growth by 50% (IC_{50}) or colony formation by 90% (IC_{90}) are determined by these experiments. When a modulator such as verapamil is combined with antitumor agents, the IC_{50} or IC_{90} values of the antitumor drugs in MDR tumor cells are decreased (Table 1). The sensitizing effect of the modulators can be expressed quantitatively as the IC_{50} (or IC_{90}) values without a modulator, divided by the IC_{50} (or IC_{90}) values with a modulator.

Since P-glycoprotein reduces the accumulation of antitumor drugs in MDR tumor cells, quantifying antitumor drugs in the resistant cells can be used to find modulators of MDR. Increased drug accumulation by

Table 1 Reversal of MDR by Verapamil and Cyclosporine[a]

Modulator	Concentration (μM)	IC_{50} (nM)			
		VCR in		ADM in	
		K562	K562/ADM	K562	K562/ADM
Verapamil	0	4.3	689	14	2480
	1	2.4	505	7.2	1020
	3	2.0	102	6.6	268
	10	2.2	21	6.1	130
Cyclosporine	0	3.3	639	23	2970
	1	1.8	460	20	3210
	3	1.6	155	17	560
	10	1.3	5.2	15	34

[a] K562 and K562/ADM cells were treated with graded concentration of vincristine (VCR) or doxorubicin (ADM) in the absence or presence of the indicated concentrations of verapamil and cyclosporine, and the concentrations of VCR and ADM necessary to inhibit the growth of tumor cells by 50% (IC_{50}) were determined.

modulators in MDR tumor cells correlates well with the reversal of drug resistance (see Table 1; Fig. 4).

Multidrug resistance modulation can also be assessed by the inhibitory effects of a modulator on the molecular function of P-glycoprotein in cell-free systems. P-glycoprotein has the ability to bind various drugs. Photoaffinity-labeling studies demonstrated that drugs, such as vinblastine (3,4), verapamil (40,41), cyclosporine (42), azidopine (43), and progesterone (44), specifically bind P-glycoprotein at a common drug-binding site. This binding occurs independently of ATP. Many modulators of MDR inhibit the specific binding of such drugs to P-glycoprotein (Fig. 5). By using membrane vesicles from MDR tumor cells that express P-glycoprotein, we could estimate the ability of drug transport by P-glycoprotein in the presence of ATP (45,46). Modulators also inhibit the transport of antitumor agents that depends on the presence of ATP.

P-glycoprotein can specifically bind ATP (47), and purified P-glycoprotein has ATPase activity (5,6). Drugs transported by P-glycoprotein stimulate its ATPase activity (48,49). Many modulators of MDR are competitive inhibitors of antitumor agent efflux (50,51) and are themselves transported by P-glycoprotein. Therefore, modulators also enhance the ATPase activity of P-glycoprotein.

The modulators found in these in vitro systems should be tested further to overcome drug resistance in animals inoculated with MDR tumors.

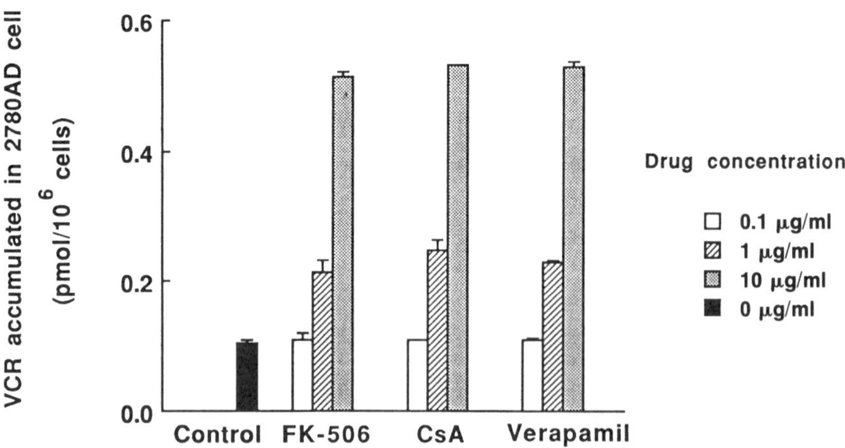

Figure 4 Increased accumulation of vincristine (VCR) in MDR tumor cells by chemosensitizers. Cellular accumulation of VCR was examined in the absence or presence of indicated concentrations of FK-506, cyclosporine, and verapamil.

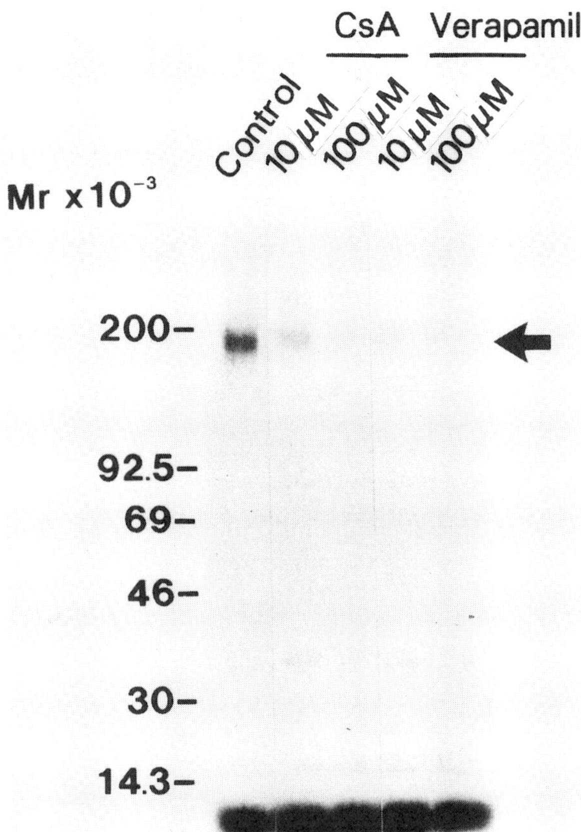

Figure 5 Inhibition of [³H]azidopine photolabeling of P-glycoprotein by cyclosporine (CsA) and verapamil. K562/ADM membrane vesicles (50 μg of protein) were incubated with 200 nM [³H]azidopine in the absence or presence of CsA or verapamil at the indicated concentrations. The photolabeled proteins were analyzed by sodium dodecyl sulfate–polyacrylamide gel electrophoresis (SDS–PAGE) followed by fluorography. The arrow on the right indicates location of P-glycoprotein.

B. In Vivo Systems

The therapeutic effects of modulators can be evaluated by experimental combination chemotherapy. Mice were inoculated with MDR tumors, such as P388/VCR and P388/ADM, and were treated with antitumor drugs combined with modulators. Administration of vincristine to mice with

Table 2 Effect of MS-073 on Antitumor Activity of VCR in P388/VCR-Bearing Mice[a]

Drug	Dosage (mg/kg)	Mean survival time (days)	T/C (%)
None (control)		10.5	100
MS-073	100	10.5	100
VCR	0.1	11.5	110
+ MS-073	3	12.5[b]	119
	10	14.5[b]	138
	30	15.5[b]	148
	100	16.0[b]	152

[a] One million P388/VCR cells were implanted i.p. and drugs were given i.p. on days 1–5.
[b] Significant difference by Student's t test.

P388/VCR tumors had only a marginal effect on the life span of the mice, whereas the same treatment showed significant increase in the life span of mice inoculated with the drug-sensitive P388 tumors. When mice with P388/VCR tumors were treated with vincristine combined with a modulator (e.g., verapamil or MS-073), the life span of the mice was significantly prolonged (Table 2) and, in some cases, tumor-free survivors were obtained. The P388/ADM cells showed higher resistance than P388/VCR cells against various antitumor drugs because the cells expressed larger amounts of P-glycoprotein, and the activity of topoisomerase II was reduced in the cells. Therefore, the therapeutic effects in P388/ADM-inoculated mice were inferior to those in P388/VCR-inoculated mice.

The combined effect of modulators was also evaluated with human MDR tumors in vivo when human tumor cells were inoculated into nude mice. Since most human leukemic tumors could not be taken up by nude mice, carcinoma cells were often used for the study.

IV. DRUGS REVERSING MDR IN TUMOR CELLS

In 1981, we reported that the calcium channel blocker verapamil (Fig. 6) inhibited active drug efflux and restored drug sensitivity in MDR cells (52). Various compounds, including calcium channel blockers and calmodulin inhibitors enhance the cytotoxic activity of various antitumor agents (Table 3; 37,52–57; for review see Refs. 58, 59). Verapamil was reported to be a good inhibitor of the photoaffinity labeling of P-glycoprotein with a vinblastine analogue (3,4) and of the transport of vinca alkaloids into

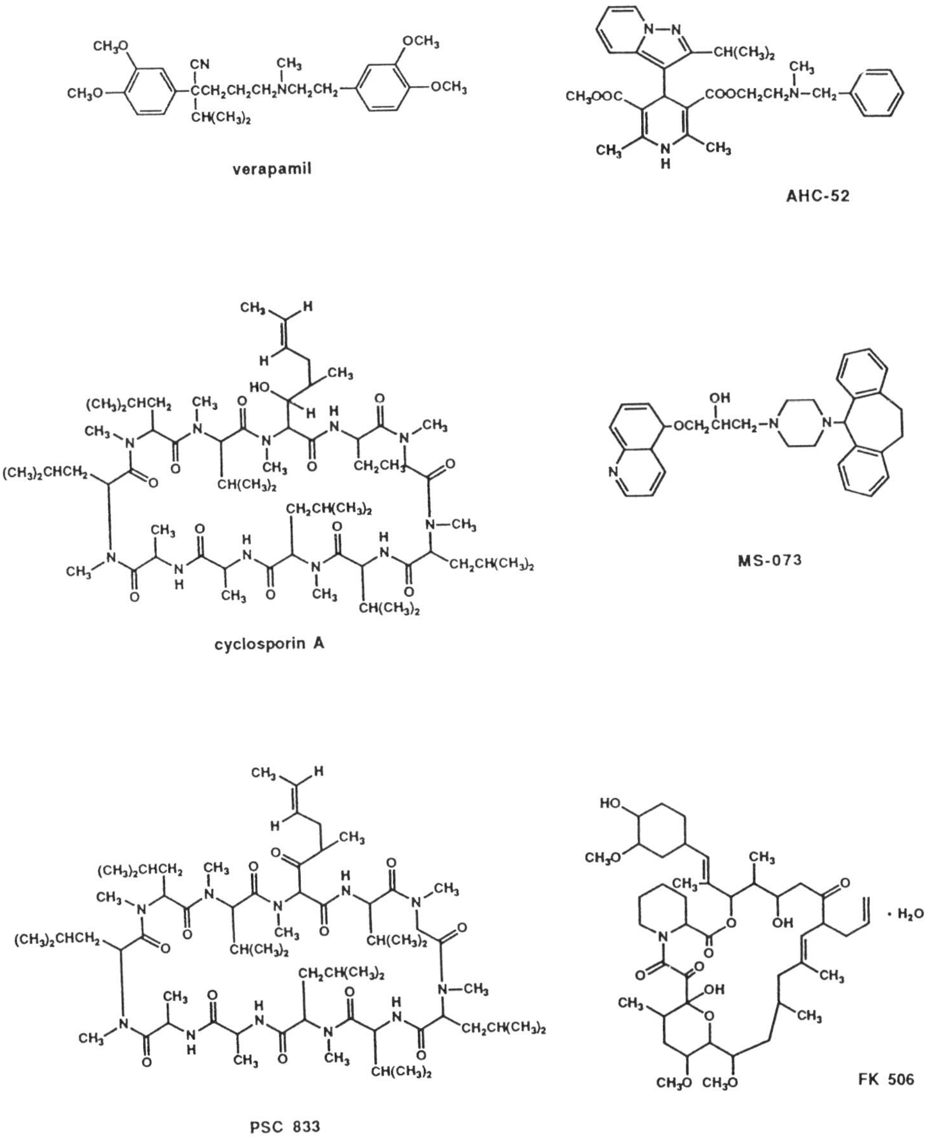

Figure 6   Structures of chemosensitizing agents that reverse MDR.

Table 3 Potentiation of Antitumor Agents by Various Agents

Antitumor agent	Potentiating agent
Vincristine, vinblastine	Verapamil and its analogues
	Trifluoperazine
	Nifedipine and its analogues
	Diltiazem
	Perhexiline
	Quinidine
	Cyclosporine and its analogues
	FK-506
Doxorubicin (Adriamycin), daunomycin	Verapamil and its analogues
	Trifluoperazine
	Nifedipine and its analogues
	Diltiazem
	Perhexiline
	Quinidine
	Cyclosporine and its analogues
	FK-506
Bleomycin, peplomycin	Verapamil
	Pimozide
	Melittin
	Chlorpromazine
Etoposide	Verapamil
	Nifedipine and its analogues
	Diltiazem
Vindesine, taxol	Verapamil
	Nifedipine and its analogues
	Diltiazem
Dactinomycin (actinomycin D), mitoxantrone	Verapamil
Aclarubicin	Nifedipine and its analogues
Mitomycin, menogarol	Diltiazem
Rhodamine	Verapamil
Cisplatin	w5, w7
	Verapamil
Chloroquine	Verapamil

vesicles from MDR cells (45,46). Direct binding of verapamil to P-glyco-protein was shown using MDR Chinese hamster lung and human K562 cells (40,41). Verapamil was actively effluxed from resistant cells (41). These findings suggest that verapamil competitively inhibits the transport of antitumor agents by P-glycoprotein, resulting in the reversal of MDR.

Preliminary clinical studies have been carried out combining calcium channel blockers with antitumor agents. Combination chemotherapy appeared promising against refractory acute lymphocytic leukemia of children, malignant lymphoma, multiple myeloma, various advanced solid tumors, and small-cell lung cancer, but had side effects such as reversible hypotension and arrhythmias (60–63).

Cyclosporine (see Fig. 6), an immunosuppressive drug, is another chemosensitizer that has been well studied (64,65) and used clinically to overcome drug resistance. Cyclosporine is also a competitive inhibitor of drug transport by P-glycoprotein (50,51). Clinical combination chemotherapy was carried out using cyclosporine on refractory multiple myeloma patients (66). Nine of 21 patients responded to combination chemotherapy with cyclosporine. Interestingly, the *MDR1* gene was detected in 12 of 15 patients tested before the treatment, and 7 patients with the gene responded to the treatment, whereas none without the gene responded. Clinical studies with verapamil and cyclosporine suggest that combination chemotherapy with chemosensitizers could help patients overcome clinical drug resistance, especially those with resistant tumors that express P-glycoprotein.

In a search for more potent chemosensitizers for MDR with less toxicity, several drugs were found to reverse MDR. Most of these chemosensitizers, as verapamil and cyclosporine, competitively inhibit the drug transport by P-glycoprotein. AHC-52 is a newly synthesized compound, with a potent activity and relatively low host toxicity (67). Although its chemical structure (see Fig. 6) partially resembles nifedipine, its calcium-antagonizing activity was 500-fold lower than that of nifedipine. AHC-52 at 0.5 μg/ml completely reversed the in vitro resistance to vincristine in P388/VCR. Of various regimens examined for the in vivo treatment of P388/VCR-bearing mice, the combination of 0.05 mg/kg of vincristine with 100 mg/kg twice a day of AHC-52 demonstrated the best result, with a 206% increase in life span. This result was comparable with that observed in parental P388-bearing mice treated with the optimal dose of vincristine alone, indicating almost complete reversal of resistance by combination VCR–AHC-52 therapy. In addition, the combination of the two agents was effective in the treatment of P388-bearing mice, with some long-term survivors.

MS-073 (see Fig. 6) is a quinoline derivative that is effective in overcoming MDR in vitro and in vivo (68). MS-073 at 0.1 μM almost completely reversed resistance to vincristine in P388/VCR in vitro. The compound also reversed the resistance in vitro against vincristine, doxorubicin, etoposide, and dactinomycin in K562/ADM cells, ADM-resistant human ovarian carcinoma A2780 cells, and colchicine-resistant human KB cells.

MS-073 administered intraperitoneally daily for 5 days with vincristine enhanced the chemotherapeutic effect of vincristine in P388/VCR-bearing mice. Increases in life span of 19–52% were obtained by the combination of 100 μg/kg of vincristine with 3–100 mg/kg of MS-073, compared with the control (see Table 2). The ability of MS-073 to reverse MDR was higher, especially at low MS-073 doses, than that of verapamil both in vitro and in vivo. MS-073 enhanced accumulation of [^{3}H]vincristine in K562/ADM cells. Photolabeling of P-glycoprotein with 200 nM [^{3}H]azidopine in K562/ADM plasma membranes was completely inhibited by 10 μM MS-073, indicating that MS-073 reverses MDR by competitively inhibiting drug binding to P-glycoprotein. MS-209, an analogue of MS-073, is now considered a promising clinical candidate because of its high oral bioavailability and its MDR-reversing effects.

FK-506 (see Fig. 6), a novel immunosuppressive agent, is an interesting compound. FK-506 at 3 μg/ml and 10 μg/ml completely reversed the resistance against vincristine in vitro in P388/VCR, P388/ADM, and doxorubicin-resistant human ovarian cancer A2780 cells (69). FK-506 also enhanced the cytotoxicity of vincristine in highly resistant human K562/ADM in vitro, and the chemotherapeutic effect of vincristine in P388/VCR-bearing mice. When 20 mg/kg of the compound was combined with 200 mg/kg of vincristine, 151% of T/C value was obtained. Under the protocol used in the study, FK-506 was more potent than cyclosporine and verapamil. FK-506 efficiently inhibited [^{3}H]azidopine binding to P-glycoprotein. The binding of vincristine to K562/ADM plasma membrane was inhibited by FK-506 as effectively as cyclosporine. Moreover, the accumulation of vincristine in doxorubicin-resistant human ovarian cancer A2780 cells was increased by FK-506 as efficiently as cyclosporine and verapamil (see Fig. 4).

PSC833 (see Fig. 6), a nonimmunosuppressive analogue of cyclosporine, is more effective than cyclosporine in overcoming MDR in vitro and in vivo (70–72). It was tenfold more effective than cyclosporine in vitro. Moreover, PSC833 surpassed cyclosporine and verapamil in prolonging life in P388/VCR-bearing mice when chemosensitizers were orally administered, and vincristine or doxorubicin was administered intraperitoneally or intravenously. PSC833, as does cyclosporine, inhibited [^{3}H]azidopine binding to P-glycoprotein, and increased cellular accumulation of vincristine and doxorubicin in resistant tumors.

Some of these chemosensitizers have progressed to clinical phase studies. In the future, new chemosensitizers will be used in patients with refractory cancers, and the combined effect of chemosensitizers and antitumor agents will be clinically evaluated.

V. MONOCLONAL ANTIBODIES AGAINST P-GLYCOPROTEIN AND THERAPEUTIC IMPLICATIONS

In an attempt to identify the changes in the plasma membrane associated with MDR and to elucidate their roles, we have developed monoclonal antibodies (MAbs) against K562/ADM. The antibodies, designated MRK16 and MRK17, recognized P-glycoprotein at an extracellular domain of the protein (73). The epitope of MRK16 was assigned to the first and fourth external domains of human P-glycoprotein (74). As of now, several monoclonal antibodies have been raised against P-glycoprotein (73,75–79; Table 4) and are used for various studies in this field.

The expression of the P-glycoprotein in normal tissues was examined with monoclonal antibodies, and P-glycoprotein was found in adrenal, gravid uterus, kidney, liver, colon, and the capillary endothelium in brain (18–24). The antibodies were used for detecting P-glycoprotein in tumor samples and in sorting multidrug-resistant cells (80). In addition to these basic research and diagnostic uses of the antibodies, promising therapeutic usefulness was also found (81). MRK16 and MRK17, given intravenously, prevented tumor development in athymic mice inoculated subcutaneously with doxorubicin-resistant human ovarian carcinoma A2780 cells (Fig. 7). Treatment with MRK16 induced rapid regression of the established, subcutaneous, resistant tumors and apparent cures of some animals. These monoclonal antibodies may thus have potential as treatment tools against MDR human tumors possessing P-glycoprotein.

The mechanisms for these therapeutic effects were examined, and MRK16 and MRK17 were shown to mediate antibody-dependent cellular cytotoxicity (ADCC) by mononuclear cells (82). When highly purified lymphocytes (>99%) and monocytes (>97%) were isolated from blood mononuclear cells, MRK16 promoted both lymphocyte- and mono-

Table 4 Monoclonal Antibodies Against P-glycoprotein

Antibodies	Ig class	Epitope in P-glycoprotein	Ref.
C219	IgG2a	Cytoplasmic	75
JSB-1	IgG1	Cytoplasmic	76
MRK16	IgG2a	Extracellular	73
HYB-241	IgG1	Extracellular	77
UIC2	IgG2a	Extracellular	78
4E3	IgG2a	Extracellular	79

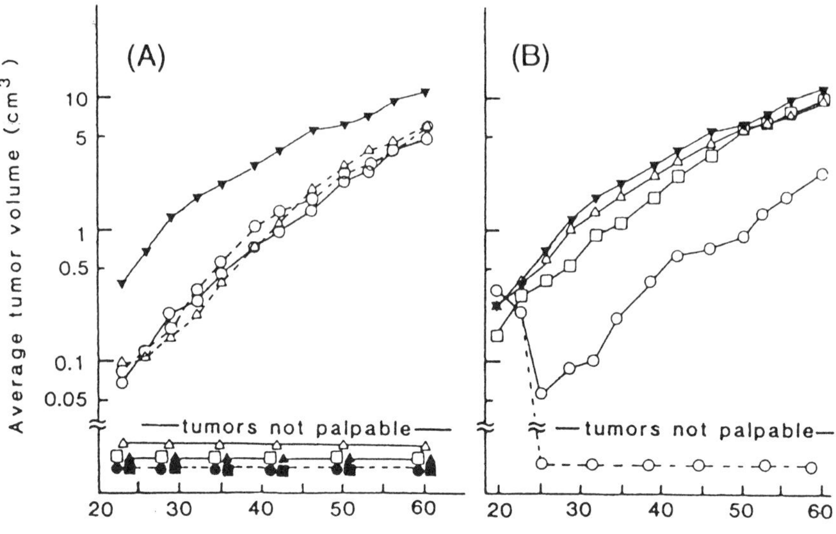

Figure 7 In vivo effects of MRK16, MRK17, and doxorubicin on the growth of drug-resistant tumor xenografts. Human ovarian carcinoma A2780 cells resistant to doxorubicin (2780AD) were used in this experiment. All of the mice were given injections of 10^7 2780AD cells s.c. on day 0. In (A), on days 2 and 7 after tumor cell inoculation, groups of animals (five nude mice per group) were treated IV with 0.001 (O), 0.01 (△), 0.03 (□), 0.1 (●), 0.3 (▲), or 1 mg (■) of MRK16 (solid line) or MRK17 (broken line) antibody. Untreated animals (▼) served as controls. In (B), mice were inoculated s.c. with 10^7 2780AD cells as above. When the tumors became palpable on day 20, mice were randomized into four groups (five mice per group). One group was untreated (▼); a second group was treated with 1 mg of MRK16 on days 20, 23, and 26 (O); a third group was treated with 1 mg of MRK17 on days 20, 23, and 26 (△); and the fourth group was treated with 6 mg/ kg, an optimal dose, of ADM on days 20, 24, and 28 (□). MRK16 treatment resulted in rapid regression of subcutaneous tumors. Thus, only one of five animals continued to bear a palpable tumor after day 23. An additional animal showed a recurrent tumor between days 42 and 60. The average tumor volume of these two mice is shown (O—O). The remaining three animals were tumor-free at day 60, as is shown in the figure (O---O).

cyte-mediated tumor cell killing, whereas MRK17 induced only a lymphocyte-mediated ADCC reaction. Recently, we have succeeded in developing a recombinant mouse–human chimeric antibody in which the antigen-recognizing variable regions of MRK16 are joined with the constant regions of human antibodies (83). The chimeric monoclonal antibody, MH162, was more effective than MRK16 in the promotion of ADCC reaction against MDR tumor cells, when human lymphocytes and monocytes were used as effector cells (84). Pretreatment of lymphocytes with interleukin-2 (IL-2) resulted in the significant potentiation of the MH162-dependent killing of MDR cells. Similarly, pretreatment of monocytes with some cytokines (IL-3, GM-CSF, and M-CSF) caused significant increase in MH162-mediated lysis of the resistant cells by the monocytes.

Another therapeutic application of the antibody is to construct the bispecific antibody. We constructed the bispecific $F(ab')_2$, which was composed of two Fab fragments; one was derived from anti-CD3 MAb (OKT3) and the other from MRK16 (85,86). This bispecific $F(ab')_2$ enhanced binding and killing activities of human peripheral blood mononuclear cells against P-glycoprotein-positive human kidney cancer cells, whereas it showed no effect on P-glycoprotein-negative cells.

Since some antibodies against P-glycoprotein inhibit its drug transport, they could be useful to modulate MDR when combined with antitumor agents. MRK16 increased cellular accumulation of vincristine, and enhanced the sensitivity of MDR tumor cells to vincristine in vitro (73). When human colon carcinoma HT-29 cells transfected with *MDR1* gene (HT-29^{mdr1}) were inoculated into athymic mice, the combined treatment of MRK16 and vincristine prolonged the survival of the tumor-bearing mice, whereas MRK16 alone or vincristine alone showed no significant effects (87).

Finally, combination of MRK16 with antitumor agents and cyclosporine also induced interesting therapeutic responses. MRK16 markedly increased the cellular accumulation of cyclosporine in MDR cells (88). As a result, cellular accumulation of vincristine and doxorubicin in K562/ADM cells was synergistically increased by MRK16 and cyclosporine (88; Fig. 8). Accordingly, MRK16 and cyclosporine synergistically enhanced the cytotoxicity of doxorubicin and vincristine in MDR tumors (88,89). Similar effects were obtained in the combination of MRK16 with PSC833, but not with verapamil. Since MRK16 alone induced regression of MDR tumors in athymic mice (81), the combined use of MRK16, cyclosporine, and antitumor agents would have clinical advantages in the treatment of resistant tumors expressing P-glycoprotein.

Although some problems still exist in the use of monoclonal antibodies in immunotherapy (81,90), the antibodies against the multidrug transporter

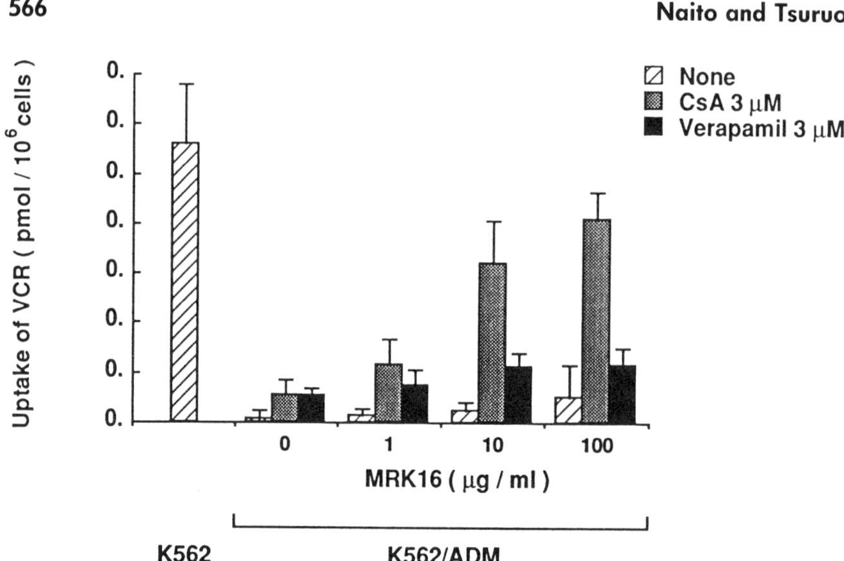

Figure 8   Synergistic enhancement of vincristine (VCR) accumulation by MRK16 and cyclosporine. Cellular accumulation of VCR was examined in the absence or presence of the indicated concentrations of MRK16 alone, MRK16 combined with 3 μM cyclosporine, and MRK16 combined with 3 μM verapamil.

P-glycoprotein could be useful agents in the treatment of human drug-resistant cancers, and further investigations are warranted.

VI. POSTTRANSLATIONAL MODIFICATION AND TRANSCRIPTIONAL CONTROL OF P-GLYCOPROTEIN

P-glycoprotein is posttranslationally modified by glycosylation and phosphorylation (91,92). Although glycosylation would not affect the function of P-glycoprotein significantly, phosphorylation could modulate it. P-glycoprotein is a basally phosphorylated protein, and the phosphorylation is stimulated by phorbol esters and verapamil (92). Protein kinase C (PKC) and other kinases phosphorylate P-glycoprotein. Some MDR tumor cells contain increased levels of PKC (93). Interestingly, treating the cells with phorbol esters increased the phosphorylation of P-glycoprotein, reduced the accumulation of antitumor agents in the cells, and increased drug resistance to some extent (93,94). When MCF-7 breast carcinoma cells, transfected with the human *MDR1* gene, were again transfected with PKCα, the resistance to doxorubicin and vincristine was increased with the enhanced phosphorylation of P-glycoprotein, and the drug accumulation was reduced in the cells (95). The treatment with phorbol dibutyrate further increased the resistance to doxorubicin. In contrast, the treatment of SW620 human colon carcinoma cells with sodium butyrate inhibited the phosphorylation of P-glycoprotein, whereas it increased the P-glycoprotein levels (96). A tight relationship was demonstrated between decreased phosphorylation of P-glycoprotein and increased vinblastine accumulation after sodium butyrate treatment (96). This evidence suggests that PKC-mediated phosphorylation could be one of the regulatory mechanisms of P-glycoprotein function, although it is not convincing. Reconstitution of the active P-glycoprotein into liposomes would elucidate the role of phosphorylation. We also need to determine if dephosphorylation of P-glycoprotein can completely inhibit its transport function.

Another attractive approach for reversing MDR is to suppress the expression of P-glycoprotein in the cells. Such expression is a crucial event that results in MDR, and many studies have reported the regulatory mechanism of *MDR1* gene expression in various cells. However, only a few studies have ever tried to suppress *MDR1* gene expression at the transcriptional level (97), and the modulation of MDR by such an approach has not been attained.

VII. CONCLUSIONS AND FUTURE DIRECTIONS

In this chapter we described therapeutic approaches to overcoming MDR in cancer cells. Several new antitumor drugs have been demonstrated to be effective for the treatment of resistant tumors in vitro and in vivo. Because P-glycoprotein plays a central role in MDR, most therapeutic approaches involve application of chemosensitizing drugs and monoclonal antibodies targeted against P-glycoprotein. Chemosensitizing drugs, such as verapamil and cyclosporine, competitively inhibit the efflux of antitumor drugs from the cells by P-glycoprotein. New chemosensitizing drugs are undergoing clinical studies in Japan, the United States, and Europe. Monoclonal antibodies against P-glycoprotein are also attractive tools for overcoming P-glycoprotein-mediated MDR. Some antibodies, such as MRK16, enhance the immune response to resistant tumors that possess P-glycoprotein. They also modulate the transport function of P-glycoprotein and could be combined with antitumor drugs and chemosensitizers.

An interesting approach is to suppress the expression of the *MDR1* gene in tumor cells at the transcriptional level, which, in turn, could suppress the emergence of MDR. This type of therapeutic approach, including antisense strategy, should be developed further in the future.

In the studies to reverse MDR mediated by P-glycoprotein, we must be concerned about the physiological functions of P-glycoprotein expressed in various normal tissues. Its expression in brain capillary endothelium could be functionally involved in the blood–brain barrier (98–100). In the adrenal gland it could be responsible for the secretion of steroid hormones (101–103). In the luminal surface of colon, brush-border of proximal tubules in kidney, and biliary canalicular surface of hepatocytes, it could contribute to the excretion of natural toxic substances into the lumen of the gastrointestinal tract, urine, and bile, respectively (104,105). In addition, multipotent stem cells in bone marrow are relatively resistant to the treatment with anticancer drugs, owing to the expression of P-glycoprotein in the cells (106). Therefore, when we intend to modulate the function of P-glycoprotein in MDR tumor cells, its function in these normal tissues could also be affected. In fact, the administration of verapamil and cyclosporine significantly altered the pharmacodynamics of antitumor drugs, and the bioavailability of antitumor drugs was enhanced severalfold (107). Accordingly, the toxicity of antitumor drugs when combined with modulators could be greater than when used alone.

The modulation of MDR is not easy to achieve and is fraught with toxicity liabilities. Nevertheless, the therapeutic approaches described here are encouraging. Further studies are needed to develop effective modalities to overcome drug resistance.

REFERENCES

1. Tsuruo T. Mechanisms of multidrug resistance and implications for therapy. Jpn J Cancer Res 1987; 79:285–296.
2. Roninson IB, ed. Molecular and Cellular Biology of Multidrug Resistance in Tumor Cells. New York: Plenum Publishing, 1989.
3. Safa AR, Glover CJ, Meyers MB, Biedler JL, Felsted RL. Vinblastine photoaffinity labeling of a high molecular weight surface membrane glycoprotein specific for multidrug-resistant cells. J Biol Chem 1986; 261:6137–6140.
4. Cornwell MM, Safa AR, Felsted RL, Gottesman MM, Pastan I. Membrane vesicles from multidrug resistant human cancer cells contain a specific 150- to 170-kDa protein detected by photoaffinity labeling. Proc Natl Acad Sci USA 1986; 83:3847–3850.
5. Hamada H, Tsuruo T. Purification of the 170- to 180-kilodalton membrane glycoprotein associated with multidrug resistance: the 170- to 180-kilodalton membrane glycoprotein is an ATPase. J Biol Chem 1988; 263:1454–1458.
6. Hamada H, Tsuruo T. Characterization of the ATPase activity of the 170- to 180-kilodalton membrane glycoprotein (P-glycoprotein) associated with multidrug resistance. Cancer Res 1988; 48:4926–4932.
7. Willingham MC, Richert ND, Cornwell MM, Tsuruo T, Hamada H, Gottes-

man MM, Pastan I. Immunocytochemical localization of P170 at the plasma membrane of multidrug-resistant human cells. J Histochem Cytochem 1987; 35:1451–1456.

8. Gros P, Neriah YB, Croop JM, Housman DE. Isolation and expression of a complementary DNA (*mdr*) that confers multidrug resistance. Nature 1986; 323:728–731.

9. Sugimoto Y, Tsuruo T. DNA mediated transfer and cloning of a human multidrug-resistant gene of Adriamycin-resistant myelogenous leukemia K562. Cancer Res 1987; 47:2620–2625.

10. Ueda K, Cardarelli C, Gottesman MM, Pastan I. Expression of a full-length cDNA for the human *mdr1* (P-glycoprotein) gene confer multidrug resistance. Proc Natl Acad Sci USA 1987; 84:3004–3008.

11. Bell DR, Gerlach JH, Kartner N, Buich RN, Ling V. Detection of P-glycoprotein in ovarian cancer: a molecular marker associated with multidrug resistance. J Clin Oncol 1985; 3:311–315.

12. Fojo AT, Ueda K, Slamon DJ, Poplack DG, Gottesman MM, Pastan I. Expression of a multidrug resistance gene in human tumors and tissues. Proc Natl Acad Sci USA 1987; 84:265–269.

13. Tsuruo T, Sugimoto Y, Hamada H, Roninson I, Okumura N, Adachi K, Morishima Y, Ohno R. Detection of multidrug resistance markers, P-glycoprotein and *mdr1* mRNA, in human leukemia cells. Jpn J Cancer Res 1987; 78:1415–1419.

14. Ishida Y, Ohtsu T, Hamada H, Sugimoto Y, Tobinai K, Minato K, Tsuruo T, Shimoyama M. Multidrug resistance in cultured human leukemia and lymphoma cell lines detected by a monoclonal antibody, MRK16. Jpn J Cancer Res 1989; 80:1006–1013.

15. Mizoguchi T, Yamada K, Furukawa T, Hidaka K, Hisatsugu T, Shimazu H, Tsuruo T, Sumizawa T, Akiyama S. Expression of the *MDR1* gene in human gastric and colorectal carcinomas. JNCI 1990; 82:1679–1683.

16. Pirker R, Wallner J, Geissler K, Linkesch W, Haas OA, Bettelheim P, Hopfner M, Scherrer R, Valent P, Havelec L, Ludwing H, Lechner K. *MDR1* gene expression and treatment outcome in acute leukemia. JNCI 1991; 83:708–712.

17. Holzmayer TA, Hilsenbeck S, Von Hoff DD, Roninson IB. Clinical correlates of *MDR1* (P-glycoprotein) gene expression in ovarian and small-cell lung carcinomas. JNCI 1992; 84:1486–1491.

18. Thiebaut F, Tsuruo T, Hamada H, Gottesman MM, Pastan I, Willingham MC. Cellular localization of the multidrug-resistance gene product P-glycoprotein in normal human tissues. Proc Natl Acad Sci USA 1987; 84:7735–7738.

19. Fairchild G, Ivy SP, Rushmore T, Lee G, Koo P, Goldsmith ME, Myers CE, Farber E, Cowan KH. Carcinogen-induced *mdr* overexpression is associated with xenobiotic resistance in rat preneoplastic liver nodules and hepatocellular carcinomas. Proc Natl Acad Sci USA 1987; 84:7701–7705.

20. Sugawara I, Kataoka I, Morishita Y, Hamada H, Tsuruo T, Itoyama S, Mori S. Tissue distribution of P-glycoprotein encoded by a multidrug resis-

tant gene as revealed by a monoclonal antibody MRK16. Cancer Res 1988; 48:1926–1929.

21. Sugawara I, Nakahama M, Hamada H, Tsuruo T, Mori S. Apparent stronger expression in the human adrenal cortex than in the human adrenal medulla of M_r 170,000–180,000 P-glycoprotein. Cancer Res 1988; 48:4611–4614.

22. Arceci RJ, Croop JM, Horwitz SB, Housman D. The gene encoding multidrug resistance is induced and expressed at high levels during pregnancy in the secretory epithelium of the uterus. Proc Natl Acad Sci USA 1988; 85:4350–4354.

23. Thiebaut F, Tsuruo T, Hamada H, Gottesman MM, Pastan I, Willingham MC. Immunohistochemical localization in normal tissues of different epitopes in the multidrug transport protein P170: evidence for localization in brain capillaries and crossreactivity of one antibody with a muscle protein. J Histochem Cytochem 1989; 37:159–164.

24. Sugawara I, Hamada H, Tsuruo T, Mori S. Specialized localization of P-glycoprotein recognized by MRK16 monoclonal antibody in endothelial cells of the brain and the spinal cord. Jpn J Cancer Res 1990; 81:727–730.

25. Watanabe M, Komeshima N, Nakajima S, Tsuruo T. MX2, a morpholino anthracycline, as a new antitumor agent against drug-sensitive and multidrug-resistant human and murine tumor cells. Cancer Res 1988; 48:6653–6657.

26. Watanabe M, Komeshima N, Naito M, Isoe T, Otake N, Tsuruo T. Cellular pharmacology of MX2, a new morpholino anthracycline, in human pleiotropic drug-resistant cells. Cancer Res 1991; 51:157–161.

27. Tsuruo T, Yusa K, Sudo Y, Takamori R, Sugimoto Y. A fluorine-containing anthracycline (ME2303) as a new antitumor agent against murine and human tumors and their multidrug-resistant sublines. Cancer Res 1989; 49:5537–5542.

28. Tsuruo T, Sato S, Yusa K. Antitumor activity of ME2303, a fluorine-containing anthracycline, against human tumors implanted in nude mice. Jpn J Cancer Res 1989; 80:686–689.

29. Tsuruo T, Oh-hara T, Iida H, Tsukagoshi S, Sato Z, Matsuda I, Iwasaki S, Okuda S, Shimizu F, Sasagawa K, Fukami M, Fukuda K, Arakawa M. Rhizoxin, a macrocyclic lactone antibiotic, as a new antitumor agent against human and murine tumor cells and their vincristine-resistant sublines. Cancer Res 1986; 46:381–385.

30. Tsuruo T, Matsuzaki T, Matsushita M, Saito H, Yokokura T. Antitumor effect of CPT-11, a new derivative of camptothecin, against pleiotropic drug-resistant tumors in vitro and in vivo. Cancer Chemother Pharmacol 1988; 21:71–74.

31. Tsuruo T, Naito M, Takamori R, Tsukahara S, Yamabe-Mitsuhashi J, Yamazaki A, Oh-hara T, Sudo Y, Nakaike S, Yamagishi T. A benzophenazine derivative, N-β-dimethylaminoetyl 9-carboxy-5-hydroxy-10-methoxybenzo[a]phenazine-6-carboxamide, as new antitumor agent against multi-

drug-resistant and sensitive tumors. Cancer Chemother Pharmacol 1990; 26:83–87.

32. Morimoto M, Ashizawa T, Ohono H, Azuma M, Kobayashi E, Okabe M, Gomi K, Kono M, Saitoh Y, Kanda Y, Arai H, Sato A, Kasai M, Tsuruo T. Antitumor activity of 7-N-{{2-{[2-(γ-L-glutamylamino)ethyl]-dithio}ethyl}}-mitomycin C. Cancer Res 1991; 51:110–115.

33. Tsuruo T, Sudo Y, Asami N, Inaba M, Morimoto M. Antitumor activity of a derivative of mitomycin, 7-N-[2-[[2-(γ-L-glutamylamino)ethyl]dithio]-ethyl]mitomycin C (KW-2149), against murine and human tumors and a mitomycin C-resistant tumor in vitro and in vivo. Cancer Chemother Pharmacol 1990; 27:89–93.

34. Lee JH, Naito M, Turuo T. Non-enzymatic reductive activation of 7-N-{{2-{[2-(γ-L-glutamylamino)ethyl]dithio}ethyl}}-mitomycin C (KW-2149) by thiol molecules: a novel mitomycin C derivative effective on mitomycin C-resistant tumor cells. Cancer Res 1994; 54:2398–2403.

35. Tsuruo T, Oh-hara T, Saito H. Characteristics of vincristine resistance in vincristine resistant human myelogenous leukemia K562. Anticancer Res 1986; 6:637–642.

36. Tsuruo T, Iida-Saito H, Kawabata H, Oh-hara T, Hamada H, Utakoji T. Characteristics of resistance to Adriamycin in human myelogenous leukemia K562 resistant to Adriamycin and in isolated clones. Jpn J Cancer Res 1986; 77:682–692.

37. Rogan AM, Hamilton TC, Young RC, Klecker RW, Ozols RF. Reversal of Adriamycin resistance by verapamil in human ovarian cancer. Science 1984; 224:994–996.

38. Akiyama S, Fojo A, Hanover JA, Pastan I, Gottesman MM. Isolation and genetic characterization of human KB cell lines resistant to multiple drugs. Somatic Cell Mol Genet 1985; 11:117–126.

39. Johnson RK, Chitnis MP, Embrey WM, Gregory EB. Characteristics in vivo of resistance and cross resistance of an Adriamycin-resistant subline of P388 leukemia. Cancer Treat Rep 1978; 62:1535–1547.

40. Safa AR. Photoaffinity labeling of the multidrug-resistance-related P-glyco-protein with photoactive analogs of verapamil. Proc Natl Acad Sci USA 1988; 85:7187–7191.

41. Yusa K, Tsuruo T. Reversal mechanism of multidrug resistance by vera-pamil: direct binding of verapamil to P-glycoprotein on specific sites and transport of verapamil outward across the plasma membrane of K562/ADM cells. Cancer Res 1989; 49:5002–5006.

42. Foxwell BMJ, Mackie A, Ling V, Ryffel B. Identification of the multidrug resistance-related P-glycoprotein as a cyclosporine binding protein. Mol Pharmacol 1989; 36:543–546.

43. Yang CPH, Mellado W, Horwitz SB. Azidopine photoaffinity labeling of multidrug resistance-associated glycoproteins. Biochem Pharmacol 1988; 37:1417–1421.

44. Qian XD, Beck WT. Progesterone photoaffinity labels P-glycoprotein in

multidrug-resistant human leukemic lymphoblasts. J Biol Chem 1990; 265:18753–18756.

45. Naito M, Hamada H, Tsuruo T. ATP/Mg^{2+}-dependent binding of vincristine to the plasma membrane of multidrug-resistant K562 cells. J Biol Chem 1988; 263:11887–11891.

46. Horio M, Gottesman MM, Pastan I. ATP-dependent transport of vinblastine in vesicles from human multidrug-resistant cells. Proc Natl Acad Sci USA 1988; 85:3580–3584.

47. Cornwell MM, Tsuruo T, Gottesman MM, Pastan I. ATP-binding properties of P-glycoprotein from multidrug-resistant KB cells. FASEB J 1987; 1:51–54.

48. Ambudkar SV, Lelong IH, Zhang J, Cardarelli CO, Gottesman MM, Pastan I. Partial purification and reconstitution of the human multidrug resistance pump: characterization of the drug-stimulatable ATP hydrolysis. Proc Natl Acad Sci USA 1992; 89:8472–8476.

49. Sarkadi B, Price EM, Boucher RC, Germann UA, Scarborugh GA. Expression of the human multidrug resistance cDNA in insect cells generates a high activity drug-stimulated membrane ATPase. J Biol Chem 1992; 267:4854–4858.

50. Natio M, Tsuruo T. Competitive inhibition by verapamil of ATP-dependent high affinity vincristine binding to the plasma membrane of multidrug-resistant K562 cells without calcium ion involvement. Cancer Res 1989; 49:1452–1455.

51. Tamai I, Safa AR. Competitive interaction of cyclosporines with vinca alkaloid-binding site of P-glycoprotein in multidrug-resistant cells. J Biol Chem 1990; 265:16509–16513.

52. Tsuruo T, Iida H, Tsukagoshi S, Sakurai Y. Overcoming of vincristine resistance in P388 leukemia, in vivo and in vitro through enhanced cytotoxicity of vincristine and vinblastine by verapamil. Cancer Res 1981; 41:1967–1972.

53. Tsuruo T, Iida H, Tsukagoshi S, Sakurai Y. Increased accumulation of vincristine and Adriamycin in drug-resistant P388 tumor cells following incubation with calcium antagonists and calmodulin inhibitors. Cancer Res 1982; 42:4730–4733.

54. Tsuruo T, Iida H, Nojiri M, Tsukagoshi S, Sakurai Y. Circumvention of vincristine and Adriamycin resistance in vitro and in vivo by calcium influx blockers. Cancer Res 1983; 43:2905–2910.

55. Slater LM, Murray SL, Wetzel MM, Wisdom RH, Du Vall EM. Verapamil restoration of daunorubicin responsiveness in daunorubicin-resistant Ehrlich ascites carcinoma. J Clin Invest 1982; 10:1131–1134.

56. Ramu A, Fuks Z, Gatt S, Glaubiger D. Reversal of acquired resistance to doxorubicin in P388 murine leukemia cells by perhexiline maleate. Cancer Res 1984; 44:144–148.

57. Ganapathi R, Grabowski D. Enhancement of sensitivity to Adriamycin in resistant P388 leukemia by the calmodulin inhibitor trifluoperazine. Cancer Res 1983; 43:3696–3699.

58. Tsuruo T. Circumvention of drug resistance with calcium channel blockers and monoclonal antibodies. In: Ozols RF, ed., Drug Resistance in Cancer Therapy. New York: Kluwer Academic Publishers 1989:73–95.
59. Tsuruo T. Reversal of multidrug resistance by calcium channel blockers and other agents. In: Roninson IB, ed. Molecular and Cellular Biology of Multidrug Resistance in Tumor Cells. New York: Plenum Publishing, 1991:349–372.
60. Bessho F, Kinumak H, Kobayashi M, Habu H, Nakamura K, Yokota S, Tsuruo T, Kobayashi N. Treatment of children with refractory acute lymphocytic leukemia with vincristine and dilitiazem. Med Pediatr Oncol 1985; 13:199–202.
61. Presant CA, Kennedy PS, Wiseman C, Gala K, Bouzaglou A, Wyres M, Naessig V. Verapamil reversal of clinical doxorubicin resistance in human cancer: a Wilshire Oncology Medical Group pilot phase I–II study. Am J Clin Oncol 1986; 9:355–357.
62. Dalton WS, Grogan TM, Meltzer PS, Scheper RJ, Durie BGM, Taylor CW, Miller TP, Salmon SE. Drug-resistance in multiple myeloma and non-Hodgkin's lymphoma: detection of P-glycoprotein and potential circumvention by addition of verapamil to chemotherapy. J Clin Oncol 1989; 7:415–424.
63. Miller TP, Grogan TM, Dalton WS, Spier CM, Scheper RJ, Salmon SE. P-glycoprotein expression in malignant lymphoma and reversal of clinical drug resistance with chemotherapy plus high-dose verapamil. J Clin Oncol 1991; 9:17–24.
64. Slater LM, Sweet P, Stupeckey M, Gupta S. Cyclosporin A reverses vincristine and daunorubicin resistance in acute lymphatic leukemia in vitro. J Clin Invest 1986; 77:1405–1408.
65. Twentyman PR, Fox NE, White DJ. Cyclosporin A and its analogues as modifiers of Adriamycin and vincristine resistance in a multi-drug resistant human lung cancer cell line. Br J Cancer 1987; 56:55–57.
66. Sonneveld P, Durie BGM, Lokhorst HM, Marie JP, Solbu G, Sucin S, Zittoun R, Löwenberg B, Nooter K. Modulation of multidrug-resistant multiple myeloma by cyclosporin. Lancet 1992; 340:255–259.
67. Shinoda H, Inaba M, Tsuruo T. In vivo circumvention of vincristine resistance in mice with P388 leukemia using a novel compound, AHC-52. Cancer Res 1989; 49:1722–1726.
68. Sato W, Fukazawa N, Suzuki T, Yusa K, Tsuruo T. Circumvention of multidrug resistance by a newly synthesized quinoline derivative, MS-073. Cancer Res 1991; 51:2420–2424.
69. Naito M, Oh-hara T, Yamazaki A, Danki T, Tsuruo T. Reversal of multidrug resistance by an immunosuppressive agent FK-506. Cancer Chemother Pharmacol 1992; 29:195–200.
70. Boesch D, Muller K, Manzanedo AP, Loor F. Restoration of daunomycin retention in multidrug-resistant P388 cells by submicromolar concentrations of SDZ PSC 833, a nonimmunosuppressive cyclosporin derivative. Exp Cell Res 1991; 196:26–32.
71. Boesch D, Gaveriaux C, Jachez B, Manzanedo PM, Bollinger P, Loor F.

In vivo circumvention of P-glycoprotein-mediated multidrug resistance of tumor cells with SDZ PSC 833. Cancer Res 1991; 51:4226–4233.

72. Watanabe T, Tsuge H, Oh-hara T, Natio M, Tsuruo T. Comparative study on reversal efficacy of SDZ PSC 833, cyclosporin A and verapamil on multidrug resistance in vitro and in vivo. Acta Oncol 1994; (in press).

73. Hamada H, Tsuruo T. Functional role for the 170- to 180-kDa glycoprotein specific to drug-resistant tumor cells as revealed by monoclonal antibodies. Proc Natl Acad Sci USA 1986; 83:7785–7789.

74. Georges E, Tsuruo T, Ling V. Topology of P-glycoprotein as determined by epitope mapping of MRK16 monoclonal antibody. J Biol Chem 1993; 268:1792–1798.

75. Kartner N, Everden-Porelle Bradle G, Ling V. Detection of P-glycoprotein in multidrug-resistant cell lines by monoclonal antibodies. Nature 1985; 316:820–823.

76. Scheper RJ, Bulte JWM, Brakkee JGP, Quak JJ, Van der Schoot E, Balm AJM, Meijer CJLM, Broxterman HJ, Kuiper CM, Lankelma J, Pinedo HM. Monoclonal antibody JSB-1 detects a highly conserved epitope on the P-glycoprotein associated with multidrug resistance. Int J Cancer 1988; 42:389–394.

77. Meyers MB, Rittman-Grauer L, O'Brien JP, Safa AR. Characterization of monoclonal antibodies recognizing an M_r 180,000 P-glycoprotein in multidrug-resistant human tumor cells. Cancer Res 1989; 49:3209–3214.

78. Merchetner EB, Roninson IB. Efficient inhibition of P-glycoprotein mediated multidrug resistance with a monoclonal antibody. Proc Natl Acad Sci USA 1992; 89:5824–5828.

79. Arceci RJ, Stieglitz K, Bras J, Schinkel A, Baas F, Croop J. Monoclonal antibody to an external epitope of the human *MDR1* P-glycoprotein. Cancer Res 1993; 53:310–317.

80. Padmanabhan R, Tsuruo T, Kane SE, Willingham MC, Howard BH, Gottesman MM, Pastan I. Magnetic-affinity cell sorting of human multidrug-resistant cells. JNCI 1991; 83:565–569.

81. Tsuruo T, Hamada H, Sato S, Heike Y. Inhibition of multidrug-resistant human tumor growth in athymic mice by anti-P-glycoprotein monoclonal antibodies. Jpn J Cancer Res 1989; 80:627–631.

82. Heike Y, Hamada H, Inamura N, Sone S, Ogura T, Tsuruo T. Monoclonal anti-P-glycoprotein antibody-dependent killing of multidrug-resistant tumor cells by human mononuclear cells. Jpn J Cancer Res 1990; 81:1155–1161.

83. Hamada H, Miura K, Ariyoshi K, Heike Y, Sato S, Kameyama K, Kurosawa Y, Tsuruo T. Mouse–human chimeric antibody against the multidrug transporter P-glycoprotein. Cancer Res 1990; 50:3167–3171.

84. Nishioka Y, Sone S, Heike Y, Hamada H, Ariyoshi K, Tsuruo T, Ogura T. Effector cell analysis of human multidrug-resistant cell killing by mouse–human chimeric antibody against P-glycoprotein. Jpn J Cancer Res 1992; 83:644–649.

85. Heike Y, Okumura K, Tsuruo T. Augmentation by bispecific F(ab')$_2$ reactive with P-glycoprotein and CD3 of cytotoxicity of human effector cells

on P-glycoprotein positive human renal cancer cells. Jpn J Cancer Res 1992; 83:366–372.

86. Duk JV, Tsuruo T, Segal DM, Bolhuis RLH, Colognol R, Van De Griend RJ, Fleuren GJ, Warnaar SO. Bispecific antibodies reactive with the multidrug-resistance-related glycoprotein and CD3 induce lysis of multidrug-resistant tumor cells. Int J Cancer 1989; 44:738–743.

87. Pearson JW, Fogler WE, Volker K, Usui N, Goldenberg SK, Gruys E, Riggs CW, Komschlies K, Wiltrout RH, Tsuruo T, Pastan I, Gottesman MM, Longo DL. Reversal of drug resistance in a human colon cancer xenograft expressing MDR1 complementary DNA by a in vivo administration of MRK16 monoclonal antibody. JNCI 1991; 83:1386–1391.

88. Naito M, Tsuge H, Kuroko C, Koyama T, Tomida A, Tatsuta T, Heike Y, Tsuruo T. Enhancement of cellular accumulation of cyclosporin A by anti-P-glycoprotein monoclonal antibody MRK16, and synergistic modulation of multidrug resistance. JNCI 1993; 85:311–316.

89. Naito M, Tsuge H, Kuroko C, Tomida A, Tsuruo T. Enhancement of reversing effect of cyclosporin A on vincristine resistance by anti-P-glycoprotein monoclonal antibody MRK16. Jpn J Cancer Res 1993; 84:489–492.

90. LoBuglio AF, Wheeler RH, Trang J, Haynes A, Rogers K, Harvey EB, Sun L, Ghrayeb J, Khazaeli MB. Mouse/human chimeric monoclonal antibody in man: kinetics and immune response. Proc Natl Acad Sci USA 1989; 86:4220–4224.

91. Greenberger LM, Williams SS, Geroges E, Ling V, Horwitz SB. Electrophoretic analysis of P-glycoproteins produced by mouse J774.2 and Chinese hamster ovary multidrug-resistant cells. JNCI 1988; 80:506–510.

92. Hamada H, Hagiwara K, Nakajima T, Tsuruo T. Phosphorylation of the M_r 170,000 to 180,000 glycoprotein specific to multidrug-resistant tumor cells: effect of verapamil, trifluoperazine, and phorbol esters. Cancer Res 1987; 47:2860–2865.

93. Fine RL, Patel J, Chabner BA. Phorbol esters induce multidrug resistance in breast cancer cells. Proc Natl Acad Sci USA 1988; 85:582–586.

94. Chambers TC, McAvoy EM, Jacobs JW, Eilon G. Protein kinase C phosphorylates P-glycoprotein in multidrug resistant human KB carcinoma cells. J Biol Chem 1990; 265:7679–7686.

95. Yu G, Ahmad S, Aquino A, Fairchild CR, Trepel JB, Ohno S, Suzuki K, Tsuruo T, Cowan KH, Glazer RI. Transfection with protein kinase Cα confers increased multidrug resistance to MCF-7 cells expressing P-glycoprotein. Cancer Commun 1991; 3:181–189.

96. Bates SE, Currier SJ, Alvarez M, Fojo AT. Modulation of P-glycoprotein phosphorylation and drug transport by sodium butyrate. Biochemistry 1992; 31:6366–6372.

97. Kioka N, Hosokawa N, Komano T, Hiroyoshi K, Nagata K, Ueda K. Quercetin, a bioflavonoid, inhibits the increase of human multidrug resistance gene (*MDR1*) expression caused by arsenite. FEBS Lett 1992; 301:307–309.

98. Tatsuta T, Naito M, Oh-hara T, Sugawara I, Tsuruo T. Functional involve-

ment of P-glycoprotein in blood–brain barrier. J Biol Chem 1992; 267:20383–20391.

99. Tsuji A, Terasaki T, Takabatake Y, Tenda Y, Tamai I, Yamashima T, Moritani S, Tsuruo T, Yamashita J. P-glycoprotein as the drug efflux pump in primary cultured bovine brain capillary endothelial cells. Life Sci 1992; 51:1427–1437.

100. Shirai A, Naito M, Tatsuta T, Dong J, Hanaoka K. Mikami K, Oh-hara T, Tsuruo T. Transport of cyclosporin A across the brain capillary endothelial cell monolayer by P-glycoprotein. Biochim Biophys Acta 1994; 1222:400–404.

101. Naito M, Yusa K, Tsuruo T. Steroid hormones inhibit binding of vinca alkaloid to multidrug resistance related P-glycoprotein. Biochem Biophys Res Commun 1989; 158:1066–1071.

102. Yang CPH, DePinho SG, Greenberger LM, Arceci R, Horwits SB. Progesterone interacts with P-glycoprotein in multidrug-resistant cells and in the endometrium of gravid uterus. J Biol Chem 1989; 264:782–788.

103. Ueda K, Okamura N, Hirai M, Tanigawara Y, Saeki T, Kioka N, Komano T, Hori R. Human P-glycoprotein transports cortisol aldosterone, and dexamethasone but not progesterone. J Biol Chem 1992; 267:24248–24252.

104. Tanigawara Y, Okamura N, Hirai M, Yasuhara M, Ueda K, Kioka N, Komano T, Hori R. Transport of digoxin by human P-glycoprotein expressed in porcine kidney epithelial cell line (LLC-PK$_1$). J Pharmacol Exp Ther 1992; 263:840–845.

105. Kamimoto Y, Gatmaitan Z, Hsu J, Arias IM. The function of Gp170, the multidrug resistance gene product, in rat liver canalicular membrane vesicles. J Biol Chem 1989; 264:11693–11698.

106. Chaudhary PM, Roninson IB. Expression and activity of P-glycoprotein, a multidrug efflux pump, in human hematopoietic stem cells. Cell 1991; 66:85–94.

107. Horton JK, Thimmaiah KN, Houghton JA, Horiwits ME, Houghton PJ. Modulation by verapamil of vincristine pharmacokinetics and toxicity in mice bearing human tumor xenografts. Biochem Pharmacol 1989; 38:1727–1736.

19

Glutathione Conjugation and ATP-Dependent Export of Anticancer Drugs

Toshihisa Ishikawa and Francis Ali-Osman
The University of Texas M. D. Anderson Cancer Center, Houston, Texas

I. CELLULAR BIOCHEMISTRY OF GLUTATHIONE

A. Biosynthesis and Regulation of Intracellular Glutathione

Glutathione (γ-Glu-Cys-Gly; GSH) is widely distributed in animals, plants, and microorganisms (1). Cellular GSH is associated with a variety of physiologically important functions in cellular defense and metabolism, including the modulation of thiol–disulfide status of cellular proteins, protection of cells from oxidative stress, detoxification of electrophilic compounds, and synthesis and transport of biologically active, endogenous substances (2–13). Moreover, GSH interacts with a wide range of drugs. Recent studies indicate that GSH is a critical determinant in the tumor cell resistance to alkylating agents, such as L-phenylalanine mustard (melphalan), bifunctional nitrosoureas, and cisplatin (14–20). This chapter features a novel aspect of GSH in drug resistance of tumor cells, in particular GSH conjugation of anticancer drugs and their ATP-dependent efflux from cells.

The research on GSH has a long history. Indeed, GSH was first discovered by de Rey-Pailhade in 1888 (21; see Ref. 22 for review), and its exact biochemical structure was later established by Harrington and Mead, in

1935 (23). The GSH molecule bears two important features in its structure, the γ-glutamate linkage and the SH-group, both of which are intimately linked to its intracellular stability and biological functions. The intracellular concentration of GSH in mammalian cells is 1–10 mM, which is even higher than the intracellular concentration of adenosine triphosphate (ATP). In many cells, GSH accounts for more than 90% of the total nonprotein sulfur. Such high intracellular concentration is made possible by the γ-glutamic acid linkage structure that protects the GSH molecule from protease cleavage. The SH-group of GSH is strongly nucleophilic and confers to the molecule the unique ability to react with a wide variety of agents, including free radicals, reactive oxygen species, heavy metals, and cytotoxic compounds, thereby functioning as a significant detoxification mechanism of living cells.

The biosynthesis of GSH takes place in the cytosol (Fig. 1). The reaction consists of two steps catalyzed by γ-glutamylcysteine synthetase and by GSH synthetase, for which each step requires one molecule of ATP. γ-Glutamylcysteine synthetase catalyzes the first step (Reaction 1) in which an amide linkage is formed between the amino group of cysteine and the γ-carboxyl group of glutamate. In the second step, GSH synthetase catalyzes the reaction between glycine and the cysteine carboxyl group of γ-glutamylcysteine:

$$\text{L-Glu} + \text{L-Cys} + \text{ATP} \rightarrow \text{γ-glutamylcysteine} + \text{ADP} + \text{Pi}$$

(Reaction 1)

$$\text{γ-Glutamylcysteine} + \text{L-Gly} + \text{ATP} \rightarrow \text{GSH} + \text{ADP} + \text{Pi}$$

(Reaction 2)

The reaction catalyzed by γ-glutamylcysteine synthetase is the rate-limiting step of the GSH synthesis and is controlled by negative-feedback from its end product, GSH, by nonallosteric competitive inhibition (24; see Fig. 1).

γ-Glutamylcysteine synthetase is effectively inhibited by a specific inhibitor, buthionine sulfoximine (25). The development of this compound evolved from earlier studies of Meister and Griffith on the inhibition of glutamine synthetase by methionine sulfoximine (26). Methionine sulfoximine inhibits both glutamine synthetase and γ-glutamylcysteine synthetase. Methionine sulfoximine, however, could not be used for the specific modulation of cellular GSH, since inhibition of brain glutamine synthetase by this agent resulted in severe convulsions and death. Specific inhibitors of γ-glutamylcysteine synthetase lacking inhibition of glutamine synthetase were developed by replacing the *S*-methyl moiety of methionine sulfoximine with larger *S*-alkyl groups. The buthionine sulfoximine thus ob-

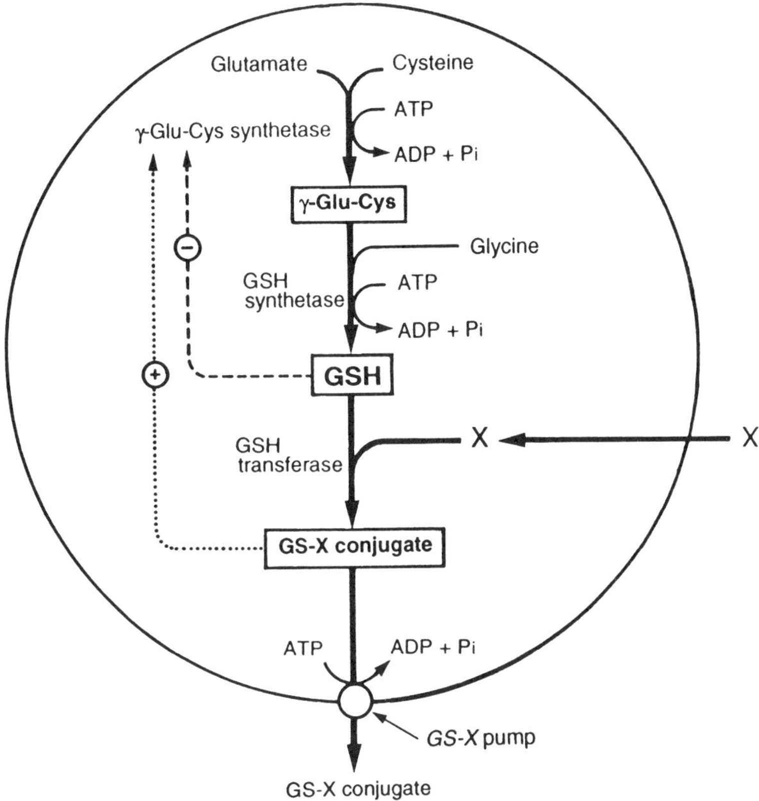

Figure 1   Schematic illustration for the biosynthesis of GSH, conjugation of GSH with electrophilic drugs (X), and ATP-dependent export of GSH conjugates from cells by the *GS-X* pump. GSH inhibits γ-glutamylcysteine synthetase (γ-Glu-Cys synthetase) and the product inhibition can be relieved by GSH conjugates (GS-X).

tained is several hundred times more potent than methionine sulfoximine in inhibiting γ-glutamylcysteine synthetase. Inhibition of γ-glutamylcysteine synthetase by buthionine sulfoximine results in a substantial (up to 95%) reduction of cellular GSH level both in cell culture and in animals (14). Accumulating evidence suggests that modulation of cellular GSH in this manner is critically important to reversing resistance to alkylating agents in tumor cells (see Sec. IV.A).

γ-Glutamylcysteine synthetase can be induced by electrophilic compounds, such as cisplatin, in human ovarian cancer cells (27) and by prostaglandin A_2 in murine leukemia L1210 cells (28). The negative-feedback inhibition of γ-glutamylcysteine synthetase by GSH was released by a glutathione S-conjugate, S-(2,4-dinitrophenyl)-glutathione (29), suggesting a potential role of GSH conjugates in stimulation of the γ-glutamylcysteine synthetase reaction (see Fig. 1). When GSH is consumed and feedback inhibition to γ-glutamylcysteine synthetase is lost, availability of cysteine as a precursor can become the limiting factor (30). To a limited degree, cysteine can be taken up from the plasma. However, since cysteine is rapidly autoxidized to cystine, its plasma concentrations are low (5–10 μM) compared with cystine levels (100–200 μM). Alternative sources of cysteine are the uptake of cystine, with subsequent intracellular reduction, and cysteine production from methionine by the cystathionine pathway (30). Cystine transport activity was significantly induced in human fibroblast cells by diethylmalate and other electrophilic agents (31).

B. Conjugation of Anticancer Drugs with Glutathione

A variety of electrophilic compounds derived from endogenous or exogenous sources are conjugated with GSH (32). There is accumulating evidence that alkylating anticancer drugs undergo GSH conjugation. In many cases, the conjugation reaction is catalyzed by cytosolic or microsomal glutathione S-transferases (GST). The GSH conjugates thus formed are actively eliminated from cells by an ATP-dependent transport system, named the *GS-X* pump (13; Fig. 1). This pump plays a key role in reducing the intracellular accumulation of GSH–drug conjugates, as well as in their further metabolism (i.e., γ-glutamyltransferase and dipeptidase reactions and mercapturic acid formation).

In vitro studies have demonstrated that intracellular GSH and GST levels are elevated in tumors resistant to alkylating anticancer drugs. Stable overexpression of γ-glutamylcysteine synthetase, a rate-limiting enzyme for GSH biosynthesis, and individual GST isozymes was observed in some human tumors. Since the elevation of intracellular GSH levels or the overexpression of GST in tumor cells is associated with non–P-glycoprotein-mediated drug resistance phenotypes, a critical role of GSH and GST has been suggested.

Several possible mechanisms have been proposed for the drug resistance associated with GSH. These include (1) enhanced inactivation of electrophilic anticancer drugs, such as cisplatin, melphalan (L-phenylalanine mustard), and chlorambucil, by direct conjugation with GSH; (2)

GSH-dependent denitrosation of nitrosoureas, which leads to a decrease in nitrosourea cytotoxicity; (3) quenching of chloroethylated–DNA mono-adducts and platinum–DNA adducts; (4) active elimination of biologically active GSH drug conjugates, such as bis(glutathionato)-platinum(II) and 2'-chloroethyl-S-glutathione.

1. Reaction of Cisplatin with Glutathione

Cisplatin is an effective antitumor agent in the treatment of solid tumors in the brain, head and neck, ovary, testicle, and bladder (33,34). The antitumor activity of this agent is attributed primarily to its ability to form interstrand platinum adducts in DNA (35–39). Despite its clinical effectiveness, cellular drug resistance is a major obstacle to long-term, sustained patient response to cisplatin-based therapy. Several potential biochemical and molecular mechanisms of cisplatin resistance have hitherto been identified. They include decreased intracellular accumulation of cisplatin (40,41), elevated cellular GSH (27) and metallothioneine content (42), and increased DNA repair (43). Importantly, the cytotoxicity of cisplatin has been significantly enhanced by the depletion of cellular GSH in some tumor lines (18,44). Glutathione can quench DNA–platinum monoadducts before their conversion to cytotoxic DNA cross-links (17), or GSH may form a complex (or complexes) with cisplatin, thereby reducing the amount of intracellular cisplatin available for interaction with DNA (45,46). Although accumulating evidence supports a significant role of GSH in tumor cisplatin resistance, the exact molecular mechanism of the reaction between cisplatin and GSH is not fully understood.

Recent studies in our laboratory have provided evidence for the direct interaction between cisplatin and GSH, both in a cell-free system as well as in cells of the L1210 murine leukemia line (20). The reaction proceeds nonenzymatically. The reaction product was isolated by QAE-Sephadex anion-exchange chromatography and identified by a combination of high-performance liquid chromatography (HPLC) and atomic absorption spectroscopy. Stoichiometric analysis showed a 2:1 molar ratio of GSH/cisplatin for the reaction (Fig. 2). The molecular mass assessed by mass spectroscopy was 809 Da, corresponding to a GS–platinum chelate complex, bis(glutathionato)–platinum, in which two GSH molecules act as bidentate chelating ligands and coordinate to the platinum through the cysteinyl sulfur and nitrogen atoms. The ^{1}H nuclear magnetic resonance (NMR) spectra of the GS–platinum complex exhibited broadened signal lines caused by an effect from the platinum atom at the center of the molecule. The GS–platinum complex exhibits a broad absorption peak at 200–400 nm, with a molar extinction coefficient of 8.05 mM^{-1} cm^{-1} at 280 nm (20).

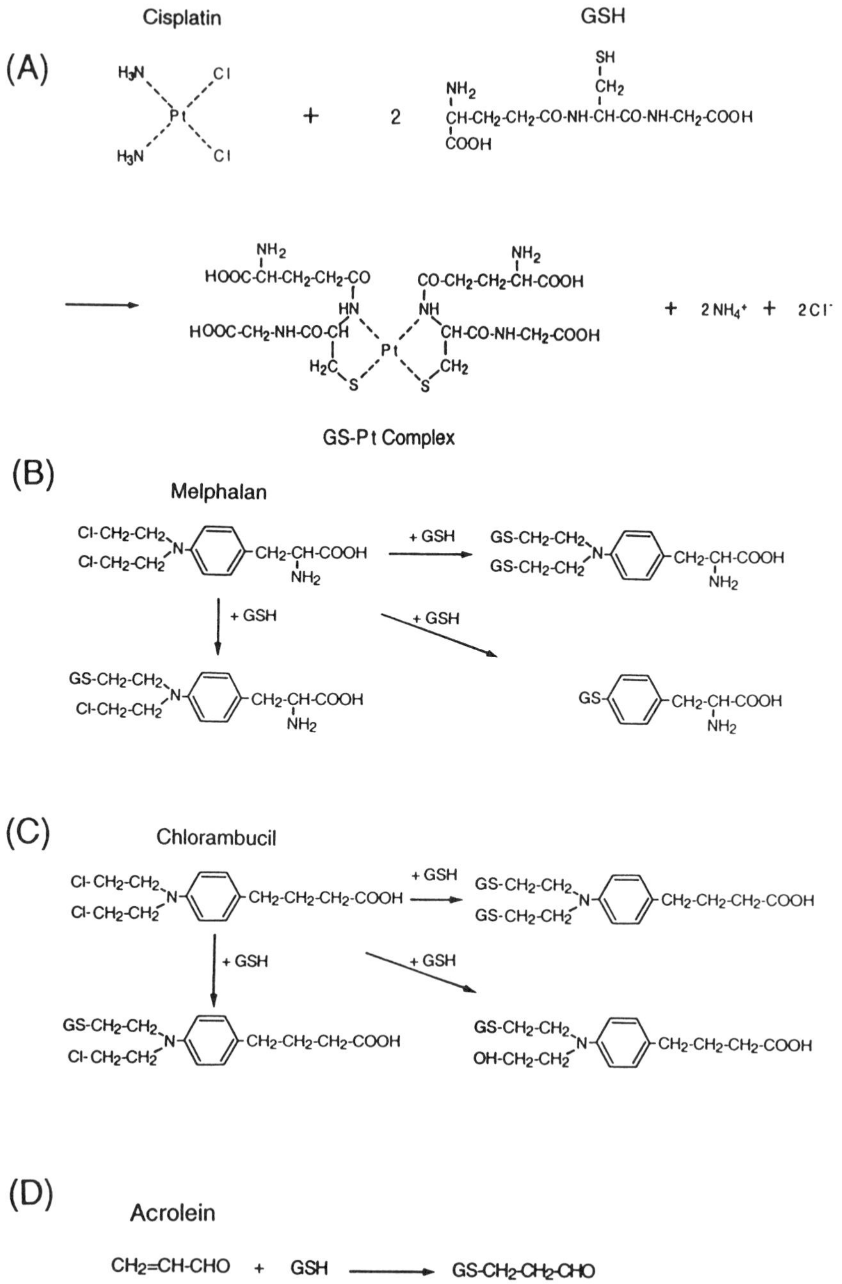

Figure 2 Reactions of GSH with (A) cisplatin, (B) melphalan, (C) chlorambucil, and (D) acrolein.

By a combination of HPLC and atomic absorption spectroscopy, the GS–platinum complex was identified as a major metabolite in L1210 leukemia cells incubated with 20 μM cisplatin. The intracellular content of the GS–platinum complex reached a maximal level (0.91 nmol $\times$ mg protein^{-1}) after 12 h, corresponding to about 60% of the intracellular platinum content (1.50 nmol $\times$ mg protein^{-1}). Thus, the formation of the GS–platinum complex is considered a significant part of the cellular metabolism of cisplatin (20).

Godwin et al. (27) have recently demonstrated that cisplatin-resistant human ovarian cancer cell lines, obtained by exposure to near continuously increasing concentrations of cisplatin, have strikingly increased (4- to 50-fold) levels of cellular GSH, compared with the original drug-sensitive cells. Increased cellular GSH levels in cisplatin-resistant variants are closely related to enhanced mRNA levels of both γ-glutamylcysteine synthetase and γ-glutamyltransferase, suggesting that the GSH-associated metabolism of cisplatin may be a significant property of cisplatin-resistant cells. In those resistant variant cells, mRNA levels of P-glycoprotein, multidrug resistance-associated protein (MRP), and topoisomerase II were unchanged (47). The cellular GSH levels in human ovarian carcinoma cell lines exhibited a significant correlation with IC$_{50}$ values for cisplatin, carboplatin, and iproplatin; however, no correlation was observed between GST activity and IC$_{50}$ values for those platinum drugs (48). Transfection studies with class π isozyme of human GST (see Sec. II.A. for nomenclature of human GST isozymes) in MCF7 human breast cancer cells and NIH 3T3 cells have shown that increased expression of the isozyme does not confer significant resistance to cisplatin (49,50). The contribution of class π GST to the reaction of cisplatin with GSH appears to be a minor determinant in those cells.

2. Glutathione Conjugation of Melphalan and Chlorambucil

Cisplatin-resistant tumor cells were often found to be cross-resistant to bifunctional nitrogen mustards, such as melphalan and chlorambucil (see Fig. 2). Vistica and co-workers first reported that murine L1210 leukemia cells resistant to melphalan contain elevated levels of both GSH and GST (51,52) and that significant reduction of GSH level conferred drug sensitivity (53). Thus, GSH was proposed to be a critical determinant for the inactivation of melphalan in tumor cells. Three GSH adducts of melphalan (see Fig. 2) were identified in reactions catalyzed by human and rabbit liver microsomal GST (54,55). These adducts were also produced by cytosolic GSTs, although the isoenzymes involved were not specified. Likewise, GSH conjugates of chlorambucil were also identified (56). In murine hepatic GSTs, class α isozyme has been suggested to represent a specific mechanism for the GSH conjugation of melphalan, whereas class μ and

π isozymes were not effective (57). Although liver cytosol contains enzymes that enhance the rate of GSH conjugation of melphalan, in human melanoma cells, GST-catalyzed conjugation appeared to be a minor determinant of the overall rate of melphalan–GSH conjugate formation (58). Spontaneous GSH conjugation takes place at significant rates even in the absence of GST. Friedman et al. pointed out that the relation between GSH levels, GST activity, and the transport of melphalan, and the resistance phenotype of human medulloblastoma cell lines was complex (59). The contribution of individual isozymes of GSTs to the GSH conjugation of melphalan in human tumor cells remains to be elucidated.

In melphalan-resistant L1210 cells, the increased cellular content of GSH was ascribed to increased synthesis of cellular GSH (52). γ-Glutamylcysteine synthetase activity increased about 1.5-fold in melphalan-resistant L1210 cells, whereas GSH synthetase activity was equivalent in both drug-sensitive and drug-resistant cells. The increase of cellular GSH in the resistant cells was accompanied by an increase in the amount of γ-glutamyltransferase, a key enzyme of GSH catabolism. It is suggested that the drug-resistant tumor cells developed an efficient mechanism for maintenance of elevated GSH that involves both γ-glutamyltransferase-initiated catabolism of GSH to cysteine and its reutilization by γ-glutamylcysteine synthetase (52). For this metabolism, efflux of GSH from cells is necessary, since γ-glutamyltransferase and dipeptidase are ectoenzymes localized at the outer surface of the plasma membrane.

3. Glutathione Conjugation of Acrolein Derived from Cyclophosphamide

Cyclophosphamide is used in the treatment of breast carcinoma, lymphoma, multiple myeloma, carcinoma of the lung, and some sarcomas. It has also been used for immunosuppression before organ transplantation, as well as the treatment of some autoimmune diseases. Cyclophosphamide per se is a prodrug, showing no alkylating activity. In vivo, cyclophosphamide is bioactivated by the microsomal mixed-function oxidase reaction which predominantly takes place in the liver. The metabolic activation of cyclophosphamide involves the formation of 4-hydroxyphosphamide, which rearranges to its isomer, aldophosphamide. Aldophosphamide, in turn, undergoes β-elimination to release acrolein and phosphamide mustard. The latter was identified as the bifunctional alkylator and is effective in chemotherapy (60–62). Acrolein, on the other hand, is a highly reactive, genotoxic aldehyde. Therefore, it must be inactivated and eliminated from cells.

Acrolein is inactivated by GSTs either by conjugation with GSH or by covalent binding to the enzymes (63). The catalytic efficiency (k_{cat}/K_m)

of human GST π is the highest among classes α, μ, and π of human GST. Acrolein ranks among the most active substrates known for GST π isozyme. The irreversible binding of acrolein to GST molecules, which takes place in the absence of GSH, results in an inactivation of the enzyme. The GST π isozyme reacted significantly more rapidly with acrolein than did other isozymes of human GSTs.

4. Glutathione-Mediated Inactivation of Chloroethylnitrosoureas

Chloroethylnitrosoureas (CENUs) are the most effective agents used in clinical therapy of brain tumors (64). Reed and May have demonstrated that those agents undergo spontaneous hydrolytic decomposition, both in aqueous buffers and under intracellular pH conditions to yield, through a diazonium hydroxide, carbamoylating organic isocyanates and bifunctional alkylating chloroethylcarbonium ions (65) (Fig. 3). The latter are the most critical intermediates that react with DNA to form cross-link adducts. The chloroethylcarbonium ions, however, are highly electrophilic and can readily react with various nucleophiles, including GSH. The reaction of GSH with the chloroethylcarbonium ions is considered to be a major pathway of inactivation of bifunctional nitrosoureas in chemotherapy. The resulting product, 2'-chloroethyl-S-glutathione, does not exhibit bifunctional activity; however, it can be converted to an episulfonium ion, a genotoxic electrophile, which reacts with the N^7 atom of guanine in DNA (66–69). The active elimination of 2'-chloroethyl-S-glutathione is considered to be an important factor in reducing its potential toxicity.

In addition to those reactions, carmustine 1,3-bis(2-chloroethyl)-1-nitrosourea (BCNU) can be inactivated by GSH-dependent denitrosation (see Fig. 2), which is catalyzed by cytosolic GSTs (70–73; see Sec. II.B).

5. Glutathione-Dependent Quenching of Chloroethylated– and Platinated–DNA Monoadducts

The formation of DNA cross-links is essential for the antitumor activity of chloroethylnitrosoureas (CENUs), as well as that of cisplatin and other platinum analogues. However, the cross-link formation of those agents can be quenched by cellular GSH (19,17). Importantly, the quenching reactions must take place in the nuclei, whereas direct interaction and inactivation of those agents by GSH may occur in both the cytoplasm and nuclei.

In the antitumor action of CENU, critical cross-links have been proposed to involve a rapid O^6-guanine chloroethylation on one DNA strand. This is subsequently followed by a rearrangement of the O^6-(2-chloroeth-

(A)

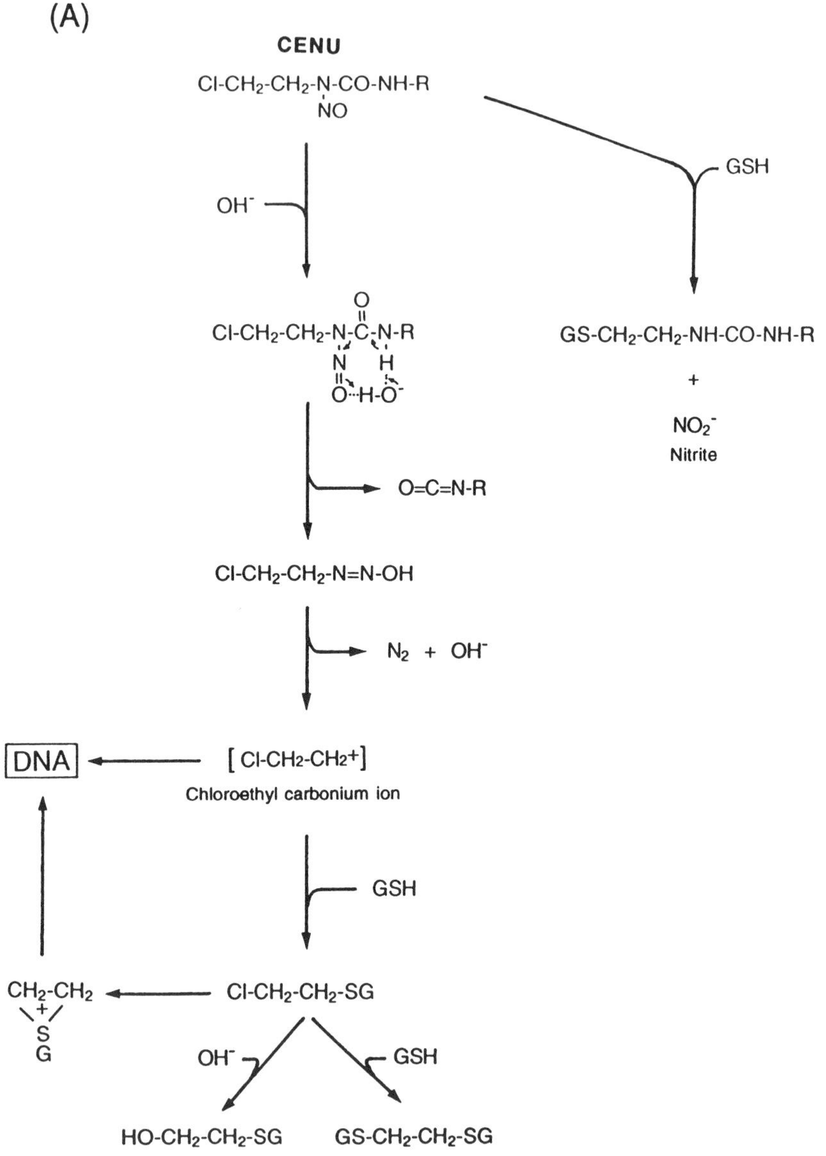

Figure 3 Reactions of GSH with (A) chloroethyl nitrosoureas (CENU) and with (B) chloroethyl–DNA monoadducts. R is 2′-chloroethyl BCNU [*N*,*N*′-bis(2-chloroethyl)-*N*-nitrosourea] or cyclohexyl CCNU [1-(2-chloroethyl)-3-(cyclohexyl)-1-nitrosourea].

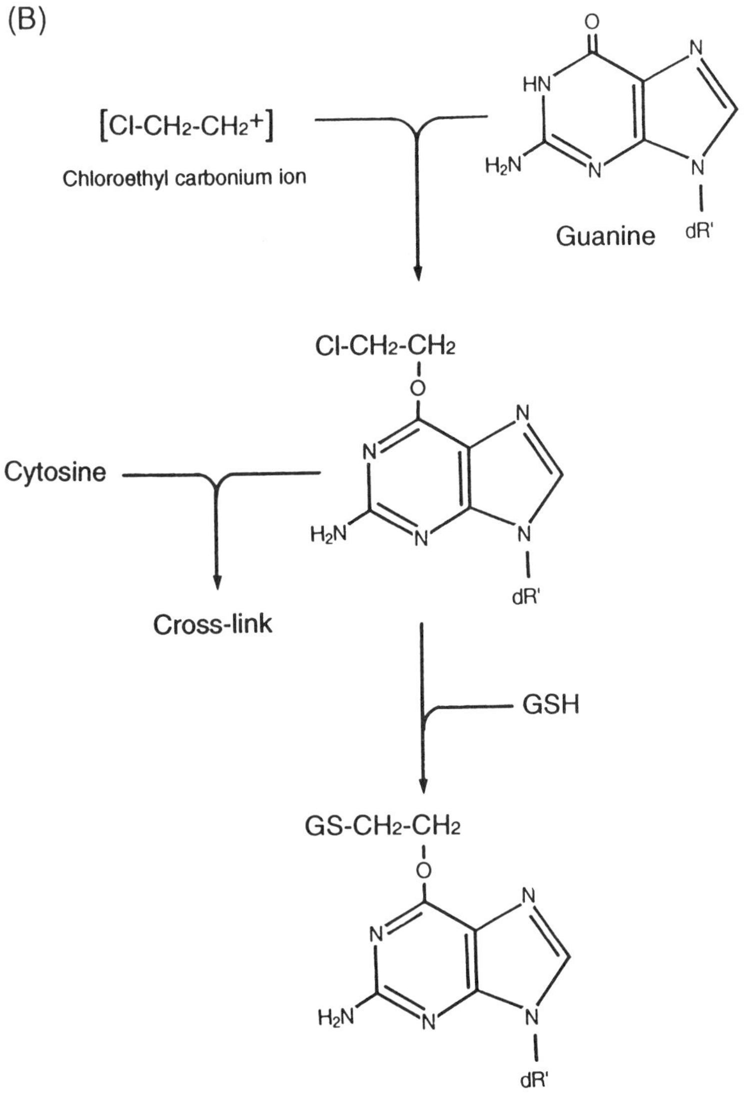

Figure 3 *(Continued)*.

yl)guanine to N^1, O^6-ethanguanine and by the reaction with the second DNA strand, in particular with cytosine, thereby forming a cross-link between two DNA strands (69) (Fig. 3). In the presence of GSH, this cross-link formation was significantly inhibited (19). The quenching was substantially dependent on the concentration of GSH and the incubation time. It was also demonstrated that 56% of the total GSH was bound to quenched 2-chloroethylated Col E1 DNA and 25% to quenched 2-chloroethylated calf thymus DNA. The GSH binding to cross-linked DNA and native DNA was insignificant. The formation of 1-(O^6-deoxyguanosyl)-2-S-glutathionylethane has been proposed as a product generated from the quenching reaction (19). The results suggest that, in addition to the direct inactivation of reactive cytotoxic CENU species, GSH can modulate cellular response to CENUs by quenching chloroethylated DNA in the nuclei, thereby decreasing the formation of potentially lethal DNA cross-links. In support of this possible reaction, a reaction product, 1-(guan-1-yl)-2-(cystein-S-yl)ethane, has recently been identified (74).

As with CENU, GSH could modulate the toxicity of cisplatin and other platinum complexes by at least two different mechanisms. First, the electrophilicity of platinum can be inactivated by directly binding to the SH-group of GSH (see Fig. 2), thereby preventing the drug from reaching the critical DNA target. Second, GSH may reduce platinum cytotoxicity by quenching DNA–Pt monoadducts before they can rearrange to toxic bifunctional adducts. The second possible mechanism was examined in an in vitro study in which DNA was treated with cis-[^{3}H]dichloro(ethylenediamine)-platinum(II) and the resulting ^{3}H-labeled platinum–DNA monoadducts were incubated with GSH (17). After digestion of DNA adducts and separation by ion-suppression reverse-phase HPLC, two hydrophilic adducts were detected. One of the adducts is most probably a GSH adduct cross-linked by platinum to N^7-deoxyguanine (17); however, the exact structure of the adduct still remains to be elucidated.

II. HUMAN GLUTATHIONE TRANSFERASES

A. Polymorphism of Human Glutathione Transferase Isozymes

The glutathione transferases (GSTs) constitute a family of isozymes that catalyze reactions between GSH and electrophilic organic compounds. Four classes of cytosolic human GSTs have been identified, α, μ, π, and θ, as well as one microsomal enzyme (75) (Table 1). Expression of GST isozyme genes is tissue-specific and genetically regulated. Despite their common biochemical function as catalysts of GSH conjugation, the differ-

Table 1 Nomenclature for Human Glutathione Transferases (GSTs)

Type	Class	Nomenclature	Chromosome
Cytosolic GST	α	GSTA1-1	6
		GSTA2-2	6
	μ	GSTM1a-1a	1
		GSTM1b-1b	1
		GSTM2-2	
		GSTM3-3	
		GSTM4-4	
		GSTM5-5	
	π	GSTP1-1[a]	11
	θ		
Microsomal GST			12

[a] Two novel variants (P1b and P1c) of GSTP1 isozyme have been identified in human brain tumors (Ali-Osman and Akande, unpublished work). GSTP1b has the same structure as GSTP1a, the previously identified form, but codon 105 has been changed from ATC (Ile) to GTC (Val); GSTP1c has ATC (Ile) at codon 105, but codon 114 has been changed from GCC (Ala) to GTG (Val).

ent GST isozymes are encoded by distinct genes, with different chromosomal localization. In recent years, the application of molecular biological techniques to elucidate GST gene structure has revealed the immense complexity of the multigene family (see Ref. 8 for a recent review). The activity of GSTs exhibits broad and overlapping substrate specificities toward structurally diverse electrophiles. This reflects their flexible capacities in the detoxification of a variety of reactive metabolites generated from endogenous and exogenous sources. In this context, the GSTs are the first line of cellular defense against cytotoxic or carcinogenic compounds. Comprehensive overviews of the biochemistry and regulation of GSTs have been summarized in excellent recent reviews (6–12).

In cancer chemotherapy, on the other hand, GST activity can be a critical determinant in certain drug-resistant phenotypes. Accumulating evidence shows that increased GST activity as well as expression levels of the isozymes are associated with acquired resistance to several anticancer drugs (76–83). However, there is still a critical gap in our knowledge concerning the direct interactions between GSTs and individual alkylating anticancer agents. Although it is assumed that electrophilic anticancer drugs, such as nitrogen mustards and nitrosoureas, are inactivated in a GSH–GST-dependent manner, this has not been fully proved. In the next section, we will discuss the direct interactions of GSTs with 1,3-bis(2-

chloroethyl)-1-nitrosourea (BCNU) and chlorambucil, introducing most recent advances in this respect.

B. Glutathione Transferases in Drug Resistance of Human Tumors

Carmustine undergoes GST-dependent denitrosation to give 2-chloro-ethyl-3-ethyl-glutathionylurea and nitrite (70–73) (Fig. 3), and this reaction may contribute to inactivation of BCNU in tumor cells. The possible involvement of human GSTs in the enzymatic denitrosation has recently been examined using two human lung cancer cell lines, U1690 and U180 (73). The U1810 cells are 3.2-fold more resistant to BCNU than are U1690 cells. This resistance phenotype was not correlated with cellular levels of GSTs P1-1 or A1-1, although U1690 cells expressed isozymes P1-1 and A1-1 1.3- and 15-fold higher in the cytosol fraction than did the U1810 cells. GST3-3, on the other hand, was detectable in U1810 cells, but not in U1690 cells. Studies with purified human GST A1-1, GST M1-1, GST M3-3, and GST P1-1 demonstrated that GST M3-3, but not the other isozymes, catalyzed the denitrosation of BCNU. These findings strongly suggest that human GST M3-3 is involved in tumor cell resistance to BCNU.

Chlorambucil (see Fig. 2) is an anticancer drug used for the treatment of Hodgkin's and non-Hodgkin's lymphoma, chronic lymphocytic leukemia, and ovarian cancer. Several lines of research suggest that tumor cell resistance to chlorambucil is associated with enhanced expression of GSTs. Lewis et al. reported that amplification of class α GST in Chinese hamster ovary cells was associated with resistance (76). Puchalski and Fahl found increased resistance to chlorambucil after transfection of mouse and monkey cells with rat GSTs 1-1 (class α), 3-3 (class μ), or human GST P1-1 (84). Johnston et al. reported an inverse correlation between both GSH and total GST activity and chlorambucil-dependent DNA adducts formed in vitro in human chronic lymphocytic leukemic lymphocytes (81). Ciaccio et al. have shown that murine GSTs of α, μ, and π classes, as well as human GSTs of α and π classes, catalyze GSH conjugation of chlorambucil in vitro at pH 6.5 (56,85). In contrast, however, the transfection of human GST P1-1 into NIH 3T3 cells failed to alter their sensitivity to chlorambucil (50). Moreover, Leyland-Jones et al. reported no significant decrease in cell sensitivity to chlorambucil in a human breast cancer cell line that was stably transfected with a human α class GST (86). These studies suggest that certain GST isozymes may contribute to drug inactivation by catalyzing the GSH conjugation in cell-free systems: however, additional mechanisms must be involved to confer resistance in living cells.

Recently, Meyers et al. (87) have investigated the GST-mediated and nonmediated conjugation reactions of chlorambucil with GSH in vitro under subphysiological conditions. They found that the mono-GSH conjugate of chlorambucil (see Fig. 2) is a pure competitive inhibitor for human GSTs A1-1 and A2-2, with K_i of as low as 1.3 and 1.2 μM, respectively. This indicates that subunits A1 and A2 have high affinities toward the mono-GSH conjugate. GSTs P1-1 and M1a-1a, on the other hand, were inhibited by the mono-GSH conjugate only at concentrations above 10 μM. Incubation of 2 μM chlorambucil, a clinically significant concentration, with 5 mM GSH at pH 7.0 showed catalysis of GSH monoconjugation by GST A1-2 (20–50 μM) to be equivalent to 18% of the spontaneous rate. The principal effect of GST A1-2 was sequestration of the mono-GSH conjugate, which reached about 75% of the total reaction products at 60 min, compared to about 30% in controls. The active site of GST A1-2 may have a high affinity toward this mono-GSH conjugate to retain the conjugate molecule, and at the same time the enzymatic activity is inhibited by the mono-GSH conjugate. Thus, the contribution of GSTs to detoxification of chlorambucil will depend on the relative molarities of chlorambucil, its mono-GSH conjugate, and GSTs, as well as on the cellular capacity to excrete the mono-GSH conjugate to relieve product inhibition (87).

III. ATP-DEPENDENT GLUTATHIONE *S*-CONJUGATE EXPORT PUMP, *GS-X* PUMP

A. The Phase III Detoxification System in Drug Metabolism and Disposition

The transmembrane export of intracellular metabolites is a critical cellular function. There is now clear evidence for the existence of an ATP-dependent export pump, the *GS-X* pump, that transports a variety of GSH conjugates and certain organic anions out of cells (88). Such an export pump becomes even more important as evidence continues to accumulate showing that the GSH conjugation reaction is a step in the detoxification of electrophilic-reactive compounds derived from exogenous and endogenous sources (89). The generated GSH conjugates are then actively exported out of cells. The *GS-X* pump plays a physiologically important role as a member of the "phase III" system in drug metabolism (13).

Drug resistance of tumors in vivo is determined not only by the properties of tumor cells themselves, but also by the drug metabolism and disposition in normal organs in the body, such as liver, kidney, and lung. Metabolism of drugs is generally referred to as phases I and II, for which phase I includes oxidation of xenobiotics, and phase II deals with the conjugation of phase I products. The oxidative metabolism in the phase I system is mediated by cytochrome P-450 or a flavin, mixed-function oxidase. In the phase II system, activated hydrophobic xenobiotics are converted into more hydrophilic forms by conjugation reactions with glucuronide, sulfate, or GSH. This phase II metabolism is considered the detoxification process of xenobiotics. For example, mitoxanthrone, a chemotherapeutic agent used in the treatment of breast cancer, is oxidized by cytochrome P-450 and, subsequently, conjugated with GSH by microsomal GST, as well as with glucuronide by 3-methylcholanthrene-inducible glucuronyl transferases (90). Cyclophosphamide is another antitumor agent that undergoes the microsomal mixed-function oxidase reaction for its bioactivation to generate aldophosphamide. Acrolein released from the aldophosphamide is genotoxic and, therefore, must be conjugated with GSH by human GSTs (63; see Sec. I.B.3).

In some cases, however, the phase II system is a critical step in the formation of genotoxic electrophiles. In addition, accumulation of the resulting metabolites in cells can lead to a decrease in the detoxification activity of the phase II system. Several GSH-conjugates inhibit both glutathione S-transferases and GSSG reductase (7,91). The binding of S-(2,4-dinitrophenyl)-glutathione at the active site of GSSG reductase was demonstrated by X-ray crystallography (91). In this context, the export of metabolites represents a critical aspect of xenobiotic metabolism and differentiates it from the reactions in phase I and phase II. The physiological importance of the elimination of GSH conjugates (phase III) is underscored in several examples for which the GSH conjugation reaction results in bioactivation, as opposed to detoxification. Dihaloethanes (e.g., dibromo- and dichloroethanes) are known to be activated by enzymatic glutathione conjugation to episulfonium ions, genotoxic electrophiles, which react with N^7 position of guanine in DNA (92). Furthermore, for some classes of alkylators, such as alkyl-N-nitro-N'-nitrosoguanidines (93), reaction with GSH increases alkylating activity, with a corresponding increase in cytotoxicity and mutagenicity (94,95). In such cases, the *GS-X* pump must serve a critical role in reducing the intracellular accumulation of such reactive GSH conjugates.

B. *GS-X* Pump in Drug Resistance

The *GS-X* pump is a novel ATP-dependent transporter, distinct from both the P-glycoprotein (MDR1) (96,97) and the multidrug resistance-associated protein (MRP) (98). The physiological role and kinetic properties of the *GS-X* pump have been intensively studied using plasma membrane vesicles prepared from different organs and cell types, such as heart (99–101), liver (101–106), erythrocytes (107,108), mastocytoma cells (109), and leukemia cells (20). Dubin-Johnson syndrome in humans, an autosomal recessive benign disorder characterized by chronic conjugated hyperbilirubinemia, is suggested to be due to a defect in the function of the export pump in the liver (110,111). The *GS-X* pump plays an important role in glutathione disulfide (GSSG) efflux in oxidative stress, cysteinyl leukotriene release in inflammation, and elimination of a variety of GSH conjugates in xenobiotic metabolism (see Refs. 13 and 89 for recent reviews).

Recently, our laboratory has obtained evidence for the active export of a GS–platinum complex from leukemia cells mediated by the *GS-X* pump (20). Elimination of the GS–platinum complex from tumor cells may represent an important mechanism that reduces the intracellular accumulation of the platinum complex. The GS–platinum, generated from the reaction of cisplatin with GSH (see Sec. I.B.1), inhibited cell-free protein synthesis in a rabbit reticulocyte lysate system using both chloramphenicol acetyltransferase mRNA and poly(A) mRNA from HL-60 human promyelocytic leukemia cells. Half-maximal inhibition of protein synthesis occurred at a concentration of 190 μM of the GS–platinum complex. The inhibition did not result in significant changes in the molecular size of the synthesized proteins, suggesting that the inhibition occurred at the initiation step of translation. These results suggest that intracellular accumulation of the GS–platinum complex may potentially modulate the antitumor action of cisplatin (i.e., DNA cross-link formation) by inhibiting protein synthesis. By using plasma membrane vesicles prepared from L1210 cells, the transport of the GS–platinum complex across the plasma membrane was shown to be an ATP-dependent process (Fig. 4). The apparent K_m values for ATP and the GS–platinum complex were 49 and 110 mM, respectively. The ATP could be replaced by other nucleotides—namely, CTP, GTP, TTP, and UTP; however, their efficiencies were less than 20% compared with that of ATP. The ATP-dependent transport of the GS–platinum complex was inhibited by vanadate (IC$_{50}$ = 35 μM) as well as by *S*-(2,4-dinitrophenyl)-glutathione, leukotriene-C$_4$, and GSSG, but not by doxorubicin, daunorubicin, or verapamil (Table 2).

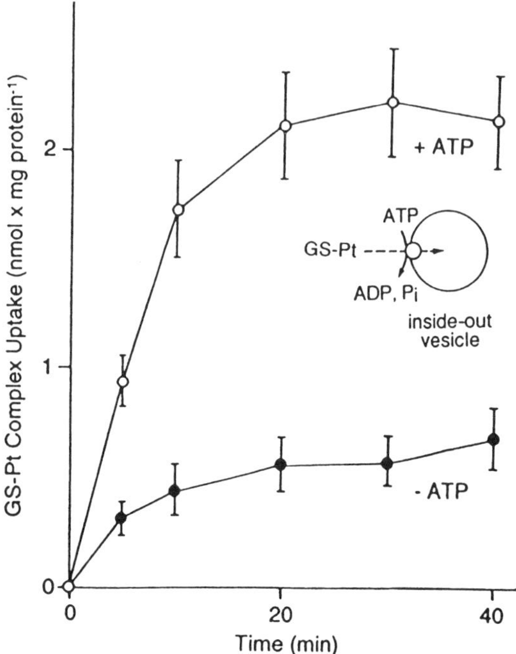

Figure 4 ATP-dependent transport of the GS–platinum complex across the plasma membrane of L1210 leukemia cells. The uptake of the [^{3}H]GS–platinum complex by inside-out vesicles of the plasma membrane from L1210 cells was stimulated by ATP (1 mM). In this experiment, plasma membrane vesicles (50 μg of protein) were incubated with 200 μM [^{3}H]GS–platinum complex at 37°C. Data are presented as mean values of triplicate measurements.

These results strongly suggest that the ATP-dependent transport of the GS–platinum complex is mediated by the *GS-X* pump, and that this active transport is a significant mechanism in reducing the intracellular accumulation of the potentially cytotoxic complex.

Furthermore, the *GS-X* pump was functionally overexpressed in cisplatin-resistant human promyelocytic leukemia HL-60 cells (HL-60/R-CP; 112). The rate of the ATP-dependent transport of the GS–Pt complex was about fourfold greater in the membrane vesicles from HL-60/R-CP cells than that of HL-60 cells, whereas the apparent K_m value for the GS–platinum complex was unchanged (130 μM for the membrane vesicle preparations from resistant and sensitive cells). In addition, ATP-dependent transport of leukotriene C$_4$, an endogenous substrate of the *GS-X* pump, was

Table 2 Effect of GSSG, DNP-SG, LTC$_4$, Verapamil, Doxorubicin, and Daunorubicin on ATP-Stimulated GS–Platinum Uptake by L1210 Plasma Membrane Vesicles[a]

Compound	Concentration (μM)	ATP-stimulated GS–platinum uptake nmol/mg protein per 10 min	%
None	0	1.26	100
GSSG	100	0.56	44
DNP-SG	100	0.15	12
	10	0.78	62
LTC$_4$	10	0.11	9
	1	0.43	34
Doxorubicin	100	1.16	92
Daunorubicin	100	1.20	95
Verapamil	100	1.31	104

[a] L1210 plasma membrane vesicles (50 μg of protein) were incubated with 200 μM [^{3}H]GS–platinum complex at 37°C for 10 min. The compounds were added into the incubation medium at the final concentrations indicated in the table. ATP-stimulated uptake was obtained from the difference in the radioactivities incorporated into the vesicles in the presence and absence of 1 mM ATP. Data are presented as mean values of triplicate measurements.

also fivefold higher in the membrane vesicles from HL-60/R-CP cells than in HL-60 cells. The cisplatin-resistant cells, HL-60/R-CP, were about tenfold more resistant to cisplatin than were their parental cells; growth IC$_{50}$ values were 10 and 0.8 μM for HL-60/R-CP and HL-60 cells, respectively. The intracellular GSH level in the resistant cells increased about sevenfold [7.52 $\pm$ 0.74 nmol/10^6 cells (n = 3) for HL-60/R-CP cells vs. 1.15 $\pm$ 0.12 nmol/10^6 cells (n = 3) for HL-60 cells]. In contrast with the remarkable increase in cisplatin-resistance in HL-60/R-CP cells, there was no significant difference between HL-60 and HL-60/R-CP cells in terms of the cellular sensitivities toward doxorubicin and vincristine, suggesting that the P-glycoprotein is not involved in the resistance mechanism.

In addition to biochemical changes, HL-60/R-CP cells exhibited a detectable morphological alteration, characterized by increased numbers of intracellular vesicles (112). Fluorescence microscopy with monochlorobimane revealed that the GSH conjugate accumulates in intracellular vesicles of the cisplatin-resistant cells in an energy-dependent manner (112). The *GS-X* pump is suggested to contribute to the vesicle-mediated excretion of GSH–drug conjugates from certain tumor cells. In many cases, drug-resistant tumor cells are more vesicular than are sensitive cells, suggesting that intracellular vesicles may sequester drugs or drug metabolites in a nontoxic site or efflux them by means of exocytosis. Such intracellular compartmentalization of drug metabolites is considered to be an important mechanism for drug resistance.

IV. ATTENUATION OF DRUG RESISTANCE

A. Modulation of Intracellular Glutathione Pool

In the 1950s, it was already noticed that the use of alkylating agents in the clinical treatment of human cancers resulted in resistance development (113,114). Since that time, an increasing number of studies have been carried out to reveal the mechanism underlying the acquired resistance. In 1960, Hirono, a Japanese pathologist, set the first milestone for our understanding of the mechanism in tumor resistance to alkylating agents (115). He succeeded in establishing resistant variants of the Yoshida ascites sarcoma and ascites hepatoma to methyl-bis(β-chlorethyl)-amine N-oxide. Chief among his findings were correlation of resistance with a significant increase in nonprotein sulfhydryl group in the resistant sublines, and the cross-resistance of resistant sublines to other alkylating reagents (115,116). Similar findings were later reported for other resistant tumor cells (117,118), and the increased nonprotein thiol was identified to be GSH (118). At that time, however, GSH was not considered to be particularly reactive toward alkylating agents. Studies in Vistica's laboratory on the effect of melphalan on resistant and sensitive leukemia cells led to the important finding that the doses of melphalan required to kill the cells varied considerably, and that this was related to the cellular GSH levels. The growth of tumor cells in media containing decreased levels of cysteine led to lower GSH levels and to increased sensitivity to melphalan (119). Thus, evidence was provided for the relation between cellular sensitivity to melphalan and the cellular GSH level, and melphalan was shown to be detoxified by conversion to nontoxic derivatives in GSH-dependent reactions (51) (Sec. I.B.2).

Buthionine sulfoximine, the specific inhibitor of γ-glutamylcysteine synthetase mentioned in Section I.A, was developed by Griffith and Meister in 1979 (26). It was expected that the inhibition of γ-glutamylcysteine synthetase by the agent makes tumor cells more susceptible to certain chemotherapeutic agents through the depletion of cellular GSH. The potential usefulness of buthionine sulfoximine in the sensitization of tumor cells was first demonstrated in studies with human lymphoid cells (120), murine mastocytoma, and lymphoma cells (121,122). During incubation with buthionine sulfoximine, cellular GSH decreased exponentially with a half-time of 4–6 h, becoming as low as 5% of the initial level after 30 h. Decrease of cellular GSH was mainly due to the efflux of GSH (or GSH equivalents) from cells (120). In those studies, the treatment of tumor cells with buthionine sulfoximine enhanced the cellular sensitivity to irradiation (120), oxidative cytolysis (121), and alkylating anticancer drugs (122). Importantly, treatment of resistant human ovarian cancer cells with buthionine sulfoximine led to the reversal of resistance to melphalan and cisplatin (18). Reduction of the cellular GSH content in melphalan-resistant L1210 cells by maintaining them with low concentration of cysteine in the culture medium also conferred drug sensitivity (53). The detoxification of melphalan positively correlates with the intracellular concentration of GSH (51).

Ozols and collaborators examined the relation between GSH level and expression of both primary drug resistance and cross-resistance in a human ovarian cancer cell line (123), as well as in an intraperitoneal model of human ovarian cancer in nude mice (124). With mice bearing resistant tumors, sensitization was achieved by continuous intraperitoneal infusion of buthionine sulfoximine. Their studies have shown the high efficiency of buthionine sulfoximine in the sensitization of human tumor cells to alkylating agents in vivo. A clinical trial of buthionine sulfoximine is currently in progress. In the protocol used for one of the several current clinical trials, the patients are given six doses of buthionine sulfoximine (1500 mg/m^2) intravenously at 12-h intervals over 3 days in the first week. In the second week, the same schedule is followed, but melphalan is given at a dose of 15 mg/m^2 as a 30-min intravenous infusion 1 h after the fifth dose of buthionine sulfoximine. Cycles of buthionine sulfoximine and melphalan administration are repeated at 3-week intervals (125).

The cellular GSH level apparently determines the degree of drug resistance of tumors to alkylating agents. However, not all of the reported findings are in accordance with this paradigm. The cellular GSH level is a dynamic factor, which can be readily affected by the cellular metabolism, including synthesis, conjugation, oxidation, and transport. The ability of cells to synthesize GSH relatively rapidly in response to stress may be even more important than the cellular GSH level itself. In addition, it is important to note the subcellular localization of GSH in mitochondria and the nuclei. In particular, nuclear GSH is suggested to play a critical role in different processes, including the protection of the SH-group of DNA-binding proteins, such as zinc-finger and cysteine-rich motifs, the regulation of chromatin compaction, and DNA synthesis. It has recently been reported that DNA repair enzymes (e.g., polymerase and ligase) are sensitive to the depletion of cellular GSH. Furthermore, nuclear GSH is known to quench platinum– or chloroethyl–DNA monoadducts (see Sec. I.B.5). The nuclear pool of GSH was found more resistant to depletion than the cytoplasmic pool (126), suggesting that nuclear GSH might be essential in protecting DNA and nuclear structures from the attack of chemicals, including alkylating antitumor agents.

B. Modulation of Glutathione Transferases

Ethacrynic acid, a substrate and inhibitor for GSTs, is a potential modulator in chemotherapy. The half-maximal inhibitory concentrations (IC_{50}) of ethacrynic acid for classes α, μ, and π of human GSTs are 6.0, 0.3, and 3.3 μM, respectively (127). Furthermore, the GSH conjugate of ethacrynic acid is a more potent inhibitor for classes α and μ, but not π, GSTs: IC_{50} values are 0.8, <0.1, and 11.0 μM for class α, μ, and π isozymes, respectively (127). Tew et al. demonstrated that ethacrynic acid potentiated the cytotoxicity of chlorambucil in human as well as rat tumor cell lines (128). Walker 256 rat breast carcinoma cells, with acquired resistance to nitrogen mustards, and human colon carcinoma cell lines, HT 29 and BE, were sensitized to chlorambucil when ethacrynic acid was administrated together with the alkylating agent. The GST activity was inhibited in cells treated with ethacrynic acid solely or in combination with chlorambucil. In addition, a depletion in intracellular GSH was also evident following the ethacrynic acid treatment. Likewise, human melanoma cells were sensitized to melphalan by ethacrynic acid (129). The induction of DNA interstrand cross-links by melphalan was 1.4-fold enhanced by ethacrynic acid (129). Thus, ethacrynic acid was suggested to be a potential sensitizer for the treatment of tumor cells resistant to alkylating agents.

In Phase I trials, O'Dwyer et al. (130) have demonstrated that tolerable doses of ethacrynic acid inhibited GST activity in previously treated cancer patients with severe neoplasms. Ethacrynic acid (25–75 mg/m^2 orally, every 6 h for three doses) and N,N',N''-triethylenethiophosphoramide (thiotepa) (30–55 mg/m^2 IV, 1 h after a second dose of ethacrynic acid) were administrated in the clinical trials. Ethacrynic acid caused diuresis at every dose, and drug combinations resulted in myelosuppression. The GST activity, monitored in peripheral mononuclear cells, declined to below 40% of control, with a time course similar to the diuretic effect. Recovery of activity was found by 12–24 h following treatment (130). The combination of thiotepa and ethacrynic acid is currently being tested in Phase II trials (131).

V. CONCLUSIONS AND FUTURE DIRECTIONS

Drug resistance is a biological response of tumor cells to chemotherapeutic agents and may represent the combined effects of different resistance determinants. Identification and modulation of these determinants is important for understanding the biological nature of drug resistance and solving the associated problems in human cancer chemotherapy. Recent studies of the multidrug resistance phenotype of tumor cells have led to the discovery of P-glycoprotein, a 170-kDa plasma membrane glycoprotein that mediates the efflux of certain anticancer drugs from cells (96,97; see Chap. 17). The overexpression of this export pump in tumor cells is closely associated with several multidrug-resistance phenotypes. More recently, another type of drug transporter, the multidrug-resistance-associated protein (MRP), has been identified in doxorubicin-resistant small-cell lung cancer in humans (98). P-glycoprotein and MRP, however, are not the only mechanisms for tumor drug resistance. As discussed in this chapter, the GSH-mediated drug metabolism and disposition contributes significantly to tumor resistance to alkylating agents.

The pathway of GSH-mediated drug inactivation is a biologically "expensive" mechanism. The synthesis of GSH and the export of GSH conjugates from cells requires at least three molecules of ATP to metabolize one molecule of drug (see Fig. 1). In cisplatin detoxification, at least five molecules of ATP are required: four molecules of ATP for the synthesis of two molecules of GSH, and at least one molecule of ATP for the export of GS–platinum complex. This compares unfavorably with the glycolytic pathway in which only two molecules of ATP are gained from one molecule of glucose. This expensive but important mechanism was developed and conserved throughout evolution of biological systems. Evidence that GSH, GST, and the *GS-X* pump (or *GS-X* pumplike transporters) exist not only in animal cells, but also in plants and yeast cells (132), strongly suggests that this GSH-associated metabolic pathway is fundamentally important for the survival of living cells.

Although much attention has hitherto been paid to the function of cellular GSH and GST as critical determinants in tumor resistance to alkylating agents, evidence is gradually accumulating for the important role of the *GS-X* pump in the mechanism of GSH-associated drug resistance. As already mentioned, certain GSH conjugates are potentially cytotoxic, since their intracellular accumulation can inhibit GST. To maintain a high efficiency of GST function in cells, continuous elimination of GSH conjugates out of cells is required. The *GS-X* pump is responsible for this task.

However, transfection of GST genes per se does not result in remarkable resistance (49,50).

The *GS-X* pump is a unique drug exporter, intimately linked to cellular GSH metabolism (13,89). The recent finding in our laboratory that the *GS-X* pump mediates the elimination of GS–platinum complex from tumor cells (20,112) indicates its physiologically significant role in the disposition of metal complexes. Metal-containing compounds are attracting interest as tools for therapy and diagnosis (133). Knowledge about the mechanisms of influx and efflux of metallocompounds, as well as their biotransformation in cells, is important for improving their efficacy. The molecular structure of the *GS-X* pump is not yet known. However, accumulating evidence suggests that it is involved in the elimination of both heavy-metal–glutathione complexes and a variety of glutathione–drug conjugates from cells (134,135). Recent studies involving cloning the Menkes' syndrome gene have revealed that a P-type ATPase is a putative export pump for copper ion (136). On the other hand, heavy-metal tolerance in the fission yeast was closely associated with the expression of an ATP-binding–cassette-type vacuolar membrane transporter (137) that is homologous to mammalian P-glycoprotein, MRP, and cystic fibrosis transmembrane conductance regulator (CFTR; 138). It is especially interesting that a 200-kDa membrane glycoprotein is overexpressed in cisplatin-resistant sublines of murine lymphoma (139), but its potential identity in relation to the *GS-X* pump remains to be elucidated.

The *GS-X* pump is functionally overexpressed in cisplatin-resistant human leukemia HL-60 cells (112). In addition to the structural characterization of the *GS-X* pump, it would be interesting and important to understand how the expression of its gene(s) is regulated in drug-resistant and drug-sensitive tumor cells. As demonstrated in a cisplatin-resistant ovarian cancer cell line, increased GSH levels are associated with elevated mRNA levels and expression of γ-glutamylcysteine synthetase and γ-glutamyl transferase. The latter is the enzyme that catalyzes the first step of the catabolism of GSH conjugates exported from cells by the *GS-X* pump. The results indicate that the expression of GSH-metabolizing enzymes involved in the biosynthesis, transport, and catabolism, is possibly regulated by certain master switches. Heat shock led to an increased expression of γ-glutamylcysteine synthetase and also enhanced efflux of a GSH conjugate, S-(2,4-dinitrophenyl)-glutathione, in K562 erythroid cells (140). Several heat-shock proteins are induced by heavy metals and certain SH-group reagents (141), including cisplatin (142). It is likely that the expression of some enzymes in GSH metabolism is modified by such stress-response elements. Studies in a variety of cisplatin-resistant cell lines, on the other hand, have suggested a potentially important role of *fos* and *ras* oncogenes in drug resistance (143–145). Elevated mRNA levels of c-*fos* and c-Ha-*ras* oncogenes have been shown in cisplatin-resistant cell lines in vitro as well as cell lines developed from patients failing cisplatin combination therapy (143–145). The observation that the gene of class π GST and the *pgp1* gene of P-glycoprotein contain an AP-1-binding site in the upstream regions suggest that Fos/Jun may play a role in coordinating gene expression of those proteins (146,147). However, evidence of a direct link between the mechanism of drug resistance and the overexpression of such oncogenes and heat-shock proteins is still missing. Biochemical pathways in which those gene products can act with critical determinants in drug-resistant mechanisms should be identified.

The molecular mechanism of drug resistance in tumor cells is complex. Figure 5 summarizes currently known mechanisms of drug resistance. It is only recently that the function of the *GS-X* pump in tumor cells has been recognized, and its potential role in drug resistance discussed (13,20). In addition, tumor necrosis factor (TNF) is known to induce oxidative

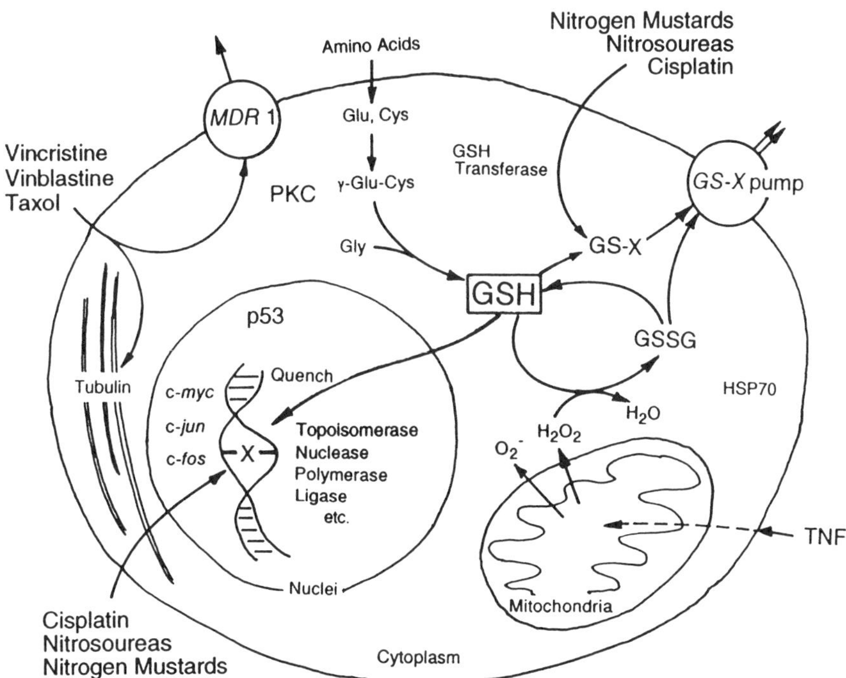

Figure 5 Schematic illustration for different mechanisms of tumor cell resistance to anticancer drugs.

stress in mitochondria (148–150), and the *GS-X* pump may play a critical role in GSSG efflux under TNF-induced oxidative stress. As previously pointed out, the *GS-X* pump mediates export of a variety of biologically active GSH conjugates associated with cell growth or signal transmission (see Ref. 13 for review). Certain biologically active, arachidonic acid metabolites (e.g. prostaglandin A_2 and leukotriene A_4) are conjugated with GSH. The *GS-X* pump mediates the transmembrane export of these endogenous metabolites. In particular, the A and J series of prostaglandins, which suppress tumor growth (151), are currently under preclinical study for the treatment of chemotherapeutically resistant ovarian cancer (152). The potential role of the *GS-X* pump in drug resistance and growth regulation of cancer cells will be examined in future studies using specific inhibitors, antibodies, or antisense nucleotides to block its function. Knowledge obtained in those studies will significantly contribute to our understanding of the molecular structure and function of the *GS-X* pump in tumor drug resistance, and to the development of new antitumor drugs that target it.

ACKNOWLEDGMENT

Studies in Ishikawa's laboratory were supported in part by a research grant from the International Life Sciences Institute Research Foundation, Washington, DC.

REFERENCES

1. Fahey RC, Sundquist AR. Evolution of glutathione metabolism. Adv Enzymol Relat Areas Mol Biol 1991; 64:1–53.
2. Kosower NS, Kosower EM. The glutathione status in cells. Int Rev Cytol 1978; 54:109–160.
3. Meister A, Anderson M. Glutathione. Annu Rev Biochem 1983; 54:305–329.
4. Ziegler DM. Role of reversible oxidation–reduction of enzyme thiols–disulfides in metabolic regulation. Annu Rev Biochem 1985; 54:305–329.
5. Dolphin D, Poulson R, Aveamovic O, eds. Glutathione: Chemical, Biochemical, and Medical Aspects. New York: John Wiley & Sons, 1989.
6. Sies H, Ketterer B, eds. Glutathione Conjugation: Mechanisms and Biological Significance. London: Academic Press, 1989.
7. Mannervik B. The isozymes of glutathione transferase. Adv Enzymol Relat Areas Mol Biol 1985; 58:357–417.
8. Pickett CB, Lu AYH. Glutathione *S*-transferases: gene structure, regulation, and biological function. Annu Rev Biochem 1989; 58:743–764.
9. Coles B, Ketterer B. The role of glutathione and glutathione transferases in chemical carcinogenesis. Crit Rev Biochem Mol Biol 1990; 25:47–70.

10. Hayes JD, Pickett CB, Mantle TJ, eds. Glutathione *S*-Transferases and Drug Resistance. London: Taylor & Francis, 1990.

11. Tshucida S, Sato K. Glutathione transferases and cancer. Crit Rev Biochem Mol Biol 1992; 27:337–384.

12. Waxman DJ. Glutathione *S*-transferases: role in alkylating agent resistance and possible target of modulation chemotherapy. Cancer Res 1990; 50:6449–6454.

13. Ishikawa T. The ATP-dependent glutathione *S*-conjugate export pump. Trends Biochem Sci 1992; 17:463–468.

14. Meister A. Glutathione deficiency produced by inhibition of its synthesis, and its reversal; applications in research and therapy. Pharmacol Ther 1991; 51:155–154.

15. Arrick BA, Nathan C. Glutathione metabolism as a determinant of therapeutic efficacy: a review. Cancer Res 1984; 44:4224–4232.

16. Somfai-Relle S, Suzukake K, Vistica DT. Glutathione-conferred resistance to antineoplastics: approaches toward its reduction. Cancer Treat Rev 1984; 11:443–54.

17. Eastman A. Cross-linking of glutathione to DNA by cancer chemotherapeutic platinum coordination complexes. Chem Biol Interact 1987; 61:241–248.

18. Hamilton TC, Winker MA, Louie KG, Batist G, Behrens BC, Tsuruo T, Grozinger KR, Mckoy WM, Young RC, Ozols RF. Augmentation of adriamycin, melphalan, and cisplatin cytotoxicity in drug-resistant and -sensitive human ovarian carcinoma cell lines by buthionine sulfoximine mediated glutathione depletion. Biochem Pharmacol 1985; 34:2583–2586.

19. Ali-Osman F. Quenching of DNA cross-link precursors of chloroethylnitrosoureas and attenuation of DNA interstrand cross-linking by glutathione. Cancer Res 1989; 49:5258–5261.

20. Ishikawa T, Ali-Osman F. Glutathione-associated *cis*-diamminedichloroplatinum(II) metabolism and ATP-dependent efflux from leukemia cells. J Biol Chem 1993; 268:20116–20125.

21. de Rey-Pailhade J. Sur un corps d'origine organique hydrgénantle soufre a froid. CR Acad Sci 1888; 106:1683–1684.

22. Meister A. On the discovery of glutathione. Trends Biochem Sci 1988; 13:185–188.

23. Harrington CR, Mead TH. CXCIV. Synthesis of glutathione. Biochem J 1935; 29:1602–1611.

24. Richman PG, Meister A. Regulation of γ-glutamyl-cysteine synthetase by nonallosteric feedback inhibition of glutathione. J Biol Chem 1975; 250:1422–1426.

25. Griffith OW, Meister A. Potent and specific inhibition of glutathione synthesis by buthionine sulfoximine (*S-n*-butyl homocysteine sulfoximine). J Biol Chem 1979; 254:7558–7560.

26. Meister A, Griffith OW. Effects of methionine sulfoximine analogs on the synthesis of glutamine and glutathione: possible chemotherapeutic implications. Cancer Treat Rep 1979; 63:1115–1121.

27. Godwin AK, Meister A, O'Dwyer P, Huang CH, Hamilton TC, Anderson M. High resistance to cisplatin in human ovarian cancer cell lines is associ-

ated with marked increase of glutathione synthesis. Proc Natl Acad Sci USA 1992; 89:3070–3074.

28. Ohno K, Hirata M. Induction of γ-glutamylcysteine synthetase by prostaglandin A₂ in L-1210 cells. Biochem Biophys Res Commun 1990; 168:551–557.

29. Kondo T, Taniguchi N, Kawakami Y. Significance of glutathione S–conjugate for glutathione metabolism in human erythrocytes. Eur J Biochem 1984; 145:131–136.

30. Bannai S. Transport of cystine and cysteine in mammalian cells. Biochim Biophys Acta 1984; 779:289–306.

31. Bannai S. Induction of cystine and glutamate transport activity in human fibroblast by diethyl malate and other electrophilic agents. J Biol Chem 1984; 259:2435–2440.

32. Chasseaud LF. The role of glutathione and glutathione S-transferases in the metabolism of chemical carcinogens and other electrophilic agents. Adv Cancer Res 1979; 29:175–275.

33. Prestayco AW, Crooke ST, Carter SK, eds. Cisplatin: Current Status and New Developments. New York: Academic Press, 1980.

34. Rosenberg B. Fundamental studies with cisplatin. Cancer 1985; 55:2303–2316.

35. Rosenberg B, van Camp L, Trosko JE, Mansour VH. Platinum compounds: new class of potent antitumor agents. Nature 1969; 222:385–386.

36. Roberts JJ, Pascoe JM. Cross-linking of complementary strands of DNA in mammalian cells by antitumor platinum compounds. Nature 1972; 235:282–284.

37. Cohen GL, Bauer WR, Barton JK, Lippard SJ. Binding of *cis*- and *trans*-dichlorodiammineplatinum(II) to DNA: evidence for unfolding and shortening of the double helix. Science 1979; 203:1014–1016.

38. Zwelling LA, Michaels S, Schwartz H, Dobson PP, Kohn KW. DNA cross-linking as an indicator of sensitivity and resistance of mouse L1210 leukemia to *cis*-diamminedichloroplatinum(II) and L-phenylalanine mustard. Cancer Res 1982; 41:640–649.

39. Eastman A. Characterization of the adducts produced in DNA by *cis*-diaminedichloroplatinum(II) and *cis*-dicloro(ethylenediamine)-platinum. Biochemistry 1983; 22:3927–3933.

40. Andrews PA, Velury S, Mann S, Howell SB. *cis*-Diamminedichloroplatinum(II) accumulation in sensitive and resistant human ovarian carcinoma cells. Cancer Res 1988; 48:68–73.

41. Kraker AJ, Moore CW. Accumulation of *cis*-diamminedichloroplatinum(II) and platinum analogues by platinum-resistant murine leukemia cells in vitro. Cancer Res 1988; 48:9–13.

42. Bakka A, Endresen L, Johnsen ABS, Emison PD, Rugstad HE. Resistance against *cis*-dichlorodiamine platinum in cultured cells with a high content of metallothionein. Toxicol Appl Pharmacol 1981; 61:215–226.

43. Eastman A, Schulte N. Enhanced DNA repair as a mechanism of resistance to *cis*-diamminedichloroplatinum(II). Biochemistry 1988; 27:4730–4734.

44. Andrews PA, Murphy MP, Howell SB. Differential sensitization of human ovarian carcinoma and mouse L1210 cells to cisplatin and melphalan by glutathione depletion. Mol Pharmacol 1986; 30:643–650.

45. Odenheimer B, Wolf W. Reaction of cisplatin with sulfur-containing amino acids and peptides I: cysteine and glutathione. Inorg Chim Acta 1982; 66:L41–L43.

46. Dedon PC, Borch RF. Characterization of the reactions of platinum antitumor agents with biologic and nonbiologic sulfur-containing nucleophiles. Biochem Pharmacol 1987; 36:1955–1964.

47. Hamaguchi K, Godwin AK, Yakushiji M, O'Dwyer P, Ozols RF, Hamilton TC. Cross-resistance to diverse drugs is associated with primary cisplatin resistance in ovarian cancer cell lines. Cancer Res 1993; 53:5225–5232.

48. Mistry P, Kelland LR, Abel S, Sidhar S, Harrap KR. The relationship between glutathione, glutathione-S-transferase and cytotoxicity of platinum drugs and melphalan in eight human ovarian carcinoma cell lines. Br J Cancer 1991; 64:215–220.

49. Moskow JA, Townsend AJ, Cowan KH. Elevation of π class glutathione S-transferase activity in human breast cancer cells by transfection of the GST π gene and its effect on sensitivity to toxins. Mol Pharmacol 1989; 36:22–28.

50. Nakagawa K, Saijo N, Tsuchida S, Sakai M, Tsunokawa Y, Yokota J, Muramatsu M, Sato K, Terada M, Tew KD. Glutathione S-transferase π as a determinant of drug resistance in transfectant cell lines. J Biol Chem 1990; 265:4296–4301.

51. Suzukake K, Vistica BP, Vistica DT. Dechlorination of L-phenylalanine mustard by sensitive and resistant tumor cells and its relationship to intracellular glutathione content. Biochem Pharmacol 1983; 32:165–167.

52. Ahmad S, Okine L, Le B, Najarian P, Vistica D. Elevation of glutathione in phenylalanine mustard-resistant murine L1210 leukemia cells. J Biol Chem 1987; 262:15048–15053.

53. Suzukake K, Petro BJ, Vistica DT. Reduction in glutathione content of L-PAM resistant L1210 cells confers drug sensitivity. Biochem Pharmacol 1982; 31:121–124.

54. Dulik DM, Fenselau C, Hilton J. Characterization of melphalan–glutathione adducts whose formation is catalyzed by glutathione transferases. Biochem Pharmacol 1986; 35:3405–3409.

55. Dulik DM, Colvin OM, Fenselau C. Characterization of glutathione conjugates of chlorambucil by fast atom bombardment and thermospray liquid chromatography/mass spectrometry. Biomed Environ Mass Spectrom 1990; 19:248–252.

56. Ciaccio PJ, Tew KD, LaCreta FP. The spontaneous and glutathione S-transferase-mediated reaction of chlorambucil with glutathione. Cancer Commun 1990; 2:279–286.

57. Bolton MG, Colvin OM, Hilton J. Specificity of isozymes of murine hepatic glutathione S-transferase for the conjugation of glutathione with L-phenylalanine mustard. Cancer Res 1991; 51:2410–2415.

58. Guenther TS, Whalen R, Jevtovic-Todorvic V. Direct measurement of melphalan conjugation with glutathione: studies with human melanoma cells and mammalian liver. J Pharm Exp Ther 1992; 260:1331–1336.

59. Friedman HS, Skapek SX, Colvin OM, Elion GB, Blum MR, Savina PM, Hilton J, Schold SC, Kurzberg J, Binger DD. Melphalan transport, glutathione levels, and glutathione-S-transferase activity in human medulloblastoma. Cancer Res 1988; 48:5397–5402.

60. Struck RF, Kirk MC, Witt MH, Laster WR. Isolation and mass spectral identification of blood metabolites of cyclophosphamide: evidence for phosphamide mustard as the biologically active metabolite. Biomed Mass Spectrom 1975; 2:46–52.

61. Colvin M, Brundrett RB, Kan M-N, Jardine I, Fenselau C. Alkylating properties of phosphoramide mustard. Cancer Res 1976; 36:1121–1126.

62. Friedman OM, Wdinsky I, Myles A. Cyclophosphamide-related phosphoramide mustards: recent advances and historical perspective. Cancer Treat Rep 1976; 60:337–346.

63. Berhane K, Mannervik, B. Inactivation of the genotoxic aldehyde acrolein by human glutathione transferases of class alpha, mu, and pi. Mol Pharmacol 1990; 37:251–254.

64. Prestayco AW, Crooke ST, Baker LH, Carter SK, Schein PS, eds. Nitrosoureas: Current Status and New Developments. London: Academic Press, 1981.

65. Reed DJ, May HE. Alkylation and carbamoylation intermediates from the carcinostatic 1-(2-chloroethyl)-3-cyclohexyl-1-nitrosourea (CCNU). Life Sci 1975; 16:1263–1270.

66. Reed DJ, Foureman GL, A comparison of the alkylating capabilities of the cysteinyl and glutathionyl conjugates of 1,2-dichloroethane. Adv Exp Biol 1986; 197:469–475.

67. Guengerich FP, Crawford WM, Dooradzki JY, McDonald T, Watanabe PG. In vitro activation of 1,2-dichloroethane by microsomal and cytosolic enzymes. Toxicol Appl Pharmacol 1980; 55:303–317.

68. Van Bladeren PJ, Van der Gen A, Breimer DD, Mohn GM. Stereoselective activation of vicinal dihalogen compounds to mutagens by glutathione conjugation. Biochem Phamacol 1979; 28:2521–2524.

69. Tong WP, Kirk MC, Ludlum DB. Formation of the cross-link, 1-[N^3-deoxycytidyl]1,2-[N^1-deoxyguanosyl]ethane, in DNA treated with N,N'-bis(2-chloroethyl)-N-nitrosourea (BCNU). Cancer Res 1982; 42:3102–3105.

70. Talcott RE, Levin VA. Glutathione-dependent denitrosation of N,N'-bis(2-chloroethyl)-N-nitrosourea (BCNU): nitrite release catalyzed by liver cytosol in vitro. Drug Metab Dispos 1983; 11:175–176.

71. Jensen DE, Stelman GJ. Evidence for cytosolic glutathione transferase-mediated denitrosation of nitrosoimetidine and 1-methyl-2-nitro-1-nitrosoguanidine. Carcinogenesis (Lond) 1987; 8:1791–1800.

72. Smith M, Evans CG, Doane-Setzer P, Castro VM, Tahir MK, Mannervik B. Denitrosation of 1,3-bis(2-chloroethyl)-1-nitrosourea by class mu gluta-

thione transferases and its role in cellular resistance in rat brain tumor cells. Cancer Res 1989; 49:2621–2625.

73. Berhane K, Hao X-Y, Egyházi S, Honsson J, Ringborg U, Mannervik B. Contribution of glutathione transferase M3-3 to 1,3-bis(2-chloroethyl)-1-nitrosourea resistance in a human non-small cell lung cancer cell line. Cancer Res 1993; 53:4257–4261.

74. Niu T, Yu D, Kirk MC, Ludlum DB. Synthesis of the prototype DNA–protein cross-link, 1-(guan-1-yl)-2-(cystein-*S*-yl)ethane, and its role in the reaction of the haloethylnitrosoureas. Carcinogenesis 1993; 14:195–198.

75. Mannervik B, Awasthi, YC, Board PG, Hayes JD, Di Ilio C, Ketterer B, Listowstky I, Morgenstern R, Muramatsu M, Pearson W, Pickett CB, Sato K, Widersten M, Wolf CR. Nomenclature for human glutathione transferases. Biochem J 1992; 282:305–308.

76. Batist G, Tulpule A, Sinha BK, Katki AG, Myers CE, Cowan K. Overexpression of a novel anionic glutathione *S*-transferase in multidrug-resistant human breast cancer cells. J Biol Chem 1986; 261:15544–15549.

77. Buller A, Clapper ML, Tew KD. Glutathione *S*-transferases in nitrogen mustard-resistant and sensitive cell lines. Mol Pharmacol 1987; 31:575–578.

78. Evans CG, Bodell WJ, Tokuda K, Doane-Setzer P, Smith MT. Glutathione and related enzymes in rat brain tumor cell resistance to 1,3-bis(2-chloroethyl)-1-nitrourea and nitrogen mustard. Cancer Res 1987; 47:2525–2530.

79. Lewis AD, Hickson ID, Robson CN, Harris AL, Hayes JD, Griffiths SA, Manson MM, Hall AE, Moss JE, Wolf CR. Amplification and increased expression of alpha class glutathione *S*-transferase-encoding genes associated with resistance to nitrogen mustards. Proc Natl Acad Sci USA 1988; 85:8511–8515.

80. Ali-Osman F, Stein D, Renwick A. Glutathione content and glutathione-*S*-transferase expression in 1,3-bis(2-chloroethyl)-1-nitrosourea-resistant human malignant astrocytoma cell lines. Cancer Res 1990; 50:6979–6980.

81. Johnston JB, Israels LG, Goldenberg GJ, Anhalt CD, Verburg L, Mowat MR, Begleiter A. Glutathione *S*-transferase activity, sulfhydryl group and glutathione levels, and DNA cross-linking activity with chlorambucil in chronic lymphocytic leukemia. JNCI 1990; 82:776–779.

82. Stelmack GL, Goldberg GJ. Increased expression of cytosolic glutathione *S*-transferases in drug-resistant L5178 murine lymphoblasts: chemical selectivity and molecular mechanisms. Cancer Res 1993; 53:3530–3535.

83. Nakagawa K, Yokota J, Wada M, Sasaki Y, Fujiwara Y, Sakai M, Muramatsu M, Terasaki T, Tsunokawa Y, Terada M, Saijo N. Levels of glutathione *S*-transferase π mRNA in human lung cancer cell lines correlate with the resistance to cisplatin and carboplatin. Jpn J Cancer Res 1988; 79:301–304.

84. Puchalski RB, Fahl WE. Expression of recombinant glutathione *S*-transferase π, Ya or Yb$_1$ confers resistance to alkylating agents. Proc Natl Acad Sci USA 1990; 87:2443–2447.

85. Ciaccio PJ, Tew KD, Lacreta FP. Enzymatic conjugation of chlorambucil

with glutathione by human glutathione S-transferase and inhibition by ethacrynic acid. Biochem Pharmacol 1991; 42:1504–1507.

86. Leyland-Jones BR, Townsend AJ, Tu C-PD, Cowan KH, Goldsmith ME. Antineoplastic drug sensitivity of human MCF-7 cancer cells stably transfected with a human α class glutathione S-transferase gene. Cancer Res 1991; 51:587–594.

87. Meyer DJ, Gilmore KS, Harris JM, Hartley JA, Ketterer B. Chlorambucil–monoglutathionyl conjugate is sequestered by human alpha class glutathione S-transferases. Br J Cancer 1992; 66:433–438.

88. Ishikawa T. Is the glutathione S–conjugate carrier an *mdr1* gene product? Trends Biochem Sci 1990; 15:219–220.

89. Ishikawa T. Glutathione S–conjugate export pump. In: Tew KD, Pickett CB, Mantle TJ, Mannervik B, Hayes JD, eds. Structure and Function of Glutathione S-transferases. Boca Raton: CRC Press, 1993:211–221.

90. Wolf CR, Macpherson JS, Smyth JF. Evidence for the metabolism of mitoxantrone by microsomal glutathione transferases and 3-methylcholanthrene-inducible glucuronosyl transferases. Biochem Pharmacol 1986; 35:1577–1581.

91. Bilzer M, Krauth-Siegel RL, Schirmer RH, Akerboom TPM, Sies H, Schulz GE. Interaction of a glutathione S–conjugate with glutathione reductase. Eur J Biochem 1984; 138:373–378.

92. Ozawa N, Guengerich FP. Evidence for formation of an S-[2-(N^7-guanyl)ethyl]glutathione adduct in glutathione-mediated binding of the carcinogen 1,2-dibromoethane to DNA. Proc Natl Acad Sci USA 1983; 80:5266–5270.

93. Lawley PD, Thatcher CJ. Methylation of deoxyribonucleic acid in cultured mammalian cells by N-methyl-N'-nitro-N-nitrosoguanidine. Biochem J 1970; 116:693–707.

94. Romert L, Jenssen D. Mechanism of N-acetylcysteine (NAC) and other thiols as both positive and negative modifiers of MNNG-induced mutagenicity in V79 Chinese hamster cells. Carcinogenesis (Lond) 1987; 8:1531–1535.

95. Schultz U, McCalla DR. Reactions of cysteine with N-methyl-N-nitroso-p-toluenesulfonamide and N-methyl-N'-nitro-N-nitrosoguanidine. Can J Chem 1969; 47:2021.

96. Endicott JA, Ling V. The biochemistry of P-glycoprotein-mediated multidrug resistance. Annu Rev Biochem 1989; 58:137–171.

97. Gottesman MM, Pastan I. The multidrug transporter, a double-edged sward. J Biol Chem 1988; 263:12163–12166.

98. Cole SPC, Bhardwaj G, Gerlach JH, Mackie JE, Grant CE, Almquist KC, Stewart AJ, Kurz EU, Duncan AMV, Deeley RG. Overexpression of a transporter gene in a multidrug-resistant human lung cancer cell line. Science 1992; 258:1650–1654.

99. Ishikawa T. ATP/Mg^{2+}-dependent cardiac transport system for glutathione S–conjugates. J Biol Chem 1989; 264:17343–17348.

100. Ishikawa T. Leukotriene C$_4$ inhibits ATP-dependent transport of glutathione S–conjugate across rat heart sarcolemma. FEBS Lett 1989; 246:177–180.

101. Ishikawa T, Kobayashi K, Sogame Y, Hayashi K. Evidence for leukotriene C_4 transport mediated by an ATP-dependent glutathione *S*–conjugate carrier in rat heart and liver plasma membranes. FEBS Lett 1989; 259: 95–98.

102. Ishikawa T, Müller M, Klünemann, Schaub T, Keppler D. ATP-dependent primary active transport of cysteinyl leukotrienes across liver canalicular membrane: role of the ATP-dependent transport system for glutathione *S*–conjugates. J Biol Chem 1990; 265:19279–19286.

103. Kobayashi K, Sogame Y, Hara H, Hayashi K. Mechanism of glutathione *S*–conjugate transport in canalicular and basolateral rat liver plasma membranes. J Biol Chem 1990; 265:7737–7741.

104. Akerboom TPM, Narayanaswami V, Kunst M, Sies H. ATP-dependent *S*-(2,4-dinitrophenyl)glutathione transport in canalicular plasma membrane vesicles from rat liver. J Biol Chem 1991; 266:13147–13152.

105. Nishida T, Hardenbrook C, Gatmaitan Z, Arias I. ATP-dependent organic anion transport system in normal and TR$^-$ rat liver canalicular membranes. Am J Physiol 1992; 262:G629–G635.

106. Fernandez-Chea JC, Takikawa H, Horie T, Ooktens M, Kaplowitz N. Canalicular transport of reduced glutathione in normal and mutant Eisai hyperbilirubinemic rats. J Biol Chem 1992; 267:1667–1673.

107. Kondo T, Murao M, Taniguchi N. Glutathione *S*–conjugate transport using inside-out vesicles from human erythrocytes. Eur J Biochem 1982; 125:551–554.

108. LaBelle EF, Singh SV, Srivastava SK, Awasthi YC. Dinitrophenyl glutathione efflux from human erythrocytes is primary active ATP-dependent transport. Biochem J 1986; 238:443–449.

109. Schaub T, Ishikawa T, Keppler D. ATP-dependent leukotriene export from mastocytoma cells. FEBS Lett 1991; 279:83–86.

110. Dubin IN, Johnson FB. Chronic idiopathic jaundice with unidentified pigment in liver cells: a clinicopathologic entity with a report of 12 cases. Medicine 1954; 33:155–197.

111. Jansen PLM. Oude Elferrink RPJ. Hereditary hyperbilirubinemias: a molecular and mechanistic approach. Semin Liver Dis 1988; 8:168–178.

112. Ishikawa T, Wright CD, Ishizuka H. '*GS-X* pump' is functionally overexpressed in cisplatin-resistant human leukemia HL-60 cell and down-regulated by cell differentiation. J Biol Chem 1994; 269:29085–29093.

113. Karnofsky DA. Differences between cancers in terms of therapeutic responses. Cancer Res 1956; 16:684–697.

114. Law LW. Evaluation of drug resistance. Cancer Res 1956; 16:698–716.

115. Hirono I. Non-protein sulphydryl group in the original strain and sub-line of the ascites tumor resistant to alkylating reagents. Nature 1960; 25:1059–1060.

116. Hirono I. Mechanism of natural and acquired resistance to methyl-bis-(b-chlorethyl)-amine *N*-oxide in ascites tumors. Jpn J Cancer Res 1961; 52:39–48.

117. Calcutt G, Connors TA, Elson LA, Ross WC. Reduction of the toxicity

of "radiomimetic" alkylating agents in rats by thiol pretreatment Part II. Mechanism and protection. Biochem Pharmacol 1963; 12:833–837.

118. Ball CR, Connors TA, Double JA, Ujhazy V, Whisson ME. Comparison of nitrogen-mustard-sensitive and -resistant Yoshida sarcomas. Int J Cancer 1966; 1:319–327.

119. Vistica DT. Cytotoxicity as an indicator for transport mechanism. Evidence that melphalan is transported by two leucine-preferring carrier systems in the L1210 murine leukemia cells. Biochim Biophys Acta 1979; 550:309–317.

120. Dethmers JK, Meister A. Glutathione export by human lymphoid cells: depletion of glutathione by inhibition of its synthesis decreases export and increases sensitivity to irradiation. Proc Natl Acad Sci USA 1981; 78:7492–7496.

121. Arrick BA, Nathan CF, Griffith OW, Cohn ZA. Glutathione depletion sensitizes tumor cells to oxidative cytolysis. J Biol Chem 1982; 257:1231–1237.

122. Arrick BA, Nathan CF, Cohn ZA. Inhibition of glutathione synthesis augments lysis of murine tumor cells by sulfhydryl-reactive antineoplastics. J Clin Invest 1983; 171:258–267.

123. Green JA, Vistica DT, Young RC, Hamilton TC, Rogan AM, Ozols RF. Melphalan resistance in human ovarian cancer: characterization of drug resistant cell lines and potentiation of melphalan cytotoxicity by glutathione depletion. Cancer Res 1984; 44:5427–5431.

124. Ozols RF, Louie KG, Plowman J, Behrens, Fine RL, Dykes D, Hamilton TC. Enhanced melphalan cytotoxicity in human ovarian cancer in vitro and in tumor-bearing nude mice by buthionine sulfoximine depletion of glutathione. Biochem Pharmacol 1987; 36:147–153.

125. O'Dwyer PJ, Hamilton TC, Young RC, LaCreta FP, Carp N, Tew KD, Padavic K, Comis RL, Ozols RF. Depletion of glutathione in normal and malignant human cells in vivo by buthionine sulfoximine: clinical and biochemical results. JNCI 1992; 84:264–267.

126. Bellomo G, Vairetti M, Stivala L, Mirabelli F, Richelmi P, Orrenius S. Demonstration of nuclear compartmentalization of glutathione in hepatocytes. Proc Natl Acad Sci USA 1992; 89:4412–4416.

127. Ploman JHTM, Van Ommen B, Van Bladeren PJ. Inhibition of rat and human glutathione S-transferase isozymes by ethacrynic acid and its glutathione conjugate. Biochem Pharmacol 1990; 40:1631–1635.

128. Tew KD, Bomber AM, Hoffman SJ. Ethacrynic acid and piriprost as enhancers of cytotoxicity in drug resistance and sensitive cells. Cancer Res 1988; 48:3622–3625.

129. Hansson J, Berhane K, Castro VM, Jungnelius U, Mannervik B, Ringborg U. Sensitization of human melanoma cells to the cytotoxic effect of melphalan by the glutathione transferase inhibitor ethacrynic acid. Cancer Res 1991; 51:94–98.

130. O'Dwyer P, LaCreta F, Nash S, Tinsley PW, Schilder R, Clapper ML, Tew KD, Panting L, Litwin S, Comis RL, Ozols RF. Phase I study of thiotepa in combination with glutathione transferase inhibitor ethacrynic acid. Cancer Res 1991; 51:6059–6065.

131. Ranganathan S, Ciccio PJ, Tew KD. Principles of drug modulation applied to glutathione S-transferases. In: Tew KD, Pickett CB, Mantle TJ, Mannervik B, Hayes JD, eds. Structure and Function of Glutathione Transferases. Boca Raton: CRC Press, 1993:249–256.

132. Martinoia E, Grill E, Tommasini R, Kreuz K, Amrhein N. ATP-dependent glutathione S–conjugate "export" pump in the vacuolar membrane of plants. Nature 1993; 364:247–249.

133. Abrams MJ, Murrer BA. Metal compounds in therapy and diagnosis. Science 1993; 261:725–730.

134. Ballatori N, Clarkson TW. Biliary transport of glutathione and methylmercury. Am J Physiol 1983; 244:G435–G441.

135. Gyurasics A, Varga F, Gregus Z. Effect of arsenicals on biliary excretion of endogenous glutathione and xenobiotics with glutathione-dependent hepatobiliary transport. Biochem Pharmacol 1991; 41:937–944.

136. Vulpe C, Levinson B, Whitney S, Packman S, Gitchir J. Isolation of a candidate gene for Menkes disease and evidence that it encodes a copper-transporting ATPase. Nature Genet 1993; 3:7–13.

137. Ortiz DF, Kreppel L, Speiser DM, Scheel G, McDonald G, Ow DW. Heavy metal tolerance in the fission yeast requires an ATP-binding cassette-type vacuolar membrane transporter. EMBO J 1992; 10:3491–3499.

138. Riodan JR, Rommers JM, Kerem B, Alon N, Rozmahel R, Grzelcak Z, Zielenski J, Lok S, Plavsic NP, Chou J-L, Drumm ML, Iannuzzi MC, Collins FS, Tsui L-C. Identification of the cystic fibrosis gene: cloning and characterization of complementary DNA. Science 1989; 245:1066–1073.

139. Kawai K, Kamatani N, Georges E, Ling V. Identification of a membrane glycoprotein overexpressed in murine lymphoma sublines resistant to cis-diamminedichloroplatinum(II). J Biol Chem 1990; 265:13137–13142.

140. Kondo T, Yoshida K, Urata Y, Goto S, Gasa S, Taniguchi N. γ-Glutamyl-cysteine synthetase and active transport of glutathione S–conjugate are responsive to heat shock in K562 erythroid cells. J Biol Chem 1993; 268:20366–20372.

141. Morimoto RI, Sarge KD, Abravaya K. Transcriptional regulation of heat shock genes. J Biol Chem 1992; 267:21987–21990.

142. Oesterreich S, Schunck H, Benndorf R, Bielka H. Cisplatin induces the small heat shock protein HSP25 and thermotolerance in Ehrlich ascites tumor cells. Biochem Biophys Res Commun 1991; 180:243–248.

143. Isonishi S, Hom DK, Thiebaut FB, Mann SC, Andrews PA, Basu A, Lazo JS, Eastman A, Howell SB. Expression of the c-Ha-*ras* oncogene in mouse NIH 3T3 cells induces resistance to cisplatin. Cancer Res 1991; 51:5903–5909.

144. Kashani-Sabet M, Wang W, Scanlon KJ. Cyclosporin A suppress cisplatin-induced c-*fos* gene expression in ovarian carcinoma cells. J Biol Chem 1990; 265:11285–11288.

145. Kashani-Sabet M, Lu Y, Leong L, Haedicke K, Scanlon KJ. Differential oncogene amplification in tumor cells from a patient treated with cisplatin and 5-fluorouracil. Eur J Cancer 1990; 26:383–390.

146. Morrow CS, Cowan KH, Doldsmith ME. Structure of the human genomic glutathione S-transferase-π gene. Gene 1989; 75:3–11.
147. Teeter LD, Eckersberg T, Tsei Y, Kuo MT. Analysis of the Chinese hamster P-glycoprotein/multi-drug resistance gene *pgp1* reveals that the AP-1 site is essential for full promoter activity. Cell Growth Differ 1991; 2:429–437.
148. Yamaguchi N, Kuriyama H, Watanabe N, Neda H, Maeda M, Niitsu Y. Intracellular hydroxyl radical production induced by recombinant human tumor necrosis factor and its implication in the killing of tumor cells in vivo. Cancer Res 1989; 49:1671–1675.
149. Schulze-Osthoff K, Bakker AC, Vanhaesebroeck B, Beyaert R, Jacob WA, Fiers W. Cytotoxic activity of tumor necrosis factor is mediated by early damage of mitochondrial functions: evidence for the involvement of mitochondrial radical generation. J Biol Chem 1992; 267:5317–5323.
150. Higuchi M, Shirotani K, Higaki N, Toyoshima S, Osawa T. Damage to mitochondrial respiration chain is related to phospholipase A_2 activation caused by tumor necrosis factor. J Immunother 1992; 12:41–49.
151. Narumiya S, Fukushima M. Site and mechanism of growth inhibition by prostaglandins. I. Active transport and intracellular accumulation of cyclopentenone prostaglandins, a relation leading to growth inhibition. J Pharmacol Exp Ther 1986; 239:500–505.
152. Noyori R, Suzuki M. Organic synthesis of prostaglandins: advancing biology. Science 1993; 259:44–45.

20

Circumventing Transport-Associated Resistance Through Drug Delivery

Alain R. Thierry
*National Cancer Institute, National Institutes of Health,
Bethesda, Maryland*

I. INTRODUCTION

The therapeutic potential of anticancer agents may be hindered by drug resistance in tumor cells (see Chap. 2). Such tumors as lung carcinoma, ovarian carcinoma, or neuroblastoma, although initially sensitive to cytostatic drugs, become resistant after a variable time. This form of resistance is known as acquired resistance. In addition, numerous adult cancers, in particular of the gastrointestinal tract, are from the start refractory to all chemotherapeutic treatments. This form of resistance is known as intrinsic resistance. Modulation of drug resistance has become an important priority in cancer chemotherapy, and the mechanisms involved have been intensively investigated. These mechanisms are multifactorial; enzymes, such as glutathione transferase (see Chap. 19) or topoisomerase II (1), play a significant role. Resistance may be not only to the initial cytostatic drug, but also to unrelated cytostatic agents that had not been previously used in the treatment (hence, the name multidrug resistance; MDR). The acquired MDR phenotype has been the subject of numerous recent studies, and the factors involved have been partly elucidated (see Chap. 17).

The MDR phenotype was first characterized by the overexpression of the *mdr1* gene, which encodes a plasma membrane glycoprotein of 170 kDa, called P-glycoprotein (Pgp; 1–3). P-glycoprotein is believed to act

"

as an energy-dependent drug-efflux pump causing reduced cellular drug accumulation. Hence, attempts to circumvent multidrug resistance often focus on inhibitors of the Pgp transport function. Several agents have been shown to inhibit the activity of the Pgp and thus to diminish drug resistance. Most prominent among them are calcium channel blockers such as verapamil, calmodulin inhibitors, and protein kinase C inhibitors (see Chap. 18). In addition to the Pgp-mediated activity, the MDR phenotype appears to be accompanied by multiple changes described in recent reports (4–8). For instance, it has been demonstrated that drug *distribution* in MDR cells is altered, showing a much higher cytoplasm/nucleus ratio than in sensitive cells (6–8). Thus, it appears that acquired MDR generally affects cellular drug transport functions. This raises the interesting possibility of using drug delivery systems to bypass transport-associated resistance.

The weak selectivity and low therapeutic index of most antitumor agents have prompted a search, not only for new drugs, but also for innovative ways to improve therapeutic use of existing drugs. Prominent among these approaches has been the use of drug delivery technology. From the vector system used in drug delivery, one can distinguish the soluble and the nonsoluble vector approach. Numerous strategies using a soluble vector for anticancer drug delivery, such as conjugation of the drug with ligand or antibodies to receptor proteins at the surface of the targeted tumor cells, have been considered (Table 1). Macromolecules present in blood, such as macroglobulin and human serum albumin, have also been used as conjugates to chemotherapeutic agents and have enhanced drug delivery. Among those soluble vectors, only antibody–drug conjugates appear to reverse MDR. For example, by using antibody–daunorubicin conjugates, enhancement of drug accumulation in a resistant HL-60 human leukemia cell line was observed (32). Antibody-drug conjugates have a different route of uptake compared with the free drug and, consequently, may escape the cellular mechanisms responsible for resistance to the free drug. An interesting off-shoot of the antibody–drug conjugate approach is to develop monoclonal antibodies to surface antigens present only on drug-resistant cells, such as the Pgp (12). Nonsoluble vectors have also been successfully used for the delivery of anticancer agents. Among those are micelles (24), virosomes (25), high-density lipoproteins (28), cyanoacrylate nanospheres (23), and liposomes (19,20,33,34). So far, only the last two have been shown to modulate multidrug resistance in MDR cell lines by increasing intracellular drug availability.

The observation of increased drug activity against resistant cells when the drug is delivered in the form of antibody–drug conjugates, nano-

Table 1 Delivery Systems Used in Antimicrobial and Anticancer Therapy

Delivery system	Drug	Ref.	Modulation of drug resistance
Soluble vector conjugates			
Macroglobulin	Peptides	9	
Human serum albumin	Doxorubicin	10	
Antibody			
Transferrin receptor	Neuropeptide	11	
Pgp	Doxorubicin	12	+
Ligand			
Transferrin	Nucleic acid	13	
	Doxorubicin	14	
Asialoglycoprotein	Oligonucleotides	15	
	DNA	16	
Cholesterol	Oligonucleotides	17	
Ferrichrome	β-Lactam antibiotics	18	
Nonsoluble vector structure			
Liposomes	Doxorubicin	19,20	+
	Methotrexate	21	+
	Taxol	22	+
Cyanoacrylate nanospheres	Doxorubicin	23	+
Micelles	Enterotoxin	24	
Virosomes	Hygromycin B	25	
Adenovirus–polylysine	Nucleic acids	26,27	
Lipoprotein (HDL, LDL)	Lipophilic drugs	28,29	
Adjuvant			
Cyclodextrin	Platinum compounds	30	
Cremophor-EL	Taxol	31	+

spheres, or liposomes, points out that drug delivery can potentially overcome transport-associated drug resistance. These drug carriers use a different route of cellular uptake than the free drug; thus, the anticancer agent delivered by them may escape the cellular mechanisms responsible for resistance to the free drug. Hence, in addition to the transport-associated benefits, drug carriers may have a biological function at the subcellular level.

II. LIPOSOMES AND LIPOSOMAL TRANSPORT

Liposomes are a broadly applicable and exciting drug delivery system. They are versatile, nontoxic, and biodegradable, and have been studied extensively in vitro and in vivo (35,36). Numerous liposomal preparations have been formulated for the transport of drugs such as antibiotics, anticancer agents, antigens, hormones, and viruses (35,36). In fact, quite a few formulations of liposome-based therapeutic products are in clinical trials for cancer, treatment of viral or fungal infections, and preparation of vaccines (35–37).

Liposomes are microscopic, closed vesicles, composed of bilayered phospholipid membranes surrounding an internal aqueous space (35,36). This vesicular structure allows encapsulation of hydrophilic drugs in the internal aqueous space and intercalation of lipophilic drugs within the membrane itself. The possibility of integrating peptides or proteins with hydrophobic domains makes possible the attachment of antibodies by the lipid bilayer or by conjugation to the outer surface of the liposome (Table 2). There are two basic liposomal structures: (1) multilamellar vesicles comprising several lipid bilayers, separated by aqueous fluid; and (2) unilamellar vesicles consisting of a single bilayer membrane surrounding the internal aqueous fluid (see Table 2). The size of liposomes greatly varies, depending on the liposomal preparation, and may range in diameter from about 10 nm to 10 μm (36). As intracellular drug release appears to be a limiting factor in liposome delivery, different types of liposomes have been developed to facilitate intracellular drug release, such as pH-sensitive or virus-coated liposomes (see Table 2). Thus, liposomes may exhibit differences in structure, size, and phospholipid composition and, consequently, each liposome-encapsulated drug is likely to display specific pharmacological properties.

Liposomes can interact with cells using such processes as lipid exchange, adsorption, fusion, and endocytosis (35). Although adsorption, lipid exchange, or fusion have been observed in in vitro experimental cell systems, it is likely that endocytosis is principally responsible for the cellular uptake after systemic administration. Consequently, cells of different endocytic activity may differ in their capacity to internalize liposomes and, thereby, influence their biodistribution following injection. Intravenously administered liposomes are rapidly and largely sequestered by mononuclear phagocytes of the reticuloendothelial system; the blood clearance rate depending on liposomal change, size, and lipid composition (35). Large neutral liposomes (>0.5 μm in diameter) are confined primarily in the intravascular space following intravenous administration and are

Table 2 Liposomal Delivery Systems Used in Antimicrobial and Anticancer Therapy

Liposome type		Methodology/composition/characteristic	Drug	Ref.
Conventional	MLV	PC:C/lower toxicity	Doxorubicin	38
		DOPS:POPC	Muramyl tripeptide	39
		Reverse-phase evaporation		40
	LUV	PC:PS:C	Doxorubicin	41
		Filter extrusion		42
	SUV	DMPC:DMPG	Amphotericin	43
		Cardiolipin/lower toxicity	Doxorubicin	44
		Phosphatidylglycerol/long circulating time	Doxorubicin	45
		Minimal volume entrapment	Oligonucleotides	46
Immuno-liposomes	SUV	Antilaminin	Doxorubicin	47
		Anti-Fc receptor	Dideoxycytidine triphosphate	48
		Anti-HLA class 1	Oligonucleotides	49
		Covalently attached proteins		50
pH-sensitive liposomes	MLV	OA:PE/increase intracellular release		51
	SUV	DOPE:DOSG/increase intracellular release	Soluble protein	52
Virus-coated liposomes	MLV	Sendai virus particles/increase intracellular release	DNA	53

Abbreviations: MLV, multilamellar vesicles; LUV, large unilamellar vesicles; SUV, small unilamellar vesicles; PC, phosphatidylcholine; C, cholesterol; DOPS, dioleoyl phosphatidylserine; POPC, palmitoyl-oleoyl phosphatidylcholine; PS, phosphatidylserine; DMPC, dimyristoyl phosphatidylcholine; DMPG, dimyristoyl phosphatidylglycerol; OA, oleic acid; PE, phosphatidylethanolamine; DOPE, dioleoyl phosphatidylethanolamine; DOSG, dioleoyl succinyl glycerol.

distributed mainly in tissues or organs containing phagocytic cells, such as the blood monocytes and the fixed tissue macrophages of the spleen, liver, and bone marrow. Alternatively, small, neutral liposomes ($<0.1\ \mu$m in diameter) can have access to cells located in the interstitial space in addition to the phagocytic cells in the intravascular space, making possible a lower blood clearance and elimination rate, compared with larger liposomes. Plasma half-life of liposomes may reach 10–15 h, depending on their lipid composition (37). The specific biodistribution of liposomes may be unfavorable for the treatment of some diseases. However, liposomal drug delivery has proved successful in cancer therapy and in the treatment of infections, showing better drug efficacy and lesser toxicity than the free drug (37). Nevertheless, clinical trials of liposomal drugs in cancer therapy currently underway seem to show that their benefits depend more closely on altered pharmacokinetics than on enhanced drug delivery to tumor, or to increased tumor responsiveness (37). Recently, liposome encapsulation of antitumor agents has been shown to inhibit drug-associated tumor cell resistance and, in particular, the MDR phenotype (19,20).

III. MODULATION OF MULTIDRUG RESISTANCE BY ENCAPSULATING DRUG

Most of the chemotherapeutic agents used in liposomal form have been doxorubicin (Dox) or cisplatin derivatives. Rahman et al. (44) developed a liposomal doxorubicin formulation with improved efficacy compared with free Dox, exhibiting antitumor activity at doses that caused fewer myocardial alterations (54). We have recently reported that this liposomal doxorubicin (Dox-lip) preparation modulates the MDR phenotype in various MDR cell lines (human ovarian, breast, and colon cancer cell lines and a Chinese hamster lung fibroblastic cell line) (19,20,55,56). The doxorubicin–liposome exhibited a partial reversal of MDR in these cells; there was a three- to ninefold increase of drug sensitivity (IC_{50}) compared with free drug. This effect was specific to MDR cells, since Dox-lip did not enhance cell sensitivity to Dox in the parental sensitive cell lines (19,20). We have shown that Dox-lip reversed drug resistance to an extent comparable with that of verapamil, one of the most potent MDR phenotype inhibitors, when used at the maximum clinically useful concentration (1.5 μM). This effect may have resulted, at least in part, from an increase in cellular drug accumulation, as presented in Figure 1. Circumvention of MDR by liposomally encapsulated doxorubicin was recently confirmed by other workers, who also demonstrated that MDR reversal could be explained by a decrease of intracellular drug concentration (33,34). However, the level of drug resistance in numerous MDR cell lines is much higher than that predicted by the differences in net drug accumulation (6,8,57). Furthermore, the increase of drug accumulation observed when MDR cells are treated by MDR modulators, such as verapamil, does not fully explain the subsequent decrease of drug resistance observed (8,19). As suggested by Deffie et al. (4), the MDR phenotype is a multifactorial phenomenon that may involve decreased DNA damage, enhanced DNA repair, altered enzyme activity (glutathione transferase, topoisomerases), in addition to decreased cellular drug accumulation caused by Pgp-mediated efflux.

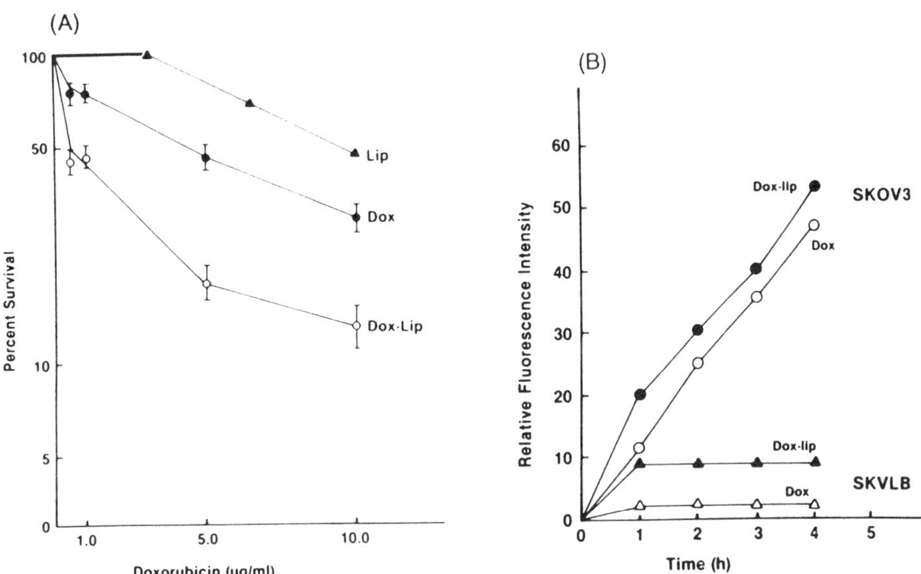

Figure 1 (A) Cytotoxicity of free doxorubicin (●), empty liposomes (▲), and liposome-encapsulated doxorubicin in human ovarian carcinoma multidrug-resistant SKVLB cells. Cells were exposed to drug for 4 h and cytotoxicity was determined using the clonogenic assay. (B) Doxorubicin accumulation in multidrug-resistant SKVLB cells and parental drug-sensitive SKOV3 cells during treatment with doxorubicin (○,△) and liposome-encapsulated doxorubicin (●,▲). Cells were incubated at a drug concentration of 5 μg/ml, and drug cell content was determined by flow cytometry. (From Ref. 56.)

We have studied the effect of Dox-lip on intracellular drug distribution in MDR cells. Doxorubicin, when presented in the free form, is mainly distributed in intracytoplasmic vesicles in human ovarian and SKVLB and human breast carcinoma MCF-7/ADR MDR cells, whereas in the parental cells, the drug is located mainly in the nucleus, where most of its action occurs (20). Hiddenburg et al. (6) and Shurhuis et al. (8) demonstrated that Dox was taken up into MDR cells mainly by the Golgi apparatus, from which the drug is then shifted to the lysosomes or mitochondria, or exocytosed. This intracellular mechanism may be responsible for a significant part of the MDR encountered in the cells tested in these studies. When presented in liposomes, Dox distribution pattern in MDR cells is altered, the drug being redistributed to nuclear compartments (20). We suggest that presentation of Dox in liposomes may alter the intracytoplasmic trafficking of the drug in MDR cells, most likely interfering with the endocytic process.

Previous work demonstrated that anticancer drugs, such as vincristine or vinblastine, bind specifically to high-affinity binding sites on the plasma membrane of resistant cells and suggested that Pgp is a drug-binding protein (1,3). We have shown that liposomes free of drug partially inhibit (by 60%) the vincristine-specific binding to Pgp-enriched membrane vesicles isolated from CH LZ cells (56). Given this observation, two hypotheses can be offered: (1) empty liposomes compete with drugs for binding to Pgp as does verapamil, or (2) liposomes modify the Pgp structure, resulting in decreased capacity or affinity for binding. Because liposomes need to be directly associated with the drug to cause reversal of Dox resistance, as previously demonstrated (20), the second hypothesis is the most likely.

Modulation of MDR in cancer cells by liposomal presentation has been demonstrated using drugs other than Dox, such as methotrexate (21) or taxol (22). In addition to its inhibitory effect on Pgp-associated drug resistance, liposomal presentation proved to be successful in modulating Pgp-unrelated drug resistance in tumor cells, such as resistance to cisplatin compounds (37,57). Drug resistance reversal caused by liposomal cisplatin preparations was mainly attributed to an increase of drug accumulation into cisplatin-resistant cells (35,37). However, so far, there is no clear elucidation of the mechanisms involved in this effect.

IV. MULTIDRUG RESISTANCE MODULATORS INTERACTING WITH BIOMEMBRANES

The physiology and composition of cell membranes are critical considerations when studying the mechanisms of cellular resistance to chemotherapeutic drugs. Since the translocation of solutes across cell membranes is influenced by the physical state of the lipid bilayer, it is reasonable to expect alterations in membrane lipids in MDR cells (58). In addition, insertion of large quantities of Pgp (up to 20% of the plasma membrane proteins) may have profound effects on the structural order of lipids in the plasma membrane of MDR cells. These changes might subsequently alter the fluidity of the cell membrane and contribute to the reduction of drug accumulation in MDR cells. Although various changes in lipid composition have been observed (59,60), an increase in membrane fluidity associated with drug resistance is neither necessary nor sufficient for the expression of the resistance (60,61). Hence, it is believed that MDR reversal is not affected by altering cell membrane fluidity.

Interestingly, hydrophobic analogues of Dox can circumvent MDR in various cell lines (62). Two different mechanisms appear to be involved in this MDR inhibitory effect: (1) the structural modification may alter the ability of the drug to interact with Pgp; (2) increased drug hydrophobicity may lead to an intracellular drug redistribution to the nucleus. This raises the question of whether hydrophobicity confers a specific affinity of membrane phospholipids for the drug, thereby inducing a specific intracellular transport. In an attempt to overcome the non–Pgp-associated class of methotrexate resistance resulting from reduced transport of this hydrophilic drug, lipid-soluble antifolates have been developed (63). These compounds modulate methotrexate resistance in some cell lines (63) and are also capable of overcoming Pgp-associated MDR. Since reversal of methotrexate resistance by lipophilic antifolates appears to be related to increased diffusion through the cell membranes, it seems reasonable to assume that this mechanism may be also involved in overcoming MDR.

Agents such as Cremophor EL surfactant, Tween 80, and Triton WR-1339 detergents or chloroquine have reversed MDR (3,31). These compounds principally act not at the plasma membrane of drug-resistant cells, but rather, in the lysosome where their accumulation results in altered lysosomal membrane phospholipids and, thereby, modified lysosomal function (2,64). Increased membrane trafficking between plasma membrane and membrane-bound intracellular organelles has been observed in MDR cells. This led us to suggest that these lysosomatropic agents perturb the cell membrane by inhibiting Pgp function and specific intracellular trafficking in MDR cells. Furthermore, it is possible that liposomes inhibit the movement of drug-containing intracellular vesicles to the membrane, thereby modifying cell physiology and drug resistance. Interestingly, these lysosomatropic agents as well as liposomes free of drug are specifically toxic to MDR cells in the absence of other agents (58) (Fig. 2). Exploiting the *collateral* sensitivity or hypersensitivity of MDR cells to several substances or conditions may be one way for counteracting insensitivity to drugs. In addition to lysosomatropic agents or liposomes, collateral sensitivity to several steroids and local anesthetics in MDR cells has been described (58). It is believed that increased drug sensitivity of MDR cells to these compounds may be due to changes in the membrane bilayer that apparently accompany the presence of large quantities of Pgp (58).

The clinical potential of substances exhibiting collateral MDR cell sensitivity, such as some local anesthetics or nonionic detergents, is low (58). Steroids may be clinically applied in combination with a cytostatic drug, as already used in many chemotherapeutic regimens, but their specific effects on tumor cell resistance have yet to be clearly demonstrated. Liposomes are nontoxic after systemic administration (35–37) and, in addition

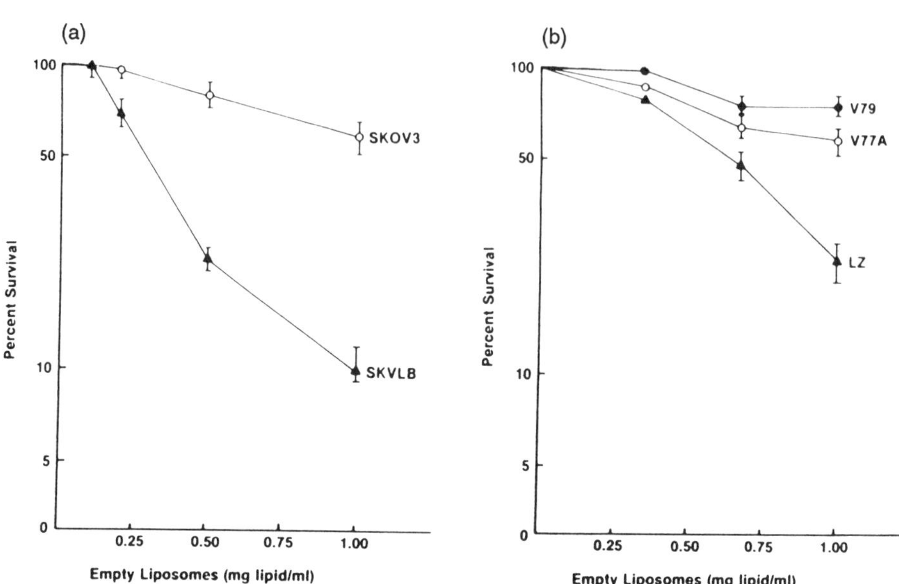

Figure 2 Cytotoxicity of empty liposomes in (a) SKOV3 and SKVLB cells and (b) CH V79, V77A, and LZ cells. Cells were treated for 4 h with increasing concentration of liposomes. SKVLB and CH LZ cell lines were established following a multistep selection process from SKOV3 and CH V79 cells, respectively, and were respectively 180- and 2000-fold more resistant than their parental counterparts. V77 is a variant with intermediate level of MDR and was derived during LZ cell line selection. The relative expression of P-glycoprotein in V77A, SKVLB, and LZ cells, determined by flow cytometric analysis of immunochemical staining (19), was estimated to be 1.0, 2.6, and 5.4, respectively. (From Ref. 56.)

to their pharmacological benefits, may hold promise for specifically killing MDR cells.

V. CONCLUSIONS AND FUTURE DIRECTIONS

The establishment and maintenance of drug resistance in mammalian cells is mediated by a variety of different mechanisms. Gottesman (65; see Chap. 17) hypothesized that Pgp acts as a "drug-vacuum cleaner" at the inner surface of the plasma cell membrane of MDR cells, the drug being extruded outside the cell after its entry by diffusion. Intracellular trafficking in MDR cells occurs by a pathway whereby drugs are trapped in acidic vesicles, which are thereafter removed from the cell by exocytosis (2,63,66). This mechanism of drug exocytosis may be part of a general mechanism by which secretory proteins or recycled membranes are transported from the Golgi apparatus to the external cell surface. This theory was supported by a recent observation showing the involvement of vacuolar H^+-ATPase activity in MDR HL-60 cells, suggesting a role for the endosomic vesicles in MDR cells (66). Hence, Pgp activity and drug exocytosis by endocytic vesicles involve cell membrane structures, and compounds or structures altering membrane behavior may have potential in overcoming MDR.

The demonstration that intracellular drug transport by membrane vesicles is associated with resistance supports the notion that the cell membrane is not a passive player, but is also a determinant of cell behavior. For example, in a recent report (67), a novel signal transduction pathway—the activation of phospholipase D—is suggested to be a second-messenger system able to regulate membrane traffic. Future advances in our understanding of the regulation of intracellular membrane trafficking may offer new ways for overcoming transport-associated drug resistance.

Liposomes formed of membrane bilayers are effective MDR modulators. First, drug encapsulated in liposomes may bypass the Pgp-mediated drug efflux. Liposomes must be associated with the drug to cause MDR reversal, consistent with the hypothesis that Pgp acts as drug vacuum cleaner, extruding a drug immediately after its entry into cells. Second, evidence shows that the presentation of drugs in liposomes may alter the intracytoplasmic vesicle transport and exocytosis of the drug in MDR cells. Endocytotic and exocytotic mechanisms are involved in the uptake and the intracellular transport of liposomes and, consequently, liposomal delivery may bypass intracellular transport by the vesicle-trafficking mechanisms involved, resulting in reduced drug concentrations reaching target sites in MDR cells.

Compounds that alter cell membrane structure or functions have reversed drug resistance, suggesting that the cell membrane may be a valid target for overcoming transport-associated drug resistance. However, toxicity considerations limit the clinical potential of these compounds. Liposomes, however, offer a nontoxic approach; liposomal delivery is already being extensively used in clinical studies. Liposomal delivery improves the therapeutic index of anticancer agents by enhancing drug bioavailability and reducing drug-associated toxicity. Recent data show that liposomal presentation of a drug may increase its intracellular concentration in MDR cells. Hence, in addition to their pharmacological benefits as a carrier system, liposomes or drug delivery in general may also affect cellular phenomena, such as transport-associated drug resistance.

REFERENCES

1. Roninson IB. Molecular and Cellular Biology of Multidrug Resistance in Tumor Cells. New York: Plenum Press, 1991.
2. Beck WT. The cell biology of multiple drug resistance. Biochem Pharmacol 1987; 36:2879–2887.
3. Endicott JA, Ling V. The biochemistry of P-glycoprotein-mediated multidrug resistance. Annu Rev Biochem 1989; 58:137–171.
4. Deffie AM, Alan T, Seneviratne C, Beenken SW, Batra JU, Shea TC, Henner WD, Goldenberg GJ. Multifactorial resistance to Adriamycin: relationship of DNA repair, glutathione transferase activity, drug efflux and P-glycoprotein in cloned cell lines of Adriamycin-sensitive and resistant P388 leukemia. Cancer Res 1988; 48:3595–3602.
5. Burres NS, Myers MT, Sartorelli AC. Evidence of multifactorial mechanisms in an Adriamycin-resistant HL-60 promyelocytic leukemia cell line. Cancer Biochem Biophys 1988; 10:47–57.
6. Hindenburg AA, Gervansoni S, Krishna S, Stewart V, Rosado M, Bhalla K, Baker M, Taub R. Intracellular distribution and pharmacokinetics of daunorubicin in anthracycline-sensitive and resistant HL-60 cells. Cancer Res 1989; 49:4607–4614.
7. Keizer H, Schuurhuis GJ, Broxterman H, Lankelma J, Schoonen W, Van Rijn J, Pinedo H, Joenje H. Correlation of multidrug resistance with decreased drug accumulation, altered subcellular drug distribution, and increased P-glycoprotein expression in cultured SW 1573 human lung tumor cells. Cancer Res 1989; 49:2988–2993.
8. Schuurhuis GJ, van Heijningen TH, Cervantes A, et al. Changes in subcellular doxorubicin distribution and cellular accumulation alone can largely account for doxorubicin resistance in SW-1573 lung cancer and MCF-7 breast cancer multidrug resistant tumour cells. Br J Cancer 1993; 68:898–908.
9. Mitsuda S, Nakagawa T, Osada T, et al. A receptor mediated delivery of an HIV-1 derived peptide vaccine. Biochem Biophys Res Commun 1993; 194:1155–1160.
10. Sett R, Sarkar K, Das PK. Macrophage-directed delivery of doxorubicin conjugated to neoglycoprotein using leishmaniasis as the model disease. J Infect Dis 1993; 168:994–999.
11. Bickel U, Yoshikawa T, Landaw EM, Faull KF, Pardridge WM. Pharmacologic effects in vivo in brain by vector-mediated peptide drug delivery. Proc Natl Acad Sci USA 1993; 90:2618–2622.
12. Vogel CW, Bredehorst R, Panneerselvam M, Splangler CJ. Potential use of monoclonal antibody–drug conjugates to prevent drug resistance. In Mechanisms of Drug Resistance in Neoplastic Cells. New York: Academic Press, 1988:371–383.
13. Curiel DT, Agarwal S, Wagner E, Cotten M. Adenovirus enhancement of transferrin-polylysine-mediated gene delivery. Proc Natl Acad Sci USA 1991; 88:8850–8854.

14. Berezi A, Ruthner M, Szuts V, Fritzer M, Goldenberg H. Influence of conjugation of doxorubicin to transferrin on the iron uptake by K562 cells via receptor-mediated endocytosis. Eur J Biochem 1993; 213:427–436.
15. Bunnell BA, Askari FK, Wilson JM. Targeted delivery of antisense oligonucleotides by molecular conjugates. Somat Cell Mol Genet 1992; 18:559–569.
16. Cristiano RJ, Smith LC, Kay MA, Brinkley BR, Woo SL. Hepatic gene therapy: efficient gene delivery and expression in primary hepatocytes utilizing a conjugated adenovirus–DNA complex. Proc Natl Acad Sci USA 1993; 90:11548–11552.
17. Ryte AS, Karamyshev VN, Nechaeva MV, Vlassov VV. Interaction of cholesterol-conjugated alkylating oligonucleotide derivatives with cellular biopolymers. FEBS Lett 1992; 299:124–126.
18. Dolence EK, Minnick AA, Lin CE, Miller MJ, Payne SM. Synthesis and siderophore and antibacterial activity of N^5-acetyl-N^5-hydroxy-L-ornithine-derived siderophore–beta-lactam conjugates: iron-transport-mediated drug delivery. J Med Chem 1991; 35:968–978.
19. Thierry AR, Jorgensen TJ, Forst D, Belli JA, Dritschilo A, Rahman A. Modulation of multidrug resistance in Chinese hamster cells by liposome-encapsulated doxorubicin. Cancer Commun 1989; 1:311–316.
20. Thierry AR, Vige D, Belli JA, Dritschilo A, Rahman A. Modulation of doxorubicin resistance in multi-drug resistant cells by liposomes. FASEB J 1993; 7:572–579.
21. Kinsky SC, Hashimoto K, Loader JE, Knight MS, Fernandes DJ. Effect of liposomes sensitized with methotrexate on cells that are resistant to methotrexate. Biochim Biophys Acta 1986; 885:129–135.
22. Sharma A, Mayhew E, Straubinger RM. Antitumor effect of taxol-containing liposomes in a taxol-resistant murine tumor model. Cancer Res 1993; 53:5877–5881.
23. Cuvier C, Roblot-Treupel L, Millot JM, Poupon MF. Doxorubicin-loaded nanospheres bypass tumor cell multidrug resistance. Biochem Pharmacol 1992; 44:509–517.
24. Kabanov AV, Slepnev VI, Kuznetsova LE, et al. Pluronic micelles as a tool for low-molecular compound vector delivery into a cell: effect of *Staphylococcus aureus* enterotoxin B on cell loading with micelle incorporated fluorescent dye. Biochem Int 1992; 26:1035–1042.
25. Bagai S, Sarkar DP. Targeted delivery of hygromycin B using reconstituted Sendai viral envelopes lacking hemagglutinin-neuraminidase. FEBS Lett 1993; 326:183–188.
26. Cotten M, Wagner E, Zatloukal K, et al. High-efficiency receptor-mediated delivery of small and large (48 kilobase) gene constructs using the endosome-disruption activity of defective or chemically inactivated adenovirus particles. Proc Natl Acad Sci USA 1992; 89:6094–6098.
27. McPhaul MJ, Deslypere JP, Allman DR, Gerard RD. The adenovirus-mediated delivery of a reporter gene permits the assessment of androgen recep-

tor function in genital skin fibroblast cultures. Stimulation of G_s and inhibition of G_0. J Biol Chem 1993; 268:26063–26066.

28. Bijsterbosch MK, Van Berkel TJ. Lactosylated high density lipoprotein: a potential carrier for the site-specific delivery of drugs to parenchymal liver cells. Mol Pharmacol 1992; 42:404–411.

29. Jori G, Reddi E. The role of lipoproteins in the delivery of tumour-targeting photosensitizers. Int J Biochem 1993; 25:1369–1375.

30. Cucinotta V, Mangano A, Nobile G, Santoro AM, Vecchio G. New platinum(II) complexes of beta-cyclodextrin diamine derivatives and their antitumor activity. J Inorg Biochem 1993; 52:183–190.

31. Webster L, Linsenmeyer M, Millward M, et al. Measurement of Cremophor EL following taxol: plasma levels sufficient to reverse drug exclusion mediated by the multidrug-resistant phenotype. JNCI 1993; 85:1685–1690.

32. Hindenburg A, Stewart VJ, Nepo AG, Taub RN, Baker MA. Circumvention of anthracycline resistance in a human leukemia cell line using daunorubicin: monoclonal antibody conjugates. Proc Am Soc Clin Oncol 1986; 5:46–51.

33. Fan D, Bucana C, O'Brian CA, Zwelling LA, Seid C, Fidler I. Enhancement of murine tumor cell sensitivity to Adriamycin by presentation of the drug in phosphatidylcholine–phosphatidylserine liposomes. Cancer Res 1990; 50:3619–3626.

34. Sadavisan R, Morgan R, Fabian C, Stephens R. Reversal of multidrug resistance in HL-60 cells by verapamil and liposome-encapsulated doxorubicin. Cancer Lett 1991; 57:165–171.

35. Ostro MJ, Cullis PR. Use of liposomes as injectable-drug delivery systems. Am J Hosp Pharm 1989; 46:1576–1586.

36. Mayhew FG. Liposomes and delivery of chemotherapeutic agents. Adv Oncol 1993; 9:3–6.

37. Sugarman SM, Perez-Soler R. Liposomes in the treatment of malignancy: a clinical perspective. Crit Rev Oncol Hematol 1992; 12:231–242.

38. Gabizon A, Dagan A, Branholz Y, Fuks Z. Liposomes as in vivo carriers of Adriamycin: reduced cardiac uptake and preserved antitumor activity in mice. Cancer Res 1982; 42:4734–4739.

39. McEwen E, Kurzman I, Rosenthal RC, Roush JK, Howard E. Therapy for osteosarcoma in dogs with intravenous injection of liposome-encapsulated muramyl tripeptide. JNCI 1989; 81:935–938.

40. Pidgeon C, McNeely S, Schmidt T, Johnson JE. Multilayered vesicles prepared by reverse-phase evaporation: liposome structure and optimum solute entrapment. Biochemistry 1987; 26:17–29.

41. Storm G, Roerdink FH, Steerenberg PA, Crommeliu DJA. Influence of lipid composition on the antitumor activity exerted by doxorubicin-containing liposomes in a rat solid tumor model. Cancer Res 1987; 47:3366–3372.

42. McDonald RC, McDonald RI, Menco BP, Hu L. Small-volume extrusion apparatus for preparation of large, unilamellar vesicles. Biochim Biophys Acta 1991; 1061:297–303.

43. Wiebe VJ, DeGregorio JW. Liposome-encapsulated amphotericin B: promis-

ing new treatment for disseminated fungal infections. Rev Infect Dis 1988; 10:1097–1101.

44. Treat J, Greenspan A, Forst D, Sanchez JA, Ferans VJ, Potkul LA, Woolley PV, Rahman, A. Antitumor activity of liposome-encapsulated doxorubicin in advanced breast cancer: Phase II study. JNCI 1990; 82:1706–1710.

45. Gabizon A, Shiota R, Papahadjopoulos D. Pharmacokinetics and tissue distribution of doxorubicin encapsulated in stable liposomes with long circulating time. JNCI 1989; 81:1484–1488.

46. Thierry AR, Rahman A, Dritschilo A. Overcoming multidrug resistance in human tumor cells using free and liposomally encapsulated antisense oligodeoxynucleotides. Biochem Biophys Res Commun 1993; 190:952–960.

47. Rahman A, Panneerselvam M, Guirguis R, Castronovo V, Daddona PE, Liotta LA. Anti-laminin receptor antibody targeting of liposomes with encapsulated doxorubicin to human breast cancer cells in vitro. JNCI 1989; 81:1784–1800.

48. Betageri GV, Black V, Wahl LM, Weinstein JN. Fc-receptor-mediated targeting of antibody-bearing liposomes containing dideoxycytidine triphosphate to human monocytes/macrophages. J Pharm Pharmacol 1993; 45:48–53.

49. Zelphati O, Zon G, Leserman L. Inhibition of HIV-1 replication in cultured cells with antisense oligonucleotides encapsulated in immunoliposomes. Antisense Res Dev 1993; 3:323–329.

50. Hutchinson FJ, Francis SE, Lyle IG, Jones M. The characterization of liposomes with covalently attached proteins. Biochim Biophys Acta 1989; 978:17–24.

51. Düzgünes N, Straubinger RM, Baldwin PA, Papahadjopoulos D. Proton-induced fusion of oleic acid–phosphatidylethanolamine liposomes. FEBS Lett 1980; 179:148–154.

52. Reddy R, Zhou F, Huang L, Rouse BT. In vivo cytotoxic T lymphocyte induction with soluble proteins administered in liposomes. J Immunol 1992; 148:1585–1589.

53. Kaneda Y, Uchida T, Kim J, Okada Y. The improved efficient method for introducing macromolecules into cells using HVJ (Sendai virus) liposomes with gangliosides. Exp Cell Res 1987; 173:56–69.

54. Herman EH, Rahman A, Ferrano VJ, et al. Prevention of chronic doxorubicin cardiotoxicity in beagles by liposomal encapsulation. Cancer Res 1983; 43:5427–5432.

55. Oudard S, Thierry A, Jorgensen TJ, Rahman A. Sensitization of multidrug resistant colon cancer cells to doxorubicin by encapsulation in liposomes. Cancer Chemother Pharmacol 1991; 28:259–265.

56. Thierry AR, Dritschilo A, Rahman A. Effect of liposomes on P-glycoprotein function in multidrug resistant cells. Biochem Biophys Res Commun 1992; 187:1098–1105.

57. Steerenberg PA, Storm G, de Groot G, et al. Liposomes as drug carrier system for cis-diamminedichloroplatinum. Cancer Chemother Pharmacol 1988; 21:299–307.

58. Cano DF, Riordan JR. Collateral sensitivity of multidrug-resistant cells. In: Roninson I, ed. Molecular and Cellular Biology of Multidrug Resistance in Tumor Cells. New York: Plenum Press, 1991:337–348.

59. Escriba PV, Ferrer-Montiel AV, Ferragut JA, Gonzalez-Ros JM. Role of membrane lipids in the interaction of daunomycin with plasma membranes from tumor cells: implications in drug-resistance phenomena. Biochemistry 1990; 29:7275–7282.

60. Alon N, Busche R, Tummler B, Riordan JR. Membrane lipids of multidrug resistant cells: chemical composition and physical state. In: Roninson IB, ed. Molecular and Cellular Biology of Multidrug Resistance in Tumor Cells. New York: Plenum Press, 1991:263–278.

61. Montaudon D, Vrignaud P, Londos-Gagliandi D, Robert J. Fluorescence anisotropy of cell membranes of doxorubicin-sensitive and resistant rodent tumoral cells. Cancer Res 1986; 46:5602–5605.

62. Lothstreim L, Wright HM, Sweatman TW, Israel M. N-Benzyladriamycin-14-valerate and drug resistance: correlation of anthracycline structural modification with intracellular accumulation and distribution in multidrug resistant cells. Oncol Res 1993; 4:341–347.

63. Assaraf YG, Molina A, Schimke RT. Cross-resistance to the lipid-soluble antifolate trimetrexate in human carcinoma cells with the multidrug-resistant phenotype. JNCI 1989; 81:290–294.

64. Sehested M, Jensen PB, Skovsgaard T, Bindslev N, Demant EFJ, Friche E, Vindelov L. Inhibition of vincristine binding to plasma membrane vesicles from daunorubicin resistant Ehrlich ascites cells by multidrug resistance modulators. Br J Cancer 1989; 60:809–814.

65. Cornwell MM, Pastan I, Gottesman MM. Binding of drugs and ATP by P-glycoprotein and transport of drugs by vesicles from human multidrug-resistant cells. In: Roninson I, ed. Molecular and Cellular Biology of Multidrug Resistance in Tumor Cells. New York: Plenum Press, 1991:229–240.

66. Marquardt D, Center MS. Involvement of vacuolar H^+-adenosine triphosphatase activity in multidrug resistance in HL-60 cells. JNCI 1991; 83:1098–1102.

67. Brown HA, Gutowski S, Moomaw CR, Slaughter C, Sternweis D. ADP-ribosylation factor, a small GTP-dependent regulatory protein stimulates phospholipase D activity. Cell 1993; 75:1137–1144.

Index

Page references to chemical structures or figures are given in **boldface**.

A 80556, **247**
ABC transporters, 29, 106, 108, 529
ABLC liposomes, 318
Acetylcholine receptor 74, 75, **77**
Acetylglucosamine, 134
Acholeplasma laidlawii, 87–88
Achromycin (*see* Tetracycline)
Acinetobacter calcoaceticus, 155,
    161
Acinetobacter spp., 10
acrA Mutants, 204, 205
Acrolein, **582,** 584, 592
Actinomycin D, **26,** 27, 526, 531,
    532, 539, 549
Active efflux (*see* Efflux)
Active pumping rate, 34
Active transport, 291, 292
ACV (*see* Acyclovir)
Acyclovir, 410, 425, 427
Adenosine, 404, 408, **409, 413,** 415,
    416–418
Adenosine deaminase, 406, 407
Adenosine kinase, 406

Adenylate cyclase, 408
ADM (*see* Doxorubicin)
Adrenocorticoids (*see* Steroids)
Adriamycin (*see* Doxorubicin)
Aerobactin, 152
AHC52, **559,** 561
AICAR transformylase (*see*
    Aminoimidazolecarboxamide
    ribonucleotide transformylase)
AIDS, 334, 337, 344
Alaphosphin, 292, 294
Albicidin, 292, 293, 299
Albomycin, 292, 293, 294
Aldophosphamide, 592
Alkylating agents, 25, 29, 580
Allopurinol, 394, 395
AM 1155, **247**
Ambisomes, 318
Amikacin, 7, **176**
Amiloride, 107
Aminocycletols (*see*
    Aminoglycosides)

About the Editor

NAFSIKA H. GEORGOPAPADAKOU is Distinguished Research Leader in the Department of Oncology at the Roche Research Center, Nutley, New Jersey. A member of the American Society for Microbiology, the American Association for Cancer Research, the American Academy of Microbiology, the American Chemical Society, and the American Society for Biochemistry and Molecular Biology, among other organizations, she is the coeditor of one book and the author or coauthor of over 100 professional papers and abstracts that reflect her research interests in antimicrobial therapy. Dr. Georgopapadakou received the B.A. degree (1971) in chemistry from Mills College, Oakland, California, and the Ph.D. degree (1975) in biochemistry from Yale University, New Haven, Connecticut.